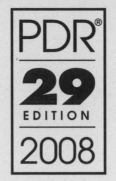

29 EDITION

2008

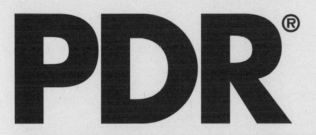

for Nonprescription Drugs,
Dietary Supplements, and Herbs

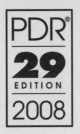

PDR®
29
EDITION
2008

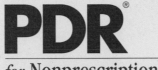

PDR®
for Nonprescription Drugs,
Dietary Supplements, and Herbs

Executive Vice President, PDR: Kevin D. Sanborn
Vice President, Client Services & Publishing:
Christopher Young
Vice President, Clinical Relations: Mukesh Mehta, RPh
Vice President, Operations: Brian Holland
Vice President, Strategic Marketing: Valerie E. Berger
Vice President, Pharmaceutical Sales: Anthony Sorce
Senior Director, Copy Sales: Bill Gaffney
Senior Product Manager: Ilyaas Meeran
National Sales Manager: Elaine Musco
Senior Solutions Manager: Debra Goldman
Solutions Manager: Lois Smith
Sales Coordinator: Janet Wallendal

Senior Director, Editorial & Publishing: Bette LaGow
Director, Database & Vendor Management:
Jeffrey D. Schaefer
Manager, Professional Services: Michael DeLuca,
PharmD, MBA
Drug Information Specialists: Anila Patel, PharmD;
Nermin Shenouda, PharmD; Greg Tallis, RPh
Project Editor: Lori Murray

Production Manager, PDR: Steven Maher
Manager, Production Purchasing: Thomas Westburgh
Senior Print Production Manager: Dawn Dubovich
Production Manager: Gayle Graizzaro
PDR Database Supervisor: Regina L. Dickerson
Index Supervisor: Noel Deloughery
Index Editor: Allison O'Hare
Format Editor: Eric Udina
Senior Production Coordinators: Gianna Caradonna,
Yasmin Hernández
Production Coordinator: Nick W. Clark
Production Specialist: Jennifer Reed
Traffic Assistant: Kim Condon
Vendor Management Specialist: Gary Lew

Manager, Art Department: Livio Udina
Electronic Publishing Designers: Deana DiVizio,
Carrie Faeth, Jamie Pinedo
Production Associate: Joan K. Akerlind
Digital Imaging Manager: Christopher Husted
Digital Imaging Coordinator: Michael Labruyere

ISBN: 1-56363-662-X

FOREWORD TO THE 29TH EDITION

Physicians' Desk Reference® has been providing unparalleled drug information to doctors and other healthcare professionals for more than 60 years. A wider variety of *PDR®* reference options than ever before is now available and in more formats—in print, on CD, on the Internet, and for PDA.

Physicians' Desk Reference® for Nonprescription Drugs, Dietary Supplements, and Herbs features five indices and a full-color Product Identification Guide followed by three distinct sections of product information. Two of the sections, *Nonprescription Drug Information* and *Generic Drug Information*, provide labeling of products marketed in compliance with the Code of Federal Regulations labeling requirements for OTC drugs.

The other product section, *Dietary and Herbal Supplement Information*, contains manufacturer-supplied labeling for nutritional supplements and herbal remedies. Please note that these products are marketed under the Dietary Supplement Health and Education Act of 1994 and therefore have not been evaluated by the Food and Drug Administration. Such products are not intended to diagnose, treat, cure, or prevent any disease.

The five indices in the book contain manufacturer contact information, product names, prescribing categories, active ingredients, and a listing of "companion" OTC drugs that may be recommended to relieve symptoms caused by prescription drug therapy.

A new feature for this edition is the inclusion of a dozen product comparison tables at the end of the book. These tables cover various OTC therapeutic categories and allow for easy comparison of active ingredients, drug strengths, and dosages.

About This Book
PDR® for Nonprescription Drugs, Dietary Supplements, and Herbs is published annually by Thomson Healthcare. The book is made possible through the courtesy of the manufacturers whose products appear in it. The information on each product described in the book has been prepared by the manufacturer and edited and approved by the manufacturer's medical department, medical director, or medical counsel. The function of the publisher is the compilation, organization, and distribution of this information. During compilation of this information, the publisher has emphasized the necessity of describing products comprehensively in order to provide all the facts necessary for sound and intelligent decision-making. Descriptions seen here include all information made available by the manufacturer.

In organizing and presenting the material in *PDR® for Nonprescription Drugs, Dietary Supplements, and Herbs*, the publisher does not warrant or guarantee any of the products described, or perform any independent analysis in connection with any of the product information contained herein. *Physicians' Desk Reference®* does not assume, and expressly disclaims, any obligation to obtain and include any information other than that provided to it by the manufacturer. It should be understood that by making this material available the publisher is not advocating the use of any product described herein, nor is the publisher responsible for misuse of a product due to typographical error. Additional information on any product may be obtained from the manufacturer.

Other Prescribing Aids from PDR
For complicated cases and special patient problems, there is no substitute for the in-depth data contained in *Physicians' Desk Reference*. But for those times when you need quick access to critical prescribing information, you may want to consult the **PDR® Monthly Prescribing Guide™**, the essential drug reference designed specifically for use at the point of care. Distilled from the pages of *PDR*, this digest-sized reference presents the key facts on more than 1,500 drug formulations, including therapeutic class, indications and contraindications, warnings and precautions, pregnancy rating, drug interactions and side effects, and adult and pediatric dosages. The guide is intended to supplement full prescribing information for Rx medications, although in certain instances OTC products are included as well. When applicable, each drug entry also gives the *PDR* page number to turn to for further information. In addition, a full-color insert of pill images allows you to correctly identify each product. Issued monthly, the guide is regularly updated with detailed descriptions of new drugs to receive FDA approval, as well as FDA-approved revisions to existing product information. You'll also find bulletins about major new developments in the pharmaceutical industry, an overview of important new agents nearing approval, and recent clinical findings on common nutritional supplements. To learn more about this useful publication and to inquire about subscription rates, call 800-232-7379.

New Evidence-Based Application for Your PDA
We are pleased to announce the launch of **Thomson Clinical Xpert™**, a powerful medical reference for Palm® OS and Pocket PC handhelds developed by Thomson Healthcare. Designed specifically for use at the point of care, this decision-support tool puts drug, disease, and laboratory information instantly into the hands of physicians and other clinical professionals via their PDA.

Much more than a quick drug lookup, Thomson Clinical Xpert provides medical references and point-of-care tools you need in your daily workflow, including:

- **Drug labeling:** Search more than 4,000 trade names

- **Interaction checker:** Check up to 32 medications at one time

- **Toxicology information:** Screen 200 of the most common poisonings and drug overdoses

- **Medical calculators:** Dosing, metric conversions, and more

- **News and alerts:** Get FDA announcements, clinical updates, and upcoming drug launches

- **Laboratory test information:** Identify and interpret details of more than 500 laboratory tests

- **Disease database:** Find current evidence-based treatment recommendations

- **Alternative medicine database:** Consult information on more than 300 popular herbs and dietary supplements

Thomson Clinical Xpert is available **free** to registered members of PDR.net, your medical professional web portal for drug information and much more. Go to *www.PDR.net* to put this clinical-decision support tool to work for you now.

Web-Based Clinical Resources
PDR.net, a web portal designed specifically for healthcare professionals, provides a wealth of clinical information, including full drug and disease monographs, specialty-specific resource centers, patient education, clinical news, and conference information. PDR.net gives prescribers online access to authoritative, evidence-based information they need to support or confirm diagnosis and treatment decisions, including:

- Daily feeds of specialty news, conference coverage, and monthly summaries

- FDA-approved and other manufacturer-provided product labeling for more than 4,000 brand-name drugs

- Multidrug interaction checker and other tools

- Extensive disease diagnosis and treatment information

- Customizable patient education

- Professional resources

PDR.net is also home to our **Clinical Resource Centers**, giving you the latest medical news and disease information all in one easy place. Log on to *www.PDR.net* to visit one of these clinical specialties:

- Allergy and Immunology

- Psychiatry

- Cardiovascular

- Pulmonology

- Dermatology

- Rheumatology

- Diabetes and Endocrinology

- Urology

- Nephrology

- Women's Health

- Neurology

- Pediatrics

- And more

Online access is **free** for U.S.-based MDs, DOs, dentists, NPs, and PAs in full-time patient practice, as well as for medical students, residents, and other select prescribing allied health professionals. Register today at *www.PDR.net*.

For more information on these or any other members of the growing family of *PDR* products, please call, toll-free, 800-232-7379 or fax 201-722-2680.

HOW TO USE THIS BOOK

The 2008 edition of *PDR® for Nonprescription Drugs, Dietary Supplements, and Herbs* features a format designed to help you find the information you need as quickly and easily as possible. Now, in addition to consulting the five indices, you can go directly to a specific product comparison table to find the relevant over-the-counter (OTC) products for a particular condition. Details of this organization are outlined below.

FIVE INDICES

- **Manufacturers' Index** lists all pharmaceutical manufacturers that provided OTC drug labeling for this edition. Each entry contains addresses, phone numbers, and emergency contacts, as well as a listing of that manufacturer's products and the corresponding page numbers for labeling information.

- **Product Name Index** provides the page number of each product description in the Nonprescription Drug Information and Dietary and Herbal Supplement Information sections. Listings appear alphabetically by brand name.

- **Product Category Index** lists all fully described products according to therapeutic or pharmaceutical drug category (e.g., acetaminophen combinations).

- **Active Ingredients Index** contains product cross-references by generic ingredient.

- **Companion Drug Index** lists OTC products that may be used in conjunction with prescription drug therapy to relieve symptoms of a particular condition or drug-induced side effects.

PRODUCT IDENTIFICATION GUIDE
Organized alphabetically by manufacturer name. This section shows full-color, actual-sized photos of tablets and capsules, plus a variety of other dosage forms and packages.

NONPRESCRIPTION DRUG INFORMATION
Organized alphabetically by manufacturer name. The product labeling in this section includes brand-name OTC drugs and other medical products marketed for home use. **Please keep in mind that the product information included herein is valid as of press time (July 2007).** Additional information, as well as updates to the product labeling, can be obtained from the manufacturer.

DIETARY AND HERBAL SUPPLEMENT INFORMATION
Organized alphabetically by manufacturer name. This section contains product labeling for dietary and herbal supplements marketed under the Dietary Supplement Health and Education Act of 1994. Be aware that these products are not federally regulated and are not intended to diagnose, treat, cure, or prevent any disease.

GENERIC DRUG INFORMATION
Organized alphabetically by product name. The product labeling in this section provides information on generic OTC drugs marketed for home use. **Please keep in mind that the product information included herein is valid as of press time (July 2007).** Additional information, as well as updates to the product labeling, can be obtained from the manufacturer.

PRODUCT COMPARISON TABLES
Organized alphabetically by therapeutic category and brand name. These tables provide a quick and easy way to compare the active ingredients and dosages of common brand-name OTC drugs. More than 10 therapeutic categories are covered, including antacid and heartburn agents; laxatives; and cough, cold, and flu products.

CONTENTS

Manufacturers' Index   **1**
Section 1
Lists all participating pharmaceutical manufacturers. Includes addresses, phone numbers, and emergency contacts. Shows each manufacturer's products and the page number of those described.

Product Name Index (Pink Pages)   **101**
Section 2
Gives the page number of each product description found in the book. Products are listed alphabetically by brand name.

Product Category Index (Blue Pages)   **201**
Section 3
Lists all fully described products by prescribing category.

Active Ingredients Index   **301**
Section 4
A cross-reference by generic ingredient of all product descriptions.

Companion Drug Index   **401**
Section 5
Lists symptoms occurring during prescription drug therapy and presents over-the-counter products that may be recommended for relief.

Poison Control Centers 411
A national directory arranged alphabetically by state and city.

Drug Information Centers 415
A national directory arranged alphabetically by state and city.

Herb/Drug Interactions 421
Arranged alphabetically by herb name.

Overview of Commonly Used Herbs 424
A quick reference guide arranged alphabetically by herb name.

Product Identification Guide   **501**
Section 6
Shows full-color, actual-sized photos of tablets and capsules, plus pictures of a variety of other dosage forms and packages. Arranged alphabetically by manufacturer.

Nonprescription Drug Information   **601**
Section 7
Provides information on hundreds of brand-name over-the-counter drugs and other medical products. Entries are arranged alphabetically by manufacturer.

Dietary and Herbal Supplement Information   **685**
Section 8
Includes manufacturers' descriptions of various products marketed under the Dietary Supplement, Health and Education Act of 1994. Entries are organized alphabetically by manufacturer.

Generic Drug Information   **707**
Section 9
Includes product descriptions of various generic over-the-counter drugs. Arranged alphabetically by product name.

NEW Product Comparison Tables

Table 1. Acne Products 715
Table 2. Allergic Rhinitis Products 719
Table 3. Analgesic Products 723
Table 4. Antacid and Heartburn Products 728
Table 5. Antidiarrheal Products 731
Table 6. Antiflatulant Products 733

Table 7. Contact Dermatitis Products 734
Table 8. Cough, Cold, and Flu Products 736
Table 9. Headache/Migraine Products 747
Table 10. Laxative Products 752
Table 11. Psoriasis Products 755
Table 12. Wound Care Products 757

SECTION 1

MANUFACTURERS' INDEX

This index lists manufacturers that have supplied information for this edition. Each company's entry includes the address, phone, and fax number of its headquarters and regional offices, as well as company contacts for inquiries, orders, and emergency information.

Products with entries in the Nonprescription Drug Information section are listed with their page numbers under the heading "OTC Products Described." Products with entries in the Dietary Supplement Information section are listed with their page numbers under the

heading "Dietary Supplements Described." Other OTC products and dietary supplements available from the manufacturer follow these two sections.

A bold page number next to the manufacturer's name shows where to find product photographs, when available.

- The ◆ symbol marks drugs shown in the Product Identification Guide.

- *Italic page numbers* signify partial information.

A&Z PHARMACEUTICAL INC.   686
180 Oser Avenue, Suite 300
Hauppauge, NY 11788
Direct Inquiries to:
(631) 952-3800

Dietary Supplements Described:
D-Cal Chewable Caplets **686**

ACTAVIS, INC.   602
7205 Windsor Boulevard
Baltimore, MD 21244
Direct Inquiries to:
Customer Service
(800) 432-8534

OTC Products Described:
Permethrin Lotion **602**

ADAMS RESPIRATORY   502, 602
THERAPEUTICS
14841 Sovereign Road
Fort Worth, TX 76155
Direct Inquiries to:
(817) 786-1200
Fax: (817) 786-1150
(866) MUCINEX

OTC Products Described:
◆ Delsym Liquid Grape Flavor **502, 602**
◆ Delsym Liquid Orange
   Flavor **502, 603**
◆ Mucinex 600mg Extended-
   Release Bi-Layer
   Tablets **502, 605**
◆ Mucinex 1200mg Extended-
   Release Bi-Layer
   Tablets **502, 606**

◆ Mucinex Cold Liquid **502, 604**
◆ Mucinex Cough Liquid **502, 603**
◆ Mucinex Mini-Melts Bubble
   Gum Flavor **502, 604**
◆ Mucinex Mini-Melts Grape
   Flavor **502, 604**
◆ Mucinex Cough Mini-Melts
   Orange Cream Flavor **502, 605**
◆ Mucinex D 600mg/60mg
   Extended-Release Bi-Layer
   Tablets **502, 606**
◆ Mucinex D 1200mg/120mg
   Extended-Release Bi-Layer
   Tablets **502, 606**
◆ Mucinex DM 600mg/30mg
   Extended-Release Bi-Layer
   Tablets **502, 607**
◆ Mucinex DM 1200mg/60mg
   Extended-Release Bi-Layer
   Tablets **502, 607**
◆ Mucinex Liquid **502, 603**

AWARENESS   502, 686
CORPORATION/dba
AWARENESS LIFE
25 South Arizona Place, Suite 500
Chandler, AZ 85225
Direct Inquiries to:
(800) 69AWARE
www.awarenesslife.net

Dietary Supplements Described:
◆ Awareness Clear Capsules **686**
◆ Daily Complete Liquid **502, 686**
◆ Experience Capsules **502, 686**
◆ Female Balance *502*
◆ Pure Gardens Cream **686**
◆ PureTrim Mediterranean
   Wellness Shake **502, 686**
◆ SynergyDefense Capsules **502, 686**

BEACH PHARMACEUTICALS   687
Division of Beach Products, Inc.
EXECUTIVE OFFICE:
5220 South Manhattan Avenue
Tampa, FL 33611
(813) 839-6565
Direct Inquiries to:
Richard Stephen Jenkins, Executive V.P.:
(813) 839-6565
Clete Harmon, Senior V.P., Regulatory
and Business Affairs:
(864) 277-7282
Manufacturing and Distribution:
1700 Perimeter Road
Greenville, SC 29605
(800) 845-8210

Dietary Supplements Described:
Beelith Tablets **687**

BEUTLICH LP,   608
PHARMACEUTICALS
1541 Shields Drive
Waukegan, IL 60085-8304
Direct Inquiries to:
(847) 473-1100
(800) 238-8542 in the U.S. and Canada
M-Th: 7:30 a.m. - 4:00 p.m. CT
FAX: (847) 473-1122
www.beutlich.com
beutlich@beutlich.com

OTC Products Described:
Hurricaine Topical Anesthetic Gel,
   1 oz. Wild Cherry, Pina Colada,
   Watermelon, and Fresh Mint,
   5.25 g. Wild Cherry **608**
Hurricaine Topical Anesthetic Liquid,
   1 oz. Wild Cherry, Pina Colada,
   0.005 fl. oz. Snap-n-Go Swabs
   Wild Cherry **608**

(◆) **Shown in Product Identification Guide**   *Italic Page Number* **Indicates Brief Listing**

BEUTLICH LP, PHARMACEUTICALS—cont.

Hurricaine Topical Anesthetic Spray,
2 oz. Wild Cherry **608**
Hurricaine Topical Anesthetic Spray
Extension Tubes (200) **608**
Hurricaine Topical Anesthetic Spray
Kit, 2 oz. Wild Cherry with
disposable Extension Tubes
(200) **608**

Dietary Supplements Described:
Peridin-C Vitamin C Supplement **687**

BOEHRINGER INGELHEIM   503, 608
CONSUMER HEALTH
CARE PRODUCTS
DIVISION

Division of Boehringer Ingelheim
Pharmaceuticals, Inc.
900 Ridgebury Road
P.O. Box 368
Ridgefield, CT 06877
Direct Inquiries to:
(888) 285-9159

OTC Products Described:
♦ Dulcolax Stool Softener **503, 609**
♦ Dulcolax Suppositories **503, 609**
♦ Dulcolax Tablets **503, 608**
♦ Zantac 75 Tablets **503, 609**
♦ Maximum Strength Zantac
150 Tablets **503, 610**
♦ Maximum Strength Zantac
150 Cool Mint Tablets **503, 610**

DANNMARIE, LLC.   687

2005 Palmer Avenue, #200
Larchmont, New York 10538
Direct Inquiries to:
(877) 425-8767
www.premcal.com
E-mail: info@premcal.com

Dietary Supplements Described:
PremCal Light, Regular, and Extra
Strength Tablets **687**

ENIVA NUTRACEUTICS   503, 687

9702 Ulysses Street NE
Minneapolis, MN 55434
Direct Inquiries to:
(763) 795-8870
FAX: (763) 795-8890
www.eniva.com

Dietary Supplements Described:
♦ Efacor Dietary Supplement **503, 687**
♦ Vibe Liquid Multi-Nutrient
Supplement **503, 688**

4LIFE RESEARCH   689

9850 South 300 West
Sandy, UT 84070
Direct Inquiries to:
(801) 562-3600
FAX: (801) 562-3699
productsupport@4life.com
www.4life.com

Dietary Supplements Described:
4Life Transfer Factor Plus Tri-Factor
Formula **689**

Other Products Available:
4Life Transfer Factor Advanced
Formula

4Life Transfer Factor Age-Defying
Effects
4Life Transfer Factor Belle Vie
4Life Transfer Factor Cardio
4Life Transfer Factor Chewable
4Life Transfer Factor énummi
4Life Transfer Factor GluCoach
4Life Transfer Factor Go Stix
4Life Transfer Factor Immune Spray
4Life Transfer Factor Kids
4Life Transfer Factor MalePro
4Life Transfer Factor ReCall
4Life Transfer Factor RenewAll
4Life Transfer Factor RioVida
4Life Transfer Factor Toothpaste

GREEK ISLAND LABS   690

7620 East McKellips Road
Suite 4 PMB 86
Scottsdale, AZ 85257
Direct Inquiries to:
www.greekislandlabs.com
(888) 841-7363

Dietary Supplements Described:
Natural Joint Capsules **690**

HYLAND'S, INC.

(See STANDARD HOMEOPATHIC
COMPANY)

MANNATECH, INC.   503, 690

600 S. Royal Lane
Suite 200
Coppell, TX 75019
Direct Inquiries to:
Customer Service
(972) 471-8111
www.mannatech.com/Country.aspx

Dietary Supplements Described:
♦ Ambrotose Capsules **503, 690**
♦ Ambrotose Powder **503, 690**
♦ Advanced Ambrotose
Capsules **503, 690**
♦ Advanced Ambrotose
Powder **503, 690**
♦ Ambrotose AO Capsules **503, 691**
♦ PLUS Caplets **503, 691**

Other Products Available:
AmbroStart Fiber and Metabolic
Dietary Supplement
CardioBALANCE Heart Care Formula
Capsules
EM•PACT Sports Drink
Emprizone Advanced Skin Care Gel
FIRM with Ambrotose Lotion
GI-Pro Probiotic Dietary Supplement
Capsules
GI-Zyme Digestive Enzyme Dietary
Supplement Capsules
Glyco•Bears Children's Chewable
Vitamin and Mineral Dietary
Supplement
GlycoLEAN Accelerator 3 Capsules
GlycoLEAN FiberSlim Capsules
GlycoLEAN GlycoSlim Drinks
ImmunoSTART Colostrum and
Glyconutritional Dietary
Supplement Chewable Tablets
MannaBAR Nutrition Bars
Manna•Bears Pectin Gums
Manna-C Capsules

MannaCLEANSE Caplets
Optimal Skin Care System
Phyt•Aloe Capsules
Phyt•Aloe Powder
PhytoMatrix Multivitamin/Mineral
Supplement
SPORT Capsules

MATRIXX INITIATIVES, INC.   503, 611

4742 North 24th Street
Suite 455
Phoenix, AZ 85016
Direct Inquiries to:
(602) 385-8888
FAX: (602) 385-8850
www.zicam.com

OTC Products Described:
♦ Nasal Comfort Moisture
Therapy Sprays - Scented
and Unscented **503, 611**
♦ Zicam Allergy Relief **504, 611**
♦ Zicam Cold Remedy
Chewables **504, 611**
♦ Zicam Cold Remedy
ChewCaps **504, 611**
♦ Zicam Cold Remedy Gel
Swabs **504, 611**
♦ Zicam Cold Remedy
Nasal Gel **504, 611**
♦ Zicam Cold Remedy
Oral Mist **504, 611**
♦ Zicam Cold Remedy
RapidMelts **504, 611**
♦ Zicam Cold Remedy
RapidMelts with
Vitamin C **504, 611**
♦ Zicam Cough Max Cough
Spray **504, 613**
♦ Zicam Cough Max Cough
Melts **504, 613**
♦ Zicam Extreme Congestion
Relief **504, 613**
♦ Zicam Intense Sinus Relief ... **504, 613**
♦ Zicam Multi-Symptom Liquid
Daytime **503, 613**
♦ Zicam Multi-Symptom Cold &
Flu Daytime To Go **503, 615**
♦ Zicam Multi-Symptom Cold &
Flu Nighttime Liquid ... **503, 614**
♦ Zicam Multi-Symptom Cold &
Flu Nighttime To Go **503, 615**
♦ Zicam Sinus Melts **504, 616**

MAYOR PHARMACEUTICAL   692
LABORATORIES

2401 South 24th Street
Phoenix, AZ 85034
Direct Inquiries to:
Medical Director
(602) 244-8899
www.vitamist.com

Dietary Supplements Described:
VitaMist Intra-Oral Spray **692**

MEMORY SECRET   504, 693

1221 Brickell Avenue
Suite 1540
Miami, FL 33131
Direct Inquiries to:
(866) 673-2738
FAX: (305) 675-2279
E-mail: intelectol@memorysecret.net

Dietary Supplements Described:
♦ Intelectol Tablets **504, 693**

MISSION PHARMACAL   **616**
COMPANY

10999 IH 10 West, Suite 1000
San Antonio, TX 78230-1355
Direct All Inquiries to:
P.O. Box 786099
San Antonio, TX 78278-6099
(800) 292-7364 Customer Service
(M-F 8:30 - 5 C.S.T.)
(210) 696-8400
FAX: (210) 696-6010

OTC Products Described:
Thera-Gesic Creme 616

Dietary Supplements Described:
Calcet Triple Calcium + Vitamin D
    Tablets 693
Citracal Caplets 693

Other Products Available:
Calcet Plus Multivitamin/Mineral
    Tablets
Citracal 250mg + D Tablets
Citracal Creamy Bites Caramel
    Chewable Pieces
Citracal Creamy Bites Chocolate
    Fudge Chewable Pieces
Citracal Creamy Bites Lemon Cream
    Chewable Pieces
Citracal Kosher Tablets
Citracal Petites Tablets
Citracal Plus Tablets
Citracal Prenatal + DHA
    (Tablets + Capsules)
Citracal Prenatal 90 + DHA
    (Tablets + Capsules)
Citracal Prenatal Rx Tablets
Compete Multivitamin/Mineral
    Tablets
Fosfree Multivitamin/Mineral
    Tablets
Iromin-G Multivitamin/Mineral
    Tablets
Maxilube Personal Lubricant
Mission Prenatal Tablets
Mission Prenatal F.A. Tablets
Mission Prenatal H.P. Tablets
Oncovite Tablets
Thera-Gesic Plus Creme

NOVARTIS CONSUMER   **504, 617**
HEALTH, INC.

200 Kimball Drive
Parsippany, NJ 07054-0622
Direct Inquiries to:
Consumer & Professional Affairs
(800) 452-0051
FAX: (800) 635-2801
Or write to the above address

OTC Products Described:
Buckley's Chest Congestion
    Mixture 618
Buckley's Cough Mixture 618
Bufferin Extra Strength Tablets 617
♦ Bufferin Regular Strength
    Tablets 504, 617
Comtrex Maximum Strength Day/
    Night Cold & Cough Caplets -
    Day Formulation 618
Comtrex Maximum Strength Day/
    Night Cold & Cough Caplets -
    Night Formulation 618
Comtrex Maximum Strength Non-
    Drowsy Cold & Cough
    Caplets 619
♦ Desenex Athlete's Foot
    Cream 505, 620

Desenex Athlete's Foot Liquid
    Spray 619
♦ Desenex Athlete's Foot Shake
    Powder 505, 619
♦ Desenex Athlete's Foot Spray
    Powder 505, 619
Desenex Jock Itch Spray Powder ... 619
♦ Excedrin Back & Body
    Caplets 505, 620
♦ Excedrin Extra Strength
    Caplets/Tablets/
    Geltabs 505, 621
♦ Excedrin Migraine Caplets/
    Tablets/Geltabs 505, 622
♦ Excedrin PM Caplets/
    Tablets 505, 623
♦ Excedrin Sinus Headache
    Caplets/Tablets 505, 623
♦ Excedrin Tension Headache
    Caplets/Tablets/
    Geltabs 505, 621
♦ Ex•Lax Chocolated Laxative
    Pieces 505, 625
♦ Ex•Lax Regular Strength
    Pills 505, 625
♦ Ex•Lax Maximum Strength
    Pills 505, 625
♦ 4-Way Fast Acting Nasal
    Spray 504, 624
4-Way Menthol Nasal Spray 624
4-Way Moisturizing Relief Nasal
    Spray 624
4-Way Saline Nasal Spray 625
♦ Gas-X Regular Strength
    Chewable Tablets 505, 626
♦ Gas-X Extra Strength
    Chewable Tablets 505, 626
♦ Gas-X Extra Strength
    Softgels 505, 626
♦ Gas X Extra Strength Thin
    Strips 505, 626
♦ Gas-X Maximum Strength
    Softgels 505, 626
♦ Gas-X with Maalox Extra
    Strength Chewable
    Tablets 506, 626
♦ Lamisil ᴬᵀ Creams (Athlete's
    Foot & Jock Itch) 506, 627
♦ Lamisil ᴬᵀ Athlete's Foot Spray
    Pump 506
♦ Lamisil ᴬᵀ Jock Itch Spray Pump 506
♦ Lamisil ᴬᶠ Defense Powders
    (Shake & Spray) 506, 627
♦ Maalox Regular Strength
    Antacid/Antigas Liquid 506, 628
♦ Maalox Maximum Strength
    Multi Symptom Antacid/
    Antigas Liquid 506, 628
♦ Maalox Maximum Strength
    Total Stomach Relief
    Liquid 506, 629
♦ Maalox Maximum Strength
    Multi Symptom Antacid/
    Antigas Chewable
    Tablets 506, 629
♦ Mineral Ice 506, 629
Theraflu Cold & Cough Hot Liquid ... 630
Theraflu Cold & Sore Throat Hot
    Liquid 630
Theraflu Flu & Chest Congestion Hot
    Liquid 631
Theraflu Flu & Sore Throat Hot
    Liquid 631
Theraflu Daytime Severe Cold
    Caplets 634
Theraflu Nighttime Severe Cold
    Caplets 635
Theraflu Daytime Severe Cold Hot
    Liquid 632

♦ Theraflu Nighttime Severe
    Cold Hot Liquid 506, 632
♦ Theraflu Thin Strips Daytime
    Cold & Cough 506, 633
♦ Theraflu Thin Strips Nighttime
    Cold & Cough 506, 633
Theraflu Warming Relief Daytime
    Severe Cold 634
♦ Theraflu Warming Relief
    Nighttime Severe Cold 506, 635
Triaminic Chest & Nasal Congestion
    Liquid 636
Triaminic Cold & Allergy Liquid 636
♦ Triaminic Day Time Cold &
    Cough Liquid 507, 637
♦ Triaminic Night Time Cold &
    Cough Liquid 507, 637
Triaminic Cough & Sore Throat
    Liquid 638
Triaminic Cough & Runny Nose
    Softchews 639
♦ Triaminic Thin Strips Day Time
    Cold & Cough 506, 640
♦ Triaminic Thin Strips Night
    Time Cold & Cough 506, 640
♦ Triaminic Thin Strips Cold with
    Stuffy Nose 506, 639
♦ Triaminic Thin Strips Cough &
    Runny Nose 506, 640
♦ Triaminic Thin Strips Long Acting
    Cough *506*
♦ Triaminic Infant & Toddler Thin
    Strips Decongestant 507, 638
♦ Triaminic Infant & Toddler Thin
    Strips Decongestant Plus
    Cough 507, 638
♦ Vagistat-1 .... 507, 641

Dietary Supplements Described:
♦ Benefiber Fiber Supplement
    Caplets 504, 694
♦ Benefiber Fiber Supplement
    Powder 504, 694
♦ Benefiber Fiber Supplement
    Sugar Free Assorted Fruit
    Chewables 504, 694
♦ Benefiber Fiber Supplement
    Sugar Free Orange Creme
    Chewables 504, 694
♦ Benefiber Fiber Supplement
    Plus B Vitamins & Folic
    Acid Caplets 504, 695
♦ Benefiber Fiber Supplement
    Plus B Vitamins & Folic
    Acid Powder 504, 695
♦ Benefiber Fiber Supplement
    Plus Calcium Chewable
    Tablets 504, 696

Other Products Available:
Lamisil ᴬᵀ Gel (Athlete's Foot & Jock
    Itch)
No-Doz Maximum Strength Caplets
Triaminic Cough & Sore Throat
    Softchews
Triaminic Flu, Cough & Fever Liquid
Triaminic Long Acting Cough Liquid
Triaminicin Tablets

PROCTER & GAMBLE   **507, 641**

P.O. Box 559
Cincinnati, OH 45201
Direct Inquiries to:
Consumer Relations
(800) 832-3064

OTC Products Described:
Head & Shoulders Intensive
    Solutions Dandruff Shampoo 641
♦ Metamucil Capsules 507, 642

PROCTER & GAMBLE—cont.

Metamucil Powder, Original Texture
Orange Flavor 642
Metamucil Powder, Original Texture
Regular Flavor 642
◆ Metamucil Smooth Texture
Powder, Orange Flavor 507, 642
Metamucil Smooth Texture Powder,
Sugar-Free, Orange Flavor ... 642
Metamucil Smooth Texture Powder,
Sugar-Free, Regular Flavor 642
◆ Metamucil Wafers, Apple Crisp
& Cinnamon Spice
Flavors 507, 642
Children's Pepto 641
◆ Pepto-Bismol Original Liquid,
Original and Cherry
Chewable Tablets &
Caplets 507, 643
Pepto-Bismol Maximum Strength
Liquid 643
◆ Prilosec OTC Tablets 507, 644
◆ ThermaCare Heat Wraps 507, 645
ThermaCare Therapeutic Heat
Wraps 647
◆ Vicks Formula 44 Cough Relief
Liquid 508, 648
◆ Vicks Formula 44D Cough &
Head Congestion Relief
Liquid 508, 649
◆ Vicks Formula 44E Cough &
Chest Congestion Relief
Liquid 508, 649
◆ Pediatric Vicks 44e Cough &
Chest Congestion Relief
Liquid 507, 654
◆ Vicks Formula 44M Cough,
Cold & Flu Relief Liquid ... 508, 649
◆ Pediatric Vicks Formula 44m
Cough & Cold Relief
Liquid 507, 655
Vicks Cough Drops, Menthol and
Cherry Flavors 650
◆ Vicks DayQuil LiquiCaps/
Liquid Multi-Symptom
Cold/Flu Relief 507, 651
◆ Vicks NyQuil LiquiCaps/Liquid
Multi-Symptom Cold/Flu
Relief 507, 653
◆ Children's Vicks NyQuil Cold/
Cough Relief 507, 650
◆ Vicks NyQuil Cough Liquid 508, 652
Vicks NyQuil D Cold & Flu Multi-
Symptom Relief Liquid 652
Vicks Sinex Nasal Spray and Ultra
Fine Mist 655
Vicks Sinex 12-Hour Nasal Spray
and Ultra Fine Mist 656
Vicks Vapor Inhaler 656
Vicks VapoRub Cream 656
Vicks VapoRub Ointment 656
Vicks VapoSteam 657

Dietary Supplements Described:
◆ Align Daily Probiotic
Supplement 507, 696
Metamucil Dietary Fiber
Supplement 696

REESE PHARMACEUTICAL   **508, 657**
COMPANY

10617 Frank Avenue
Cleveland, OH 44106
Direct Inquiries to:
Voice: (800) 321-7178
FAX: (216) 231-6444
www.reesepharmaceutical.com

OTC Products Described:
◆ Reese's Pinworm
Treatments 508, 657

Other Products Available:
Dentapaine Oral Pain Reliever
Double Tussin DM Intense Strength
Cough Reliever
Refenesen Chest Congestion Relief
Products

SCHERING-PLOUGH   **508, 658**
HEALTHCARE PRODUCTS

556 Morris Avenue
Summit, NJ 07901-1330
Direct Product Requests to:
Schering-Plough HealthCare Products
556 Morris Avenue
Summit, NJ 07901-1330
For Medical Emergencies Contact:
Consumer Relations Department
P.O. Box 377
Memphis, TN 38151
(901) 320-2988 (Business Hours)
(901) 320-2364 (After Hours)

OTC Products Described:
◆ Claritin-D Non-Drowsy 12 Hour
Tablets 508, 658
◆ Claritin-D Non-Drowsy 24 Hour
Tablets 508, 658
◆ Claritin Children's 24 Hour
Non-Drowsy Chewables ... 508, 659
◆ Claritin Children's 24 Hour
Non-Drowsy Allergy
Syrup 508, 659
◆ Claritin Non-Drowsy 24 Hour
Tablets 508, 659
◆ Claritin Reditabs 24 Hour Non-
Drowsy Tablets 508, 659

STANDARD HOMEOPATHIC   **660**
COMPANY

Hyland's
210 West 131st Street
Box 61067
Los Angeles, CA 90061
Direct Inquiries to:
Jay Borneman
(800) 624-9659, Ext. 20

OTC Products Described:
Hyland's BackAche with Arnica
Caplets 660
Hyland's Calms Forté Tablets and
Caplets 660
Hyland's Calms Forté 4 Kids
Tablets 661
Hyland's Colic Tablets 661
Hyland's Earache Drops 661
Hyland's Earache Tablets 661
Hyland's Leg Cramps with Quinine
Tablets and Caplets 661
Hyland's Migraine Headache Relief
Tablets 662
Hyland's Nerve Tonic Tablets and
Caplets 662
Hyland's Restful Legs Tablets 662
Hyland's Sniffles 'N Sneezes 4 Kids
Tablets 662
Hyland's Teething Gel 663
Hyland's Teething Tablets 663
Ivy Block 663
Smile's Prid Salve 662

TAHITIAN NONI   **508, 698**
INTERNATIONAL

333 West River Park Drive
Provo, UT 84604
Direct Inquiries to:
(801) 234-1000
www.tahitiannoni.com

Dietary Supplements Described:
◆ Tahitian Noni Leaf Serum
Soothing Gel 508, 698
◆ Tahitian Noni Liquid 508, 698
◆ Tahitian Noni Seed Oil 508, 699

TOPICAL BIOMEDICS, INC.   **508, 700**

P.O. Box 494
Rhinebeck, NY 12572-0494
Direct Inquiries to:
Aurora Paradise
(845) 871-4900
FAX: (845) 876-0818
Aparadise@topicalbiomedics.com

Dietary Supplements Described:
◆ Topricin Cream 508, 700

UAS LABORATORIES   **663**

9953 Valley View Road
Eden Prairie, MN 55344
Direct Inquiries to:
Dr. S.K. Dash
(952) 935-1707
FAX: (952) 935-1650

OTC Products Described:
DDS-Acidophilus Capsules, Tablets,
and Powder 663

UPSHER-SMITH   **663**
LABORATORIES, INC

6701 Evenstad Drive
Maple Grove, MN 55369
Direct Inquiries to:
Professional Services:
(800) 654-2299

OTC Products Described:
Amlactin Moisturizing Lotion and
Cream *663*
Amlactin AP Anti-Itch Moisturizing
Cream *664*
Amlactin XL Moisturizing Lotion *664*

WELLNESS INTERNATIONAL   **664**
NETWORK, LTD.

5800 Democracy Drive
Plano, TX 75024
Direct Inquiries to:
Product Inquiries
(972) 312-1100
E-mail: winproducts@winltd.com
Branch Office:
WIN Worldwide BV
Kruisweg 583-2132 NA Hoofdoorp,
The Netherlands
Tel: 31-20-446-46-46
FAX: 31-20-446-4647

OTC Products Described:
BioLean Accelerator Tablets 664
BioLean Free Tablets 665
BioLean II Tablets 664
BioLean LipoTrim Capsules 665

BioLean Mass Appeal Tablets 665
BioLean ProXtreme Dietary
     Supplement 666
DHEA Plus Capsules 666
Food for Thought Dietary
     Supplement 666
Phyto-Vite Tablets 667
Satiete Tablets 667
WINOmeg3Complex Capsules 667

Dietary Supplements Described:
BioLean Sure2Endure Tablets 703
Sleep-Tite Caplets 700
StePHan Clarity Capsules 700
StePHan Elasticity Capsules 701
StePHan Elixir Capsules 701
StePHan Essential Capsules 701
StePHan Feminine Capsules 701
StePHan Flexibility Capsules 701
StePHan Lovpil Capsules 702
StePHan Masculine Capsules 702
StePHan Protector Capsules 702
StePHan Relief Capsules 702
StePHan Tranquility Capsules 702
Winrgy Dietary Supplement 703

Other Products Available:
WINSalon Collection
WINSpa Collection

WYETH CONSUMER HEALTHCARE 668

Wyeth
Five Giralda Farms
Madison, NJ 07940-0871
Direct Inquiries to:
Wyeth Consumer Healthcare
(800) 322-3129 (9-5 E.S.T.)

OTC Products Described:
Advil Caplets 668
Advil Gel Caplets 668
Advil Liqui-Gels 668
Advil Tablets 668
Advil Allergy Sinus Caplets 669
Children's Advil Oral Suspension ... 670
Advil Cold & Sinus Caplets 669
Advil Cold & Sinus Liqui-Gels 669
Infants' Advil Concentrated Drops -
     White Grape (Dye-Free) 672
Advil Multi-Symptom Cold
     Caplets 669
Advil PM Caplets 671

Advil PM Liqui-Gels 671
Alavert Allergy & Sinus D-12 Hour
     Tablets 673
Alavert Orally Disintegrating
     Tablets 673
Anbesol Cold Sore Therapy
     Ointment 674
Baby Anbesol Gel 673
Anbesol Junior Gel 673
Anbesol Maximum Strength Gel 673
Anbesol Maximum Strength
     Liquid 673
Children's Dimetapp Cold & Allergy
     Elixir 674
Children's Dimetapp Cold & Allergy
     Chewable Tablets 676
Children's Dimetapp DM Cold &
     Cough Elixir 675
Children's Dimetapp Long Acting
     Cough Plus Cold Syrup 675
Toddler's Dimetapp Cold and Cough
     Drops 676
FiberCon Caplets 676
Preparation H Maximum Strength
     Cream 677
Preparation H Ointment 677
Preparation H Suppositories 677
Preparation H Medicated Wipes 678
Primatene Mist 678
Robitussin Chest Congestion
     Liquid 679
Robitussin Cough & Allergy Syrup ... 680
Robitussin Cough & Cold CF
     Liquid 682
Robitussin Cough & Cold CF
     Pediatric Drops 682
Robitussin Cough & Cold Long-
     Acting Liquid 682
Robitussin Pediatric Cough & Cold
     Long-Acting Liquid 682
Robitussin Cough & Congestion
     Liquid 681
Robitussin Cough Gels Long-
     Acting 680
Robitussin Cough Long Acting
     Liquid 681
Robitussin Pediatric Cough Long
     Acting Liquid 681
Robitussin Sugar Free Cough
     Syrup 681
Robitussin Cough DM Syrup 681
Robitussin Cough DM Infant
     Drops 681

Robitussin Cough Drops Menthol,
     Cherry, and Honey 679
Robitussin Honey Cough Drops 679
Robitussin Sugar Free Throat
     Drops 679
Robitussin Head & Chest
     Congestion PE Syrup 680
Robitussin Night Time Cough & Cold
     Syrup 683
Robitussin Night Time Pediatric
     Cough & Cold Syrup 683

Dietary Supplements Described:
Caltrate 600 + D Tablets 704
Caltrate 600 + D PLUS Minerals
     Chewables 704
Caltrate 600 + D PLUS Minerals
     Tablets 704
Centrum Tablets 704
Centrum Kids Complete Children's
     Chewables 705
Centrum Performance Multivitamin/
     Multimineral Supplement 705
Centrum Silver Tablets 706

Other Products Available:
Junior Strength Advil Chewable
     Tablets
Regular Strength Anbesol Gel
Regular Strength Anbesol Liquid
Axid AR
Caltrate 600 Tablets
Centrum Liquid
Centrum Chewable Tablets
Centrum Silver Chewables
ChapStick 100% Natural
ChapStick Cold Sore Therapy
ChapStick Flava-Craze
ChapStick Lip Balm
ChapStick Lip Moisturizer
ChapStick Medicated
ChapStick OverNight Lip Treatment
ChapStick Ultra SPF 30
Children's Dimetapp ND Orally
     Dissolving Tablets
Toddler's Dimetapp Cold Drops
Children's Dimetapp Nighttime Flu
     Syrup
Dristan 12 Hour Nasal Spray
Dristan Cold Multi-Symptom Tablets
Primatene Tablets
Robitussin Cold & Congestion
     Tablets
Robitussin Sunny Orange and
     Raspberry Vitamin C Supplement
     Drops

SECTION 2

PRODUCT NAME INDEX

This index includes all entries in the Product Information sections. Products are listed alphabetically by brand name.

If an entry in the index lists multiple page numbers, the first one shown refers to the photograph of the

product, the last one to its prescribing information.

- **Bold page numbers** indicate that the entry contains full product information.

- *Italic page numbers* signify partial information.

A

Adult Strength products
(see base product name)
Advil Caplets (Wyeth) **668**
Advil Gel Caplets (Wyeth) **668**
Advil Liqui-Gels (Wyeth) **668**
Advil Tablets (Wyeth) **668**
Advil Allergy Sinus Caplets
(Wyeth) **669**
Children's Advil Oral Suspension
(Wyeth) **670**
Advil Cold & Sinus Caplets (Wyeth) ... **669**
Advil Cold & Sinus Liqui-Gels
(Wyeth) **669**
Infants' Advil Concentrated Drops -
White Grape (Dye-Free) (Wyeth) ... **672**
Advil Multi-Symptom Cold Caplets
(Wyeth) **669**
Advil PM Caplets (Wyeth) **671**
Advil PM Liqui-Gels (Wyeth) **671**
Alavert Allergy & Sinus D-12 Hour
Tablets (Wyeth) **673**
Alavert Orally Disintegrating Tablets
(Wyeth) **673**
Align Daily Probiotic
Supplement (Procter &
Gamble) **507, 696**
Allergy Antihistamine Capsules
(Generic) **708**
Ambrotose Capsules
(Mannatech) **503, 690**
Ambrotose Powder
(Mannatech) **503, 690**
Advanced Ambrotose Capsules
(Mannatech) **503, 690**
Advanced Ambrotose Powder
(Mannatech) **503, 690**
Ambrotose AO Capsules
(Mannatech) **503, 691**

Amlactin AP Anti-Itch Moisturizing
Cream (Upsher-Smith) *664*
Amlactin Moisturizing Lotion and
Cream (Upsher-Smith) *663*
Amlactin XL Moisturizing Lotion
(Upsher-Smith) *664*
Anbesol Cold Sore Therapy Ointment
(Wyeth) **674**
Baby Anbesol Gel (Wyeth) **673**
Anbesol Junior Gel (Wyeth) **673**
Anbesol Maximum Strength Gel
(Wyeth) **673**
Anbesol Maximum Strength Liquid
(Wyeth) **673**
Anti-Diarrheal Caplets (Generic) **708**
Awareness Clear Capsules
(Awareness Corporation/
Awareness Life) **686**

B

Beelith Tablets (Beach) **687**
Benefiber Fiber Supplement
Caplets (Novartis
Consumer) **504, 694**
Benefiber Fiber Supplement
Powder (Novartis
Consumer) **504, 694**
Benefiber Fiber Supplement
Sugar Free Assorted Fruit
Chewables (Novartis
Consumer) **504, 694**
Benefiber Fiber Supplement
Sugar Free Orange Creme
Chewables (Novartis
Consumer) **504, 694**
Benefiber Fiber Supplement
Plus B Vitamins & Folic
Acid Caplets (Novartis
Consumer) **504, 695**

Benefiber Fiber Supplement
Plus B Vitamins & Folic
Acid Powder (Novartis
Consumer) **504, 695**
Benefiber Fiber Supplement
Plus Calcium Chewable
Tablets (Novartis
Consumer) **504, 696**
BioLean Accelerator Tablets
(Wellness International) **664**
BioLean Free Tablets (Wellness
International) **665**
BioLean II Tablets (Wellness
International) **664**
BioLean LipoTrim Capsules (Wellness
International) **665**
BioLean Mass Appeal Tablets
(Wellness International) **665**
BioLean ProXtreme Dietary
Supplement (Wellness
International) **666**
BioLean Sure2Endure Tablets
(Wellness International) **703**
Buckley's Chest Congestion Mixture
(Novartis Consumer) **618**
Buckley's Cough Mixture (Novartis
Consumer) **618**
Bufferin Extra Strength Tablets
(Novartis Consumer) **617**
Bufferin Regular Strength
Tablets (Novartis
Consumer) **504, 617**

C

Calcet Triple Calcium + Vitamin D
Tablets (Mission) **693**
Calcium Antacid Tablets (Generic) **708**
Caltrate 600 + D Tablets (Wyeth) **704**
Caltrate 600 + D PLUS Minerals
Chewables (Wyeth) **704**

Caltrate 600 + D PLUS Minerals
Tablets (Wyeth) 704
Centrum Tablets (Wyeth) 704
Centrum Kids Complete Children's
Chewables (Wyeth) 705
Centrum Performance Multivitamin/
Multimineral Supplement
(Wyeth) 705
Centrum Silver Tablets (Wyeth) 706
Children's Strength products
(see base product name)
Citracal Caplets (Mission) 693
Claritin Children's 24 Hour Non-
Drowsy Chewables
(Schering-Plough) 508, 659
Claritin Children's 24 Hour Non-
Drowsy Allergy Syrup
(Schering-Plough) 508, 659
Claritin Non-Drowsy 24 Hour
Tablets (Schering-Plough) 508, 659
Claritin Reditabs 24 Hour Non-
Drowsy Tablets (Schering-
Plough) 508, 659
Claritin-D Non-Drowsy 12 Hour
Tablets (Schering-Plough) 508, 658
Claritin-D Non-Drowsy 24 Hour
Tablets (Schering-Plough) 508, 658
Comtrex Maximum Strength Day/
Night Cold & Cough Caplets - Day
Formulation (Novartis Consumer) .. 618
Comtrex Maximum Strength Day/
Night Cold & Cough Caplets -
Night Formulation (Novartis
Consumer) 618
Comtrex Maximum Strength Non-
Drowsy Cold & Cough Caplets
(Novartis Consumer) 619

D

Daily Complete Liquid
(Awareness Corporation/
Awareness Life) 502, 686
D-Cal Chewable Caplets (A&Z
Pharm) 686
DDS-Acidophilus Capsules, Tablets,
and Powder (UAS Labs) 663
Delsym Liquid Grape Flavor
(Adams) 502, 602
Delsym Liquid Orange Flavor
(Adams) 502, 603
Desenex Athlete's Foot Cream
(Novartis Consumer) 505, 620
Desenex Athlete's Foot Liquid Spray
(Novartis Consumer) 619
Desenex Athlete's Foot Shake
Powder (Novartis
Consumer) 505, 619
Desenex Athlete's Foot Spray
Powder (Novartis
Consumer) 505, 619
Desenex Jock Itch Spray Powder
(Novartis Consumer) 619
DHEA Plus Capsules (Wellness
International) 666
Children's Dimetapp Cold & Allergy
Elixir (Wyeth) 674
Children's Dimetapp Cold & Allergy
Chewable Tablets (Wyeth) 676
Children's Dimetapp DM Cold &
Cough Elixir (Wyeth) 675
Children's Dimetapp Long Acting
Cough Plus Cold Syrup (Wyeth) ... 675
Toddler's Dimetapp Cold and Cough
Drops (Wyeth) 676
Dulcolax Stool Softener
(Boehringer Ingelheim) 503, 609

Dulcolax Suppositories
(Boehringer Ingelheim) 503, 609
Dulcolax Tablets (Boehringer
Ingelheim) 503, 608

E

Efacor Dietary Supplement
(Eniva) 503, 687
Excedrin Back & Body Caplets
(Novartis Consumer) 505, 620
Excedrin Extra Strength
Caplets/Tablets/Geltabs
(Novartis Consumer) 505, 621
Excedrin Migraine Caplets/
Tablets/Geltabs (Novartis
Consumer) 505, 622
Excedrin PM Caplets/Tablets
(Novartis Consumer) 505, 623
Excedrin Sinus Headache
Caplets/Tablets (Novartis
Consumer) 505, 623
Excedrin Tension Headache
Caplets/Tablets/Geltabs
(Novartis Consumer) 505, 621
Ex•Lax Chocolated Laxative
Pieces (Novartis Consumer) .. 505, 625
Ex•Lax Regular Strength Pills
(Novartis Consumer) 505, 625
Ex•Lax Maximum Strength Pills
(Novartis Consumer) 505, 625
Experience Capsules
(Awareness Corporation/
Awareness Life) 502, 686
Extra Strength products
(see base product name)

F

Female Balance (Awareness
Corporation/Awareness Life) *502*
FiberCon Caplets (Wyeth) 676
Food for Thought Dietary Supplement
(Wellness International) 666
4Life Transfer Factor Plus Tri-Factor
Formula (4Life) 689
4-Way Fast Acting Nasal Spray
(Novartis Consumer) 504, 624
4-Way Menthol Nasal Spray (Novartis
Consumer) 624
4-Way Moisturizing Relief Nasal
Spray (Novartis Consumer) 624
4-Way Saline Nasal Spray (Novartis
Consumer) 625

G

Gas-X Regular Strength
Chewable Tablets (Novartis
Consumer) 505, 626
Gas-X Extra Strength Chewable
Tablets (Novartis
Consumer) 505, 626
Gas-X Extra Strength Softgels
(Novartis Consumer) 505, 626
Gas-X Extra Strength Thin
Strips (Novartis Consumer) ... 505, 626
Gas-X Maximum Strength
Softgels (Novartis
Consumer) 505, 626
Gas-X with Maalox Extra
Strength Chewable Tablets
(Novartis Consumer) 506, 626

H

Head & Shoulders Intensive
Solutions Dandruff Shampoo
(Procter & Gamble) 641
Heartburn Relief, Acid Reducer
Tablets (Generic) 709

Hurricaine Topical Anesthetic Gel,
1 oz. Wild Cherry, Pina Colada,
Watermelon, and Fresh Mint,
5.25 g. Wild Cherry (Beutlich) 608
Hurricaine Topical Anesthetic Liquid,
1 oz. Wild Cherry, Pina Colada,
0.005 fl. oz. Snap-n-Go Swabs
Wild Cherry (Beutlich) 608
Hurricaine Topical Anesthetic Spray,
2 oz. Wild Cherry (Beutlich) 608
Hurricaine Topical Anesthetic Spray
Extension Tubes (200) (Beutlich) .. 608
Hurricaine Topical Anesthetic Spray
Kit, 2 oz. Wild Cherry with
disposable Extension Tubes (200)
(Beutlich) 608
Hyland's BackAche with Arnica
Caplets (Standard Homeopathic) ... 660
Hyland's Calms Forté Tablets and
Caplets (Standard Homeopathic) ... 660
Hyland's Calms Forté 4 Kids Tablets
(Standard Homeopathic) 661
Hyland's Colic Tablets (Standard
Homeopathic) 661
Hyland's Earache Drops (Standard
Homeopathic) 661
Hyland's Earache Tablets (Standard
Homeopathic) 661
Hyland's Leg Cramps with Quinine
Tablets and Caplets (Standard
Homeopathic) 661
Hyland's Migraine Headache Relief
Tablets (Standard Homeopathic) 662
Hyland's Nerve Tonic Tablets and
Caplets (Standard Homeopathic) ... 662
Hyland's Restful Legs Tablets
(Standard Homeopathic) 662
Hyland's Sniffles 'N Sneezes 4 Kids
Tablets (Standard Homeopathic) 662
Hyland's Teething Gel (Standard
Homeopathic) 663
Hyland's Teething Tablets (Standard
Homeopathic) 663

I

Infants' Strength products
(see base product name)
Intelectol Tablets (Memory
Secret) 504, 693
Ivy Block (Standard Homeopathic) 663

J

Junior Strength products
(see base product name)

L

Lamisil^AT Creams (Athlete's
Foot & Jock Itch) (Novartis
Consumer) 506, 627
Lamisil^AT Athlete's Foot Spray Pump
(Novartis Consumer) *506*
Lamisil^AT Jock Itch Spray Pump
(Novartis Consumer) *506*
Lamisil^AF Defense Powders
(Shake & Spray) (Novartis
Consumer) 506, 627

M

Maalox Regular Strength
Antacid/Antigas Liquid
(Novartis Consumer) 506, 628
Maalox Maximum Strength
Multi Symptom Antacid/
Antigas Liquid (Novartis
Consumer) 506, 628

Maalox Maximum Strength
    Total Stomach Relief Liquid
    (Novartis Consumer) 506, 629
Maalox Maximum Strength
    Multi Symptom Antacid/
    Antigas Chewable Tablets
    (Novartis Consumer) 506, 629
Maximum Strength products
    (see base product name)
Metamucil Capsules (Procter &
    Gamble) 507, 642
Metamucil Dietary Fiber Supplement
    (Procter & Gamble) 696
Metamucil Powder, Original Texture
    Orange Flavor (Procter &
    Gamble) 642
Metamucil Powder, Original Texture
    Regular Flavor (Procter &
    Gamble) 642
Metamucil Smooth Texture
    Powder, Orange Flavor
    (Procter & Gamble) 507, 642
Metamucil Smooth Texture Powder,
    Sugar-Free, Orange Flavor (Procter
    & Gamble) 642
Metamucil Smooth Texture Powder,
    Sugar-Free, Regular Flavor
    (Procter & Gamble) 642
Metamucil Wafers, Apple Crisp
    & Cinnamon Spice Flavors
    (Procter & Gamble) 507, 642
Mineral Ice (Novartis
    Consumer) 506, 629
Mucinex 600mg Extended-
    Release Bi-Layer Tablets
    (Adams) 502, 605
Mucinex 1200mg Extended-
    Release Bi-Layer Tablets
    (Adams) 502, 606
Mucinex Cold Liquid (Adams) ... 502, 604
Mucinex Cough Liquid
    (Adams) 502, 603
Mucinex Mini-Melts Bubble
    Gum Flavor (Adams) 502, 604
Mucinex Mini-Melts Grape
    Flavor (Adams) 502, 604
Mucinex Cough Mini-Melts
    Orange Cream Flavor
    (Adams) 502, 605
Mucinex D 600mg/60mg
    Extended-Release Bi-Layer
    Tablets (Adams) 502, 606
Mucinex D 1200mg/120mg
    Extended-Release Bi-Layer
    Tablets (Adams) 502, 606
Mucinex DM 600mg/30mg
    Extended-Release Bi-Layer
    Tablets (Adams) 502, 607
Mucinex DM 1200mg/60mg
    Extended-Release Bi-Layer
    Tablets (Adams) 502, 607
Mucinex Liquid (Adams) 502, 603

N
Nasal Comfort Moisture
    Therapy Sprays - Scented
    and Unscented (Matrixx) 503, 611
Non-Drowsy Nasal Decongestant
    Maximum Strength Tablets
    (Generic) 710
Non-Drowsy Nasal Decongestant PE
    Tablets (Generic) 711
Natural Joint Capsules (Greek Island
    Labs) 690
Nicotine Gum, Stop Smoking Aid
    (Generic) 709
Nicotine Transdermal System Patch,
    Stop Smoking Aid (Generic) 710

O
Original Strength products
    (see base product name)

P
Children's Pepto (Procter & Gamble) ... 641
Pepto-Bismol Original Liquid,
    Original and Cherry
    Chewable Tablets & Caplets
    (Procter & Gamble) 507, 643
Pepto-Bismol Maximum Strength
    Liquid (Procter & Gamble) 643
Peridin-C Vitamin C Supplement
    (Beutlich) 687
Permethrin Lotion (Actavis) 602
Phyto-Vite Tablets (Wellness
    International) 667
PLUS Caplets (Mannatech) 503, 691
PremCal Light, Regular, and Extra
    Strength Tablets (Dannmarie) 687
Preparation H Maximum Strength
    Cream (Wyeth) 677
Preparation H Ointment (Wyeth) 677
Preparation H Suppositories
    (Wyeth) 677
Preparation H Medicated Wipes
    (Wyeth) 678
Prilosec OTC Tablets (Procter &
    Gamble) 507, 644
Primatene Mist (Wyeth) 678
Pure Gardens Cream (Awareness
    Corporation/Awareness Life) 686
PureTrim Mediterranean
    Wellness Shake (Awareness
    Corporation/Awareness Life) .. 502, 686

R
Reese's Pinworm Treatments
    (Reese) 508, 657
Regular Strength Pain Relief Tablets
    (Generic) 711
Regular Strength products
    (see base product name)
Robitussin Chest Congestion Liquid
    (Wyeth) 679
Robitussin Cough & Allergy Syrup
    (Wyeth) 680
Robitussin Cough & Cold CF Liquid
    (Wyeth) 682
Robitussin Cough & Cold CF
    Pediatric Drops (Wyeth) 682
Robitussin Cough & Cold Long-Acting
    Liquid (Wyeth) 682
Robitussin Pediatric Cough & Cold
    Long-Acting Liquid (Wyeth) 682
Robitussin Cough & Congestion
    Liquid (Wyeth) 681
Robitussin Cough Gels Long-Acting
    (Wyeth) 680
Robitussin Cough Long Acting Liquid
    (Wyeth) 681
Robitussin Pediatric Cough Long
    Acting Liquid (Wyeth) 681
Robitussin Sugar Free Cough Syrup
    (Wyeth) 681
Robitussin Cough DM Syrup (Wyeth) .. 681
Robitussin Cough DM Infant Drops
    (Wyeth) 681
Robitussin Cough Drops Menthol,
    Cherry, and Honey (Wyeth) 679
Robitussin Honey Cough Drops
    (Wyeth) 679
Robitussin Sugar Free Throat Drops
    (Wyeth) 679
Robitussin Head & Chest Congestion
    PE Syrup (Wyeth) 680
Robitussin Night Time Cough & Cold
    Syrup (Wyeth) 683

Robitussin Night Time Pediatric
    Cough & Cold Syrup (Wyeth) 683

S
Satiete Tablets (Wellness
    International) 667
Sleep-Tite Caplets (Wellness
    International) 700
Smile's Prid Salve (Standard
    Homeopathic) 662
StePHan Clarity Capsules (Wellness
    International) 700
StePHan Elasticity Capsules
    (Wellness International) 701
StePHan Elixir Capsules (Wellness
    International) 701
StePHan Essential Capsules
    (Wellness International) 701
StePHan Feminine Capsules
    (Wellness International) 701
StePHan Flexibility Capsules
    (Wellness International) 701
StePHan Lovpil Capsules (Wellness
    International) 702
StePHan Masculine Capsules
    (Wellness International) 702
StePHan Protector Capsules
    (Wellness International) 702
StePHan Relief Capsules (Wellness
    International) 702
StePHan Tranquility Capsules
    (Wellness International) 702
SynergyDefense Capsules
    (Awareness Corporation/
    Awareness Life) 502, 686

T
Tahitian Noni Leaf Serum
    Soothing Gel (Tahitian Noni
    International) 508, 698
Tahitian Noni Liquid (Tahitian
    Noni International) 508, 698
Tahitian Noni Seed Oil (Tahitian
    Noni International) 508, 699
Theraflu Cold & Cough Hot Liquid
    (Novartis Consumer) 630
Theraflu Cold & Sore Throat Hot
    Liquid (Novartis Consumer) 630
Theraflu Flu & Chest Congestion Hot
    Liquid (Novartis Consumer) 631
Theraflu Flu & Sore Throat Hot Liquid
    (Novartis Consumer) 631
Theraflu Daytime Severe Cold
    Caplets (Novartis Consumer) 634
Theraflu Nighttime Severe Cold
    Caplets (Novartis Consumer) 635
Theraflu Daytime Severe Cold Hot
    Liquid (Novartis Consumer) 632
Theraflu Nighttime Severe Cold
    Hot Liquid (Novartis
    Consumer) 506, 632
Theraflu Thin Strips Daytime
    Cold & Cough (Novartis
    Consumer) 506, 633
Theraflu Thin Strips Nighttime
    Cold & Cough (Novartis
    Consumer) 506, 633
Theraflu Warming Relief Daytime
    Severe Cold (Novartis Consumer) .. 634
Theraflu Warming Relief
    Nighttime Severe Cold
    (Novartis Consumer) 506, 635
Thera-Gesic Creme (Mission) 616
ThermaCare Heat Wraps
    (Procter & Gamble) 507, 645
ThermaCare Therapeutic Heat Wraps
    (Procter & Gamble) 647

Topricin Cream (Topical
  BioMedics) **508, 700**
**Triaminic Chest & Nasal Congestion
  Liquid** (Novartis Consumer) **636**
Triaminic Cold & Allergy Liquid
  (Novartis Consumer) **636**
**Triaminic Day Time Cold &
  Cough Liquid** (Novartis
  Consumer) **507, 637**
**Triaminic Night Time Cold &
  Cough Liquid** (Novartis
  Consumer) **507, 637**
Triaminic Cough & Sore Throat Liquid
  (Novartis Consumer) **638**
**Triaminic Cough & Runny Nose
  Softchews** (Novartis Consumer) **639**
**Triaminic Thin Strips Day Time
  Cold & Cough** (Novartis
  Consumer) **506, 640**
**Triaminic Thin Strips Night Time
  Cold & Cough** (Novartis
  Consumer) **506, 640**
**Triaminic Thin Strips Cold with
  Stuffy Nose** (Novartis
  Consumer) **506, 639**
**Triaminic Thin Strips Cough &
  Runny Nose** (Novartis
  Consumer) **506, 640**
**Triaminic Thin Strips Long Acting
  Cough** (Novartis Consumer) *506*
**Triaminic Infant & Toddler Thin
  Strips Decongestant**
  (Novartis Consumer) **507, 638**
**Triaminic Infant & Toddler Thin
  Strips Decongestant Plus
  Cough** (Novartis Consumer) .. **507, 638**

V

Vagistat-1 (Novartis Consumer) .. **507, 641**
**Vibe Liquid Multi-Nutrient
  Supplement** (Eniva) **503, 688**
**Vicks Formula 44 Cough Relief
  Liquid** (Procter & Gamble) **508, 648**
**Vicks Formula 44D Cough &
  Head Congestion Relief
  Liquid** (Procter & Gamble) **508, 649**

**Vicks Formula 44E Cough &
  Chest Congestion Relief
  Liquid** (Procter & Gamble) **508, 649**
**Pediatric Vicks 44e Cough &
  Chest Congestion Relief
  Liquid** (Procter & Gamble) **507, 654**
**Vicks Formula 44M Cough, Cold
  & Flu Relief Liquid** (Procter &
  Gamble) **508, 649**
**Pediatric Vicks Formula 44m
  Cough & Cold Relief Liquid**
  (Procter & Gamble) **507, 655**
**Vicks Cough Drops, Menthol and
  Cherry Flavors** (Procter &
  Gamble) **650**
**Vicks DayQuil LiquiCaps/Liquid
  Multi-Symptom Cold/Flu
  Relief** (Procter & Gamble) ... **507, 651**
**Vicks NyQuil LiquiCaps/Liquid
  Multi-Symptom Cold/Flu
  Relief** (Procter & Gamble) **507, 653**
**Children's Vicks NyQuil Cold/
  Cough Relief** (Procter &
  Gamble) **507, 650**
Vicks NyQuil Cough Liquid
  (Procter & Gamble) **508, 652**
**Vicks NyQuil D Cold & Flu
  Multi-Symptom Relief Liquid**
  (Procter & Gamble) **652**
**Vicks Sinex Nasal Spray and Ultra
  Fine Mist** (Procter & Gamble) **655**
**Vicks Sinex 12-Hour Nasal Spray
  and Ultra Fine Mist** (Procter &
  Gamble) **656**
Vicks Vapor Inhaler (Procter &
  Gamble) **656**
Vicks VapoRub Cream (Procter &
  Gamble) **656**
Vicks VapoRub Ointment (Procter &
  Gamble) **656**
Vicks VapoSteam (Procter &
  Gamble) **657**
VitaMist Intra-Oral Spray (Mayor) **692**

W

WINOmeg3Complex Capsules
  (Wellness International) **667**

Winrgy Dietary Supplement (Wellness
  International) **703**

Z

Zantac 75 Tablets (Boehringer
  Ingelheim) **503, 609**
**Maximum Strength Zantac 150
  Tablets** (Boehringer
  Ingelheim) **503, 610**
**Maximum Strength Zantac 150
  Cool Mint Tablets**
  (Boehringer Ingelheim) **503, 610**
Zicam Allergy Relief (Matrixx) ... **504, 611**
Zicam Cold Remedy Chewables
  (Matrixx) **504, 611**
Zicam Cold Remedy ChewCaps
  (Matrixx) **504, 611**
Zicam Cold Remedy Gel Swabs
  (Matrixx) **504, 611**
Zicam Cold Remedy Nasal Gel
  (Matrixx) **504, 611**
Zicam Cold Remedy Oral Mist
  (Matrixx) **504, 611**
Zicam Cold Remedy RapidMelts
  (Matrixx) **504, 611**
**Zicam Cold Remedy RapidMelts
  with Vitamin C** (Matrixx) **504, 611**
Zicam Cough Max Cough Spray
  (Matrixx) **504, 613**
Zicam Cough Max Cough Melts
  (Matrixx) **504, 613**
**Zicam Extreme Congestion
  Relief** (Matrixx) **504, 613**
Zicam Intense Sinus Relief
  (Matrixx) **504, 613**
**Zicam Multi-Symptom Liquid
  Daytime** (Matrixx) **503, 613**
**Zicam Multi-Symptom Cold &
  Flu Daytime To Go**
  (Matrixx) **503, 615**
**Zicam Multi-Symptom Cold &
  Flu Nightitime Liquid**
  (Matrixx) **503, 614**
**Zicam Multi-Symptom Cold &
  Flu Nighttime To Go**
  (Matrixx) **503, 615**
Zicam Sinus Melts (Matrixx) **504, 616**

SECTION 3

PRODUCT CATEGORY INDEX

This index cross-references each brand by pharmaceutical category. All fully described products in the Product Information sections are included.

If an entry in the index lists multiple page numbers, the first one shown refers to the photograph of the product,

the last one to its prescribing information.

The classification of each product is determined by the publisher in cooperation with the product's manufacturer or, when necessary, by the publisher alone.

A

ACNE PREPARATIONS
(see under:
  SKIN & MUCOUS MEMBRANE AGENTS
    ACNE PREPARATIONS)

ALTERNATIVE MEDICINE
(see under:
  HOMEOPATHIC REMEDIES)

AMINO ACIDS
(see under:
  DIETARY SUPPLEMENTS
    AMINO ACIDS & COMBINATIONS
    NUTRITIONAL THERAPY, ENTERAL
      AMINO ACIDS & COMBINATIONS)

ANALEPTIC AGENTS
(see under:
  CENTRAL NERVOUS SYSTEM STIMULANTS)

ANALGESICS
(see under:
  MIGRAINE PREPARATIONS
  RESPIRATORY AGENTS
    MISCELLANEOUS COLD & COUGH PRODUCTS WITH ANALGESICS
  SKIN & MUCOUS MEMBRANE AGENTS
    ANALGESICS & COMBINATIONS
    ANESTHETICS & COMBINATIONS)

ACETAMINOPHEN & COMBINATIONS
(see also under:
  ANTIHISTAMINES & COMBINATIONS
  RESPIRATORY AGENTS
    DECONGESTANTS & COMBINATIONS)

Comtrex Maximum Strength Day/Night
  Cold & Cough Caplets - Day
  Formulation (Novartis Consumer) **618**
Comtrex Maximum Strength Day/Night
  Cold & Cough Caplets - Night
  Formulation (Novartis Consumer) **618**
Comtrex Maximum Strength Non-Drowsy
  Cold & Cough Caplets (Novartis
  Consumer) **619**

Excedrin Back & Body Caplets
  (Novartis Consumer) **505, 620**
Excedrin Extra Strength Caplets/
  Tablets/Geltabs (Novartis
  Consumer) **505, 621**
Excedrin Migraine Caplets/
  Tablets/Geltabs (Novartis
  Consumer) **505, 622**
Excedrin PM Caplets/Tablets
  (Novartis Consumer) **505, 623**
Excedrin Sinus Headache Caplets/
  Tablets (Novartis
  Consumer) **505, 623**
Excedrin Tension Headache
  Caplets/Tablets/Geltabs
  (Novartis Consumer) **505, 621**
Regular Strength Pain Relief Tablets
  (Generic) **711**
Theraflu Cold & Sore Throat Hot Liquid
  (Novartis Consumer) **630**
Theraflu Flu & Chest Congestion Hot
  Liquid (Novartis Consumer) **631**
Theraflu Flu & Sore Throat Hot Liquid
  (Novartis Consumer) **631**
Theraflu Daytime Severe Cold Caplets
  (Novartis Consumer) **634**
Theraflu Nighttime Severe Cold Caplets
  (Novartis Consumer) **635**
Theraflu Daytime Severe Cold Hot Liquid
  (Novartis Consumer) **632**
Theraflu Nighttime Severe Cold Hot
  Liquid (Novartis
  Consumer) **506, 632**
Theraflu Warming Relief Daytime Severe
  Cold (Novartis Consumer) **634**
Theraflu Warming Relief Nighttime
  Severe Cold (Novartis
  Consumer) **506, 635**

Triaminic Cough & Sore Throat Liquid
  (Novartis Consumer) **638**
Vicks Formula 44M Cough, Cold &
  Flu Relief Liquid (Procter &
  Gamble) **508, 649**
Vicks DayQuil LiquiCaps/Liquid
  Multi-Symptom Cold/Flu Relief
  (Procter & Gamble) **507, 651**
Vicks NyQuil LiquiCaps/Liquid
  Multi-Symptom Cold/Flu Relief
  (Procter & Gamble) **507, 653**
Vicks NyQuil D Cold & Flu Multi-
  Symptom Relief Liquid (Procter &
  Gamble) **652**
Zicam Multi-Symptom Liquid
  Daytime (Matrixx) **503, 613**
Zicam Multi-Symptom Cold & Flu
  Daytime To Go (Matrixx) **503, 615**
Zicam Multi-Symptom Cold & Flu
  Nightitime Liquid (Matrixx) **503, 614**
Zicam Multi-Symptom Cold & Flu
  Nighttime To Go (Matrixx) **503, 615**
Zicam Sinus Melts (Matrixx) **504, 616**

MISCELLANEOUS ANALGESIC AGENTS
ThermaCare Heat Wraps (Procter &
  Gamble) **507, 645**
ThermaCare Therapeutic Heat Wraps
  (Procter & Gamble) **647**

**NONSTEROIDAL ANTI-INFLAMMATORY DRUGS
  (NSAIDS) & COMBINATIONS**
Advil Caplets (Wyeth) **668**
Advil Gel Caplets (Wyeth) **668**
Advil Liqui-Gels (Wyeth) **668**
Advil Tablets (Wyeth) **668**
Advil Allergy Sinus Caplets (Wyeth) **669**
Children's Advil Oral Suspension
  (Wyeth) **670**
Advil Cold & Sinus Caplets (Wyeth) **669**
Advil Cold & Sinus Liqui-Gels (Wyeth) **669**

ANALGESICS—cont.
NONSTEROIDAL ANTI-INFLAMMATORY DRUGS (NSAIDS) & COMBINATIONS—cont.
Infants' Advil Concentrated Drops - White Grape (Dye-Free) (Wyeth) 672
Advil Multi-Symptom Cold Caplets (Wyeth) 669
Advil PM Caplets (Wyeth) 671
Advil PM Liqui-Gels (Wyeth) 671
SALICYLATES
ASPIRIN & COMBINATIONS
Bufferin Extra Strength Tablets (Novartis Consumer) 617
Bufferin Regular Strength Tablets (Novartis Consumer) 504, 617
Excedrin Back & Body Caplets (Novartis Consumer) 505, 620
Excedrin Extra Strength Caplets/ Tablets/Geltabs (Novartis Consumer) 505, 621
Excedrin Migraine Caplets/ Tablets/Geltabs (Novartis Consumer) 505, 622
ANESTHETICS
(see under:
SKIN & MUCOUS MEMBRANE AGENTS
ANESTHETICS & COMBINATIONS)
ANORECTAL PRODUCTS
(see under:
SKIN & MUCOUS MEMBRANE AGENTS
ANORECTAL PREPARATIONS)
ANTACIDS
(see under:
GASTROINTESTINAL AGENTS
ANTACID & ANTIFLATULENT COMBINATIONS
ANTACIDS)
ANTHELMINTICS
(see under:
ANTI-INFECTIVE AGENTS, SYSTEMIC
ANTHELMINTICS)
ANTIARTHRITICS
(see under:
ANALGESICS
NONSTEROIDAL ANTI-INFLAMMATORY DRUGS (NSAIDS) & COMBINATIONS
SALICYLATES
SKIN & MUCOUS MEMBRANE AGENTS
ANALGESICS & COMBINATIONS)
ANTIEMETICS
(see under:
GASTROINTESTINAL AGENTS
ANTIEMETICS)
ANTIFLATULENTS
(see under:
GASTROINTESTINAL AGENTS
ANTACID & ANTIFLATULENT COMBINATIONS
ANTIFLATULENTS)
ANTIFUNGALS
(see under:
SKIN & MUCOUS MEMBRANE AGENTS
ANTI-INFECTIVES
ANTIFUNGALS & COMBINATIONS
VAGINAL PREPARATIONS
ANTI-INFECTIVES
ANTIFUNGALS & COMBINATIONS)
ANTIHISTAMINES & COMBINATIONS
Advil Allergy Sinus Caplets (Wyeth) 669
Advil Multi-Symptom Cold Caplets (Wyeth) 669
Advil PM Caplets (Wyeth) 671
Advil PM Liqui-Gels (Wyeth) 671
Alavert Allergy & Sinus D-12 Hour Tablets (Wyeth) 673
Alavert Orally Disintegrating Tablets (Wyeth) 673
Allergy Antihistamine Capsules (Generic) 708

Claritin Children's 24 Hour Non-Drowsy Chewables (Schering-Plough) 508, 659
Claritin Children's 24 Hour Non-Drowsy Allergy Syrup (Schering-Plough) 508, 659
Claritin Non-Drowsy 24 Hour Tablets (Schering-Plough) 508, 659
Claritin Reditabs 24 Hour Non-Drowsy Tablets (Schering-Plough) 508, 659
Claritin-D Non-Drowsy 12 Hour Tablets (Schering-Plough) 508, 658
Claritin-D Non-Drowsy 24 Hour Tablets (Schering-Plough) 508, 658
Comtrex Maximum Strength Day/Night Cold & Cough Caplets - Night Formulation (Novartis Consumer) 618
Children's Dimetapp Cold & Allergy Elixir (Wyeth) 674
Children's Dimetapp Cold & Allergy Chewable Tablets (Wyeth) 676
Children's Dimetapp DM Cold & Cough Elixir (Wyeth) 675
Children's Dimetapp Long Acting Cough Plus Cold Syrup (Wyeth) 675
Excedrin PM Caplets/Tablets (Novartis Consumer) 505, 623
Robitussin Cough & Allergy Syrup (Wyeth) 680
Robitussin Cough & Cold Long-Acting Liquid (Wyeth) 682
Robitussin Pediatric Cough & Cold Long-Acting Liquid (Wyeth) 682
Robitussin Night Time Cough & Cold Syrup (Wyeth) 683
Robitussin Night Time Pediatric Cough & Cold Syrup (Wyeth) 683
Theraflu Cold & Cough Hot Liquid (Novartis Consumer) 630
Theraflu Cold & Sore Throat Hot Liquid (Novartis Consumer) 630
Theraflu Flu & Sore Throat Hot Liquid (Novartis Consumer) 631
Theraflu Nighttime Severe Cold Caplets (Novartis Consumer) 635
Theraflu Nighttime Severe Cold Hot Liquid (Novartis Consumer) 506, 632
Theraflu Thin Strips Nighttime Cold & Cough (Novartis Consumer) 506, 633
Theraflu Warming Relief Nighttime Severe Cold (Novartis Consumer) 506, 635
Triaminic Cold & Allergy Liquid (Novartis Consumer) 636
Triaminic Night Time Cold & Cough Liquid (Novartis Consumer) 507, 637
Triaminic Cough & Runny Nose Softchews (Novartis Consumer) 639
Triaminic Thin Strips Night Time Cold & Cough (Novartis Consumer) 506, 640
Triaminic Thin Strips Cough & Runny Nose (Novartis Consumer) 506, 640
Vicks Formula 44M Cough, Cold & Flu Relief Liquid (Procter & Gamble) 508, 649
Pediatric Vicks Formula 44m Cough & Cold Relief Liquid (Procter & Gamble) 507, 655

Vicks NyQuil LiquiCaps/Liquid Multi-Symptom Cold/Flu Relief (Procter & Gamble) 507, 653
Children's Vicks NyQuil Cold/ Cough Relief (Procter & Gamble) 507, 650
Vicks NyQuil Cough Liquid (Procter & Gamble) 508, 652
Vicks NyQuil D Cold & Flu Multi-Symptom Relief Liquid (Procter & Gamble) 652
Zicam Multi-Symptom Cold & Flu Daytime To Go (Matrixx) 503, 615
Zicam Multi-Symptom Cold & Flu Nighttime Liquid (Matrixx) 503, 614
Zicam Multi-Symptom Cold & Flu Nighttime To Go (Matrixx) 503, 615
ANTI-INFECTIVE AGENTS
(see under:
ANTI-INFECTIVE AGENTS, SYSTEMIC
SKIN & MUCOUS MEMBRANE AGENTS
ANTI-INFECTIVES
VAGINAL PREPARATIONS)
ANTI-INFECTIVE AGENTS, SYSTEMIC
ANTHELMINTICS
Reese's Pinworm Treatments (Reese) 508, 657
ANTI-INFECTIVES, NON-SYSTEMIC
SCABICIDES & PEDICULICIDES
(see under:
SKIN & MUCOUS MEMBRANE AGENTS
ANTI-INFECTIVES
SCABICIDES & PEDICULICIDES)
ANTI-INFLAMMATORY AGENTS
(see under:
ANALGESICS
NONSTEROIDAL ANTI-INFLAMMATORY DRUGS (NSAIDS) & COMBINATIONS
SALICYLATES)
ANTIMYCOTICS
(see under:
SKIN & MUCOUS MEMBRANE AGENTS
ANTI-INFECTIVES
ANTIFUNGALS & COMBINATIONS
VAGINAL PREPARATIONS
ANTI-INFECTIVES
ANTIFUNGALS & COMBINATIONS)
ANTIPRURITICS
(see under:
ANTIHISTAMINES & COMBINATIONS)
ANTIPYRETICS
(see under:
ANALGESICS
ACETAMINOPHEN & COMBINATIONS
NONSTEROIDAL ANTI-INFLAMMATORY DRUGS (NSAIDS) & COMBINATIONS
SALICYLATES)
ANTITUSSIVES
(see under:
RESPIRATORY AGENTS
ANTITUSSIVES)
ARTHRITIS MEDICATIONS
(see under:
ANALGESICS
NONSTEROIDAL ANTI-INFLAMMATORY DRUGS (NSAIDS) & COMBINATIONS
SALICYLATES
SKIN & MUCOUS MEMBRANE AGENTS
ANALGESICS & COMBINATIONS)
ASTHMA PREPARATIONS
(see under:
RESPIRATORY AGENTS
BRONCHODILATORS)

B

BRONCHIAL DILATORS
(see under:
RESPIRATORY AGENTS
BRONCHODILATORS)

C

CALCIUM SUPPLEMENTS
(see under:
DIETARY SUPPLEMENTS
MINERALS & ELECTROLYTES
CALCIUM & COMBINATIONS)

CANKER SORE PREPARATIONS
(see under:
SKIN & MUCOUS MEMBRANE AGENTS
MOUTH & THROAT PRODUCTS
CANKER SORE PREPARATIONS)

CENTRAL NERVOUS SYSTEM AGENTS
(see under:
ANALGESICS
CENTRAL NERVOUS SYSTEM STIMULANTS
GASTROINTESTINAL AGENTS
ANTIEMETICS)

CENTRAL NERVOUS SYSTEM STIMULANTS
MISCELLANEOUS CENTRAL NERVOUS SYSTEM STIMULANTS
Excedrin Extra Strength Caplets/
Tablets/Geltabs (Novartis
Consumer) **505, 621**
Excedrin Migraine Caplets/
Tablets/Geltabs (Novartis
Consumer) **505, 622**
Excedrin Tension Headache
Caplets/Tablets/Geltabs
(Novartis Consumer) **505, 621**

COLD & COUGH PREPARATIONS
(see under:
ANTIHISTAMINES & COMBINATIONS
NASAL PREPARATIONS
SYMPATHOMIMETICS & COMBINATIONS
RESPIRATORY AGENTS
ANTITUSSIVES
DECONGESTANTS & COMBINATIONS
DECONGESTANTS, EXPECTORANTS & COMBINATIONS
EXPECTORANTS & COMBINATIONS
MISCELLANEOUS COLD & COUGH PRODUCTS WITH ANALGESICS
MISCELLANEOUS RESPIRATORY AGENTS
SKIN & MUCOUS MEMBRANE AGENTS
MOUTH & THROAT PRODUCTS
LOZENGES & SPRAYS)

COLD SORE PREPARATIONS
(see under:
SKIN & MUCOUS MEMBRANE AGENTS
MOUTH & THROAT PRODUCTS
COLD SORE PREPARATIONS)

CONSTIPATION AIDS
(see under:
GASTROINTESTINAL AGENTS
LAXATIVES)

COUGH PREPARATIONS
(see under:
RESPIRATORY AGENTS
ANTITUSSIVES
DECONGESTANTS, EXPECTORANTS & COMBINATIONS
EXPECTORANTS & COMBINATIONS
MISCELLANEOUS COLD & COUGH PRODUCTS WITH ANALGESICS)

D

DECONGESTANTS
(see under:
NASAL PREPARATIONS
SYMPATHOMIMETICS & COMBINATIONS
RESPIRATORY AGENTS
DECONGESTANTS & COMBINATIONS
DECONGESTANTS, EXPECTORANTS & COMBINATIONS)

DENTAL PREPARATIONS
(see under:
SKIN & MUCOUS MEMBRANE AGENTS
MOUTH & THROAT PRODUCTS
DENTAL PREPARATIONS)

DERMATOLOGICALS
(see under:
SKIN & MUCOUS MEMBRANE AGENTS)

DIARRHEA MEDICATIONS
(see under:
GASTROINTESTINAL AGENTS
ANTIDIARRHEALS)

DIET AIDS
(see under:
DIETARY SUPPLEMENTS)

DIETARY SUPPLEMENTS
AMINO ACIDS & COMBINATIONS
(see also under:
DIETARY SUPPLEMENTS
NUTRITIONAL THERAPY, ENTERAL
AMINO ACIDS & COMBINATIONS)
BioLean Mass Appeal Tablets (Wellness
International) **665**
BioLean ProXtreme Dietary Supplement
(Wellness International) **666**
Food for Thought Dietary Supplement
(Wellness International) **666**
StePHan Feminine Capsules (Wellness
International) **701**
StePHan Flexibility Capsules (Wellness
International) **701**
VitaMist Intra-Oral Spray (Mayor) **692**
Winrgy Dietary Supplement (Wellness
International) **703**

AMINO ACIDS & HERBAL COMBINATIONS
BioLean Accelerator Tablets (Wellness
International) **664**
BioLean Free Tablets (Wellness
International) **665**
BioLean II Tablets (Wellness
International) **664**
PLUS Caplets (Mannatech) **503, 691**
Satiete Tablets (Wellness
International) **667**
StePHan Clarity Capsules (Wellness
International) **700**
StePHan Elasticity Capsules (Wellness
International) **701**
StePHan Elixir Capsules (Wellness
International) **701**
StePHan Essential Capsules (Wellness
International) **701**
StePHan Lovpil Capsules (Wellness
International) **702**
StePHan Masculine Capsules (Wellness
International) **702**
StePHan Protector Capsules (Wellness
International) **702**
StePHan Relief Capsules (Wellness
International) **702**
StePHan Tranquility Capsules (Wellness
International) **702**
Vibe Liquid Multi-Nutrient
Supplement (Eniva) **503, 688**

DIGESTIVE AIDS
Align Daily Probiotic Supplement
(Procter & Gamble) **507, 696**
DDS-Acidophilus Capsules, Tablets, and
Powder (UAS Labs) **663**

ESSENTIAL FATTY ACIDS
Efacor Dietary Supplement
(Eniva) **503, 687**

FIBER SUPPLEMENTS
Benefiber Fiber Supplement
Powder (Novartis
Consumer) **504, 694**
Benefiber Fiber Supplement Sugar
Free Assorted Fruit Chewables
(Novartis Consumer) **504, 694**
Benefiber Fiber Supplement Sugar
Free Orange Creme Chewables
(Novartis Consumer) **504, 694**
Benefiber Fiber Supplement Plus B
Vitamins & Folic Acid Caplets
(Novartis Consumer) **504, 695**
Benefiber Fiber Supplement Plus B
Vitamins & Folic Acid Powder
(Novartis Consumer) **504, 695**
Benefiber Fiber Supplement Plus
Calcium Chewable Tablets
(Novartis Consumer) **504, 696**
Metamucil Dietary Fiber Supplement
(Procter & Gamble) **696**

HERBAL COMBINATIONS
DHEA & COMBINATIONS
DHEA Plus Capsules (Wellness
International) **666**
GINKGO BILOBA & COMBINATIONS
BioLean Free Tablets (Wellness
International) **665**
DHEA Plus Capsules (Wellness
International) **666**
VitaMist Intra-Oral Spray (Mayor) **692**
GINSENG & COMBINATIONS
BioLean Free Tablets (Wellness
International) **665**
HYPERICUM & COMBINATIONS
VitaMist Intra-Oral Spray (Mayor) **692**
MISCELLANEOUS HERBAL COMBINATIONS
Ambrotose Capsules
(Mannatech) **503, 690**
Ambrotose Powder
(Mannatech) **503, 690**
Advanced Ambrotose Capsules
(Mannatech) **503, 690**
Advanced Ambrotose Powder
(Mannatech) **503, 690**
Awareness Clear Capsules
(Awareness Corporation/
Awareness Life) **686**
Experience Capsules (Awareness
Corporation/
Awareness Life) **502, 686**
Tahitian Noni Liquid (Tahitian
Noni International) **508, 698**

HERBAL & MINERAL COMBINATIONS
BioLean LipoTrim Capsules (Wellness
International) **665**
Sleep-Tite Caplets (Wellness
International) **700**
StePHan Masculine Capsules (Wellness
International) **702**
StePHan Protector Capsules (Wellness
International) **702**

HERBAL & VITAMIN COMBINATIONS
Ambrotose AO Capsules
(Mannatech) **503, 691**

HERBAL, MINERAL & VITAMIN COMBINATIONS
BioLean Free Tablets (Wellness
International) **665**
BioLean Sure2Endure Tablets (Wellness
International) **703**
Centrum Performance Multivitamin/
Multimineral Supplement
(Wyeth) **705**
Daily Complete Liquid (Awareness
Corporation/
Awareness Life) **502, 686**
Phyto-Vite Tablets (Wellness
International) **667**
Satiete Tablets (Wellness
International) **667**
StePHan Clarity Capsules (Wellness
International) **700**
StePHan Elasticity Capsules (Wellness
International) **701**

DIETARY SUPPLEMENTS—cont.
HERBAL, MINERAL & VITAMIN COMBINATIONS—cont.
StePHan Elixir Capsules (Wellness International) **701**
StePHan Essential Capsules (Wellness International) **701**
StePHan Lovpil Capsules (Wellness International) **702**
StePHan Tranquility Capsules (Wellness International) **702**
Vibe Liquid Multi-Nutrient Supplement (Eniva) **503, 688**
VitaMist Intra-Oral Spray (Mayor) **692**
IMMUNE SYSTEM SUPPORT
Ambrotose Capsules (Mannatech) **503, 690**
Ambrotose Powder (Mannatech) **503, 690**
Advanced Ambrotose Capsules (Mannatech) **503, 690**
Advanced Ambrotose Powder (Mannatech) **503, 690**
Ambrotose AO Capsules (Mannatech) **503, 691**
Efacor Dietary Supplement (Eniva) **503, 687**
4Life Transfer Factor Plus Tri-Factor Formula (4Life) **689**
PLUS Caplets (Mannatech) **503, 691**
SynergyDefense Capsules (Awareness Corporation/ Awareness Life) **502, 686**
MINERALS & ELECTROLYTES
CALCIUM & COMBINATIONS
Benefiber Fiber Supplement Plus Calcium Chewable Tablets (Novartis Consumer) **504, 696**
Calcet Triple Calcium + Vitamin D Tablets (Mission) **693**
Caltrate 600 + D Tablets (Wyeth) **704**
Caltrate 600 + D PLUS Minerals Chewables (Wyeth) **704**
Caltrate 600 + D PLUS Minerals Tablets (Wyeth) **704**
Citracal Caplets (Mission) **693**
D-Cal Chewable Caplets (A&Z Pharm) **686**
PremCal Light, Regular, and Extra Strength Tablets (Dannmarie) **687**
MAGNESIUM & COMBINATIONS
Beelith Tablets (Beach) **687**
StePHan Feminine Capsules (Wellness International) **701**
MULTIMINERALS & COMBINATIONS
StePHan Feminine Capsules (Wellness International) **701**
MISCELLANEOUS DIETARY SUPPLEMENTS
Efacor Dietary Supplement (Eniva) **503, 687**
Hyland's Calms Forté 4 Kids Tablets (Standard Homeopathic) **661**
Intelectol Tablets (Memory Secret) **504, 693**
Natural Joint Capsules (Greek Island Labs) **690**
Pure Gardens Cream (Awareness Corporation/Awareness Life) **686**
PureTrim Mediterranean Wellness Shake (Awareness Corporation/ Awareness Life) **502, 686**
Tahitian Noni Liquid (Tahitian Noni International) **508, 698**

WINOmeg3Complex Capsules (Wellness International) **667**
NUTRITIONAL THERAPY, ENTERAL
AMINO ACIDS & COMBINATIONS
BioLean ProXtreme Dietary Supplement (Wellness International) **666**
LOW PROTEIN
BioLean ProXtreme Dietary Supplement (Wellness International) **666**
VITAMINS & COMBINATIONS
GERIATRIC FORMULATIONS
Centrum Silver Tablets (Wyeth) **706**
MULTIVITAMINS & COMBINATIONS
Vibe Liquid Multi-Nutrient Supplement (Eniva) **503, 688**
MULTIVITAMINS WITH MINERALS
BioLean ProXtreme Dietary Supplement (Wellness International) **666**
Centrum Tablets (Wyeth) **704**
Centrum Performance Multivitamin/ Multimineral Supplement (Wyeth) **705**
Centrum Silver Tablets (Wyeth) **706**
Food for Thought Dietary Supplement (Wellness International) **666**
StePHan Flexibility Capsules (Wellness International) **701**
Vibe Liquid Multi-Nutrient Supplement (Eniva) **503, 688**
VitaMist Intra-Oral Spray (Mayor) **692**
Winrgy Dietary Supplement (Wellness International) **703**
PEDIATRIC FORMULATIONS
Centrum Kids Complete Children's Chewables (Wyeth) **705**
VITAMIN A & COMBINATIONS
Phyto-Vite Tablets (Wellness International) **667**
B VITAMINS & COMBINATIONS
Benefiber Fiber Supplement Plus B Vitamins & Folic Acid Caplets (Novartis Consumer) **504, 695**
Benefiber Fiber Supplement Plus B Vitamins & Folic Acid Powder (Novartis Consumer) **504, 695**
Food for Thought Dietary Supplement (Wellness International) **666**
Winrgy Dietary Supplement (Wellness International) **703**
VITAMIN C & COMBINATIONS
Peridin-C Vitamin C Supplement (Beutlich) **687**
Phyto-Vite Tablets (Wellness International) **667**
Winrgy Dietary Supplement (Wellness International) **703**
VITAMIN D ANALOGUES & COMBINATIONS
Calcet Triple Calcium + Vitamin D Tablets (Mission) **693**
Citracal Caplets (Mission) **693**
PremCal Light, Regular, and Extra Strength Tablets (Dannmarie) **687**
VITAMIN E & COMBINATIONS
Phyto-Vite Tablets (Wellness International) **667**

E
ELECTROLYTES
(see under:
DIETARY SUPPLEMENTS
MINERALS & ELECTROLYTES)

EXPECTORANTS
(see under:
RESPIRATORY AGENTS
DECONGESTANTS, EXPECTORANTS & COMBINATIONS
EXPECTORANTS & COMBINATIONS)

F
FEVER PREPARATIONS
(see under:
ANALGESICS
ACETAMINOPHEN & COMBINATIONS
NONSTEROIDAL ANTI-INFLAMMATORY DRUGS (NSAIDS) & COMBINATIONS
SALICYLATES)
FOODS
(see under:
DIETARY SUPPLEMENTS
NUTRITIONAL THERAPY, ENTERAL)
FUNGAL MEDICATIONS
(see under:
SKIN & MUCOUS MEMBRANE AGENTS
ANTI-INFECTIVES
ANTIFUNGALS & COMBINATIONS
VAGINAL PREPARATIONS
ANTI-INFECTIVES
ANTIFUNGALS & COMBINATIONS)

G
GASTROINTESTINAL AGENTS
ANTACIDS
CALCIUM ANTACIDS & COMBINATIONS
Calcium Antacid Tablets (Generic) **708**
Gas-X with Maalox Extra Strength Chewable Tablets (Novartis Consumer) **506, 626**
Maalox Maximum Strength Multi Symptom Antacid/Antigas Chewable Tablets (Novartis Consumer) **506, 629**
MISCELLANEOUS ANTACID PREPARATIONS
Maalox Maximum Strength Total Stomach Relief Liquid (Novartis Consumer) **506, 629**
Children's Pepto (Procter & Gamble) **641**
ANTACID & ANTIFLATULENT COMBINATIONS
Gas-X with Maalox Extra Strength Chewable Tablets (Novartis Consumer) **506, 626**
Maalox Regular Strength Antacid/ Antigas Liquid (Novartis Consumer) **506, 628**
Maalox Maximum Strength Multi Symptom Antacid/Antigas Liquid (Novartis Consumer) **506, 628**
Maalox Maximum Strength Multi Symptom Antacid/Antigas Chewable Tablets (Novartis Consumer) **506, 629**
ANTIDIARRHEALS
Anti-Diarrheal Caplets (Generic) **708**
Maalox Maximum Strength Total Stomach Relief Liquid (Novartis Consumer) **506, 629**
Pepto-Bismol Original Liquid, Original and Cherry Chewable Tablets & Caplets (Procter & Gamble) **507, 643**
Pepto-Bismol Maximum Strength Liquid (Procter & Gamble) **643**
ANTIEMETICS
Maalox Maximum Strength Total Stomach Relief Liquid (Novartis Consumer) **506, 629**

Pepto-Bismol Original Liquid, Original and Cherry Chewable Tablets & Caplets (Procter & Gamble) **507, 643**

Pepto-Bismol Maximum Strength Liquid (Procter & Gamble) **643**

ANTIFLATULENTS

Gas-X Regular Strength Chewable Tablets (Novartis Consumer) **505, 626**

Gas-X Extra Strength Chewable Tablets (Novartis Consumer) **505, 626**

Gas-X Extra Strength Softgels (Novartis Consumer) **505, 626**

Gas-X Extra Strength Thin Strips (Novartis Consumer) **505, 626**

Gas-X Maximum Strength Softgels (Novartis Consumer) **505, 626**

HISTAMINE (H2) RECEPTOR ANTAGONISTS

Heartburn Relief, Acid Reducer Tablets (Generic) **709**

Zantac 75 Tablets (Boehringer Ingelheim) **503, 609**

Maximum Strength Zantac 150 Tablets (Boehringer Ingelheim) **503, 610**

Maximum Strength Zantac 150 Cool Mint Tablets (Boehringer Ingelheim) **503, 610**

LAXATIVES

BULK-PRODUCING LAXATIVES

Benefiber Fiber Supplement Caplets (Novartis Consumer) **504, 694**

Benefiber Fiber Supplement Plus B Vitamins & Folic Acid Caplets (Novartis Consumer) **504, 695**

Benefiber Fiber Supplement Plus B Vitamins & Folic Acid Powder (Novartis Consumer) **504, 695**

Benefiber Fiber Supplement Plus Calcium Chewable Tablets (Novartis Consumer) **504, 696**

FiberCon Caplets (Wyeth) **676**

Metamucil Capsules (Procter & Gamble) **507, 642**

Metamucil Powder, Original Texture Orange Flavor (Procter & Gamble) **642**

Metamucil Powder, Original Texture Regular Flavor (Procter & Gamble) **642**

Metamucil Smooth Texture Powder, Orange Flavor (Procter & Gamble) **507, 642**

Metamucil Smooth Texture Powder, Sugar-Free, Orange Flavor (Procter & Gamble) **642**

Metamucil Smooth Texture Powder, Sugar-Free, Regular Flavor (Procter & Gamble) **642**

Metamucil Wafers, Apple Crisp & Cinnamon Spice Flavors (Procter & Gamble) **507, 642**

FECAL SOFTENERS & COMBINATIONS

Dulcolax Stool Softener (Boehringer Ingelheim) **503, 609**

STIMULANT LAXATIVES & COMBINATIONS

Dulcolax Suppositories (Boehringer Ingelheim) **503, 609**

Dulcolax Tablets (Boehringer Ingelheim) **503, 608**

Ex•Lax Chocolated Laxative Pieces (Novartis Consumer) **505, 625**

Ex•Lax Regular Strength Pills (Novartis Consumer) **505, 625**

Ex•Lax Maximum Strength Pills (Novartis Consumer) **505, 625**

PROTON PUMP INHIBITORS

Prilosec OTC Tablets (Procter & Gamble) **507, 644**

H

HEAD LICE RELIEF
(*see under:*
SKIN & MUCOUS MEMBRANE AGENTS
ANTI-INFECTIVES
SCABICIDES & PEDICULICIDES)

HEMORRHOIDAL PREPARATIONS
(*see under:*
SKIN & MUCOUS MEMBRANE AGENTS
ANORECTAL PREPARATIONS)

HERBAL COMBINATIONS
HERBAL, MINERAL & VITAMIN COMBINATIONS
Vibe Liquid Multi-Nutrient Supplement (Eniva) **503, 688**

HERPES TREATMENT
(*see under:*
SKIN & MUCOUS MEMBRANE AGENTS
MOUTH & THROAT PRODUCTS
COLD SORE PREPARATIONS)

HISTAMINE (H2) RECEPTOR ANTAGONISTS
(*see under:*
GASTROINTESTINAL AGENTS
HISTAMINE (H2) RECEPTOR ANTAGONISTS)

HOMEOPATHIC REMEDIES
ALLERGY TREATMENT
Zicam Allergy Relief (Matrixx) **504, 611**

COLD & FLU PRODUCTS
Zicam Cold Remedy Chewables (Matrixx) **504, 611**

Zicam Cold Remedy ChewCaps (Matrixx) **504, 611**

Zicam Cold Remedy Gel Swabs (Matrixx) **504, 611**

Zicam Cold Remedy Nasal Gel (Matrixx) **504, 611**

Zicam Cold Remedy Oral Mist (Matrixx) **504, 611**

Zicam Cold Remedy RapidMelts (Matrixx) **504, 611**

Zicam Cold Remedy RapidMelts with Vitamin C (Matrixx) **504, 611**

GASTROINTESTINAL AGENTS
Hyland's Colic Tablets (Standard Homeopathic) **661**

MISCELLANEOUS HOMEOPATHIC REMEDIES
Hyland's Calms Forté Tablets and Caplets (Standard Homeopathic) **660**

Hyland's Earache Drops (Standard Homeopathic) **661**

Hyland's Nerve Tonic Tablets and Caplets (Standard Homeopathic) **662**

Hyland's Restful Legs Tablets (Standard Homeopathic) **662**

Tahitian Noni Seed Oil (Tahitian Noni International) **508, 699**

PAIN RELIEVERS
Hyland's BackAche with Arnica Caplets (Standard Homeopathic) **660**

Hyland's Earache Tablets (Standard Homeopathic) **661**

Hyland's Leg Cramps with Quinine Tablets and Caplets (Standard Homeopathic) **661**

Hyland's Migraine Headache Relief Tablets (Standard Homeopathic) **662**

Smile's Prid Salve (Standard Homeopathic) **662**

Topricin Cream (Topical BioMedics) **508, 700**

TEETHING REMEDIES
Hyland's Teething Gel (Standard Homeopathic) **663**

Hyland's Teething Tablets (Standard Homeopathic) **663**

I

IMMUNE SYSTEM SUPPORT
(*see also under:*
DIETARY SUPPLEMENTS
IMMUNE SYSTEM SUPPORT)
Efacor Dietary Supplement (Eniva) **503, 687**

L

LAXATIVES
(*see under:*
GASTROINTESTINAL AGENTS
LAXATIVES)

LICE TREATMENTS
(*see under:*
SKIN & MUCOUS MEMBRANE AGENTS
ANTI-INFECTIVES
SCABICIDES & PEDICULICIDES)

LUBRICANTS
(*see under:*
NASAL PREPARATIONS
SALINE
SKIN & MUCOUS MEMBRANE AGENTS
EMOLLIENTS & MOISTURIZERS)

M

MAGNESIUM PREPARATIONS
(*see under:*
DIETARY SUPPLEMENTS
MINERALS & ELECTROLYTES
MAGNESIUM & COMBINATIONS)

MIGRAINE PREPARATIONS
MISCELLANEOUS MIGRAINE PREPARATIONS
Hyland's Migraine Headache Relief Tablets (Standard Homeopathic) **662**

MINERALS
(*see under:*
DIETARY SUPPLEMENTS
MINERALS & ELECTROLYTES)

MINERALS & COMBINATIONS
MULTIMINERALS & COMBINATIONS
Vibe Liquid Multi-Nutrient Supplement (Eniva) **503, 688**

MOISTURIZERS
(*see under:*
SKIN & MUCOUS MEMBRANE AGENTS
EMOLLIENTS & MOISTURIZERS)

MOUTH & THROAT PRODUCTS
(*see under:*
SKIN & MUCOUS MEMBRANE AGENTS
MOUTH & THROAT PRODUCTS)

MUCOLYTICS
(*see under:*
RESPIRATORY AGENTS
DECONGESTANTS, EXPECTORANTS & COMBINATIONS
EXPECTORANTS & COMBINATIONS)

N

NAIL PREPARATIONS
(*see under:*
SKIN & MUCOUS MEMBRANE AGENTS)

NASAL PREPARATIONS
SALINE
4-Way Saline Nasal Spray (Novartis Consumer) **625**

NASAL PREPARATIONS—*cont.*
SALINE—*cont.*
Nasal Comfort Moisture Therapy
Sprays - Scented and
Unscented (Matrixx) **503, 611**
SYMPATHOMIMETICS & COMBINATIONS
4-Way Fast Acting Nasal Spray
(Novartis Consumer) **504, 624**
4-Way Menthol Nasal Spray (Novartis
Consumer) **624**
4-Way Moisturizing Relief Nasal Spray
(Novartis Consumer) **624**
Vicks Sinex Nasal Spray and Ultra Fine
Mist (Procter & Gamble) **655**
Vicks Sinex 12-Hour Nasal Spray and
Ultra Fine Mist (Procter &
Gamble) **656**
Vicks Vapor Inhaler (Procter &
Gamble) **656**
Zicam Extreme Congestion Relief
(Matrixx) **504, 613**
Zicam Intense Sinus Relief
(Matrixx) **504, 613**

NAUSEA MEDICATIONS
(*see under:*
GASTROINTESTINAL AGENTS
ANTIEMETICS)

**NONSTEROIDAL ANTI-INFLAMMATORY
AGENTS (NSAIDS)**
(*see under:*
ANALGESICS
**NONSTEROIDAL ANTI-INFLAMMATORY DRUGS
(NSAIDS) & COMBINATIONS**)

NSAIDS
(*see under:*
ANALGESICS
**NONSTEROIDAL ANTI-INFLAMMATORY DRUGS
(NSAIDS) & COMBINATIONS**
AMINO ACIDS & COMBINATIONS
Vibe Liquid Multi-Nutrient
Supplement (Eniva) **503, 688**

NUTRITIONAL THERAPY, ENTERAL
AMINO ACIDS & COMBINATIONS
Vibe Liquid Multi-Nutrient
Supplement (Envia) **503, 688**

NUTRITIONALS
(*see under:*
DIETARY SUPPLEMENTS)

O

ORAL HYGIENE PRODUCTS
(*see under:*
SKIN & MUCOUS MEMBRANE AGENTS
MOUTH & THROAT PRODUCTS)

P

PAIN RELIEVERS
(*see under:*
ANALGESICS)

PEDICULICIDES
(*see under:*
SKIN & MUCOUS MEMBRANE AGENTS
ANTI-INFECTIVES
SCABICIDES & PEDICULICIDES)

POISON IVY, OAK OR SUMAC PRODUCTS
(*see under:*
SKIN & MUCOUS MEMBRANE AGENTS
POISON IVY, OAK OR SUMAC PRODUCTS)

PROTON PUMP INHIBITORS
(*see under:*
GASTROINTESTINAL AGENTS
PROTON PUMP INHIBITORS)

PRURITUS MEDICATIONS
(*see under:*
ANTIHISTAMINES & COMBINATIONS)

PSYCHOSTIMULANTS
(*see under:*
CENTRAL NERVOUS SYSTEM STIMULANTS)

PSYCHOTHERAPEUTIC AGENTS
(*see under:*
CENTRAL NERVOUS SYSTEM STIMULANTS)

R

RESPIRATORY AGENTS
(*see also under:*
ANTIHISTAMINES & COMBINATIONS
NASAL PREPARATIONS)
ANTITUSSIVES
**NON-NARCOTIC ANTITUSSIVES &
COMBINATIONS**
Buckley's Cough Mixture (Novartis
Consumer) **618**
Comtrex Maximum Strength Day/Night
Cold & Cough Caplets - Day
Formulation (Novartis
Consumer) **618**
Comtrex Maximum Strength Day/Night
Cold & Cough Caplets - Night
Formulation (Novartis
Consumer) **618**
Comtrex Maximum Strength Non-
Drowsy Cold & Cough Caplets
(Novartis Consumer) **619**
Delsym Liquid Grape Flavor
(Adams) **502, 602**
Delsym Liquid Orange Flavor
(Adams) **502, 603**
Children's Dimetapp DM Cold &
Cough Elixir (Wyeth) **675**
Children's Dimetapp Long Acting Cough
Plus Cold Syrup (Wyeth) **675**
Toddler's Dimetapp Cold and Cough
Drops (Wyeth) **676**
Mucinex Cough Liquid
(Adams) **502, 603**
Mucinex Cough Mini-Melts
Orange Cream Flavor
(Adams) **502, 605**
Mucinex DM 600mg/30mg
Extended-Release Bi-Layer
Tablets (Adams) **502, 607**
Mucinex DM 1200mg/60mg
Extended-Release Bi-Layer
Tablets (Adams) **502, 607**
Robitussin Cough & Allergy Syrup
(Wyeth) **680**
Robitussin Cough & Cold CF Liquid
(Wyeth) **682**
Robitussin Cough & Cold CF Pediatric
Drops (Wyeth) **682**
Robitussin Cough & Cold Long-Acting
Liquid (Wyeth) **682**
Robitussin Pediatric Cough & Cold
Long-Acting Liquid (Wyeth) **682**
Robitussin Cough & Congestion Liquid
(Wyeth) **681**
Robitussin Cough Gels Long-Acting
(Wyeth) **680**
Robitussin Cough Long Acting Liquid
(Wyeth) **681**
Robitussin Pediatric Cough Long Acting
Liquid (Wyeth) **681**
Robitussin Sugar Free Cough Syrup
(Wyeth) **681**
Robitussin Cough DM Syrup
(Wyeth) **681**
Robitussin Cough DM Infant Drops
(Wyeth) **681**
Robitussin Cough Drops Menthol,
Cherry, and Honey (Wyeth) **679**
Robitussin Honey Cough Drops
(Wyeth) **679**
Robitussin Sugar Free Throat Drops
(Wyeth) **679**

Theraflu Cold & Cough Hot Liquid
(Novartis Consumer) **630**
Theraflu Daytime Severe Cold Caplets
(Novartis Consumer) **634**
Theraflu Nighttime Severe Cold Caplets
(Novartis Consumer) **635**
Theraflu Thin Strips Daytime Cold
& Cough (Novartis
Consumer) **506, 633**
Theraflu Warming Relief Daytime
Severe Cold (Novartis
Consumer) **634**
Triaminic Day Time Cold & Cough
Liquid (Novartis
Consumer) **507, 637**
Triaminic Cough & Sore Throat Liquid
(Novartis Consumer) **638**
Triaminic Cough & Runny Nose
Softchews (Novartis
Consumer) **639**
Triaminic Thin Strips Day Time
Cold & Cough (Novartis
Consumer) **506, 640**
Triaminic Infant & Toddler Thin
Strips Decongestant Plus
Cough (Novartis
Consumer) **507, 638**
Vicks Formula 44 Cough Relief
Liquid (Procter &
Gamble) **508, 648**
Vicks Formula 44D Cough &
Head Congestion Relief
Liquid (Procter &
Gamble) **508, 649**
Vicks Formula 44E Cough &
Chest Congestion Relief
Liquid (Procter &
Gamble) **508, 649**
Pediatric Vicks 44e Cough &
Chest Congestion Relief
Liquid (Procter &
Gamble) **507, 654**
Vicks Formula 44M Cough, Cold
& Flu Relief Liquid (Procter &
Gamble) **508, 649**
Pediatric Vicks Formula 44m
Cough & Cold Relief Liquid
(Procter & Gamble) **507, 655**
Vicks Cough Drops, Menthol and
Cherry Flavors (Procter &
Gamble) **650**
Vicks DayQuil LiquiCaps/Liquid
Multi-Symptom Cold/Flu
Relief (Procter &
Gamble) **507, 651**
Vicks NyQuil LiquiCaps/Liquid
Multi-Symptom Cold/Flu
Relief (Procter &
Gamble) **507, 653**
Children's Vicks NyQuil Cold/
Cough Relief (Procter &
Gamble) **507, 650**
Vicks NyQuil Cough Liquid
(Procter & Gamble) **508, 652**
Vicks NyQuil D Cold & Flu Multi-
Symptom Relief Liquid (Procter &
Gamble) **652**
Vicks VapoRub Cream (Procter &
Gamble) **656**
Vicks VapoRub Ointment (Procter &
Gamble) **656**
Vicks VapoSteam (Procter &
Gamble) **657**
Zicam Cough Max Cough Spray
(Matrixx) **504, 613**

Zicam Cough Max Cough Melts
(Matrixx) **504, 613**
Zicam Multi-Symptom Liquid
Daytime (Matrixx) **503, 613**
Zicam Multi-Symptom Cold & Flu
Daytime To Go (Matrixx) **503, 615**
Zicam Multi-Symptom Cold & Flu
Nightitime Liquid
(Matrixx) **503, 614**
Zicam Multi-Symptom Cold & Flu
Nighttime To Go
(Matrixx) **503, 615**

BRONCHODILATORS

SYMPATHOMIMETICS & COMBINATIONS
Primatene Mist (Wyeth) **678**

DECONGESTANTS & COMBINATIONS
Advil Allergy Sinus Caplets (Wyeth) **669**
Advil Cold & Sinus Caplets (Wyeth) **669**
Advil Cold & Sinus Liqui-Gels (Wyeth) **669**
Advil Multi-Symptom Cold Caplets
(Wyeth) **669**
Alavert Allergy & Sinus D-12 Hour Tablets
(Wyeth) **673**
Claritin-D Non-Drowsy 12 Hour
Tablets (Schering-Plough) **508, 658**
Claritin-D Non-Drowsy 24 Hour
Tablets (Schering-Plough) **508, 658**
Comtrex Maximum Strength Non-
Drowsy Cold & Cough Caplets
(Novartis Consumer) **619**
Children's Dimetapp Cold & Allergy Elixir
(Wyeth) **674**
Children's Dimetapp Cold & Allergy
Chewable Tablets (Wyeth) **676**
Children's Dimetapp DM Cold & Cough
Elixir (Wyeth) **675**
Toddler's Dimetapp Cold and Cough
Drops (Wyeth) **676**
Excedrin Sinus Headache Caplets/
Tablets (Novartis
Consumer) **505, 623**
4-Way Menthol Nasal Spray (Novartis
Consumer) **624**
4-Way Moisturizing Relief Nasal Spray
(Novartis Consumer) **624**
Non-Drowsy Nasal Decongestant
Maximum Strength Tablets
(Generic) **710**
Non-Drowsy Nasal Decongestant PE
Tablets (Generic) **711**
Robitussin Cough & Allergy Syrup
(Wyeth) **680**
Robitussin Head & Chest Congestion PE
Syrup (Wyeth) **680**
Robitussin Night Time Cough & Cold
Syrup (Wyeth) **683**
Robitussin Night Time Pediatric Cough &
Cold Syrup (Wyeth) **683**
Theraflu Cold & Cough Hot Liquid
(Novartis Consumer) **630**
Theraflu Cold & Sore Throat Hot Liquid
(Novartis Consumer) **630**
Theraflu Flu & Sore Throat Hot Liquid
(Novartis Consumer) **631**
Theraflu Daytime Severe Cold Caplets
(Novartis Consumer) **634**
Theraflu Nighttime Severe Cold Caplets
(Novartis Consumer) **635**
Theraflu Daytime Severe Cold Hot Liquid
(Novartis Consumer) **632**
Theraflu Nighttime Severe Cold Hot
Liquid (Novartis
Consumer) **506, 632**

Theraflu Thin Strips Daytime Cold
& Cough (Novartis
Consumer) **506, 633**
Theraflu Thin Strips Nighttime Cold
& Cough (Novartis
Consumer) **506, 633**
Theraflu Warming Relief Daytime
Severe Cold (Novartis Consumer) **634**
Theraflu Warming Relief Nighttime
Severe Cold (Novartis
Consumer) **506, 635**
Triaminic Cold & Allergy Liquid
(Novartis Consumer) **636**
Triaminic Day Time Cold & Cough
Liquid (Novartis
Consumer) **507, 637**
Triaminic Night Time Cold & Cough
Liquid (Novartis
Consumer) **507, 637**
Triaminic Thin Strips Day Time
Cold & Cough (Novartis
Consumer) **506, 640**
Triaminic Thin Strips Night Time
Cold & Cough (Novartis
Consumer) **506, 640**
Triaminic Thin Strips Cold with
Stuffy Nose (Novartis
Consumer) **506, 639**
Triaminic Infant & Toddler Thin
Strips Decongestant (Novartis
Consumer) **507, 638**
Triaminic Infant & Toddler Thin
Strips Decongestant Plus
Cough (Novartis
Consumer) **507, 638**
Vicks Formula 44D Cough & Head
Congestion Relief Liquid
(Procter & Gamble) **508, 649**
Vicks DayQuil LiquiCaps/Liquid
Multi-Symptom Cold/Flu Relief
(Procter & Gamble) **507, 651**
Vicks NyQuil D Cold & Flu Multi-
Symptom Relief Liquid (Procter &
Gamble) **652**
Vicks Vapor Inhaler (Procter &
Gamble) **656**
Zicam Multi-Symptom Cold & Flu
Daytime To Go (Matrixx) **503, 615**
Zicam Multi-Symptom Cold & Flu
Nighttime To Go (Matrixx) **503, 615**
Zicam Sinus Melts (Matrixx) **504, 616**

**DECONGESTANTS, EXPECTORANTS &
COMBINATIONS**
Comtrex Maximum Strength Day/Night
Cold & Cough Caplets - Day
Formulation (Novartis Consumer) **618**
Comtrex Maximum Strength Day/Night
Cold & Cough Caplets - Night
Formulation (Novartis Consumer) **618**
Mucinex Cold Liquid (Adams) **502, 604**
Mucinex D 600mg/60mg
Extended-Release Bi-Layer
Tablets (Adams) **502, 606**
Mucinex D 1200mg/120mg
Extended-Release Bi-Layer
Tablets (Adams) **502, 606**
Robitussin Cough & Cold CF Liquid
(Wyeth) **682**
Robitussin Cough & Cold CF Pediatric
Drops (Wyeth) **682**
Triaminic Chest & Nasal Congestion
Liquid (Novartis Consumer) **636**

EXPECTORANTS & COMBINATIONS
Buckley's Chest Congestion Mixture
(Novartis Consumer) **618**
Mucinex 600mg Extended-Release
Bi-Layer Tablets (Adams) **502, 605**

Mucinex 1200mg Extended-
Release Bi-Layer Tablets
(Adams) **502, 606**
Mucinex Cough Liquid
(Adams) **502, 603**
Mucinex Mini-Melts Bubble Gum
Flavor (Adams) **502, 604**
Mucinex Mini-Melts Grape Flavor
(Adams) **502, 604**
Mucinex Cough Mini-Melts Orange
Cream Flavor (Adams) **502, 605**
Mucinex DM 600mg/30mg
Extended-Release Bi-Layer
Tablets (Adams) **502, 607**
Mucinex DM 1200mg/60mg
Extended-Release Bi-Layer
Tablets (Adams) **502, 607**
Mucinex Liquid (Adams) **502, 603**
Robitussin Chest Congestion Liquid
(Wyeth) **679**
Robitussin Cough & Congestion Liquid
(Wyeth) **681**
Robitussin Sugar Free Cough Syrup
(Wyeth) **681**
Robitussin Cough DM Syrup (Wyeth) **681**
Robitussin Cough DM Infant Drops
(Wyeth) **681**
Robitussin Head & Chest Congestion PE
Syrup (Wyeth) **680**
Theraflu Flu & Chest Congestion Hot
Liquid (Novartis Consumer) **631**
Vicks Formula 44E Cough & Chest
Congestion Relief Liquid
(Procter & Gamble) **508, 649**
Pediatric Vicks 44e Cough & Chest
Congestion Relief Liquid
(Procter & Gamble) **507, 654**
Zicam Multi-Symptom Liquid
Daytime (Matrixx) **503, 613**

MISCELLANEOUS COLD & COUGH PRODUCTS
Robitussin Cough & Cold Long-Acting
Liquid (Wyeth) **682**
Robitussin Pediatric Cough & Cold Long-
Acting Liquid (Wyeth) **682**
Triaminic Day Time Cold & Cough
Liquid (Novartis
Consumer) **507, 637**
Triaminic Cough & Runny Nose
Softchews (Novartis Consumer) **639**

**MISCELLANEOUS COLD & COUGH PRODUCTS
WITH ANALGESICS**
Theraflu Daytime Severe Cold Caplets
(Novartis Consumer) **634**
Theraflu Daytime Severe Cold Hot Liquid
(Novartis Consumer) **632**
Triaminic Cough & Sore Throat Liquid
(Novartis Consumer) **638**
Vicks Formula 44M Cough, Cold &
Flu Relief Liquid (Procter &
Gamble) **508, 649**
Vicks DayQuil LiquiCaps/Liquid
Multi-Symptom Cold/Flu Relief
(Procter & Gamble) **507, 651**
Vicks NyQuil LiquiCaps/Liquid
Multi-Symptom Cold/Flu Relief
(Procter & Gamble) **507, 653**
Vicks NyQuil D Cold & Flu Multi-
Symptom Relief Liquid (Procter &
Gamble) **652**
Zicam Multi-Symptom Liquid
Daytime (Matrixx) **503, 613**
Zicam Multi-Symptom Cold & Flu
Daytime To Go (Matrixx) **503, 615**
Zicam Multi-Symptom Cold & Flu
Nightitime Liquid (Matrixx) **503, 614**
Zicam Multi-Symptom Cold & Flu
Nighttime To Go (Matrixx) **503, 615**

RESPIRATORY AGENTS—cont.

MISCELLANEOUS RESPIRATORY AGENTS

Hyland's Sniffles 'N Sneezes 4 Kids
Tablets (Standard Homeopathic) **662**

Robitussin Sugar Free Throat Drops
(Wyeth) **679**

S

SCABICIDES
(see under:

SKIN & MUCOUS MEMBRANE AGENTS
ANTI-INFECTIVES
SCABICIDES & PEDICULICIDES)

SHAMPOOS
(see under:

SKIN & MUCOUS MEMBRANE AGENTS
SHAMPOOS)

SKIN & MUCOUS MEMBRANE AGENTS

ACNE PREPARATIONS

DDS-Acidophilus Capsules, Tablets, and
Powder (UAS Labs) **663**

ANALGESICS & COMBINATIONS

Mineral Ice (Novartis
Consumer) **506, 629**

Thera-Gesic Creme (Mission) **616**

ThermaCare Therapeutic Heat Wraps
(Procter & Gamble) **647**

Vicks VapoRub Cream (Procter &
Gamble) **656**

Vicks VapoRub Ointment (Procter &
Gamble) **656**

ANESTHETICS & COMBINATIONS

Baby Anbesol Gel (Wyeth) **673**

Anbesol Junior Gel (Wyeth) **673**

Anbesol Maximum Strength Gel
(Wyeth) **673**

Anbesol Maximum Strength Liquid
(Wyeth) **673**

Hurricaine Topical Anesthetic Gel, 1 oz.
Wild Cherry, Pina Colada,
Watermelon, and Fresh Mint, 5.25 g.
Wild Cherry (Beutlich) **608**

Hurricaine Topical Anesthetic Liquid,
1 oz. Wild Cherry, Pina Colada,
0.005 fl. oz. Snap-n-Go Swabs Wild
Cherry (Beutlich) **608**

Hurricaine Topical Anesthetic Spray,
2 oz. Wild Cherry (Beutlich) **608**

Hurricaine Topical Anesthetic Spray
Extension Tubes (200) (Beutlich) **608**

Hurricaine Topical Anesthetic Spray Kit,
2 oz. Wild Cherry with disposable
Extension Tubes (200) (Beutlich) **608**

ANORECTAL PREPARATIONS

Preparation H Maximum Strength Cream
(Wyeth) **677**

Preparation H Ointment (Wyeth) **677**

Preparation H Suppositories (Wyeth) **677**

Preparation H Medicated Wipes
(Wyeth) **678**

ANTI-INFECTIVES

ANTIFUNGALS & COMBINATIONS

Desenex Athlete's Foot Cream
(Novartis Consumer) **505, 620**

Desenex Athlete's Foot Liquid
Spray (Novartis Consumer) **619**

Desenex Athlete's Foot Shake
Powder (Novartis
Consumer) **505, 619**

Desenex Athlete's Foot Spray
Powder (Novartis
Consumer) **505, 619**

Desenex Jock Itch Spray Powder
(Novartis Consumer) **619**

LamisilᴬᵀCreams (Athlete's Foot
& Jock Itch) (Novartis
Consumer) **506, 627**

Lamisilᴬᶠ Defense Powders
(Shake & Spray) (Novartis
Consumer) **506, 627**

SCABICIDES & PEDICULICIDES

Permethrin Lotion (Actavis) **602**

EMOLLIENTS & MOISTURIZERS

Tahitian Noni Leaf Serum Soothing
Gel (Tahitian Noni
International) **508, 698**

MOUTH & THROAT PRODUCTS

ANTIFUNGALS
(see under:

SKIN & MUCOUS MEMBRANE AGENTS
ANTI-INFECTIVES
ANTIFUNGALS & COMBINATIONS)

CANKER SORE PREPARATIONS

Anbesol Junior Gel (Wyeth) **673**

Anbesol Maximum Strength Gel
(Wyeth) **673**

Anbesol Maximum Strength Liquid
(Wyeth) **673**

Hurricaine Topical Anesthetic Gel, 1 oz.
Wild Cherry, Pina Colada,
Watermelon, and Fresh Mint,
5.25 g. Wild Cherry (Beutlich) **608**

Hurricaine Topical Anesthetic Liquid,
1 oz. Wild Cherry, Pina Colada,
0.005 fl. oz. Snap-n-Go Swabs Wild
Cherry (Beutlich) **608**

Hurricaine Topical Anesthetic Spray,
2 oz. Wild Cherry (Beutlich) **608**

Hurricaine Topical Anesthetic Spray
Extension Tubes (200)
(Beutlich) **608**

Hurricaine Topical Anesthetic Spray Kit,
2 oz. Wild Cherry with disposable
Extension Tubes (200)
(Beutlich) **608**

COLD SORE PREPARATIONS

Anbesol Cold Sore Therapy Ointment
(Wyeth) **674**

DENTAL PREPARATIONS

Anbesol Junior Gel (Wyeth) **673**

Anbesol Maximum Strength Gel
(Wyeth) **673**

Anbesol Maximum Strength Liquid
(Wyeth) **673**

Hurricaine Topical Anesthetic Gel, 1 oz.
Wild Cherry, Pina Colada,
Watermelon, and Fresh Mint,
5.25 g. Wild Cherry (Beutlich) **608**

Hurricaine Topical Anesthetic Liquid,
1 oz. Wild Cherry, Pina Colada,
0.005 fl. oz. Snap-n-Go Swabs Wild
Cherry (Beutlich) **608**

Hurricaine Topical Anesthetic Spray,
2 oz. Wild Cherry (Beutlich) **608**

Hurricaine Topical Anesthetic Spray
Extension Tubes (200)
(Beutlich) **608**

Hurricaine Topical Anesthetic Spray Kit,
2 oz. Wild Cherry with disposable
Extension Tubes (200)
(Beutlich) **608**

LOZENGES & SPRAYS

Vicks Cough Drops, Menthol and
Cherry Flavors (Procter &
Gamble) **650**

TEETHING REMEDIES

Baby Anbesol Gel (Wyeth) **673**

POISON IVY, OAK OR SUMAC PRODUCTS

Ivy Block (Standard Homeopathic) **663**

SHAMPOOS

Head & Shoulders Intensive Solutions
Dandruff Shampoo (Procter &
Gamble) **641**

VAGINAL PRODUCTS
(see under:

VAGINAL PREPARATIONS)

SKIN CARE PRODUCTS
(see under:

SKIN & MUCOUS MEMBRANE AGENTS)

SMOKING CESSATION AIDS

Nicotine Gum, Stop Smoking Aid
(Generic) **709**

Nicotine Transdermal System Patch,
Stop Smoking Aid (Generic) **710**

SUPPLEMENTS
(see under:

DIETARY SUPPLEMENTS)

SYMPATHOMIMETICS
(see under:

NASAL PREPARATIONS
SYMPATHOMIMETICS & COMBINATIONS
RESPIRATORY AGENTS
BRONCHODILATORS
SYMPATHOMIMETICS & COMBINATIONS
DECONGESTANTS & COMBINATIONS
DECONGESTANTS, EXPECTORANTS &
COMBINATIONS)

T

TEETHING REMEDIES
(see under:

SKIN & MUCOUS MEMBRANE AGENTS
MOUTH & THROAT PRODUCTS
TEETHING REMEDIES
HOMEOPATHIC REMEDIES
TEETHING REMEDIES)

THROAT LOZENGES
(see under:

SKIN & MUCOUS MEMBRANE AGENTS
MOUTH & THROAT PRODUCTS
LOZENGES & SPRAYS)

TOPICAL PREPARATIONS
(see under:

NASAL PREPARATIONS
SKIN & MUCOUS MEMBRANE AGENTS
VAGINAL PREPARATIONS)

V

VAGINAL PREPARATIONS

ANTI-INFECTIVES

ANTIFUNGALS & COMBINATIONS

Vagistat-1 (Novartis
Consumer) **507, 641**

CLEANSERS AND DOUCHES

Preparation H Medicated Wipes
(Wyeth) **678**

VITAMIN D ANALOGUES
(see under:

DIETARY SUPPLEMENTS
VITAMINS & COMBINATIONS
VITAMIN D ANALOGUES & COMBINATIONS)

VITAMINS
(see under:

DIETARY SUPPLEMENTS
VITAMINS & COMBINATIONS)

VITAMINS & COMBINATIONS

MULTIMINERALS & COMBINATIONS

Vibe Liquid Multi-Nutrient
Supplement (Eniva) **503, 688**

MULTIVITAMINS & COMBINATIONS

Vibe Liquid Multi-Nutrient
Supplement (Eniva) **503, 688**

MULTIVITAMINS WITH MINERALS

Vibe Liquid Multi-Nutrient
Supplement (Eniva) **503, 688**

W

WEIGHT CONTROL PREPARATIONS
(see under:

DIETARY SUPPLEMENTS
NUTRITIONAL THERAPY, ENTERAL)

SECTION 4

ACTIVE INGREDIENTS INDEX

This index cross-references each brand by its generic ingredients. All entries in the Product Information sections are included. Under each generic heading, all fully described products are listed first, followed by those with only partial descriptions.

If an entry in the index lists multiple page numbers, the first one shown refers to the photograph of the product, the last one to its prescribing information.

- **Bold page numbers** indicate full product information.
- *Italic page numbers* signify partial information.

Classification of products under these headings has been determined in cooperation with the products' manufacturers or, if necessary, by the publisher alone.

A

ACETAMINOPHEN
Comtrex Maximum Strength Day/Night Cold & Cough Caplets - Day Formulation (Novartis Consumer) **618**
Comtrex Maximum Strength Day/Night Cold & Cough Caplets - Night Formulation (Novartis Consumer) **618**
Comtrex Maximum Strength Non-Drowsy Cold & Cough Caplets (Novartis Consumer) **619**
Excedrin Back & Body Caplets (Novartis Consumer) **505, 620**
Excedrin Extra Strength Caplets/ Tablets/Geltabs (Novartis Consumer) **505, 621**
Excedrin Migraine Caplets/ Tablets/Geltabs (Novartis Consumer) **505, 622**
Excedrin PM Caplets/Tablets (Novartis Consumer) **505, 623**
Excedrin Sinus Headache Caplets/ Tablets (Novartis Consumer) **505, 623**
Excedrin Tension Headache Caplets/Tablets/Geltabs (Novartis Consumer) **505, 621**
Regular Strength Pain Relief Tablets (Generic) **711**
Theraflu Cold & Sore Throat Hot Liquid (Novartis Consumer) **630**
Theraflu Flu & Chest Congestion Hot Liquid (Novartis Consumer) **631**
Theraflu Flu & Sore Throat Hot Liquid (Novartis Consumer) **631**
Theraflu Daytime Severe Cold Caplets (Novartis Consumer) **634**
Theraflu Nighttime Severe Cold Caplets (Novartis Consumer) **635**

Theraflu Daytime Severe Cold Hot Liquid (Novartis Consumer) **632**
Theraflu Nighttime Severe Cold Hot Liquid (Novartis Consumer) **506, 632**
Theraflu Warming Relief Daytime Severe Cold (Novartis Consumer) **634**
Theraflu Warming Relief Nighttime Severe Cold (Novartis Consumer) **506, 635**
Triaminic Cough & Sore Throat Liquid (Novartis Consumer) **638**
Vicks Formula 44M Cough, Cold & Flu Relief Liquid (Procter & Gamble) **508, 649**
Vicks DayQuil LiquiCaps/Liquid Multi-Symptom Cold/Flu Relief (Procter & Gamble) **507, 651**
Vicks NyQuil LiquiCaps/Liquid Multi-Symptom Cold/Flu Relief (Procter & Gamble) **507, 653**
Vicks NyQuil D Cold & Flu Multi-Symptom Relief Liquid (Procter & Gamble) **652**
Zicam Multi-Symptom Liquid Daytime (Matrixx) **503, 613**
Zicam Multi-Symptom Cold & Flu Daytime To Go (Matrixx) **503, 615**
Zicam Multi-Symptom Cold & Flu Nighttime Liquid (Matrixx) **503, 614**
Zicam Multi-Symptom Cold & Flu Nighttime To Go (Matrixx) **503, 615**
Zicam Sinus Melts (Matrixx) **504, 616**

ACETYLSALICYLIC ACID
(*see under:* **ASPIRIN**)

ALLANTOIN
Anbesol Cold Sore Therapy Ointment (Wyeth) **674**

ALOE VERA
Daily Complete Liquid (Awareness Corporation/ Awareness Life) **502, 686**
Vibe Liquid Multi-Nutrient Supplement (Fniva) **503, 688**

ALPHA TOCOPHERAL ACETATE
(*see under:* **VITAMIN E**)

ALPHA-HYDROXY
Amlactin XL Moisturizing Lotion (Upsher-Smith) *664*

ALUMINUM HYDROXIDE
Maalox Regular Strength Antacid/ Antigas Liquid (Novartis Consumer) **506, 628**
Maalox Maximum Strength Multi Symptom Antacid/Antigas Liquid (Novartis Consumer) **506, 628**

AMINO ACID PREPARATIONS
BioLean Accelerator Tablets (Wellness International) **664**
BioLean Free Tablets (Wellness International) **665**
BioLean II Tablets (Wellness International) **664**
BioLean Mass Appeal Tablets (Wellness International) **665**
BioLean ProXtreme Dietary Supplement (Wellness International) **666**
Daily Complete Liquid (Awareness Corporation/ Awareness Life) **502, 686**
Food for Thought Dietary Supplement (Wellness International) **666**
4Life Transfer Factor Plus Tri-Factor Formula (4Life) **689**
PLUS Caplets (Mannatech) **503, 691**

AMINO ACID PREPARATIONS—cont.

Satiete Tablets (Wellness
International) **667**
StePHan Clarity Capsules (Wellness
International) **700**
StePHan Elasticity Capsules (Wellness
International) **701**
StePHan Elixir Capsules (Wellness
International) **701**
StePHan Essential Capsules (Wellness
International) **701**
StePHan Feminine Capsules (Wellness
International) **701**
StePHan Flexibility Capsules (Wellness
International) **701**
StePHan Lovpil Capsules (Wellness
International) **702**
StePHan Masculinc Capsules (Wellness
International) **702**
StePHan Protector Capsules (Wellness
International) **702**
StePHan Relief Capsules (Wellness
International) **702**
StePHan Tranquility Capsules (Wellness
International) **702**
Vibe Liquid Multi-Nutrient
Supplement (Eniva) **503, 688**
VitaMist Intra-Oral Spray (Mayor) **692**
Winrgy Dietary Supplement (Wellness
International) **703**
ANTIOXIDANTS
Daily Complete Liquid (Awareness
Corporation/
Awareness Life) **502, 686**
Phyto-Vite Tablets (Wellness
International) **667**
PureTrim Mediterranean Wellness
Shake (Awareness
Corporation/
Awareness Life) **502, 686**
Vibe Liquid Multi-Nutrient
Supplement (Eniva) **503, 688**
ASCORBIC ACID
(*see under:* **VITAMIN C**)
ASPIRIN
Excedrin Extra Strength Caplets/
Tablets/Geltabs (Novartis
Consumer) **505, 621**
Excedrin Migraine Caplets/
Tablets/Geltabs (Novartis
Consumer) **505, 622**
ASPIRIN BUFFERED
Bufferin Extra Strength Tablets (Novartis
Consumer) **617**
Bufferin Regular Strength Tablets
(Novartis Consumer) **504, 617**
Excedrin Back & Body Caplets
(Novartis Consumer) **505, 620**
ASTRAGALUS
StePHan Protector Capsules (Wellness
International) **702**

B

B VITAMINS
Benefiber Fiber Supplement Plus B
Vitamins & Folic Acid Caplets
(Novartis Consumer) **504, 695**
Benefiber Fiber Supplement Plus B
Vitamins & Folic Acid Powder
(Novartis Consumer) **504, 695**
BEE POLLEN
StePHan Clarity Capsules (Wellness
International) **700**
StePHan Elixir Capsules (Wellness
International) **701**
StePHan Masculine Capsules (Wellness
International) **702**

BELLADONNA
Hyland's Migraine Headache Relief
Tablets (Standard Homeopathic) **662**
BELLADONNA ALKALOIDS
Hyland's Earache Tablets (Standard
Homeopathic) **661**
Hyland's Teething Gel (Standard
Homeopathic) **663**
Hyland's Teething Tablets (Standard
Homeopathic) **663**
BENTOQUATAM
Ivy Block (Standard Homeopathic) **663**
BENZOCAINE
Anbesol Cold Sore Therapy Ointment
(Wyeth) **674**
Baby Anbesol Gel (Wyeth) **673**
Anbesol Junior Gel (Wyeth) **673**
Anbesol Maximum Strength Gel
(Wyeth) **673**
Anbesol Maximum Strength Liquid
(Wyeth) **673**
Hurricaine Topical Anesthetic Gel, 1 oz.
Wild Cherry, Pina Colada,
Watermelon, and Fresh Mint, 5.25 g.
Wild Cherry (Beutlich) **608**
Hurricaine Topical Anesthetic Liquid,
1 oz. Wild Cherry, Pina Colada,
0.005 fl. oz. Snap-n-Go Swabs Wild
Cherry (Beutlich) **608**
Hurricaine Topical Anesthetic Spray,
2 oz. Wild Cherry (Beutlich) **608**
Hurricaine Topical Anesthetic Spray
Extension Tubes (200) (Beutlich) **608**
Hurricaine Topical Anesthetic Spray Kit,
2 oz. Wild Cherry with disposable
Extension Tubes (200) (Beutlich) **608**
BIFIDOBACTERIA
Align Daily Probiotic Supplement
(Procter & Gamble) **507, 696**
BIOFLAVONOIDS
Peridin-C Vitamin C Supplement
(Beutlich) **687**
Phyto-Vite Tablets (Wellness
International) **667**
Vibe Liquid Multi-Nutrient
Supplement (Eniva) **503, 688**
BISACODYL
Dulcolax Suppositories (Boehringer
Ingelheim) **503, 609**
Dulcolax Tablets (Boehringer
Ingelheim) **503, 608**
BISMUTH SUBSALICYLATE
Maalox Maximum Strength Total
Stomach Relief Liquid
(Novartis Consumer) **506, 629**
Pepto-Bismol Original Liquid,
Original and Cherry Chewable
Tablets & Caplets (Procter &
Gamble) **507, 643**
Pepto-Bismol Maximum Strength Liquid
(Procter & Gamble) **643**
BROMPHENIRAMINE MALEATE
Children's Dimetapp Cold & Allergy Elixir
(Wyeth) **674**
Children's Dimetapp Cold & Allergy
Chewable Tablets (Wyeth) **676**
Children's Dimetapp DM Cold & Cough
Elixir (Wyeth) **675**

C

CAFFEINE
Excedrin Extra Strength Caplets/
Tablets/Geltabs (Novartis
Consumer) **505, 621**

Excedrin Migraine Caplets/
Tablets/Geltabs (Novartis
Consumer) **505, 622**
Excedrin Tension Headache
Caplets/Tablets/Geltabs
(Novartis Consumer) **505, 621**
Winrgy Dietary Supplement (Wellness
International) **703**
CALCIUM
Vibe Liquid Multi-Nutrient
Supplement (Eniva) **503, 688**
CALCIUM CARBONATE
Benefiber Fiber Supplement Plus
Calcium Chewable Tablets
(Novartis Consumer) **504, 696**
Calcet Triple Calcium + Vitamin D
Tablets (Mission) **693**
Calcium Antacid Tablets (Generic) **708**
Caltrate 600 + D Tablets (Wyeth) **704**
Caltrate 600 + D PLUS Minerals
Chewables (Wyeth) **704**
Caltrate 600 + D PLUS Minerals Tablets
(Wyeth) **704**
D-Cal Chewable Caplets
(A&Z Pharm) **686**
Gas-X with Maalox Extra Strength
Chewable Tablets (Novartis
Consumer) **506, 626**
Maalox Maximum Strength Multi
Symptom Antacid/Antigas
Chewable Tablets (Novartis
Consumer) **506, 629**
Children's Pepto (Procter & Gamble) **641**
PremCal Light, Regular, and Extra
Strength Tablets (Dannmarie) **687**
StePHan Elixir Capsules (Wellness
International) **701**
CALCIUM CITRATE
Citracal Caplets (Mission) **693**
CALCIUM GLUCONATE
Calcet Triple Calcium + Vitamin D
Tablets (Mission) **693**
CALCIUM LACTATE
Calcet Triple Calcium + Vitamin D
Tablets (Mission) **693**
CALCIUM POLYCARBOPHIL
FiberCon Caplets (Wyeth) **676**
CAMPHOR
Anbesol Cold Sore Therapy Ointment
(Wyeth) **674**
Vicks VapoRub Cream (Procter &
Gamble) **656**
Vicks VapoRub Ointment (Procter &
Gamble) **656**
Vicks VapoSteam (Procter &
Gamble) **657**
CELLULOSE
StePHan Protector Capsules (Wellness
International) **702**
CHAMOMILLA
Hyland's Colic Tablets (Standard
Homeopathic) **661**
CHLORPHENIRAMINE MALEATE
Advil Allergy Sinus Caplets (Wyeth) **669**
Advil Multi-Symptom Cold Caplets
(Wyeth) **669**
Comtrex Maximum Strength Day/Night
Cold & Cough Caplets - Night
Formulation (Novartis Consumer) **618**
Children's Dimetapp Long Acting Cough
Plus Cold Syrup (Wyeth) **675**

Italic Page Number **Indicates Brief Listing**

Robitussin Cough & Allergy Syrup
(Wyeth) **680**
Robitussin Cough & Cold Long-Acting
Liquid (Wyeth) **682**
Robitussin Pediatric Cough & Cold
Long-Acting Liquid (Wyeth) **682**
Theraflu Nighttime Severe Cold Caplets
(Novartis Consumer) **635**
Triaminic Cold & Allergy Liquid (Novartis
Consumer) **636**
Triaminic Cough & Runny Nose
Softchews (Novartis Consumer) **639**
Vicks Formula 44M Cough, Cold &
Flu Relief Liquid (Procter &
Gamble) **508, 649**
Pediatric Vicks Formula 44m
Cough & Cold Relief Liquid
(Procter & Gamble) **507, 655**
Children's Vicks NyQuil Cold/
Cough Relief (Procter &
Gamble) **507, 650**
Zicam Multi-Symptom Cold & Flu
Daytime To Go (Matrixx) **503, 615**

CHOLECALCIFEROL
Calcet Triple Calcium + Vitamin D
Tablets (Mission) **693**
Citracal Caplets (Mission) **693**

CIMETIDINE
Heartburn Relief, Acid Reducer Tablets
(Generic) **709**

CLOTRIMAZOLE
Desenex Athlete's Foot Cream
(Novartis Consumer) **505, 620**

COCOA BUTTER
Preparation H Suppositories (Wyeth) **677**

COENZYME Q-10
VitaMist Intra-Oral Spray (Mayor) **692**

COLOCYNTHIS
Hyland's Colic Tablets (Standard
Homeopathic) **661**

CYANOCOBALAMIN
(see under: **VITAMIN B₁₂**)

D

DEVICE
ThermaCare Heat Wraps (Procter &
Gamble) **507, 645**
ThermaCare Therapeutic Heat Wraps
(Procter & Gamble) **647**

DEXTROMETHORPHAN HYDROBROMIDE
Buckley's Cough Mixture (Novartis
Consumer) **618**
Comtrex Maximum Strength Day/Night
Cold & Cough Caplets - Day
Formulation (Novartis Consumer) **618**
Comtrex Maximum Strength Day/Night
Cold & Cough Caplets - Night
Formulation (Novartis Consumer) **618**
Comtrex Maximum Strength Non-Drowsy
Cold & Cough Caplets (Novartis
Consumer) **619**
Children's Dimetapp DM Cold & Cough
Elixir (Wyeth) **675**
Children's Dimetapp Long Acting Cough
Plus Cold Syrup (Wyeth) **675**
Toddler's Dimetapp Cold and Cough
Drops (Wyeth) **676**
Mucinex Cough Liquid
(Adams) **502, 603**
Mucinex Cough Mini-Melts Orange
Cream Flavor (Adams) **502, 605**

Mucinex DM 600mg/30mg
Extended-Release Bi-Layer
Tablets (Adams) **502, 607**
Mucinex DM 1200mg/60mg
Extended-Release Bi-Layer
Tablets (Adams) **502, 607**
Robitussin Cough & Allergy Syrup
(Wyeth) **680**
Robitussin Cough & Cold CF Liquid
(Wyeth) **682**
Robitussin Cough & Cold CF Pediatric
Drops (Wyeth) **682**
Robitussin Cough & Cold Long-Acting
Liquid (Wyeth) **682**
Robitussin Pediatric Cough & Cold Long-
Acting Liquid (Wyeth) **682**
Robitussin Cough & Congestion Liquid
(Wyeth) **681**
Robitussin Cough Gels Long-Acting
(Wyeth) **680**
Robitussin Cough Long Acting Liquid
(Wyeth) **681**
Robitussin Pediatric Cough Long Acting
Liquid (Wyeth) **681**
Robitussin Sugar Free Cough Syrup
(Wyeth) **681**
Robitussin Cough DM Syrup (Wyeth) **681**
Robitussin Cough DM Infant Drops
(Wyeth) **681**
Theraflu Cold & Cough Hot Liquid
(Novartis Consumer) **630**
Theraflu Daytime Severe Cold Caplets
(Novartis Consumer) **634**
Theraflu Nighttime Severe Cold Caplets
(Novartis Consumer) **635**
Theraflu Thin Strips Daytime Cold
& Cough (Novartis
Consumer) **506, 633**
Theraflu Warming Relief Daytime Severe
Cold (Novartis Consumer) **634**
Triaminic Day Time Cold & Cough
Liquid (Novartis
Consumer) **507, 637**
Triaminic Cough & Sore Throat Liquid
(Novartis Consumer) **638**
Triaminic Cough & Runny Nose
Softchews (Novartis Consumer) **639**
Triaminic Thin Strips Day Time
Cold & Cough (Novartis
Consumer) **506, 640**
Triaminic Infant & Toddler Thin
Strips Decongestant Plus
Cough (Novartis
Consumer) **507, 638**
Vicks Formula 44 Cough Relief
Liquid (Procter & Gamble) **508, 648**
Vicks Formula 44D Cough & Head
Congestion Relief Liquid
(Procter & Gamble) **508, 649**
Vicks Formula 44E Cough & Chest
Congestion Relief Liquid
(Procter & Gamble) **508, 649**
Pediatric Vicks 44e Cough & Chest
Congestion Relief Liquid
(Procter & Gamble) **507, 654**
Vicks Formula 44M Cough, Cold &
Flu Relief Liquid (Procter &
Gamble) **508, 649**
Pediatric Vicks Formula 44m
Cough & Cold Relief Liquid
(Procter & Gamble) **507, 655**
Vicks DayQuil LiquiCaps/Liquid
Multi-Symptom Cold/Flu Relief
(Procter & Gamble) **507, 651**

Vicks NyQuil LiquiCaps/Liquid
Multi-Symptom Cold/Flu Relief
(Procter & Gamble) **507, 653**
Children's Vicks NyQuil Cold/
Cough Relief (Procter &
Gamble) **507, 650**
Vicks NyQuil Cough Liquid (Procter
& Gamble) **508, 652**
Vicks NyQuil D Cold & Flu Multi-Symptom
Relief Liquid (Procter & Gamble) **652**
Zicam Cough Max Cough Spray
(Matrixx) **504, 613**
Zicam Cough Max Cough Melts
(Matrixx) **504, 613**
Zicam Multi-Symptom Liquid
Daytime (Matrixx) **503, 613**
Zicam Multi-Symptom Cold & Flu
Daytime To Go (Matrixx) **503, 615**
Zicam Multi-Symptom Cold & Flu
Nighttime Liquid (Matrixx) **503, 614**
Zicam Multi-Symptom Cold & Flu
Nighttime To Go (Matrixx) **503, 615**

DEXTROMETHORPHAN POLISTIREX
Delsym Liquid Grape Flavor
(Adams) **502, 602**
Delsym Liquid Orange Flavor
(Adams) **502, 603**

DHA (DOCOSAHEXAENOIC ACID)
(see under: **DOCOSAHEXAENOIC ACID (DHA)**)

DHEA
(see under: **DIHYDROEPIANDROSTERONE
(DHEA)**)

DIETARY SUPPLEMENT
Efacor Dietary Supplement
(Eniva) **503, 687**
Hyland's Sniffles 'N Sneezes 4 Kids
Tablets (Standard Homeopathic) **662**
Natural Joint Capsules (Greek Island
Labs) **690**
Tahitian Noni Liquid (Tahitian Noni
International) **508, 698**
Vibe Liquid Multi-Nutrient
Supplement (Eniva) **503, 688**

DIHYDROEPIANDROSTERONE (DHEA)
DHEA Plus Capsules (Wellness
International) **666**
VitaMist Intra-Oral Spray (Mayor) **692**

DIOCTYL SODIUM SULFOSUCCINATE
(see under: **DOCUSATE SODIUM**)

DIPHENHYDRAMINE CITRATE
Advil PM Caplets (Wyeth) **671**
Excedrin PM Caplets/Tablets
(Novartis Consumer) **505, 623**

DIPHENHYDRAMINE HYDROCHLORIDE
Advil PM Liqui-Gels (Wyeth) **671**
Allergy Antihistamine Capsules
(Generic) **708**
Robitussin Night Time Cough & Cold
Syrup (Wyeth) **683**
Robitussin Night Time Pediatric Cough &
Cold Syrup (Wyeth) **683**
Theraflu Thin Strips Nighttime Cold
& Cough (Novartis
Consumer) **506, 633**
Theraflu Warming Relief Nighttime
Severe Cold (Novartis
Consumer) **506, 635**
Triaminic Night Time Cold & Cough
Liquid (Novartis
Consumer) **507, 637**
Triaminic Thin Strips Night Time
Cold & Cough (Novartis
Consumer) **506, 640**
Triaminic Thin Strips Cough &
Runny Nose (Novartis
Consumer) **506, 640**

DISOCOREA
Hyland's Colic Tablets (Standard
Homeopathic) **661**

DOCOSAHEXAENOIC ACID (DHA)
Efacor Dietary Supplement
(Eniva) **503, 687**
WINOmeg3Complex Capsules (Wellness
International) **667**

DOCUSATE SODIUM
Dulcolax Stool Softener
(Boehringer Ingelheim) **503, 609**

DOXYLAMINE SUCCINATE
Vicks NyQuil LiquiCaps/Liquid
Multi-Symptom Cold/Flu Relief
(Procter & Gamble) **507, 653**
Vicks NyQuil Cough Liquid (Procter
& Gamble) **508, 652**
Vicks NyQuil D Cold & Flu Multi-Symptom
Relief Liquid (Procter & Gamble) **652**
Zicam Multi-Symptom Cold & Flu
Nightitime Liquid (Matrixx) **503, 614**
Zicam Multi-Symptom Cold & Flu
Nighttime To Go (Matrixx) **503, 615**

E

ECHINACEA ANGUSTIFOLIA
VitaMist Intra-Oral Spray (Mayor) **692**

EICOSAPENTAENOIC ACID (EPA)
Efacor Dietary Supplement
(Eniva) **503, 687**
WINOmeg3Complex Capsules (Wellness
International) **667**

EPINEPHRINE
Primatene Mist (Wyeth) **678**

ESSENTIAL FATTY ACIDS
Efacor Dietary Supplement
(Eniva) **503, 687**

ETHYL AMINOBENZOATE
(*see under:* BENZOCAINE)

EUCALYPTUS, OIL OF
Vicks VapoRub Cream (Procter &
Gamble) **656**
Vicks VapoRub Ointment (Procter &
Gamble) **656**

F

FATTY ACIDS
PureTrim Mediterranean Wellness
Shake (Awareness
Corporation/
Awareness Life) **502, 686**

FIBER, DIETARY
Benefiber Fiber Supplement
Caplets (Novartis
Consumer) **504, 694**
Benefiber Fiber Supplement
Powder (Novartis
Consumer) **504, 694**
Benefiber Fiber Supplement Sugar
Free Assorted Fruit Chewables
(Novartis Consumer) **504, 694**
Benefiber Fiber Supplement Sugar
Free Orange Creme Chewables
(Novartis Consumer) **504, 694**
Benefiber Fiber Supplement Plus B
Vitamins & Folic Acid Caplets
(Novartis Consumer) **504, 695**

Benefiber Fiber Supplement Plus B
Vitamins & Folic Acid Powder
(Novartis Consumer) **504, 695**
Benefiber Fiber Supplement Plus
Calcium Chewable Tablets
(Novartis Consumer) **504, 696**

FISH OILS
Efacor Dietary Supplement
(Eniva) **503, 687**

FOLIC ACID
Benefiber Fiber Supplement Plus B
Vitamins & Folic Acid Caplets
(Novartis Consumer) **504, 695**
Benefiber Fiber Supplement Plus B
Vitamins & Folic Acid Powder
(Novartis Consumer) **504, 695**
Saticte Tablets (Wellness
International) **667**
StePHan Elixir Capsules (Wellness
International) **701**
Vibe Liquid Multi-Nutrient
Supplement (Eniva) **503, 688**
VitaMist Intra-Oral Spray (Mayor) **692**

G

GALPHIMIA GLAUCA
Zicam Allergy Relief (Matrixx) **504, 611**

GARLIC EXTRACT
VitaMist Intra-Oral Spray (Mayor) **692**

GELSEMLUM
Hyland's Migraine Headache Relief
Tablets (Standard Homeopathic) **662**

GINKGO BILOBA
BioLean Free Tablets (Wellness
International) **665**
Centrum Performance Multivitamin/
Multimineral Supplement
(Wyeth) **705**
DHEA Plus Capsules (Wellness
International) **666**
Phyto-Vite Tablets (Wellness
International) **667**
Satiete Tablets (Wellness
International) **667**
StePHan Clarity Capsules (Wellness
International) **700**
StePHan Elixir Capsules (Wellness
International) **701**
VitaMist Intra-Oral Spray (Mayor) **692**

GINSENG
BioLean Free Tablets (Wellness
International) **665**
Centrum Performance Multivitamin/
Multimineral Supplement
(Wyeth) **705**

GLONOINUM
Hyland's Migraine Headache Relief
Tablets (Standard Homeopathic) **662**

GLUCOSAMINE HYDROCHLORIDE
Ambrotose Powder
(Mannatech) **503, 690**
Advanced Ambrotose Capsules
(Mannatech) **503, 690**
Advanced Ambrotose Powder
(Mannatech) **503, 690**
BioLean Sure2Endure Tablets (Wellness
International) **703**

GLUCOSAMINE SULFATE
VitaMist Intra-Oral Spray (Mayor) **692**

GLYCERIN
Preparation H Maximum Strength Cream
(Wyeth) **677**

GLYCERYL GUAIACOLATE
(*see under:* GUAIFENESIN)

GREEN TEA EXTRACT
Vibe Liquid Multi-Nutrient
Supplement (Eniva) **503, 688**

GUAIFENESIN
Buckley's Chest Congestion Mixture
(Novartis Consumer) **618**
Mucinex 600mg Extended-Release
Bi-Layer Tablets (Adams) **502, 605**
Mucinex 1200mg Extended-
Release Bi-Layer Tablets
(Adams) **502, 606**
Mucinex Cold Liquid (Adams) **502, 604**
Mucinex Cough Liquid
(Adams) **502, 603**
Mucinex Mini-Melts Bubble Gum
Flavor (Adams) **502, 604**
Mucinex Mini-Melts Grape Flavor
(Adams) **502, 604**
Mucinex Cough Mini-Melts Orange
Cream Flavor (Adams) **502, 605**
Mucinex D 600mg/60mg
Extended-Release Bi-Layer
Tablets (Adams) **502, 606**
Mucinex D 1200mg/120mg
Extended-Release Bi-Layer
Tablets (Adams) **502, 606**
Mucinex DM 600mg/30mg
Extended-Release Bi-Layer
Tablets (Adams) **502, 607**
Mucinex DM 1200mg/60mg
Extended-Release Bi-Layer
Tablets (Adams) **502, 607**
Mucinex Liquid (Adams) **502, 603**
Robitussin Chest Congestion Liquid
(Wyeth) **679**
Robitussin Cough & Cold CF Liquid
(Wyeth) **682**
Robitussin Cough & Cold CF Pediatric
Drops (Wyeth) **682**
Robitussin Cough & Congestion Liquid
(Wyeth) **681**
Robitussin Sugar Free Cough Syrup
(Wyeth) **681**
Robitussin Cough DM Syrup (Wyeth) **681**
Robitussin Cough DM Infant Drops
(Wyeth) **681**
Robitussin Head & Chest Congestion PE
Syrup (Wyeth) **680**
Theraflu Flu & Chest Congestion Hot
Liquid (Novartis Consumer) **631**
Triaminic Chest & Nasal Congestion
Liquid (Novartis Consumer) **636**
Vicks Formula 44E Cough & Chest
Congestion Relief Liquid
(Procter & Gamble) **508, 649**
Pediatric Vicks 44e Cough & Chest
Congestion Relief Liquid
(Procter & Gamble) **507, 654**
Zicam Multi-Symptom Liquid
Daytime (Matrixx) **503, 613**

H

HERBAL MEDICINES, UNSPECIFIED
Tahitian Noni Leaf Serum Soothing
Gel (Tahitian Noni
International) **508, 698**
Tahitian Noni Seed Oil (Tahitian
Noni International) **508, 699**

HERBALS, MULTIPLE
Ambrotose Capsules
(Mannatech) **503, 690**

Ambrotose Powder
(Mannatech) **503, 690**
Advanced Ambrotose Capsules
(Mannatech) **503, 690**
Advanced Ambrotose Powder
(Mannatech) **503, 690**
Awareness Clear Capsules (Awareness
Corporation/Awareness Life) **686**
BioLean Accelerator Tablets (Wellness
International) **664**
BioLean II Tablets (Wellness
International) **664**
Experience Capsules (Awareness
Corporation/
Awareness Life) **502, 686**
Hyland's Earache Drops (Standard
Homeopathic) **661**
StePHan Protector Capsules (Wellness
International) **702**
SynergyDefense Capsules
(Awareness Corporation/
Awareness Life) **502, 686**
Vibe Liquid Multi-Nutrient
Supplement (Eniva) **503, 688**
VltaMist Intra-Oral Spray (Mayor) **692**

HERBALS WITH MINERALS
BioLean LipoTrim Capsules (Wellness
International) **665**
Sleep-Tite Caplets (Wellness
International) **700**
StePHan Masculine Capsules (Wellness
International) **702**
Vibe Liquid Multi-Nutrient
Supplement (Eniva) **503, 688**

HERBALS WITH VITAMINS
Ambrotose AO Capsules
(Mannatech) **503, 691**
Pure Gardens Cream (Awareness
Corporation/Awareness Life) **686**
StePHan Relief Capsules (Wellness
International) **702**
Vibe Liquid Multi-Nutrient
Supplement (Eniva) **503, 688**
VitaMist Intra-Oral Spray (Mayor) **692**

HERBALS WITH VITAMINS & MINERALS
BioLean Free Tablets (Wellness
International) **665**
BioLean Sure2Endure Tablets (Wellness
International) **703**
Centrum Performance Multivitamin/
Multimineral Supplement
(Wyeth) **705**
Daily Complete Liquid (Awareness
Corporation/
Awareness Life) **502, 686**
Phyto-Vite Tablets (Wellness
International) **667**
Satiete Tablets (Wellness
International) **667**
StePHan Clarity Capsules (Wellness
International) **700**
StePHan Elasticity Capsules (Wellness
International) **701**
StePHan Elixir Capsules (Wellness
International) **701**
StePHan Essential Capsules (Wellness
International) **701**
StePHan Lovpil Capsules (Wellness
International) **702**
StePHan Tranquility Capsules (Wellness
International) **702**
Vibe Liquid Multi-Nutrient
Supplement (Eniva) **503, 688**
VitaMist Intra-Oral Spray (Mayor) **692**

HESPERIDIN COMPLEX
Peridin-C Vitamin C Supplement
(Beutlich) **687**

HESPERIDIN METHYL CHALCONE
Peridin-C Vitamin C Supplement
(Beutlich) **687**

HISTANIUM HYDROCHLORICUM
Zicam Allergy Relief (Matrixx) **504, 611**

HOMEOPATHIC FORMULATIONS
Hyland's BackAche with Arnica Caplets
(Standard Homeopathic) **660**
Hyland's Calms Forté Tablets and
Caplets (Standard Homeopathic) **660**
Hyland's Calms Forté 4 Kids Tablets
(Standard Homeopathic) **661**
Hyland's Colic Tablets (Standard
Homeopathic) **661**
Hyland's Earache Tablets (Standard
Homeopathic) **661**
Hyland's Leg Cramps with Quinine
Tablets and Caplets (Standard
Homeopathic) **661**
Hyland's Nerve Tonic Tablets and
Caplets (Standard Homeopathic) **662**
Hyland's Restful Legs Tablets (Standard
Homeopathic) **662**
Hyland's Teething Gel (Standard
Homeopathic) **663**
Hyland's Teething Tablets (Standard
Homeopathic) **663**
Smile's Prid Salve (Standard
Homeopathic) **662**
Topricin Cream (Topical
BioMedics) **508, 700**

HYDROXYPROPYL METHYLCELLULOSE
StePHan Clarity Capsules (Wellness
International) **700**
StePHan Essential Capsules (Wellness
International) **701**
StePHan Feminine Capsules (Wellness
International) **701**
StePHan Flexibility Capsules (Wellness
International) **701**
StePHan Masculine Capsules (Wellness
International) **702**
StePHan Protector Capsules (Wellness
International) **702**

HYPERICUM
Satiete Tablets (Wellness
International) **667**
VitaMist Intra-Oral Spray (Mayor) **692**

I

IBUPROFEN
Advil Caplets (Wyeth) **668**
Advil Gel Caplets (Wyeth) **668**
Advil Liqui-Gels (Wyeth) **668**
Advil Tablets (Wyeth) **668**
Advil Allergy Sinus Caplets (Wyeth) **669**
Children's Advil Oral Suspension
(Wyeth) **670**
Advil Cold & Sinus Caplets (Wyeth) **669**
Advil Cold & Sinus Liqui-Gels (Wyeth) **669**
Infants' Advil Concentrated Drops - White
Grape (Dye-Free) (Wyeth) **672**
Advil Multi-Symptom Cold Caplets
(Wyeth) **669**
Advil PM Caplets (Wyeth) **671**
Advil PM Liqui-Gels (Wyeth) **671**

IRIS VERSICOLOR
Hyland's Migraine Headache Relief
Tablets (Standard Homeopathic) **662**
IRON AMINO ACID CHELATE
StePHan Elixir Capsules (Wellness
International) **701**

K

KAVA-KAVA
VitaMist Intra-Oral Spray (Mayor) **692**

L

LACTIC ACID
Amlactin AP Anti-Itch Moisturizing Cream
(Upsher-Smith) *664*
Amlactin Moisturizing Lotion and Cream
(Upsher-Smith) *663*
LACTOBACILLUS ACIDOPHILUS
DDS-Acidophilus Capsules, Tablets, and
Powder (UAS Labs) **663**
LECITHIN
StePHan Clarity Capsules (Wellness
International) **700**
LEVMETAMFETAMINE
Vicks Vapor Inhaler (Procter &
Gamble) **656**
LOPERAMIDE HYDROCHLORIDE
Anti-Diarrheal Caplets (Generic) **708**
LORATADINE
Alavert Allergy & Sinus D-12 Hour Tablets
(Wyeth) **673**
Alavert Orally Disintegrating Tablets
(Wyeth) **673**
Claritin Children's 24 Hour Non-
Drowsy Chewables (Schering-
Plough) **508, 659**
Claritin Children's 24 Hour Non-
Drowsy Allergy Syrup (Schering-
Plough) **508, 659**
Claritin Non-Drowsy 24 Hour
Tablets (Schering-Plough) **508, 659**
Claritin Reditabs 24 Hour Non-
Drowsy Tablets (Schering-
Plough) **508, 659**
Claritin-D Non-Drowsy 12 Hour
Tablets (Schering-Plough) **508, 658**
Claritin-D Non-Drowsy 24 Hour
Tablets (Schering-Plough) **508, 658**
LUFFA OPERCULATA
Zicam Allergy Relief (Matrixx) **504, 611**

M

MAGNESIUM
StePHan Protector Capsules (Wellness
International) **702**
Vibe Liquid Multi-Nutrient
Supplement (Eniva) **503, 688**
MAGNESIUM HYDROXIDE
Maalox Regular Strength Antacid/
Antigas Liquid (Novartis
Consumer) **506, 628**
Maalox Maximum Strength Multi
Symptom Antacid/Antigas
Liquid (Novartis
Consumer) **506, 628**
MAGNESIUM OXIDE
Beelith Tablets (Beach) **687**
PremCal Light, Regular, and Extra
Strength Tablets (Dannmarie) **687**
MELATONIN
VitaMist Intra-Oral Spray (Mayor) **692**

MENTHOL
4-Way Menthol Nasal Spray (Novartis
　Consumer) **624**
Mineral Ice (Novartis
　Consumer) **506, 629**
Robitussin Cough Drops Menthol, Cherry,
　and Honey (Wyeth) **679**
Robitussin Honey Cough Drops
　(Wyeth) **679**
Robitussin Sugar Free Throat Drops
　(Wyeth) **679**
Thera-Gesic Creme (Mission) **616**
Vicks Cough Drops, Menthol and Cherry
　Flavors (Procter & Gamble) **650**
Vicks VapoRub Cream (Procter &
　Gamble) **656**
Vicks VapoRub Ointment (Procter &
　Gamble) **656**

METHYL SALICYLATE
Thera-Gesic Creme (Mission) **616**

MICONAZOLE NITRATE
Desenex Athlete's Foot Liquid Spray
　(Novartis Consumer) **619**
Desenex Athlete's Foot Shake
　Powder (Novartis
　Consumer) **505, 619**
Desenex Athlete's Foot Spray
　Powder (Novartis
　Consumer) **505, 619**
Desenex Jock Itch Spray Powder
　(Novartis Consumer) **619**

MILK OF MAGNESIA
(*see under:* **MAGNESIUM HYDROXIDE**)

MINERAL OIL
Preparation H Ointment (Wyeth) **677**

MINERALS
BioLean Mass Appeal Tablets (Wellness
　International) **665**
Vibe Liquid Multi-Nutrient
　Supplement (Eniva) **503, 688**

MINERALS, MULTIPLE
Caltrate 600 + D PLUS Minerals
　Chewables (Wyeth) **704**
Caltrate 600 + D PLUS Minerals Tablets
　(Wyeth) **704**
StePHan Feminine Capsules (Wellness
　International) **701**
Vibe Liquid Multi-Nutrient
　Supplement (Eniva) **503, 688**
VitaMist Intra-Oral Spray (Mayor) **692**

MULTIMINERALS
(*see under:* **VITAMINS WITH MINERALS**)

MULTIVITAMINS
(*see under:* **VITAMINS, MULTIPLE**)

MULTIVITAMINS WITH MINERALS
(*see under:* **VITAMINS WITH MINERALS**)

N

NIACIN
VitaMist Intra-Oral Spray (Mayor) **692**

NICOTINE
Nicotine Transdermal System Patch,
　Stop Smoking Aid (Generic) **710**

NICOTINE POLACRILEX
Nicotine Gum, Stop Smoking Aid
　(Generic) **709**

NICOTINIC ACID
(*see under:* **NIACIN**)

NUX VOMICA
Hyland's Migraine Headache Relief
　Tablets (Standard Homeopathic) **662**

O

OMEGA-3-ACID ETHYL ESTERS
WINOmeg3Complex Capsules (Wellness
　International) **667**

OMEGA-3 ACIDS
Efacor Dietary Supplement
　(Eniva) **503, 687**
WINOmeg3Complex Capsules (Wellness
　International) **667**

OMEGA-3 POLYUNSATURATES
(*see under:* **FATTY ACIDS**)

OMEGA-6 POLYUNSATURATES
WINOmeg3Complex Capsules (Wellness
　International) **667**

OMEPRAZOLE MAGNESIUM
Prilosec OTC Tablets (Procter &
　Gamble) **507, 644**

OXYMETAZOLINE HYDROCHLORIDE
Vicks Sinex 12-Hour Nasal Spray and
　Ultra Fine Mist (Procter &
　Gamble) **656**
Zicam Extreme Congestion Relief
　(Matrixx) **504, 613**
Zicam Intense Sinus Relief
　(Matrixx) **504, 613**

P

PERMETHRIN
Permethrin Lotion (Actavis) **602**

PETROLATUM
Preparation H Maximum Strength Cream
　(Wyeth) **677**
Preparation H Ointment (Wyeth) **677**

PETROLATUM, WHITE
Anbesol Cold Sore Therapy Ointment
　(Wyeth) **674**

PHENIRAMINE MALEATE
Theraflu Cold & Cough Hot Liquid
　(Novartis Consumer) **630**
Theraflu Cold & Sore Throat Hot Liquid
　(Novartis Consumer) **630**
Theraflu Flu & Sore Throat Hot Liquid
　(Novartis Consumer) **631**
Theraflu Nighttime Severe Cold Hot
　Liquid (Novartis
　Consumer) **506, 632**

PHENYLEPHRINE HYDROCHLORIDE
Comtrex Maximum Strength Non-Drowsy
　Cold & Cough Caplets (Novartis
　Consumer) **619**
Children's Dimetapp Cold & Allergy Elixir
　(Wyeth) **674**
Children's Dimetapp Cold & Allergy
　Chewable Tablets (Wyeth) **676**
Children's Dimetapp DM Cold & Cough
　Elixir (Wyeth) **675**
Toddler's Dimetapp Cold and Cough
　Drops (Wyeth) **676**
Excedrin Sinus Headache Caplets/
　Tablets (Novartis
　Consumer) **505, 623**
4-Way Fast Acting Nasal Spray
　(Novartis Consumer) **504, 624**
4-Way Menthol Nasal Spray (Novartis
　Consumer) **624**
Mucinex Cold Liquid (Adams) **502, 604**
Non-Drowsy Nasal Decongestant PE
　Tablets (Generic) **711**
Preparation H Maximum Strength Cream
　(Wyeth) **677**
Preparation H Ointment (Wyeth) **677**

Preparation H Suppositories (Wyeth) **677**
Robitussin Cough & Allergy Syrup
　(Wyeth) **680**
Robitussin Head & Chest Congestion PE
　Syrup (Wyeth) **680**
Robitussin Night Time Cough & Cold
　Syrup (Wyeth) **683**
Robitussin Night Time Pediatric Cough &
　Cold Syrup (Wyeth) **683**
Theraflu Cold & Cough Hot Liquid
　(Novartis Consumer) **630**
Theraflu Cold & Sore Throat Hot Liquid
　(Novartis Consumer) **630**
Theraflu Flu & Sore Throat Hot Liquid
　(Novartis Consumer) **631**
Theraflu Daytime Severe Cold Caplets
　(Novartis Consumer) **634**
Theraflu Nighttime Severe Cold Caplets
　(Novartis Consumer) **635**
Theraflu Daytime Severe Cold Hot Liquid
　(Novartis Consumer) **632**
Theraflu Nighttime Severe Cold Hot
　Liquid (Novartis
　Consumer) **506, 632**
Theraflu Thin Strips Daytime Cold
　& Cough (Novartis
　Consumer) **506, 633**
Theraflu Thin Strips Nighttime Cold
　& Cough (Novartis
　Consumer) **506, 633**
Theraflu Warming Relief Daytime Severe
　Cold (Novartis Consumer) **634**
Theraflu Warming Relief Nighttime
　Severe Cold (Novartis
　Consumer) **506, 635**
Triaminic Chest & Nasal Congestion
　Liquid (Novartis Consumer) **636**
Triaminic Cold & Allergy Liquid (Novartis
　Consumer) **636**
Triaminic Day Time Cold & Cough
　Liquid (Novartis
　Consumer) **507, 637**
Triaminic Night Time Cold & Cough
　Liquid (Novartis
　Consumer) **507, 637**
Triaminic Thin Strips Day Time
　Cold & Cough (Novartis
　Consumer) **506, 640**
Triaminic Thin Strips Night Time
　Cold & Cough (Novartis
　Consumer) **506, 640**
Triaminic Thin Strips Cold with
　Stuffy Nose (Novartis
　Consumer) **506, 639**
Triaminic Infant & Toddler Thin
　Strips Decongestant (Novartis
　Consumer) **507, 638**
Triaminic Infant & Toddler Thin
　Strips Decongestant Plus
　Cough (Novartis
　Consumer) **507, 638**
Vicks Formula 44D Cough & Head
　Congestion Relief Liquid
　(Procter & Gamble) **508, 649**
Vicks DayQuil LiquiCaps/Liquid
　Multi-Symptom Cold/Flu Relief
　(Procter & Gamble) **507, 651**
Vicks Sinex Nasal Spray and Ultra Fine
　Mist (Procter & Gamble) **655**
Zicam Multi-Symptom Cold & Flu
　Daytime To Go (Matrixx) **503, 615**
Zicam Multi-Symptom Cold & Flu
　Nighttime To Go (Matrixx) **503, 615**
Zicam Sinus Melts (Matrixx) **504, 616**

PHYTONUTRIENTS
Phyto-Vite Tablets (Wellness
International) **667**
Vibe Liquid Multi-Nutrient
Supplement (Eniva) **503, 688**

POTASSIUM
Vibe Liquid Multi-Nutrient
Supplement (Eniva) **503, 688**

PRAMOXINE HYDROCHLORIDE
Amlactin AP Anti-Itch Moisturizing Cream
(Upsher-Smith) *664*
Preparation H Maximum Strength Cream
(Wyeth) **677**

PROTEIN PREPARATIONS
BioLean ProXtreme Dietary Supplement
(Wellness International) **666**

PSEUDOEPHEDRINE HYDROCHLORIDE
Advil Allergy Sinus Caplets (Wyeth) **669**
Advil Cold & Sinus Caplets (Wyeth) **669**
Advil Cold & Sinus Liqui-Gels (Wyeth) **669**
Advil Multi-Symptom Cold Caplets
(Wyeth) **669**
Comtrex Maximum Strength Day/Night
Cold & Cough Caplets - Day
Formulation (Novartis Consumer) **618**
Comtrex Maximum Strength Day/Night
Cold & Cough Caplets - Night
Formulation (Novartis Consumer) **618**
Mucinex D 600mg/60mg
Extended-Release Bi-Layer
Tablets (Adams) **502, 606**
Mucinex D 1200mg/120mg
Extended-Release Bi-Layer
Tablets (Adams) **502, 606**
Non-Drowsy Nasal Decongestant
Maximum Strength Tablets
(Generic) **710**
Robitussin Cough & Cold CF Liquid
(Wyeth) **682**
Robitussin Cough & Cold CF Pediatric
Drops (Wyeth) **682**
Vicks NyQuil D Cold & Flu Multi-Symptom
Relief Liquid (Procter & Gamble) **652**

PSEUDOEPHEDRINE SULFATE
Alavert Allergy & Sinus D-12 Hour Tablets
(Wyeth) **673**
Claritin-D Non-Drowsy 12 Hour
Tablets (Schering-Plough) **508, 658**
Claritin-D Non-Drowsy 24 Hour
Tablets (Schering-Plough) **508, 658**

PSYLLIUM PREPARATIONS
Experience Capsules (Awareness
Corporation/
Awareness Life) **502, 686**
Metamucil Capsules (Procter &
Gamble) **507, 642**
Metamucil Dietary Fiber Supplement
(Procter & Gamble) **696**
Metamucil Powder, Original Texture
Orange Flavor (Procter &
Gamble) **642**
Metamucil Powder, Original Texture
Regular Flavor (Procter &
Gamble) **642**
Metamucil Smooth Texture
Powder, Orange Flavor (Procter
& Gamble) **507, 642**
Metamucil Smooth Texture Powder,
Sugar-Free, Orange Flavor (Procter &
Gamble) **642**

Metamucil Smooth Texture Powder,
Sugar-Free, Regular Flavor (Procter &
Gamble) **642**
Metamucil Wafers, Apple Crisp &
Cinnamon Spice Flavors
(Procter & Gamble) **507, 642**
StePHan Relief Capsules (Wellness
International) **702**

PYRANTEL PAMOATE
Reese's Pinworm Treatments
(Reese) **508, 657**

PYRIDOXINE HYDROCHLORIDE
(*see under:* **VITAMIN B₆**)

PYRITHIONE ZINC
Head & Shoulders Intensive Solutions
Dandruff Shampoo (Procter &
Gamble) **641**

Q

QUININE
Hyland's Leg Cramps with Quinine
Tablets and Caplets (Standard
Homeopathic) **661**

R

RANITIDINE HYDROCHLORIDE
Zantac 75 Tablets (Boehringer
Ingelheim) **503, 609**
Maximum Strength Zantac 150
Tablets (Boehringer
Ingelheim) **503, 610**
Maximum Strength Zantac 150
Cool Mint Tablets (Boehringer
Ingelheim) **503, 610**

RICE PROTEIN
PureTrim Mediterranean Wellness
Shake (Awareness
Corporation/
Awareness Life) **502, 686**

S

SANGUINARIA CANADENSIS
Hyland's Migraine Headache Relief
Tablets (Standard Homeopathic) **662**

SENNOSIDES
Ex•Lax Chocolated Laxative Pieces
(Novartis Consumer) **505, 625**
Ex•Lax Regular Strength Pills
(Novartis Consumer) **505, 625**
Ex•Lax Maximum Strength Pills
(Novartis Consumer) **505, 625**

SHARK LIVER OIL
Preparation H Ointment (Wyeth) **677**
Preparation H Suppositories (Wyeth) **677**

SILICON DIOXIDE
StePHan Protector Capsules (Wellness
International) **702**

SIMETHICONE
Gas-X Regular Strength Chewable
Tablets (Novartis
Consumer) **505, 626**
Gas-X Extra Strength Chewable
Tablets (Novartis
Consumer) **505, 626**
Gas-X Extra Strength Softgels
(Novartis Consumer) **505, 626**
Gas-X Extra Strength Thin Strips
(Novartis Consumer) **505, 626**
Gas-X Maximum Strength Softgels
(Novartis Consumer) **505, 626**

Gas-X with Maalox Extra Strength
Chewable Tablets (Novartis
Consumer) **506, 626**
Maalox Regular Strength Antacid/
Antigas Liquid (Novartis
Consumer) **506, 628**
Maalox Maximum Strength Multi
Symptom Antacid/Antigas
Liquid (Novartis
Consumer) **506, 628**
Maalox Maximum Strength Multi
Symptom Antacid/Antigas
Chewable Tablets (Novartis
Consumer) **506, 629**

SODIUM CHLORIDE
4-Way Saline Nasal Spray (Novartis
Consumer) **625**
Nasal Comfort Moisture Therapy
Sprays - Scented and
Unscented (Matrixx) **503, 611**

SOY-CONTAINING DIETARY SUPPLEMENTS
StePHan Essential Capsules (Wellness
International) **701**
StePHan Feminine Capsules (Wellness
International) **701**
StePHan Lovpil Capsules (Wellness
International) **702**
StePHan Protector Capsules (Wellness
International) **702**
StePHan Tranquility Capsules (Wellness
International) **702**

ST. JOHN'S WORT
(*see under:* **HYPERICUM**)

STEARIC ACID
StePHan Protector Capsules (Wellness
International) **702**

SULFUR
Hyland's Calms Forté 4 Kids Tablets
(Standard Homeopathic) **661**
Zicam Allergy Relief (Matrixx) **504, 611**

T

TERBINAFINE HYDROCHLORIDE
Lamisil^AT Creams (Athlete's Foot &
Jock Itch) (Novartis
Consumer) **506, 627**
Lamisil^AT Athlete's Foot Spray Pump
(Novartis Consumer) *506*
Lamisil^AT Jock Itch Spray Pump (Novartis
Consumer) *506*

TIOCONAZOLE
Vagistat-1 (Novartis
Consumer) **507, 641**

TOLNAFTATE
Lamisil^AF Defense Powders (Shake
& Spray) (Novartis
Consumer) **506, 627**

V

VALERIANA OFFICINALIS
StePHan Tranquility Capsules (Wellness
International) **702**

VINPOCETINE
Intelectol Tablets (Memory
Secret) **504, 693**

VITAMIN A
VitaMist Intra-Oral Spray (Mayor) **692**

VITAMIN B₃
(*see under:* **NIACIN**)

VITAMIN B₆
Beelith Tablets (Beach) **687**

VITAMIN B$_6$—cont.
Vibe Liquid Multi-Nutrient
    Supplement (Eniva) **503, 688**
VitaMist Intra-Oral Spray (Mayor) **692**

VITAMIN B$_{12}$
VitaMist Intra-Oral Spray (Mayor) **692**

VITAMIN B COMPLEX
VitaMist Intra-Oral Spray (Mayor) **692**

VITAMIN C
Peridin-C Vitamin C Supplement
    (Beutlich) **687**
Vibe Liquid Multl-Nutrient
    Supplement (Eniva) **503, 688**
VitaMist Intra-Oral Spray (Mayor) **692**

VITAMIN D
Caltrate 600 + D Tablets (Wyeth) **704**
Caltrate 600 + D PLUS Minerals
    Chewables (Wyeth) **704**
Caltrate 600 + D PLUS Minerals Tablets
    (Wyeth) **704**
D-Cal Chewable Caplets
    (A&Z Pharm) **686**
VitaMist Intra-Oral Spray (Mayor) **692**

VITAMIN D$_3$
PremCal Light, Regular, and Extra
    Strength Tablets (Dannmarie) **687**

VITAMIN E
Vibe Liquid Multi-Nutrient
    Supplement (Eniva) **503, 688**
VitaMist Intra-Oral Spray (Mayor) **692**

VITAMINS, MULTIPLE
Vibe Liquid Multi-Nutrient
    Supplement (Eniva) **503, 688**
VitaMist Intra-Oral Spray (Mayor) **692**

VITAMINS WITH MINERALS
BioLean ProXtreme Dietary Supplement
    (Wellness International) **666**

Centrum Tablets (Wyeth) **704**
Centrum Kids Complete Children's
    Chewables (Wyeth) **705**
Centrum Performance Multivitamin/
    Multimineral Supplement
    (Wyeth) **705**
Centrum Silver Tablets (Wyeth) **706**
Food for Thought Dietary Supplement
    (Wellness International) **666**
StePHan Flexibility Capsules (Wellness
    International) **701**
Vibe Liquid Multi-Nutrient
    Supplement (Eniva) **503, 688**
VitaMist Intra-Oral Spray (Mayor) **692**
Winrgy Dietary Supplement (Wellness
    International) **703**

W

WHITE PETROLATUM
(*see under:* **PETROLATUM, WHITE**)
WITCH HAZEL
Preparation H Medicated Wipes
    (Wyeth) **678**

X

XYLOMETAZOLINE HYDROCHLORIDE
4-Way Moisturizing Relief Nasal Spray
    (Novartis Consumer) **624**

Z

ZINC
Vibe Liquid Multi-Nutrient
    Supplement (Eniva) **503, 688**
VitaMist Intra-Oral Spray (Mayor) **692**

ZINC PYRITHIONE
(*see under:* **PYRITHIONE ZINC**)

ZINC SULFATE
Zicam Cold Remedy Chewables
    (Matrixx) **504, 611**
Zicam Cold Remedy ChewCaps
    (Matrixx) **504, 611**
Zicam Cold Remedy Oral Mist
    (Matrixx) **504, 611**
Zicam Cold Remedy RapidMelts
    (Matrixx) **504, 611**
Zicam Cold Remedy RapidMelts
    with Vitamin C (Matrixx) **504, 611**

ZINCUM ACETICUM
Zicam Cold Remedy ChewCaps
    (Matrixx) **504, 611**
Zicam Cold Remedy Chewables
    (Matrixx) **504, 611**
Zicam Cold Remedy Oral Mist
    (Matrixx) **504, 611**
Zicam Cold Remedy RapidMelts
    (Matrixx) **504, 611**
Zicam Cold Remedy RapidMelts
    with Vitamin C (Matrixx) **504, 611**

ZINCUM GLUCONICUM
Zicam Cold Remedy Chewables
    (Matrixx) **504, 611**
Zicam Cold Remedy ChewCaps
    (Matrixx) **504, 611**
Zicam Cold Remedy Gel Swabs
    (Matrixx) **504, 611**
Zicam Cold Remedy Nasal Gel
    (Matrixx) **504, 611**
Zicam Cold Remedy Oral Mist
    (Matrixx) **504, 611**
Zicam Cold Remedy RapidMelts
    (Matrixx) **504, 611**
Zicam Cold Remedy RapidMelts
    with Vitamin C (Matrixx) **504, 611**

COMPANION DRUG INDEX

This index is a quick-reference guide to OTC products that may be used in conjunction with prescription drug therapy to reverse drug-induced side effects, relieve symptoms of the illness itself, or treat sequelae of the initial disease. All entries are derived from the FDA-approved prescribing information published by *PDR*.

The products listed are generally considered effective for temporary symptomatic relief. They may not, however, be appropriate for sustained therapy, and each case must be approached on an individual basis. Certain common side effects may be harbingers of more serious reactions. When making a recommendation, be sure to adjust for the patient's age, concurrent medical conditions, and complete drug regimen. Consider timing as well, since simultaneous ingestion may not be recommended in all instances.

Please note that only products fully described in *Physicians' Desk Reference* and its companion volumes are included in this index. The publisher therefore cannot guarantee that all entries are totally accurate or complete. Keep in mind, too, that although a given OTC product is usually an appropriate companion for an entire class of prescription medications, certain drugs within the class may be exceptions. If you have any doubt about the suitability of a particular OTC product in a given situation, be sure to check the underlying *PDR* prescribing information and the relevant medical literature.

ACNE MEDICAMENTOSA
May result from the use of haloperidol, oral contraceptives containing norethindrone or norgestrel, phenytoin, thyroid hormones, azathioprine, dantrolene sodium, ethionamide, halothane, isoniazid, lithium carbonate, lithium citrate or trimethadione. The following products may be recommended:
Efacor Dietary Supplement..................**687**
Tahitian Noni Seed Oil **699**

ACUTE MOUNTAIN SICKNESS, HEADACHE SECONDARY TO
Acute mountain sickness may be treated with acetazolamide. The following products may be recommended for relief of headache:
Advil Caplets **668**
Advil Gel Caplets **668**
Advil Liqui-Gels **668**
Advil Tablets **668**
Children's Advil Oral Suspension **670**
Infants' Advil Concentrated Drops -
White Grape (Dye-Free)....................**672**

ALCOHOLISM, HYPOCALCEMIA SECONDARY TO
Alcoholism may be treated with disulfiram or naltrexone hydrochloride. The following products may be recommended for relief of hypocalcemia:
Benefiber Fiber Supplement Plus Calcium
Chewable Tablets.............................**696**
Calcium Antacid Tablets **708**
Caltrate 600 + D Tablets **704**
Caltrate 600 + D PLUS Minerals
Chewables **704**
Caltrate 600 + D PLUS Minerals
Tablets..**704**
Citracal Caplets...................................**693**

ALCOHOLISM, HYPOMAGNESEMIA SECONDARY TO
Alcoholism may be treated with disulfiram or naltrexone hydrochloride. The following products may be recommended for relief of hypomagnesemia:
Beelith Tablets **687**
D-Cal Chewable Capsules **686**

ALCOHOLISM, VITAMINS AND MINERALS DEFICIENCY SECONDARY TO
Alcoholism may be treated with disulfiram or naltrexone hydrochloride. The following products may be recommended for relief of vitamins and minerals deficiency:
BioLean Accelerator Tablets **664**
BioLean Free Tablets **665**

BioLean II Tablets................................**664**
BioLean LipoTrim Capsules **665**
BioLean Mass Appeal Tablets...............**665**
BioLean ProXtreme Dietary
Supplement......................................**666**
BioLean Sure2Endure Tablets...............**703**
Centrum Tablets...................................**704**
Centrum Performance Multivitamin/
Multimineral Supplement..................**705**
Centrum Silver Tablets.........................**706**
Daily Complete Liquid **686**
DHEA Plus Capsules............................**666**
Food for Thought Dietary
Supplement......................................**666**
Peridin-C Vitamin C Supplement **687**
Phyto-Vite Tablets................................**667**
Satiete Tablets **667**
StePHan Clarity Capsules **700**
StePHan Elasticity Capsules.................**701**
StePHan Elixir Capsules.......................**701**
StePHan Essential Capsules **701**
StePHan Feminine Capsules.................**701**
StePHan Flexibility Capsules.................**701**
StePHan Lovpil Capsules **702**
StePHan Tranquility Capsules...............**702**
Vibe Liquid Multi-Nutrient
Supplement......................................**688**
Winrgy Dietary Supplement **703**

ARTHRITIS
May be treated with corticosteroids or nonsteroidal anti-inflammatory drugs. The following products may be recommended for relief of symptoms:
Bufferin Extra Strength Tablets **617**
Bufferin Regular Strength Tablets **617**
Efacor Dietary Supplement....................**687**
Excedrin Back & Body Caplets..............**620**
Excedrin Extra Strength
Caplets/Tablets/Geltabs **621**
Mineral Ice..**629**
Natural Joint Capsules.........................**690**
StePHan Flexibility Capsules **701**
Thera-Gesic Creme **616**
ThermaCare Heat Wraps......................**645**
ThermaCare Therapeutic Heat Wraps....**647**
Topricin Cream **700**
Vicks VapoRub Cream..........................**656**
Vicks VapoRub Ointment......................**656**

BRONCHITIS, CHRONIC, ACUTE EXACERBATION OF
May be treated with quinolones, sulfamethoxazole-trimethoprim, cefixime, cefpodoxime proxetil, cefprozil, ceftibuten dihydrate, cefuroxime axetil, cilastatin sodium, clarithromycin, imipenem or loracarbef. The following products may be recommended for relief of symptoms:
Comtrex Maximum Strength
Non-Drowsy Cold & Cough Caplets....**619**
Delsym Liquid Grape Flavor..................**602**
Delsym Liquid Orange Flavor **603**
Children's Dimetapp Long Acting
Cough Plus Cold Syrup.....................**675**
Mucinex 1200mg Extended-Release
Bi-Layer Tablets **606**
Mucinex Cold Liquid **604**
Mucinex Cough Liquid..........................**603**
Mucinex Mini-Melts Bubble Gum
Flavor..**604**
Mucinex Mini-Melts Grape Flavor **604**
Mucinex Cough Mini-Melts
Orange Cream Flavor........................**605**
Mucinex D 600mg/60mg
Extended-Release Bi-Layer Tablets **606**
Mucinex DM 600mg/30mg
Extended-Release Bi-Layer Tablets **607**
Mucinex DM 1200mg/60mg
Extended-Release Bi-Layer Tablets **607**
Mucinex Liquid **603**
Robitussin Chest Congestion Liquid.......**679**
Robitussin Cough & Cold CF
Pediatric Drops.................................**682**
Robitussin Cough & Cold
Long-Acting Liquid............................**682**
Robitussin Pediatric Cough & Cold
Long-Acting Liquid **682**
Robitussin Cough & Congestion
Liquid **681**
Robitussin Sugar Free Cough Syrup......**681**
Robitussin Cough DM Syrup.................**681**
Robitussin Cough DM Infant Drops **681**
Robitussin Head & Chest
Congestion PE Syrup........................**680**
Theraflu Thin Strips Daytime
Cold & Cough **633**
Theraflu Thin Strips Nighttime
Cold & Cough **633**
Triaminic Chest & Nasal Congestion
Liquid **636**

BRONCHITIS, CHRONIC, ACUTE EXACERBATION OF—CONT.

Triaminic Day Time Cold & Cough Liquid 637
Triaminic Night Time Cold & Cough Liquid 637
Triaminic Cough & Sore Throat Liquid 638
Triaminic Cough & Runny Nose Softchews 639
Triaminic Thin Strips Cough & Runny Nose................................640
Vicks Nyquil D Cold & Flu Multi-Symptom Relief Liquid 652
Vicks VapoRub Cream.........................656
Vicks VapoRub Ointment 656
Vicks VapoSteam.................................657
Zicam Cough Max Cough Spray 613
Zicam Cough Max Cough Melts 613
Zicam Multi-Symptom Liquid Daytime....613
Zicam Multi-Symptom Cold & Flu Daytime To Go................................615
Zicam Multi-Symptom Cold & Flu Nighttime Liquid............................614
Zicam Multi-Symptom Cold & Flu Nighttime To Go...........................615

BURN INFECTIONS, SEVERE, NUTRIENTS DEFICIENCY SECONDARY TO

Severe burn infections may be treated with anti-infectives. The following products may be recommended for relief of nutrients deficiency:
BioLean Accelerator Tablets 664
BioLean Free Tablets 665
BioLean II Tablets................................664
BioLean LipoTrim Capsules 665
BioLean Mass Appeal Tablets...............665
BioLean ProXtreme Dietary Supplement 666
BioLean Sure2Endure Tablets...............703
Centrum Tablets...................................704
Centrum Kids Complete Children's Chewables 705
Centrum Performance Multivitamin/ Multimineral Supplement..................705
Centrum Silver Tablets.........................706
Daily Complete Liquid 686
DHEA Plus Capsules.............................666
Food for Thought Dietary Supplement....................................666
Phyto-Vite Tablets 667
Satiete Tablets.....................................667
StePHan Clarity Capsules 700
StePHan Elasticity Capsules.................701
StePHan Elixir Capsules........................701
StePHan Essential Capsules 701
StePHan Feminine Capsules 701
StePHan Flexibility Capsules 701
StePHan Lovpil Capsules 702
StePHan Tranquility Capsules...............702
Vibe Liquid Multi-Nutrient Supplement....................................688
Winrgy Dietary Supplement 703

CANCER, NUTRIENTS DEFICIENCY SECONDARY TO

Cancer may be treated with chemotherapeutic agents. The following products may be recommended for relief of nutrients deficiency:
BioLean Accelerator Tablets 664
BioLean Free Tablets 665
BioLean II Tablets................................664
BioLean LipoTrim Capsules 665
BioLean Mass Appeal Tablets...............665
BioLean ProXtreme Dietary Supplement 666
BioLean Sure2Endure Tablets...............703
Centrum Tablets...................................704

Centrum Kids Complete Children's Chewables 705
Centrum Performance Multivitamin/ Multimineral Supplement..................705
Centrum Silver Tablets.........................706
Daily Complete Liquid 686
DHEA Plus Capsules.............................666
Food for Thought Dietary Supplement 666
Phyto-Vite Tablets 667
Satiete Tablets.....................................667
StePHan Clarity Capsules 700
StePHan Elasticity Capsules.................701
StePHan Elixir Capsules........................701
StePHan Essential Capsules 701
StePHan Feminine Capsules 701
StePHan Flexibility Capsules 701
StePHan Lovpil Capsules 702
StePHan Tranquility Capsules...............702
Vibe Liquid Multi-Nutrient Supplement....................................688
Winrgy Dietary Supplement 703

CANDIDIASIS, VAGINAL

May be treated with antifungal agents. The following products may be recommended for relief of symptoms:
Vagistat-1 641

CONGESTIVE HEART FAILURE, NUTRIENTS DEFICIENCY SECONDARY TO

Congestive heart failure may be treated with ace inhibitors, cardiac glycosides or diuretics. The following products may be recommended for relief of nutrients deficiency:
BioLean Accelerator Tablets 664
BioLean Free Tablets 665
BioLean II Tablets................................664
BioLean LipoTrim Capsules 665
BioLean Mass Appeal Tablets...............665
BioLean ProXtreme Dietary Supplement 666
BioLean Sure2Endure Tablets...............703
Centrum Tablets...................................704
Centrum Performance Multivitamin/ Multimineral Supplement..................705
Centrum Silver Tablets.........................706
Daily Complete Liquid 686
DHEA Plus Capsules.............................666
Food for Thought Dietary Supplement 666
Phyto-Vite Tablets 667
Satiete Tablets.....................................667
StePHan Clarity Capsules 700
StePHan Elasticity Capsules.................701
StePHan Elixir Capsules........................701
StePHan Essential Capsules 701
StePHan Feminine Capsules 701
StePHan Flexibility Capsules 701
StePHan Lovpil Capsules 702
StePHan Tranquility Capsules...............702
Vibe Liquid Multi-Nutrient Supplement....................................688
Winrgy Dietary Supplement 703

CONSTIPATION

May result from the use of ace inhibitors, hmg-coa reductase inhibitors, anticholinergics, anticonvulsants, antidepressants, beta blockers, bile acid sequestrants, butyrophenones, calcium and aluminum-containing antacids, calcium channel blockers, ganglionic blockers, hematinics, monoamine oxidase inhibitors, narcotic analgesics, nonsteroidal anti-inflammatory drugs or phenothiazines. The following products may be recommended:
Align Daily Probiotic Supplement 696
Benefiber Fiber Supplement Caplets 694
Benefiber Fiber Supplement Powder......694

Benefiber Fiber Supplement Sugar Free Assorted Fruit Chewables 694
Benefiber Fiber Supplement Sugar Free Orange Creme Chewables 694
Benefiber Fiber Supplement Plus B Vitamins & Folic Acid Caplets 695
Benefiber Fiber Supplement Plus B Vitamins & Folic Acid Powder 695
Benefiber Fiber Supplement Plus Calcium Chewable Tablets................696
Dulcolax Stool Softener 609
Dulcolax Suppositories 609
Dulcolax Tablets 608
Efacor Dietary Supplement....................687
Ex•Lax Chocolated Laxative Pieces 625
Ex•Lax Regular Strength Pills 625
Ex•Lax Maximum Strength Pills............625
FiberCon Caplets 676
Metamucil Capsules 642
Metamucil Powder, Original Texture Orange Flavor...........642
Metamucil Powder, Original Texture Regular Flavor.........642
Metamucil Smooth Texture Powder, Orange Flavor 642
Metamucil Smooth Texture Powder, Sugar-Free, Orange Flavor...............642
Metamucil Smooth Texture Powder, Sugar-Free, Regular Flavor 642
Metamucil Wafers, Apple Crisp & Cinnamon Spice Flavors 642
Vibe Liquid Multi-Nutrient Supplement....................................688

CYSTIC FIBROSIS, NUTRIENTS DEFICIENCY SECONDARY TO

Cystic fibrosis may be treated with dornase alfa. The following products may be recommended for relief of nutrients deficiency:
BioLean Accelerator Tablets 664
BioLean Free Tablets 665
BioLean II Tablets................................664
BioLean LipoTrim Capsules 665
BioLean Mass Appeal Tablets...............665
BioLean ProXtreme Dietary Supplement 666
BioLean Sure2Endure Tablets...............703
Centrum Tablets...................................704
Centrum Kids Complete Children's Chewables 705
Centrum Performance Multivitamin/ Multimineral Supplement..................705
Centrum Silver Tablets.........................706
Daily Complete Liquid 686
DHEA Plus Capsules.............................666
Efacor Dietary Supplement....................687
Food for Thought Dietary Supplement 666
Phyto-Vite Tablets 667
Satiete Tablets.....................................667
StePHan Clarity Capsules 700
StePHan Elasticity Capsules.................701
StePHan Elixir Capsules........................701
StePHan Essential Capsules 701
StePHan Feminine Capsules 701
StePHan Flexibility Capsules 701
StePHan Lovpil Capsules 702
StePHan Tranquility Capsules...............702
Vibe Liquid Multi-Nutrient Supplement....................................688
Winrgy Dietary Supplement 703

DIABETES MELLITUS, CONSTIPATION SECONDARY TO

Diabetes mellitus may be treated with insulins or oral hypoglycemic agents. The following products may be recommended for relief of constipation:
Benefiber Fiber Supplement Powder......694
Benefiber Fiber Supplement Sugar Free Assorted Fruit Chewables..............................694

Benefiber Fiber Supplement
Sugar Free Orange Creme
Chewables **694**
Benefiber Fiber Supplement Plus B
Vitamins & Folic Acid Caplets **695**
Benefiber Fiber Supplement Plus B
Vitamins & Folic Acid Powder **695**
Benefiber Fiber Supplement Plus
Calcium Chewable Tablets **696**
Dulcolax Stool Softener **609**
Dulcolax Suppositories **609**
Dulcolax Tablets **608**
Ex•Lax Chocolated Laxative Pieces **625**
Ex•Lax Regular Strength Pills **625**
Ex•Lax Maximum Strength Pills **625**
FiberCon Caplets **676**
Metamucil Capsules **642**
Metamucil Powder, Original Texture
Orange Flavor **642**
Metamucil Powder, Original Texture
Regular Flavor **642**
Metamucil Smooth Texture Powder,
Orange Flavor **642**
Metamucil Smooth Texture Powder,
Sugar-Free, Orange Flavor **642**
Metamucil Smooth Texture Powder,
Sugar-Free, Regular Flavor **642**
Metamucil Wafers, Apple Crisp &
Cinnamon Spice Flavors **642**

DIABETES MELLITUS, POORLY CONTROLLED, CANDIDAL VULVOVAGINITIS SECONDARY TO

Diabetes mellitus may be treated with insulins or oral hypoglycemic agents. The following products may be recommended for relief of candidal vulvovaginitis:

Vagistat-1 ....**641**

DIABETES MELLITUS, POORLY CONTROLLED, VITAMINS AND MINERALS DEFICIENCY SECONDARY TO

Diabetes mellitus may be treated with insulins or oral hypoglycemic agents. The following products may be recommended for relief of vitamins and minerals deficiency:

BioLean Accelerator Tablets **664**
BioLean Free Tablets **665**
BioLean II Tablets **664**
BioLean Mass Appeal Tablets..............**665**
Centrum Tablets **704**
Centrum Kids Complete Children's
Chewables **705**
Centrum Performance Multivitamin/
Multimineral Supplement................**705**
Centrum Silver Tablets........................**706**
Daily Complete Liquid **686**
Food for Thought Dietary Supplement ...**666**
Peridin-C Vitamin C Supplement **687**
Phyto-Vite Tablets **667**
Satiete Tablets **667**
StePHan Clarity Capsules **700**
StePHan Elasticity Capsules................**701**
StePHan Essential Capsules **701**
StePHan Feminine Capsules **701**
StePHan Flexibility Capsules **701**
StePHan Tranquility Capsules..............**702**
Vibe Liquid Multi-Nutrient
Supplement............................**688**

DIARRHEA

May result from the use of ace inhibitors, beta blockers, cardiac glycosides, chemotherapeutic agents, diuretics, magnesium-containing antacids, nonsteroidal anti-inflammatory drugs, potassium supplements, acarbose, alprazolam, colchicine, divalproex sodium, ethosuximide, fluoxetine hydrochloride, guanethidine monosulfate, hydralazine hydrochloride, levodopa, lithium carbonate, lithium citrate, mesna, metformin hydrochloride, misoprostol, olsalazine sodium, pancrelipase, procainamide

hydrochloride, reserpine, succimer, ticlopidine hydrochloride or valproic acid. The following products may be recommended:

Align Daily Probiotic Supplement **696**
Maalox Maximum Strength
Total Stomach Relief Liquid **629**
Pepto-Bismol Original Liquid,
Original and Cherry Chewable
Tablets & Caplets **643**
Pepto-Bismol Maximum Strength
Liquid **643**

DIARRHEA, INFECTIOUS

May be treated with sulfamethoxazole-trimethoprim, ciprofloxacin or furazolidone. The following products may be recommended for relief of symptoms:

Maalox Maximum Strength Total
Stomach Relief Liquid **629**
Pepto-Bismol Original Liquid,
Original and Cherry Chewable
Tablets & Caplets **643**
Pepto-Bismol Maximum Strength
Liquid **643**

DYSPEPSIA

May result from the use of chronic systemic corticosteroid therapy, nonsteroidal anti-inflammatory drugs, ulcerogenic medications or mexiletine hydrochloride. The following products may be recommended:

Calcium Antacid Tablets **708**
Gas-X with Maalox Extra Strength
Chewable Tablets............................**626**
Maalox Regular Strength
Antacid/Antigas Liquid **628**
Maalox Maximum Strength
Multi Symptom Antacid/
Antigas Liquid **628**
Maalox Maximum Strength
Multi Symptom Antacid/
Antigas Chewable Tablets................**629**
Children's Pepto..................................**641**
Prilosec OTC Tablets **644**

FEVER

May result from the use of immunization. The following products may be recommended:

Advil Caplets......................................**668**
Advil Gel Caplets **668**
Advil Liqui-Gels **668**
Advil Tablets **668**
Children's Advil Oral Suspension **670**
Advil Cold & Sinus Caplets..................**669**
Advil Cold & Sinus Liqui-Gels..............**669**
Infants' Advil Concentrated Drops -
White Grape (Dye-Free)....................**672**
Bufferin Extra Strength Tablets **617**
Bufferin Regular Strength Tablets **617**
Comtrex Maximum Strength Day/
Night Cold & Cough Caplets -
Day Formulation **618**
Comtrex Maximum Strength Day/
Night Cold & Cough Caplets -
Night Formulation **618**
Comtrex Maximum Strength
Non-Drowsy Cold & Cough Caplets....**619**
Theraflu Cold & Sore Throat
Hot Liquid **630**
Theraflu Flu & Chest Congestion
Hot Liquid **631**
Theraflu Flu & Sore Throat
Hot Liquid **631**
Theraflu Daytime Severe Cold
Caplets **634**
Theraflu Nighttime Severe Cold
Caplets **635**
Theraflu Daytime Severe Cold Hot
Liquid **632**
Theraflu Nighttime Severe Cold Hot
Liquid **632**

TheraFlu Severe Cold Non-Drowsy
Theraflu Warming Relief Daytime
Severe Cold....................................**634**
Theraflu Warming Relief Nighttime
Severe Cold....................................**635**
Vicks Formula 44M Cough,
Cold & Flu Relief Liquid..................**649**
Vicks DayQuil LiquiCaps/Liquid
Multi-Symptom Cold/Flu Relief..........**651**
Vicks NyQuil LiquiCaps/Liquid
Multi-Symptom Cold/Flu Relief..........**653**
Vicks Nyquil D Cold & Flu
Multi-Symptom Relief Liquid **652**
Zicam Multi-Symptom Liquid Daytime....**613**
Zicam Multi-Symptom Cold & Flu
Daytime To Go **615**
Zicam Multi-Symptom Cold & Flu
Nighttime Liquid..............................**614**
Zicam Multi-Symptom Cold & Flu
Nighttime To Go **615**

FLATULENCE

May result from the use of nonsteroidal anti-inflammatory drugs, potassium supplements, acarbose, cisapride, guanadrel sulfate, mesalamine, metformin hydrochloride, methyldopa, octreotide acetate or ursodiol. The following products may be recommended:

Align Daily Probiotic Supplement **696**
Gas-X Regular Strength
Chewable Tablets............................**626**
Gas-X Extra Strength
Chewable Tablets............................**626**
Gas-X Extra Strength Softgels..............**626**
Gas-X Extra Strength Thin Strips..........**626**
Gas-X Maximum Strength Softgels........**626**
Gas-X with Maalox Extra Strength
Chewable Tablets............................**626**
Hyland's Colic Tablets..........................**661**
Maalox Regular Strength
Antacid/Antigas Liquid **628**
Maalox Maximum Strength
Total Stomach Relief Liquid **629**

FLU-LIKE SYNDROME

May result from the use of gemcitabine hydrochloride, interferon alfa-2b, recombinant, interferon alfa-n3 (human leukocyte derived), interferon beta-1b, interferon gamma-1b or succimer. The following products may be recommended:

Advil Caplets......................................**668**
Advil Gel Caplets **668**
Advil Liqui-Gels **668**
Advil Tablets **668**
Advil Allergy Sinus Caplets **669**
Children's Advil Oral Suspension **670**
Advil Cold & Sinus Caplets..................**669**
Advil Cold & Sinus Liqui-Gels..............**669**
Infants' Advil Concentrated Drops -
White Grape (Dye-Free)....................**672**
Advil Multi-Symptom Cold Caplets........**669**
Allergy Antihistamine Capsules............**708**
Bufferin Extra Strength Tablets **617**
Bufferin Regular Strength Tablets **617**
Claritin Children's 24 Hour
Non-Drowsy Chewables **659**
Claritin Children's 24 Hour
Non-Drowsy Allergy Syrup **659**
Claritin-D Non-Drowsy
12 Hour Tablets..............................**658**
Claritin-D Non-Drowsy
24 Hour Tablets..............................**658**
Comtrex Maximum Strength
Day/Night Cold & Cough Caplets -
Day Formulation **618**
Comtrex Maximum Strength
Day/Night Cold & Cough Caplets -
Night Formulation **618**
Children's Dimetapp
Cold & Allergy Elixir........................**674**

FLU-LIKE SYNDROME—CONT.

Children's Dimetapp
Cold & Allergy Chewable Tablets **676**

Children's Dimetapp DM
Cold & Cough Elixir **675**

Children's Dimetapp Long Acting
Cough Plus Cold Syrup....................**675**

Toddler's Dimetapp
Cold and Cough Drops **676**

Excedrin Extra Strength
Caplets/Tablets/Geltabs **621**

Excedrin Sinus Headache
Caplets/Tablets..................................**623**

4-Way Fast Acting Nasal Spray **624**

4-Way Menthol Nasal Spray...................**624**

4-Way Moisturizing Relief
Nasal Spray.......................................**624**

Non-Drowsy Nasal Decongestant
Maximum Strength Tablets **710**

Non-Drowsy Nasal Decongestant PE
Tablets...**711**

Robitussin Night Time
Cough & Cold Syrup.........................**683**

Robitussin Night Time
Pediatric Cough & Cold Syrup **683**

Theraflu Cold & Sore Throat
Hot Liquid **630**

Theraflu Flu & Chest Congestion
Hot Liquid **631**

Theraflu Flu & Sore Throat
Hot Liquid **631**

Theraflu Daytime Severe Cold
Caplets **634**

Theraflu Nighttime Severe Cold
Caplets **635**

Theraflu Daytime Severe Cold
Hot Liquid **632**

Theraflu Nighttime Severe Cold
Hot Liquid **632**

Theraflu Thin Strips Daytime
Cold & Cough **633**

Theraflu Thin Strips Nighttime
Cold & Cough **633**

Theraflu Warming Relief Daytime
Severe Cold.......................................**634**

Theraflu Warming Relief Nighttime
Severe Cold.......................................**635**

Triaminic Cold & Allergy Liquid..............**636**

Triaminic Day Time
Cold & Cough Liquid **637**

Triaminic Night Time
Cold & Cough Liquid **637**

Triaminic Thin Strips Day Time
Cold & Cough **640**

Triaminic Thin Strips Night Time
Cold & Cough **640**

Triaminic Thin Strips Cold with
Stuffy Nose.......................................**639**

Triaminic Thin Strips Cough &
Runny Nose.......................................**640**

Triaminic Infant & Toddler Thin Strips
Decongestant.....................................**638**

Triaminic Infant & Toddler Thin Strips
Decongestant Plus Cough **638**

Pediatric Vicks 44e Cough & Chest
Congestion Relief Liquid....................**654**

Vicks Formula 44M Cough,
Cold & Flu Relief Liquid....................**649**

Pediatric Vicks Formula 44m
Cough & Cold Relief Liquid **655**

Vicks DayQuil LiquiCaps/Liquid
Multi-Symptom Cold/Flu Relief..........**651**

Vicks NyQuil LiquiCaps/Liquid
Multi-Symptom Cold/Flu Relief..........**653**

Children's Vicks NyQuil
Cold/Cough Relief **650**

Vicks Vapor Inhaler................................**656**

Zicam Cold Remedy ChewCaps **611**

Zicam Cold Remedy RapidMelts **611**

Zicam Cold Remedy RapidMelts
with Vitamin C **611**

FLUSHING EPISODES

May result from the use of lipid lowering doses of niacin. The following products may be recommended:

Advil Liqui-Gels....................................**668**

GASTROESOPHAGEAL REFLUX DISEASE

May be treated with histamine h2 receptor antagonists, proton pump inhibitors or sucralfate. The following products may be recommended for relief of symptoms:

Calcium Antacid Tablets **708**

Gas-X with Maalox Extra Strength
Chewable Tablets..............................**626**

Maalox Regular Strength
Antacid/Antigas Liquid **628**

Maalox Maximum Strength
Multi Symptom Antacid/Antigas
Liquid **628**

Maalox Maximum Strength
Total Stomach Relief Liquid **629**

Maalox Maximum Strength
Multi Symptom Antacid/Antigas
Chewable Tablets..............................**629**

Children's Pepto...................................**641**

Pepto-Bismol Original Liquid,
Original and Cherry Chewable
Tablets & Caplets..............................**643**

Pepto-Bismol Maximum Strength
Liquid **643**

Vibe Liquid Multi-Nutrient
Supplement..**688**

Zantac 75 Tablets.................................**609**

Maximum Strength Zantac 150
Tablets...**610**

Maximum Strength Zantac 150
Cool Mint Tablets..............................**610**

HUMAN IMMUNODEFICIENCY VIRUS (HIV) INFECTIONS, NUTRIENTS DEFICIENCY SECONDARY TO

HIV infections may be treated with non-nucleoside reverse transcriptase inhibitors, nucleoside reverse transcriptase inhibitors or protease inhibitors. The following products may be recommended for relief of nutrients deficiency:

BioLean Accelerator Tablets **664**

BioLean Free Tablets **665**

BioLean II Tablets.................................**664**

BioLean LipoTrim Capsules **665**

BioLean Mass Appeal Tablets...............**665**

BioLean ProXtreme Dietary
Supplement..**666**

BioLean Sure2Endure Tablets...............**703**

Centrum Tablets....................................**704**

Centrum Kids Complete Children's
Chewables **705**

Centrum Performance Multivitamin/
Multimineral Supplement...................**705**

Centrum Silver Tablets..........................**706**

Daily Complete Liquid **686**

DHEA Plus Capsules............................**666**

Efacor Dietary Supplement....................**687**

Food for Thought Dietary
Supplement..**666**

Phyto-Vite Tablets **667**

PureTrim Mediterranean
Wellness Shake..................................**686**

Satiete Tablets......................................**667**

StePHan Clarity Capsules **700**

StePHan Elasticity Capsules..................**701**

StePHan Elixir Capsules........................**701**

StePHan Essential Capsules **701**

StePHan Feminine Capsules **701**

StePHan Flexibility Capsules.................**701**

StePHan Lovpil Capsules......................**702**

StePHan Tranquility Capsules...............**702**

Vibe Liquid Multi-Nutrient
Supplement..**688**

Winrgy Dietary Supplement **703**

HUMAN IMMUNODEFICIENCY VIRUS (HIV) INFECTIONS, XERODERMA SECONDARY TO

HIV infections may be treated with non-nucleoside reverse transcriptase inhibitors, nucleoside reverse transcriptase inhibitors or protease inhibitors. The following products may be recommended for relief of xeroderma:

Tahitian Noni Seed Oil **699**

HYPERPARATHYROIDISM, NUTRIENTS DEFICIENCY SECONDARY TO

Hyperthyroidism may be treated with methimazole. The following products may be recommended for relief of nutrients deficiency:

BioLean Accelerator Tablets **664**

BioLean Free Tablets **665**

BioLean II Tablets.................................**664**

BioLean LipoTrim Capsules **665**

BioLean Mass Appeal Tablets...............**665**

BioLean ProXtreme Dietary
Supplement..**666**

BioLean Sure2Endure Tablets...............**703**

Centrum Tablets....................................**704**

Centrum Kids Complete
Children's Chewables.........................**705**

Centrum Performance Multivitamin/
Multimineral Supplement...................**705**

Centrum Silver Tablets..........................**706**

Daily Complete Liquid **686**

DHEA Plus Capsules............................**666**

Food for Thought
Dietary Supplement **666**

Phyto-Vite Tablets **667**

PureTrim Mediterranean
Wellness Shake..................................**686**

Satiete Tablets......................................**667**

StePHan Clarity Capsules **700**

StePHan Elasticity Capsules..................**701**

StePHan Elixir Capsules........................**701**

StePHan Essential Capsules **701**

StePHan Feminine Capsules **701**

StePHan Flexibility Capsules.................**701**

StePHan Lovpil Capsules......................**702**

StePHan Tranquility Capsules...............**702**

Winrgy Dietary Supplement **703**

HYPERTHYROIDISM, NUTRIENTS DEFICIENCY SECONDARY TO

Hyperthyroidism may be treated with methimazole. The following products may be recommended for relief of nutrients deficiency:

BioLean Accelerator Tablets **664**

BioLean Free Tablets **665**

BioLean II Tablets.................................**664**

BioLean LipoTrim Capsules **665**

BioLean Mass Appeal Tablets...............**665**

BioLean ProXtreme Dietary
Supplement..**666**

BioLean Sure2Endure Tablets...............**703**

Centrum Tablets....................................**704**

Centrum Kids Complete
Children's Chewables.........................**705**

Centrum Performance Multivitamin/
Multimineral Supplement...................**705**

Centrum Silver Tablets..........................**706**

Daily Complete Liquid **686**

DHEA Plus Capsules............................**666**

Food for Thought
Dietary Supplement **666**

Phyto-Vite Tablets **667**

PureTrim Mediterranean
Wellness Shake..................................**686**

Satiete Tablets......................................**667**

StePHan Clarity Capsules **700**

StePHan Elasticity Capsules..................**701**

StePHan Elixir Capsules........................**701**

StePHan Essential Capsules **701**

StePHan Feminine Capsules **701**

StePHan Flexibility Capsules.................**701**

StePHan Lovpil Capsules......................**702**

StePHan Tranquility Capsules...............**702**

Vibe Liquid Multi-Nutrient
Supplement **688**
Winrgy Dietary Supplement **703**

HYPOKALEMIA
May result from the use of corticosteroids,
diuretics, diuretics, thiazides, thiazides,
aldesleukin, amphotericin b, carboplatin,
etretinate, foscarnet sodium, mycophenolate
mofetil, pamidronate disodium or tacrolimus.
The following products may be recommended:
Vibe Liquid Multi-Nutrient
Supplement **688**

HYPOMAGNESEMIA
May result from the use of aldesleukin, aminoglycosides, amphotericin b, caroboplatin, cisplatin,
cyclosporine, diuretics, foscarnet, pamidronate,
sargramostim or tacrolimus. The following products
may be recommended:
Beelith Tablets **687**
Vibe Liquid Multi-Nutrient
Supplement **688**

HYPOPARATHYROIDISM
May be treated with vitamin d sterols. The following
products may be recommended for relief of
symptoms:
Calcium Antacid Tablets **708**
Caltrate 600 + D Tablets **704**
Caltrate 600 + D PLUS Minerals
Chewables **704**
Caltrate 600 + D PLUS Minerals
Tablets **704**
Citracal Caplets **693**
D-Cal Chewable Caplets **686**

**HYPOTHYROIDISM, CONSTIPATION
SECONDARY TO**
Hypothyroidism may be treated with thyroid
hormones. The following products may be
recommended for relief of constipation:
Benefiber Fiber Supplement Powder......**694**
Benefiber Fiber Supplement
Sugar Free Assorted Fruit
Chewables **694**
Benefiber Fiber Supplement
Sugar Free Orange Creme
Chewables **694**
Benefiber Fiber Supplement Plus
B Vitamins & Folic Acid Caplets **695**
Benefiber Fiber Supplement
Plus B Vitamins & Folic Acid
Powder **695**
Benefiber Fiber Supplement Plus
Calcium Chewable Tablets **696**
Dulcolax Stool Softener **609**
Dulcolax Suppositories **609**
Ex•Lax Chocolated Laxative Pieces **625**
Ex•Lax Regular Strength Pills **625**
Ex•Lax Maximum Strength Pills............**625**
FiberCon Caplets **676**
Metamucil Capsules **642**
Metamucil Powder, Original Texture
Orange Flavor **642**
Metamucil Powder, Original Texture
Regular Flavor **642**
Metamucil Smooth Texture Powder,
Orange Flavor **642**
Metamucil Smooth Texture Powder,
Sugar-Free, Orange Flavor.................**642**
Metamucil Smooth Texture Powder,
Sugar-Free, Regular Flavor **642**
Metamucil Wafers, Apple Crisp &
Cinnamon Spice Flavors **642**

**INFECTIONS, BACTERIAL, UPPER RESPIRATORY
TRACT**
May be treated with amoxicillin-clavulanate,
cephalosporins, doxycycline, erythromycin,
macrolide antibiotics, penicillins or minocycline
hydrochloride. The following products may be
recommended for relief of symptoms:
Advil Caplets **668**
Advil Gel Caplets **668**

Advil Liqui-Gels **668**
Advil Tablets **668**
Advil Allergy Sinus Caplets **669**
Children's Advil Oral Suspension **670**
Advil Cold & Sinus Caplets..................**669**
Advil Cold & Sinus Liqui-Gels..............**669**
Infants' Advil Concentrated Drops -
White Grape (Dye-Free)....................**672**
Advil Multi-Symptom Cold Caplets........**669**
Allergy Antihistamine Capsules............**708**
Claritin-D Non-Drowsy 12 Hour
Tablets **658**
Claritin-D Non-Drowsy 24 Hour
Tablets **658**
Comtrex Maximum Strength
Day/Night Cold & Cough Caplets -
Day Formulation **618**
Comtrex Maximum Strength
Day/Night Cold & Cough Caplets -
Night Formulation **618**
Comtrex Maximum Strength
Non-Drowsy Cold & Cough Caplets....**619**
Delsym Liquid Grape Flavor **602**
Delsym Liquid Orange Flavor **603**
Children's Dimetapp
Cold & Allergy Elixir........................**674**
Children's Dimetapp
Cold & Allergy Chewable Tablets **676**
Children's Dimetapp DM
Cold & Cough Elixir **675**
Children's Dimetapp Long Acting
Cough Plus Cold Syrup....................**675**
Toddler's Dimetapp
Cold and Cough Drops **676**
Excedrin Extra Strength
Caplets/Tablets/Geltabs **621**
4-Way Fast Acting Nasal Spray **624**
4-Way Moisturizing Relief
Nasal Spray....................................**624**
Mucinex 1200mg Extended-Release
Bi-Layer Tablets **606**
Mucinex Cold Liquid **604**
Mucinex Cough Liquid........................**603**
Mucinex Mini-Melts
Bubble Gum Flavor..........................**604**
Mucinex Mini-Melts Grape Flavor **604**
Mucinex Cough Mini-Melts
Orange Cream Flavor.......................**605**
Mucinex D 1200mg/120mg
Extended-Release Bi-Layer Tablets **606**
Mucinex DM 600mg/30mg
Extended-Release Bi-Layer Tablets **607**
Mucinex DM 1200mg/60mg
Extended-Release Bi-Layer Tablets **607**
Mucinex Liquid **603**
Non-Drowsy Nasal Decongestant
Maximum Strength Tablets **710**
Non-Drowsy Nasal Decongestant PE
Tablets..**711**
Robitussin Cough & Allergy Syrup.........**680**
Robitussin Cough & Cold CF Liquid.......**682**
Robitussin Cough & Cold CF
Pediatric Drops...............................**682**
Robitussin Cough & Cold
Long-Acting Liquid..........................**682**
Robitussin Pediatric Cough & Cold
Long-Acting Liquid..........................**682**
Robitussin Cough & Congestion
Liquid **681**
Robitussin Cough Gels Long-Acting.......**680**
Robitussin Cough Long Acting Liquid **681**
Robitussin Pediatric Cough
Long Acting Liquid..........................**681**
Robitussin Sugar Free Cough Syrup......**681**
Robitussin Cough DM Syrup................**681**
Robitussin Cough DM Infant Drops.......**681**
Robitussin Cough Drops
Menthol, Cherry, and Honey **679**

Robitussin Honey Cough Drops **679**
Robitussin Sugar Free Throat Drops **679**
Robitussin Head & Chest
Congestion PE Syrup........................**680**
Robitussin Night Time
Cough & Cold Syrup........................**683**
Robitussin Night Time
Pediatric Cough & Cold Syrup **683**
Theraflu Cold & Sore Throat
Hot Liquid **630**
Theraflu Flu & Chest Congestion
Hot Liquid **631**
Theraflu Flu & Sore Throat
Hot Liquid **631**
Theraflu Daytime Severe Cold
Caplets..**634**
Theraflu Nighttime Severe Cold
Caplets..**635**
Theraflu Daytime Severe Cold
Hot Liquid **632**
Theraflu Nighttime Severe Cold
Hot Liquid **632**
Theraflu Thin Strips Daytime
Cold & Cough **633**
Theraflu Thin Strips Nighttime
Cold & Cough **633**
Theraflu Warming Relief Daytime
Severe Cold....................................**634**
Theraflu Warming Relief Nighttime
Severe Cold....................................**635**
Triaminic Chest & Nasal Congestion
Liquid **636**
Triaminic Cold & Allergy Liquid.............**636**
Triaminic Day Time
Cold & Cough Liquid **637**
Triaminic Cough & Sore Throat
Liquid **638**
Triaminic Cough & Runny Nose
Softchews **639**
Triaminic Thin Strips Day Time
Cold & Cough **640**
Triaminic Thin Strips Night Time
Cold & Cough **640**
Triaminic Thin Strips Cold with
Stuffy Nose **639**
Triaminic Thin Strips
Cough & Runny Nose **640**
Triaminic Infant & Toddler
Thin Strips Decongestant **638**
Triaminic Infant & Toddler
Thin Strips Decongestant
Plus Cough **638**
Vicks Formula 44 Cough Relief
Liquid **648**
Vicks Formula 44D Cough & Head
Congestion Relief Liquid...................**649**
Vicks Formula 44E Cough & Chest
Congestion Relief Liquid...................**649**
Pediatric Vicks 44e Cough & Chest
Congestion Relief Liquid...................**654**
Vicks Formula 44M Cough,
Cold & Flu Relief Liquid...................**649**
Pediatric Vicks Formula 44m
Cough & Cold Relief Liquid...............**655**
Vicks Cough Drops, Menthol and
Cherry Flavors **650**
Vicks DayQuil LiquiCaps/Liquid
Multi-Symptom Cold/Flu Relief...........**651**
Vicks NyQuil LiquiCaps/Liquid
Multi-Symptom Cold/Flu Relief...........**653**
Children's Vicks NyQuil
Cold/Cough Relief **650**
Vicks NyQuil Cough Liquid..................**652**
Vicks NyQuil D Cold & Flu
Multi-Symptom Relief Liquid **652**
Vicks Sinex Nasal Spray and
Ultra Fine Mist................................**655**
Vicks Sinex 12-Hour
Nasal Spray and Ultra Fine Mist........**656**

**INFECTIONS, BACTERIAL,
UPPER RESPIRATORY TRACT—CONT.**

Vicks Vapor Inhaler.................................**656**
Vicks VapoRub Cream............................**656**
Vicks VapoRub Ointment.......................**656**
Vicks VapoSteam...................................**657**
Zicam Cold Remedy Chewables............**611**
Zicam Cold Remedy ChewCaps............**611**
Zicam Cold Remedy Gel Swabs............**611**
Zicam Cold Remedy Nasal Gel..............**611**
Zicam Cold Remedy Oral Mist..............**611**
Zicam Cold Remedy RapidMelts............**611**
Zicam Cold Remedy RapidMelts
   with Vitamin C.................................**611**
Zicam Multi-Symptom Liquid Daytime....**613**
Zicam Multi-Symptom
   Cold & Flu Daytime To Go...............**615**
Zicam Multi-Symptom
   Cold & Flu Nighttime Liquid.............**614**
Zicam Multi-Symptom
   Cold & Flu Nighttime To Go.............**615**

INFECTIONS, SKIN AND SKIN STRUCTURE
May be treated with aminoglycosides, amoxicillin, amoxicillin-clavulanate, cephalosporins, doxycycline, erythromycin, macrolide antibiotics, penicillins or quinolones. The following products may be recommended for relief of symptoms:

Desenex Athlete's Foot Cream **620**
Lamisil[AF] Defense Powders
   (Shake & Spray) **627**

IRRITABLE BOWEL SYNDROME
May be treated with anticholinergic combinations, dicyclomine hydrochloride or hyoscyamine sulfate. The following products may be recommended for relief of symptoms:

Align Daily Probiotic Supplement **696**
Benefiber Fiber Supplement
   Sugar Free Assorted Fruit
   Chewables **694**
Benefiber Fiber Supplement
   Sugar Free Orange Creme
   Chewables **694**
FiberCon Caplets..................................**676**
Gas-X Regular Strength
   Chewable Tablets............................**626**
Gas-X Extra Strength
   Chewable Tablets............................**626**
Gas-X Extra Strength Softgels.............**626**
Gas-X Maximum Strength Softgels........**626**
Gas-X with Maalox Extra Strength
   Chewable Tablets............................**626**
Maalox Maximum Strength
   Total Stomach Relief Liquid **629**
Metamucil Capsules.............................**642**
Metamucil Powder, Original Texture
   Orange Flavor **642**
Metamucil Powder, Original Texture
   Regular Flavor **642**
Metamucil Smooth Texture Powder,
   Orange Flavor **642**
Metamucil Smooth Texture Powder,
   Sugar-Free, Orange Flavor...............**642**
Metamucil Smooth Texture Powder,
   Sugar-Free, Regular Flavor...............**642**
Metamucil Wafers, Apple Crisp &
   Cinnamon Spice Flavors...................**642**

KERATOCONJUNCTIVITIS, VERNAL
May be treated with ophthalmic mast cell stabilizers. The following products may be recommended for relief of symptoms:

Allergy Antihistamine Capsules.............**708**
Triaminic Thin Strips
   Cough & Runny Nose **640**

NASAL POLYPS, RHINORRHEA SECONDARY TO
Nasal polyps may be treated with nasal steroidal anti-inflammatory agents. The following products may be recommended for relief of rhinorrhea:

Advil Allergy Sinus Caplets **669**
Advil Multi-Symptom Cold Caplets.........**669**

Alavert Allergy & Sinus D-12 Hour
   Tablets...**673**
Alavert Orally Disintegrating Tablets......**673**
Allergy Antihistamine Capsules.............**708**
Claritin Children's 24 Hour
   Non-Drowsy Chewables **659**
Claritin Children's 24 Hour
   Non-Drowsy Allergy Syrup................**659**
Claritin Non-Drowsy 24 Hour Tablets.....**659**
Claritin Reditabs 24 Hour
   Non-Drowsy Tablets.........................**659**
Claritin-D Non-Drowsy 12 Hour
   Tablets...**658**
Claritin-D Non-Drowsy 24 Hour
   Tablets...**658**
Children's Dimetapp
   Cold & Allergy Elixir.........................**674**
Children's Dimetapp
   Cold & Allergy Chewable Tablets.......**676**
Excedrin Sinus Headache
   Caplets/Tablets...............................**623**
4-Way Menthol Nasal Spray.................**624**
Hyland's Sniffles 'N Sneezes 4 Kids
   Tablets...**662**
Robitussin Cough & Allergy Syrup.........**680**
Robitussin Cough & Cold
   Long-Acting Liquid..........................**682**
Robitussin Pediatric Cough & Cold
   Long-Acting Liquid..........................**682**
Robitussin Night Time
   Cough & Cold Syrup........................**683**
Robitussin Night Time Pediatric
   Cough & Cold Syrup........................**683**
Theraflu Cold & Cough Hot Liquid.........**630**
Theraflu Cold & Sore Throat
   Hot Liquid **630**
Theraflu Flu & Chest Congestion
   Hot Liquid **631**
Theraflu Flu & Sore Throat
   Hot Liquid **631**
Theraflu Daytime Severe Cold
   Caplets...**634**
Theraflu Nighttime Severe Cold
   Caplets...**635**
Theraflu Daytime Severe Cold
   Hot Liquid **632**
Theraflu Nighttime Severe Cold
   Hot Liquid **632**
Theraflu Thin Strips Nighttime
   Cold & Cough **633**
Theraflu Warming Relief Daytime
   Severe Cold....................................**634**
Theraflu Warming Relief Nighttime
   Severe Cold....................................**635**
Triaminic Cold & Allergy Liquid.............**636**
Triaminic Cough & Runny Nose
   Softchews **639**
Vicks Formula 44M Cough,
   Cold & Flu Relief Liquid....................**649**
Pediatric Vicks Formula 44m
   Cough & Cold Relief Liquid...............**655**
Vicks NyQuil LiquiCaps/Liquid
   Multi-Symptom Cold/Flu Relief.........**653**
Children's Vicks NyQuil
   Cold/Cough Relief **650**
Zicam Cold Remedy ChewCaps............**611**
Zicam Cold Remedy RapidMelts............**611**
Zicam Cold Remedy RapidMelts
   with Vitamin C.................................**611**

OSTEOPOROSIS
May be treated with biphosphonates, calcitonin or estrogens. The following products may be recommended for relief of symptoms:

Benefiber Fiber Supplement Plus
   Calcium Chewable Tablets................**696**
Calcet Triple Calcium + Vitamin D
   Tablets...**693**
Calcium Antacid Tablets.......................**708**
Caltrate 600 + D Tablets **704**

Caltrate 600 + D PLUS Minerals
   Chewables **704**
Caltrate 600 + D PLUS Minerals
   Tablets...**704**
Citracal Caplets...................................**693**
D-Cal Chewable Caplets.......................**686**
Natural Joint Capsules.........................**690**
PremCal Light, Regular, and
   Extra Strength Tablets......................**687**
StePHan Feminine Capsules **701**
Vibe Liquid Multi-Nutrient
   Supplement.....................................**688**

OSTEOPOROSIS, SECONDARY
May result from the use of chemotherapeutic agents, phenytoin, prolonged glucocorticoid therapy, thyroid hormones, carbamazepine or methotrexate sodium. The following products may be recommended:

Benefiber Fiber Supplement Plus
   Calcium Chewable Tablets................**696**
Calcet Triple Calcium + Vitamin D
   Tablets...**693**
Calcium Antacid Tablets.......................**708**
Caltrate 600 + D Tablets **704**
Caltrate 600 + D PLUS Minerals
   Chewables **704**
Caltrate 600 + D PLUS Minerals
   Tablets...**704**
Citracal Caplets...................................**693**
D-Cal Chewable Caplets.......................**686**
Natural Joint Capsules.........................**690**
PremCal Light, Regular, and
   Extra Strength Tablets......................**687**
StePHan Feminine Capsules **701**

OTITIS MEDIA, ACUTE
May be treated with amoxicillin, amoxicillin-clavulanate, cephalosporins, erythromycin-sulfisoxazole, macrolide antibiotics or sulfamethoxazole-trimethoprim. The following products may be recommended for relief of symptoms:

Advil Caplets......................................**668**
Advil Gel Caplets **668**
Advil Liqui-Gels..................................**668**
Advil Tablets.......................................**668**
Children's Advil Oral Suspension **670**
Advil Cold & Sinus Caplets...................**669**
Advil Cold & Sinus Liqui-Gels...............**669**
Infants' Advil Concentrated Drops -
   White Grape (Dye-Free).....................**672**
Hyland's Earache Tablets......................**661**
Theraflu Daytime Severe Cold
   Caplets...**634**
Theraflu Daytime Severe Cold
   Hot Liquid **632**

**PANCREATIC INSUFFICIENCY, NUTRIENTS
DEFICIENCY SECONDARY TO**
Pancreatic insufficiency may be treated with pancrelipase. The following products may be recommended for relief of nutrients deficiency:

BioLean Accelerator Tablets **664**
BioLean Free Tablets **665**
BioLean II Tablets................................**664**
BioLean LipoTrim Capsules **665**
BioLean Mass Appeal Tablets...............**665**
BioLean ProXtreme
   Dietary Supplement **666**
BioLean Sure2Endure Tablets...............**703**
Centrum Tablets..................................**704**
Centrum Kids Complete Children's
   Chewables **705**
Centrum Performance Multivitamin/
   Multimineral Supplement..................**705**
Centrum Silver Tablets.........................**706**
Daily Complete Liquid **686**
DHEA Plus Capsules............................**666**
Food for Thought Dietary Supplement...**666**
Phyto-Vite Tablets...............................**667**
Satiete Tablets **667**
StePHan Clarity Capsules **700**

StePHan Elasticity Capsules.................**701**
StePHan Elixir Capsules.......................**701**
StePHan Essential Capsules **701**
StePHan Feminine Capsules **701**
StePHan Flexibility Capsules **701**
StePHan Lovpil Capsules......................**702**
StePHan Tranquility Capsules...............**702**
Vibe Liquid Multi-Nutrient
   Supplement..................................**688**
Winrgy Dietary Supplement **703**

**PARKINSON'S DISEASE, CONSTIPATION
SECONDARY TO**
Parkinson's disease may be treated with centrally
active anticholinergic agents, dopaminergic agents
or selective inhibitor of mao type b. The following
products may be recommended for relief of
constipation:
Benefiber Fiber Supplement Powder......**694**
Benefiber Fiber Supplement
   Sugar Free Assorted Fruit
   Chewables **694**
Benefiber Fiber Supplement
   Sugar Free Orange Creme
   Chewables **694**
Dulcolax Stool Softener **609**
Dulcolax Suppositories **609**
Dulcolax Tablets **608**
Ex•Lax Chocolated Laxative Pieces **625**
Ex•Lax Regular Strength Pills...............**625**
Ex•Lax Maximum Strength Pills............**625**
FiberCon Caplets **676**
Metamucil Capsules **642**
Metamucil Powder, Original Texture
   Orange Flavor **642**
Metamucil Powder, Original Texture
   Regular Flavor **642**
Metamucil Smooth Texture Powder,
   Orange Flavor **642**
Metamucil Smooth Texture Powder,
   Sugar-Free, Orange Flavor................**642**
Metamucil Smooth Texture Powder,
   Sugar-Free, Regular Flavor **642**
Metamucil Wafers, Apple Crisp &
   Cinnamon Spice Flavors **642**
Vibe Liquid Multi-Nutrient
   Supplement..................................**688**

PEPTIC ULCER DISEASE
May be treated with histamine h2 receptor
antagonists, proton pump inhibitors or sucralfate.
The following products may be recommended for
relief of symptoms:
Calcium Antacid Tablets **708**
Gas-X with Maalox Extra Strength
   Chewable Tablets...........................**626**
Maalox Regular Strength
   Antacid/Antigas Liquid **628**
Maalox Maximum Strength
   Multi Symptom Antacid/Antigas
   Liquid **628**
Maalox Maximum Strength
   Multi Symptom Antacid/Antigas
   Chewable Tablets **629**
Pepto-Bismol Original Liquid,
   Original and Cherry Chewable
   Tablets & Caplets **643**
Pepto-Bismol Maximum Strength
   Liquid **643**
Prilosec OTC Tablets **644**
Zantac 75 Tablets **609**
Maximum Strength Zantac 150
   Tablets **610**
Maximum Strength Zantac 150
   Cool Mint Tablets...........................**610**

PHARYNGITIS
May be treated with cephalosporins, macrolide
antibiotics or penicillins. The following products
may be recommended for relief of symptoms:
Advil Caplets **668**
Advil Gel Caplets **668**
Advil Liqui-Gels.................................**668**

Advil Tablets.....................................**668**
Advil Allergy Sinus Caplets **669**
Children's Advil Oral Suspension **670**
Advil Cold & Sinus Caplets **669**
Advil Cold & Sinus Liqui-Gels...............**669**
Infants' Advil Concentrated Drops -
   White Grape (Dye-Free)...................**672**
Advil Multi-Symptom Cold Caplets........**669**
Comtrex Maximum Strength
   Day/Night Cold & Cough Caplets -
   Day Formulation **618**
Comtrex Maximum Strength
   Day/Night Cold & Cough Caplets -
   Night Formulation **618**
Comtrex Maximum Strength
   Non-Drowsy Cold & Cough Caplets ...**619**
Delsym Liquid Grape Flavor..................**602**
Delsym Liquid Orange Flavor **603**
Children's Dimetapp DM
   Cold & Cough Elixir **675**
Children's Dimetapp Long Acting
   Cough Plus Cold Syrup **675**
Toddler's Dimetapp
   Cold and Cough Drops **676**
Hurricaine Topical Anesthetic Gel,
   1 oz. Wild Cherry, Pina Colada,
   Watermelon, and Fresh Mint,
   5.25 g. Wild Cherry **608**
Hurricaine Topical Anesthetic Liquid,
   1 oz. Wild Cherry, Pina Colada,
   0.005 fl. oz. Snap-n-Go Swabs
   Wild Cherry **608**
Hurricaine Topical Anesthetic Spray
   Extension Tubes (200) **608**
Hurricaine Topical Anesthetic
   Spray Kit, 2 oz. Wild Cherry with
   disposable Extension
   Tubes (200) **608**
Hurricaine Topical Anesthetic
   Spray, 2 oz. Wild Cherry..................**608**
Mucinex DM 600mg/30mg
   Extended-Release Bi-Layer Tablets **607**
Mucinex DM 1200mg/60mg
   Extended-Release Bi-Layer Tablets **607**
Robitussin Cough & Cold CF Liquid.......**682**
Robitussin Cough & Cold CF
   Pediatric Drops.............................**682**
Robitussin Cough & Cold
   Long-Acting Liquid.........................**682**
Robitussin Pediatric Cough & Cold
   Long-Acting Liquid.........................**682**
Robitussin Cough & Congestion
   Liquid **681**
Robitussin Cough Long Acting
   Liquid **681**
Robitussin Pediatric Cough
   Long Acting Liquid.........................**681**
Robitussin Sugar Free Cough Syrup **681**
Robitussin Cough DM Syrup **681**
Robitussin Cough DM Infant Drops **681**
Robitussin Cough Drops Menthol,
   Cherry, and Honey **679**
Robitussin Honey Cough Drops **679**
Robitussin Sugar Free Throat Drops **679**
Theraflu Cold & Sore Throat
   Hot Liquid **630**
Theraflu Flu & Chest Congestion
   Hot Liquid **631**
Theraflu Flu & Sore Throat
   Hot Liquid **631**
Theraflu Daytime Severe Cold
   Caplets **634**
Theraflu Nighttime Severe Cold
   Caplets **635**
Theraflu Daytime Severe Cold
   Hot Liquid **632**
Theraflu Nighttime Severe Cold
   Hot Liquid **632**
Theraflu Thin Strips Daytime
   Cold & Cough **633**

Theraflu Thin Strips Nighttime
   Cold & Cough **633**
Triaminic Day Time
   Cold & Cough Liquid **637**
Triaminic Night Time
   Cold & Cough Liquid **637**
Triaminic Cough & Sore Throat
   Liquid **638**
Triaminic Thin Strips Day Time
   Cold & Cough **640**
Triaminic Infant & Toddler Thin Strips
   Decongestant Plus Cough **638**
Vicks Formula 44 Cough
   Relief Liquid **648**
Vicks Formula 44M Cough,
   Cold & Flu Relief Liquid **649**
Pediatric Vicks Formula 44m
   Cough & Cold Relief Liquid..............**655**
Vicks Cough Drops, Menthol and
   Cherry Flavors **650**
Vicks DayQuil LiquiCaps/Liquid
   Multi-Symptom Cold/Flu Relief..........**651**
Vicks NyQuil LiquiCaps/Liquid
   Multi-Symptom Cold/Flu Relief..........**653**
Children's Vicks NyQuil
   Cold/Cough Relief **650**
Vicks NyQuil Cough Liquid...................**652**
Vicks NyQuil D Cold & Flu
   Multi-Symptom Relief Liquid **652**
Vicks VapoRub Cream **656**
Vicks VapoRub Ointment **656**
Vicks VapoSteam...............................**657**
Zicam Multi-Symptom Liquid Daytime....**613**
Zicam Multi-Symptom
   Cold & Flu Daytime To Go................**615**
Zicam Multi-Symptom
   Cold & Flu Nightitime Liquid **614**
Zicam Multi-Symptom
   Cold & Flu Nighttime To Go..............**615**

**RENAL OSTEODYSTROPHY, HYPOCALCEMIA
SECONDARY TO**
Renal osteodystrophy may be treated with
vitamin d sterols. The following products may be
recommended for relief of hypocalcemia:
Benefiber Fiber Supplement Plus Calcium
   Chewable Tablets...........................**696**
Calcium Antacid Tablets **708**
Caltrate 600 + D Tablets **704**
Caltrate 600 + D PLUS Minerals
   Chewables **704**
Caltrate 600 + D PLUS Minerals
   Tablets **704**
Citracal Caplets.................................**693**
D-Cal Chewable Caplets **686**

**RESPIRATORY TRACT ILLNESS, INFLUENZA A
VIRUS-INDUCED**
May be treated with amantadine hydrochloride or
rimantadine hydrochloride. The following products
may be recommended for relief of symptoms:
Advil Liqui-Gels.................................**668**
Advil Allergy Sinus Caplets **669**
Advil Multi-Symptom Cold Caplets........**669**
Allergy Antihistamine Capsules.............**708**
Claritin-D Non-Drowsy 12 Hour
   Tablets **658**
Claritin-D Non-Drowsy
   24 Hour Tablets.............................**658**
Comtrex Maximum Strength
   Day/Night Cold & Cough Caplets -
   Day Formulation **618**
Comtrex Maximum Strength
   Day/Night Cold & Cough Caplets -
   Night Formulation **618**
Comtrex Maximum Strength
   Non-Drowsy Cold & Cough Caplets ...**619**
Delsym Liquid Grape Flavor..................**602**
Delsym Liquid Orange Flavor **603**
Children's Dimetapp
   Cold & Allergy Elixir.......................**674**

RESPIRATORY TRACT ILLNESS, INFLUENZA A VIRUS-INDUCED—CONT.

Children's Dimetapp
  Cold & Allergy Chewable Tablets **676**
Children's Dimetapp DM
  Cold & Cough Elixir **675**
Children's Dimetapp Long Acting
  Cough Plus Cold Syrup.....................**675**
Mucinex 1200mg Extended-Release
  Bi-Layer Tablets.............................**606**
Mucinex Cold Liquid **604**
Mucinex Cough Liquid...........................**603**
Mucinex Mini-Melts Bubble Gum
  Flavor..**604**
Mucinex Mini-Melts Grape Flavor **604**
Mucinex Cough Mini-Melts
  Orange Cream Flavor.......................**605**
Mucinex D 1200mg/120mg
  Extended-Release Bi-Layer Tablets **606**
Mucinex DM 600mg/30mg
  Extended-Release Bi-Layer Tablets **607**
Mucinex DM 1200mg/60mg
  Extended-Release Bi-Layer Tablets **607**
Mucinex Liquid **603**
Robitussin Cough & Allergy Syrup.........**680**
Robitussin Cough & Cold CF Liquid **682**
Robitussin Cough & Cold CF
  Pediatric Drops..............................**682**
Robitussin Cough & Cold
  Long-Acting Liquid..........................**682**
Robitussin Pediatric Cough & Cold
  Long-Acting Liquid..........................**682**
Robitussin Cough & Congestion
  Liquid **681**
Robitussin Cough Long Acting Liquid **681**
Robitussin Pediatric Cough
  Long Acting Liquid...........................**681**
Robitussin Sugar Free Cough Syrup......**681**
Robitussin Cough DM Syrup..................**681**
Robitussin Cough DM Infant Drops **681**
Robitussin Cough Drops Menthol,
  Cherry, and Honey **679**
Robitussin Honey Cough Drops **679**
Robitussin Sugar Free Throat Drops **679**
Robitussin Head & Chest
  Congestion PE Syrup........................**680**
Robitussin Night Time
  Cough & Cold Syrup.........................**683**
Robitussin Night Time
  Pediatric Cough & Cold Syrup **683**
Theraflu Cold & Sore Throat
  Hot Liquid **630**
Theraflu Flu & Chest Congestion
  Hot Liquid **631**
Theraflu Flu & Sore Throat
  Hot Liquid **631**
Theraflu Daytime Severe Cold
  Caplets...**634**
Theraflu Nighttime Severe Cold
  Caplets...**635**
Theraflu Daytime Severe Cold
  Hot Liquid **632**
Theraflu Nighttime Severe Cold
  Hot Liquid **632**
Theraflu Thin Strips Daytime
  Cold & Cough.................................**633**
Theraflu Thin Strips Nighttime
  Cold & Cough.................................**633**
Triaminic Chest & Nasal Congestion
  Liquid **636**
Triaminic Cold & Allergy Liquid.............**636**
Triaminic Day Time Cold & Cough
  Liquid **637**
Triaminic Cough & Sore Throat
  Liquid **638**
Vicks Formula 44 Cough Relief
  Liquid **648**
Vicks Formula 44D Cough &
  Head Congestion Relief Liquid **649**

Vicks Formula 44E Cough &
  Chest Congestion Relief Liquid **649**
Pediatric Vicks 44e Cough &
  Chest Congestion Relief Liquid **654**
Vicks Formula 44M Cough,
  Cold & Flu Relief Liquid **649**
Pediatric Vicks Formula 44m
  Cough & Cold Relief Liquid **655**
Vicks Cough Drops, Menthol and
  Cherry Flavors................................**650**
Vicks DayQuil LiquiCaps/Liquid
  Multi-Symptom Cold/Flu Relief..........**651**
Vicks NyQuil LiquiCaps/Liquid
  Multi-Symptom Cold/Flu Relief..........**653**
Children's Vicks NyQuil
  Cold/Cough Relief **650**
Vicks NyQuil Cough Liquid....................**652**
Vicks NyQuil D Cold & Flu
  Multi-Symptom Relief Liquid **652**
Vicks Sinex Nasal Spray and
  Ultra Fine Mist...............................**655**
Vicks Sinex 12-Hour Nasal Spray
  and Ultra Fine Mist **656**
Vicks Vapor Inhaler.............................**656**
Vicks VapoRub Cream..........................**656**
Vicks VapoRub Ointment **656**
Vicks VapoSteam.................................**657**
Zicam Cold Remedy ChewCaps **611**
Zicam Cold Remedy RapidMelts **611**
Zicam Cold Remedy RapidMelts
  with Vitamin C **611**
Zicam Multi-Symptom Liquid Daytime....**613**
Zicam Multi-Symptom
  Cold & Flu Daytime To Go.................**615**
Zicam Multi-Symptom
  Cold & Flu Nighttime Liquid **614**
Zicam Multi-Symptom
  Cold & Flu Nighttime To Go..............**615**

RHEUMATOID ARTHRITIS, KERATOCONJUNCTIVITIS SICCA SECONDARY TO

Rheumatoid arthritis may be treated with corticosteroids, nonsteroidal anti-inflammatory drugs or azathioprine. The following products may be recommended for relief of keratoconjunctivitis sicca:
StePHan Flexibility Capsules **701**

RHINITIS, NONALLERGIC

May be treated with nasal steroids or ipratropium bromide. The following products may be recommended for relief of symptoms:
Advil Caplets **668**
Advil Gel Caplets **668**
Advil Tablets.......................................**668**
Advil Allergy Sinus Caplets **669**
Children's Advil Oral Suspension **670**
Advil Cold & Sinus Caplets...................**669**
Advil Cold & Sinus Liqui-Gels...............**669**
Infants' Advil Concentrated Drops -
  White Grape (Dye-Free)....................**672**
Advil Multi-Symptom Cold Caplets.........**669**
Allergy Antihistamine Capsules.............**708**
Comtrex Maximum Strength
  Day/Night Cold & Cough Caplets -
  Night Formulation **618**
Comtrex Maximum Strength
  Non-Drowsy Cold & Cough Caplets....**619**
Children's Dimetapp
  Cold & Allergy Elixir.........................**674**
Children's Dimetapp
  Cold & Allergy Chewable Tablets **676**
Toddler's Dimetapp Cold and
  Cough Drops..................................**676**
4-Way Fast Acting Nasal Spray **624**
Hyland's Sniffles 'N Sneezes 4 Kids
  Tablets..**662**
Mucinex Cold Liquid **604**
Mucinex D 600mg/60mg
  Extended-Release Bi-Layer Tablets **606**

Nasal Comfort Moisture
  Therapy Sprays - Scented and
  Unscented **611**
Robitussin Cough & Cold
  Long-Acting Liquid..........................**682**
Robitussin Pediatric
  Cough & Cold Long-Acting Liquid.......**682**
Robitussin Night Time
  Cough & Cold Syrup.........................**683**
Robitussin Night Time Pediatric
  Cough & Cold Syrup.........................**683**
Theraflu Cold & Cough Hot Liquid **630**
Theraflu Cold & Sore Throat
  Hot Liquid **630**
Theraflu Flu & Chest Congestion
  Hot Liquid **631**
Theraflu Flu & Sore Throat
  Hot Liquid **631**
Theraflu Daytime Severe Cold
  Caplets...**634**
Theraflu Nighttime Severe Cold
  Caplets...**635**
Theraflu Daytime Severe Cold
  Hot Liquid **632**
Theraflu Nighttime Severe Cold
  Hot Liquid **632**
Theraflu Thin Strips Nighttime
  Cold & Cough.................................**633**
Theraflu Warming Relief Daytime
  Severe Cold...................................**634**
Theraflu Warming Relief Nighttime
  Severe Cold...................................**635**
Triaminic Cold & Allergy Liquid.............**636**
Triaminic Day Time Cold & Cough
  Liquid **637**
Triaminic Cough & Runny Nose
  Softchews......................................**639**
Triaminic Thin Strips Day Time
  Cold & Cough.................................**640**
Triaminic Thin Strips Night Time
  Cold & Cough.................................**640**
Triaminic Thin Strips Cold with
  Stuffy Nose....................................**639**
Triaminic Infant & Toddler Thin Strips
  Decongestant.................................**638**
Triaminic Infant & Toddler Thin Strips
  Decongestant Plus Cough **638**
Vicks Formula 44M Cough,
  Cold & Flu Relief Liquid **649**
Pediatric Vicks Formula 44m
  Cough & Cold Relief Liquid **655**
Vicks DayQuil LiquiCaps/Liquid
  Multi-Symptom Cold/Flu Relief..........**651**
Vicks NyQuil LiquiCaps/Liquid
  Multi-Symptom Cold/Flu Relief..........**653**
Children's Vicks NyQuil
  Cold/Cough Relief **650**
Vicks NyQuil D Cold & Flu
  Multi-Symptom Relief Liquid **652**
Zicam Cold Remedy ChewCaps **611**
Zicam Cold Remedy RapidMelts **611**
Zicam Cold Remedy RapidMelts
  with Vitamin C **611**
Zicam Multi-Symptom Cold & Flu
  Daytime To Go **615**
Zicam Multi-Symptom Cold & Flu
  Nighttime Liquid **614**
Zicam Multi-Symptom Cold & Flu
  Nighttime To Go **615**
Zicam Sinus Melts...............................**616**

SERUM-SICKNESSLIKE REACTIONS

May result from the use of amoxicillin, amoxicillin-clavulanate, penicillins, sulfamethoxazole-trimethoprim, antivenin (crotalidae) polyvalent, antivenin (micrurus fulvius), metronidazole, ofloxacin, streptomycin sulfate, sulfadoxine, sulfamethoxazole or sulfasalazine. The following products may be recommended:
Allergy Antihistamine Capsules.............**708**

SINUSITIS

May be treated with amoxicillin, amoxicillin-clavulanate, cefprozil, cefuroxime axetil, clarithromycin or loracarbef. The following products may be recommended for relief of symptoms:

Advil Caplets **668**
Advil Gel Caplets **668**
Advil Liqui-Gels **668**
Advil Tablets **668**
Advil Allergy Sinus Caplets **669**
Children's Advil Oral Suspension **670**
Advil Cold & Sinus Caplets..................**669**
Advil Cold & Sinus Liqui-Gels...............**669**
Infants' Advil Concentrated Drops -
   White Grape (Dye-Free) **672**
Advil Multi-Symptom Cold Caplets........**669**
Claritin-D Non-Drowsy 12 Hour
   Tablets...**658**
Claritin-D Non-Drowsy 24 Hour
   Tablets...**658**
Comtrex Maximum Strength
   Day/Night Cold & Cough Caplets -
   Day Formulation **618**
Comtrex Maximum Strength
   Day/Night Cold & Cough Caplets -
   Night Formulation **618**
Comtrex Maximum Strength
   Non-Drowsy Cold & Cough Caplets....**619**
Children's Dimetapp
   Cold & Allergy Elixir.......................**674**
Children's Dimetapp
   Cold & Allergy Chewable Tablets.....**676**
Children's Dimetapp DM
   Cold & Cough Elixir **675**
Children's Dimetapp Long Acting
   Cough Plus Cold Syrup...................**675**
Toddler's Dimetapp
   Cold and Cough Drops **676**
Excedrin Extra Strength
   Caplets/Tablets/Geltabs.................**621**
Excedrin Sinus Headache
   Caplets/Tablets..............................**623**
4-Way Fast Acting Nasal Spray **624**
4-Way Menthol Nasal Spray.................**624**
4-Way Moisturizing Relief Nasal Spray...**624**
Hyland's Sniffles 'N Sneezes 4 Kids
   Tablets...**662**
Mucinex Cold Liquid **604**
Mucinex D 600mg/60mg
   Extended-Release Bi-Layer Tablets **606**
Non-Drowsy Nasal Decongestant
   Maximum Strength Tablets **710**
Non-Drowsy Nasal Decongestant PE
   Tablets...**711**
Robitussin Cough & Allergy Syrup........**680**
Robitussin Cough & Cold
   Long-Acting Liquid.........................**682**
Robitussin Pediatric Cough & Cold
   Long-Acting Liquid.........................**682**
Robitussin Night Time
   Cough & Cold Syrup **683**
Robitussin Night Time Pediatric
   Cough & Cold Syrup **683**
Theraflu Cold & Cough Hot Liquid........**630**
Theraflu Cold & Sore Throat
   Hot Liquid **630**
Theraflu Flu & Chest Congestion
   Hot Liquid **631**
Theraflu Flu & Sore Throat
   Hot Liquid **631**
Theraflu Daytime Severe Cold
   Caplets..**634**
Theraflu Nighttime Severe Cold
   Caplets..**635**
Theraflu Daytime Severe Cold
   Hot Liquid **632**
Theraflu Nighttime Severe Cold
   Hot Liquid **632**
Theraflu Thin Strips Daytime
   Cold & Cough **633**

Theraflu Thin Strips Nighttime
   Cold & Cough **633**
Theraflu Warming Relief Daytime
   Severe Cold....................................**634**
Theraflu Warming Relief Nighttime
   Severe Cold....................................**635**
Triaminic Chest & Nasal Congestion
   Liquid **636**
Triaminic Cold & Allergy Liquid..............**636**
Triaminic Day Time
   Cold & Cough Liquid **637**
Triaminic Night Time
   Cold & Cough Liquid **637**
Triaminic Cough & Sore Throat
   Liquid **638**
Triaminic Thin Strips Day Time
   Cold & Cough **640**
Triaminic Thin Strips Night Time
   Cold & Cough **640**
Triaminic Thin Strips Cold with
   Stuffy Nose **639**
Triaminic Infant & Toddler Thin Strips
   Decongestant **638**
Triaminic Infant & Toddler Thin Strips
   Decongestant Plus Cough **638**
Vicks Formula 44D Cough &
   Head Congestion Relief Liquid **649**
Pediatric Vicks Formula 44m
   Cough & Cold Relief Liquid **655**
Vicks DayQuil LiquiCaps/Liquid
   Multi-Symptom Cold/Flu Relief.........**651**
Vicks NyQuil LiquiCaps/Liquid
   Multi-Symptom Cold/Flu Relief.........**653**
Children's Vicks NyQuil
   Cold/Cough Relief **650**
Vicks NyQuil D Cold & Flu
   Multi-Symptom Relief Liquid **652**
Vicks Sinex Nasal Spray
   and Ultra Fine Mist **655**
Vicks Sinex 12-Hour Nasal Spray
   and Ultra Fine Mist **656**
Vicks Vapor Inhaler.............................**656**
Zicam Cold Remedy ChewCaps **611**
Zicam Cold Remedy RapidMelts **611**
Zicam Cold Remedy RapidMelts
   with Vitamin C **611**
Zicam Multi-Symptom Liquid Daytime....**613**
Zicam Multi-Symptom Cold & Flu
   Daytime To Go **615**
Zicam Multi-Symptom Cold & Flu
   Nightitime Liquid.............................**614**
Zicam Multi-Symptom Cold & Flu
   Nighttime To Go.............................**615**
Zicam Sinus Melts...............................**616**

SKIN IRRITATION

May result from the use of transdermal drug delivery systems. The following products may be recommended:

Desenex Athlete's Foot Cream **620**
Efacor Dietary Supplement...................**687**
Lamisil^AF Defense Powders
   (Shake & Spray) **627**
Tahitian Noni Leaf Serum
   Soothing Gel **698**

STOMATITIS, APHTHOUS

May result from the use of selective serotonin reuptake inhibitors, aldesleukin, clomipramine hydrochloride, didanosine, foscarnet sodium, indinavir sulfate, indomethacin, interferon alfa-2b, recombinant, methotrexate sodium, naproxen, naproxen sodium, nicotine polacrilex or stavudine. The following products may be recommended:

Hurricaine Topical Anesthetic Gel,
   1 oz. Wild Cherry, Pina Colada,
   Watermelon, and Fresh Mint,
   5.25 g. Wild Cherry **608**

Hurricaine Topical Anesthetic Liquid,
   1 oz. Wild Cherry, Pina Colada,
   0.005 fl. oz. Snap-n-Go Swabs
   Wild Cherry **608**
Hurricaine Topical Anesthetic
   Spray Extension Tubes (200)...........**608**
Hurricaine Topical Anesthetic
   Spray Kit, 2 oz. Wild Cherry with
   disposable Extension
   Tubes (200)...................................**608**
Hurricaine Topical Anesthetic
   Spray, 2 oz. Wild Cherry **608**

TUBERCULOSIS, NUTRIENTS DEFICIENCY SECONDARY TO

Tuberculosis may be treated with capreomycin sulfate, ethambutol hydrochloride, ethionamide, isoniazid, pyrazinamide, rifampin or streptomycin sulfate. The following products may be recommended for relief of nutrients deficiency:

BioLean Accelerator Tablets **664**
BioLean Free Tablets **665**
BioLean II Tablets **664**
BioLean LipoTrim Capsules **665**
BioLean Mass Appeal Tablets...............**665**
BioLean ProXtreme
   Dietary Supplement **666**
BioLean Sure2Endure Tablets...............**703**
Centrum Tablets..................................**704**
Centrum Kids Complete Children's
   Chewables **705**
Centrum Performance Multivitamin/
   Multimineral Supplement **705**
Centrum Silver Tablets.........................**706**
Daily Complete Liquid **686**
DHEA Plus Capsules **666**
Efacor Dietary Supplement...................**687**
Food for Thought
   Dietary Supplement **666**
Phyto-Vite Tablets **667**
Satiete Tablets **667**
StePHan Clarity Capsules **700**
StePHan Elasticity Capsules.................**701**
StePHan Elixir Capsules.......................**701**
StePHan Essential Capsules.................**701**
StePHan Feminine Capsules.................**701**
StePHan Flexibility Capsules.................**701**
StePHan Lovpil Capsules **702**
StePHan Tranquility Capsules...............**702**
Vibe Liquid Multi-Nutrient
   Supplement....................................**688**
Winrgy Dietary Supplement **703**

VULVOVAGINITIS, CANDIDAL

May result from the use of estrogen-containing oral contraceptives, immunosuppressants or recent broad-spectrum antibiotic therapy. The following products may be recommended:

Vagistat-1..**641**

XERODERMA

May result from the use of aldesleukin, protease inhibitors, retinoids, topical acne preparations, topical corticosteroids, topical retinoids, benzoyl peroxide, clofazimine, interferon alfa-2a, recombinant, interferon alfa-2b, recombinant or pentostatin. The following products may be recommended:

Head & Shoulders Intensive Solutions
   Dandruff Shampoo **641**
Tahitian Noni Seed Oil **699**

XEROMYCTERIA

May result from the use of anticholinergics, antihistamines, retinoids, apraclonidine hydrochloride, clonidine, etretinate, ipratropium bromide, isotretinoin or Iodoxamide tromethamine. The following products may be recommended:

4-Way Moisturizing Relief Nasal Spray...**624**
Nasal Comfort Moisture Therapy
   Sprays - Scented and Unscented **611**

POISON CONTROL CENTERS

The American Association of Poison Control Centers (AAPCC) uses a single, nationwide emergency number to automatically link callers with their regional poison center. This toll-free number, **800-222-1222**, also works for **teletype lines (TTY)** for the hearing-impaired and **telecommunication devices (TTD)** for individuals who are deaf. However, a few local poison centers and the ASPCA/Animal Poison Control Center are not part of this nationwide system and continue to use separate numbers.

Most of the centers listed below are certified by the AAPCC. **Certified centers are marked by an asterisk after the name.**

Each has to meet certain criteria. It must, for example, serve a large geographic area; it must be open 24 hours a day and provide direct-dial or toll-free access; it must be supervised by a medical director; and it must have registered pharmacists or nurses available to answer questions from the public.

Within each state, centers are listed alphabetically by city. Some state poison centers also list their original emergency numbers (including TTY/TDD) that only work within that state. For these listings, callers may use either the state number or the nationwide 800 number.

ALABAMA

BIRMINGHAM

Regional Poison Control Center, The Children's Hospital of Alabama (*)

1600 7th Ave. South
Birmingham, AL 35233-1711
Business: 205-939-9201
Emergency: 800-222-1222
www.chsys.org

TUSCALOOSA

Alabama Poison Center (*)

2503 Phoenix Dr.
Tuscaloosa, AL 35405
Business: 205-345-0600
Emergency: 800-222-1222
              800-462-0800 (AL)
www.alapoisoncenter.org

ALASKA

JUNEAU

Alaska Poison Control System

Section of Community
Health and EMS
410 Willoughby Ave., Room 103
Box 110616
Juneau, AK 99811-0616
Business: 907-465-3027
Emergency: 800-222-1222
www.chems.alaska.gov

(PORTLAND, OR)

Oregon Poison Center (*)
Oregon Health Sciences University

3181 SW Sam Jackson Park Rd.
CB550
Portland, OR 97239
Business: 503-494-8311
Emergency: 800-222-1222
www.oregonpoison.com

ARIZONA

PHOENIX

Banner Poison Control Center (*)
Banner Good Samaritan Medical Center

901 E. Willetta St.
Room 2701
Phoenix, AZ 85006
Business: 602-495-4884
Emergency: 800-222-1222
www.bannerpoisoncontrol.com

TUCSON

Arizona Poison and Drug Information Center (*)
Arizona Health Sciences Center

1501 N. Campbell Ave.
Room 1156
Tucson, AZ 85724
Business: 520-626-7899
Emergency: 800-222-1222

ARKANSAS

LITTLE ROCK

Arkansas Poison and Drug Information Center
College of Pharmacy - UAMS

4301 West Markham St.
Mail Slot 522-2
Little Rock, AR 72205-7122
Business: 501-686-5540
Emergency: 800-222-1222
              800-376-4766 (AR)
TDD/TTY: 800-641-3805

ASPCA/ANIMAL POISON CONTROL CENTER

1717 South Philo Rd.
Suite 36
Urbana, IL 61802
Business: 217-337-5030
Emergency: 888-426-4435
              800-548-2423
www.napcc.aspca.org

CALIFORNIA

FRESNO/MADERA

California Poison Control System-Fresno/Madera Div.(*)
Children's Hospital of Central California

9300 Valley Children's Place
MB 15
Madera, CA 93638-8762
Business: 559-622-2300
Emergency: 800-222-1222
              800-876-4766 (CA)
TDD/TTY: 800-972-3323
www.calpoison.org

SACRAMENTO

California Poison Control System-Sacramento Div.(*)
UC Davis Medical Center

Room HSF 1024
2315 Stockton Blvd.
Sacramento, CA 95817
Business: 916-227-1400
Emergency: 800-222-1222
              800-876-4766 (CA)
TDD/TTY: 800-972-3323
www.calpoison.org

SAN DIEGO

California Poison Control System-San Diego Div. (*)
UC San Diego Medical Center

200 West Arbor Dr.
San Diego, CA 92103-8925
Business: 858-715-6300
Emergency: 800-222-1222
              800-876-4766 (CA)
TDD/TTY: 800-972-3323
www.calpoison.org

SAN FRANCISCO

California Poison Control System-San Francisco Div.(*)
San Francisco General Hospital University of California San Francisco

Box 1369
San Francisco, CA 94143-1369
Business: 415-502-6000
Emergency: 800-222-1222
              800-876-4766 (CA)
TDD/TTY: 800-972-3323
www.calpoison.org

COLORADO

DENVER

Rocky Mountain Poison and Drug Center (*)

777 Bannock St.
Mail Code 0180
Denver, CO 80204-4507
Business: 303-739-1100
Emergency: 800-222-1222
TDD/TTY: 303-739-1127 (CO)
www.RMPDC.org

CONNECTICUT

FARMINGTON

Connecticut Regional Poison Control Center (*)
University of Connecticut Health Center

263 Farmington Ave.
Farmington, CT 06030-5365
Business: 860-679-4540
Emergency: 800-222-1222
TDD/TTY: 866-218-5372
http://poisoncontrol.uchc.edu

DELAWARE

(PHILADELPHIA, PA)

The Poison Control Center (*)
Children's Hospital of Philadelphia

34th St. & Civic Center Blvd.
Philadelphia, PA 19104-4303
Business: 215-590-2003
Emergency: 800-222-1222
              800-722-7112 (DE)
TDD/TTY: 215-590-8789
www.poisoncontrol.chop.edu

DISTRICT OF COLUMBIA

WASHINGTON, DC

National Capital Poison Center (*)

3201 New Mexico Ave., NW
Suite 310
Washington, DC 20016
Business: 202-362-3867
Emergency: 800-222-1222
www.poison.org

FLORIDA

JACKSONVILLE

Florida Poison Information Center-Jacksonville (*)
SHANDS Hospital

655 West 8th St.
Jacksonville, FL 32209
Business: 904-244-4465
Emergency: 800-222-1222
http://fpicjax.org

POISON CONTROL CENTERS (cont.)

MIAMI

Florida Poison Information Center-Miami (*)
University of Miami–Department of Pediatrics

P.O. Box 016960 (R-131)
Miami, FL 33101
Business: 305-585-5250
Emergency: 800-222-1222
www.miami.edu/poison-center

TAMPA

Florida Poison Information Center-Tampa (*)
Tampa General Hospital

P.O. Box 1289
Tampa, FL 33601-1289
Business: 813-844-7044
Emergency: 800-222-1222
www.poisoncentertampa.org

GEORGIA

ATLANTA

Georgia Poison Center (*)
Hughes Spalding Children's Hospital, Grady Health System

80 Jesse Hill Jr. Dr., SE
P.O. Box 26066
Atlanta, GA 30303-3050
Business: 404-616-9237
Emergency: 800-222-1222
                 404-616-9000
                 (Atlanta)
TDD: 404-616-9287
www.georgiapoisoncenter.org

HAWAII

(DENVER, CO)

Rocky Mountain Poison and Drug Center (*)

777 Bannock St.
Mail Code 0180
Denver, CO 80204-4507
Business: 303-739-1100
Emergency: 800-222-1222
www.RMPDC.org

IDAHO

(DENVER, CO)

Rocky Mountain Poison and Drug Center (*)

777 Bannock St.
Mail Code 0180
Denver, CO 80204-4507
Business: 303-739-1100
Emergency: 800-222-1222
www.RMPDC.org

ILLINOIS

CHICAGO

Illinois Poison Center (*)

222 South Riverside Plaza
Suite 1900
Chicago, IL 60606
Business: 312-906-6136
Emergency: 800-222-1222
TDD/TTY: 312-906-6185
www.illinoispoisoncenter.org

INDIANA

INDIANAPOLIS

Indiana Poison Control Center (*)
Clarian Health Partners
Methodist Hospital

I-65 at 21st St.
Indianapolis, IN 46206-1367
Business: 317-962-2335
Emergency: 800-222-1222
                 800-382-9097
                 317-962-2323
                 (Indianapolis)
TTY: 317-962-2336
www.clarian.org/poisoncontrol

IOWA

SIOUX CITY

Iowa Statewide Poison Control Center
Iowa Health System and the University of Iowa Hospitals and Clinics

401 Douglas St., Suite 402
Sioux City, IA 51101
Business: 712-279-3710
Emergency: 800-222-1222
                 712-277-2222 (IA)
www.iowapoison.org

KANSAS

KANSAS CITY

Mid-America Poison Control Center
University of Kansas Medical Center

3901 Rainbow Blvd.
Room B-400
Kansas City, KS 66160-7231
Business   913-588-6638
Emergency: 800-222-1222
                 800-332-6633 (KS)
TDD: 913-588-6639
www.kumc.edu/poison

KENTUCKY

LOUISVILLE

Kentucky Regional Poison Center (*)

P.O. Box 35070
Louisville, KY 40232-5070
Business: 502-629-7264
Emergency: 800-222-1222
                 502-589-8222
                 (Louisville)
www.krpc.com

LOUISIANA

MONROE

Louisiana Drug and Poison Information Center (*)
University of Louisiana at Monroe

700 University Ave.
Monroe, LA 71209-6430
Business: 318-342-3648
Emergency: 800-222-1222
www.lapcc.org

MAINE

PORTLAND

Northern New England Poison Center

Maine Medical Center
22 Bramhall St.
Portland, ME 04102
Business: 207-662-7220
Emergency: 800-222-1222
                 207-871-2879 (ME)
TDD/TTY: 877-299-4447 (ME)
                 207-871-2879 (ME)
www.nnepc.org

MARYLAND

BALTIMORE

Maryland Poison Center (*)
University of Maryland at Baltimore
School of Pharmacy

20 North Pine St., PH 772
Baltimore, MD 21201
Business: 410-706-7604
Emergency: 800-222-1222
TDD: 410-706-1858
www.mdpoison.com

(WASHINGTON, DC)

National Capital Poison Center (*)

3201 New Mexico Ave., NW
Suite 310
Washington, DC 20016
Business: 202-362-3867
Emergency: 800-222-1222
TDD/TTY: 202-362-8563 (MD)
www.poison.org

MASSACHUSETTS

BOSTON

Regional Center for Poison Control and Prevention (*)
(Serving Massachusetts and Rhode Island)

300 Longwood Ave.
Boston, MA 02115
Business: 617-355-6609
Emergency: 800-222-1222
TDD/TTY: 888-244-5313
www.maripoisoncenter.com

MICHIGAN

DETROIT

Regional Poison Control Center (*)
Children's Hospital of Michigan

4160 John R. Harper
Professional Office Bldg.
Suite 616
Detroit, MI 48201
Business: 313-745-5335
Emergency: 800-222-1222
TDD/TTY: 800-356-3232
www.mitoxic.org/pcc

GRAND RAPIDS

DeVos Children's Hospital Regional Poison Center (*)

100 Michigan St., NE
Grand Rapids, MI 49503
Business: 616-391-3690
Emergency: 800-222-1222
http://poisoncenter.
        devoschildrens.org

MINNESOTA

MINNEAPOLIS

Minnesota Poison Control System (*)
Hennepin County Medical Center

701 Park Ave.
Mail Code RL
Minneapolis, MN 55415
Business: 612-873-3144
Emergency: 800-222-1222
www.mnpoison.org

MISSISSIPPI

JACKSON

Mississippi Regional Poison Control Center, University of Mississippi Medical Center

2500 North State St.
Jackson, MS 39216
Business: 601-984-1680
Emergency: 800-222-1222

POISON CONTROL CENTERS (cont.)

MISSOURI

ST. LOUIS

Missouri Regional Poison Center (*) Cardinal Glennon Children's Hospital

7980 Clayton Rd.
Suite 200
St. Louis, MO 63117
Business: 314-772-5200
Emergency: 800-222-1222
TDD/TTY: 314-612-5705
www.cardinalglennon.com

MONTANA

(DENVER, CO)

Rocky Mountain Poison and Drug Center (*)

777 Bannock St.
Mail Code 0180
Denver, CO 80204-4507
Business: 303-739-1100
Emergency: 800-222-1222
TDD/TTY: 303-739-1127
www.RMPDC.org

NEBRASKA

OMAHA

The Poison Center (*) Children's Hospital

8401 W. Dodge St., Suite 115
Omaha, NE 68114
Business: 402-955-5555
Emergency: 800-222-1222
www.nebraskapoison.com

NEVADA

(DENVER, CO)

Rocky Mountain Poison and Drug Center (*)

777 Bannock St.
Mail Code 0180
Denver, CO 80204-4507
Business: 303-739-1100
Emergency: 800-222-1222
www.RMPDC.org

(PORTLAND, OR)

Oregon Poison Center (*) Oregon Health Sciences University

3181 SW Sam Jackson Park Rd.
Portland, OR 97201
Business: 503-494-8600
Emergency: 800-222-1222
www.oregonpoison.com

NEW HAMPSHIRE

(PORTLAND, ME)

Northern New England Poison Center

Maine Medical Center
22 Bramhall St.
Portland, ME 04102
Business: 207-662-7220
Emergency: 800-222-1222
www.nnepc.org

NEW JERSEY

NEWARK

New Jersey Poison Information and Education System (*) UMDNJ

65 Bergen St.
Newark, NJ 07101
Business: 973-972-9280
Emergency: 800-222-1222
TDD/TTY: 973-926-8008
www.njpies.org

NEW MEXICO

ALBUQUERQUE

New Mexico Poison and Drug Information Center (*)

MSC09-5080
1 University of New Mexico
Albuquerque, NM 87131-0001
Business: 505-272-4261
Emergency: 800-222-1222
http://HSC.UNM.edu/pharmacy/
    poison

NEW YORK

BUFFALO

Western New York Regional Poison Control Center (*) Children's Hospital of Buffalo

219 Bryant St.
Buffalo, NY 14222
Business: 716-878-7654
Emergency: 800-222-1222
www.fingerlakespoison.org

MINEOLA

Long Island Regional Poison and Drug Information Center (*) Winthrop University Hospital

259 First St.
Mineola, NY 11501
Business: 516-663-2650
Emergency: 800-222-1222
TDD: 516-747-3323
    (Nassau)
    516-924-8811
    (Suffolk)
www.lirpdic.org

NEW YORK CITY

New York City Poison Control Center (*) NYC Dept. of Health

455 First Ave., Room 123
New York, NY 10016
Business: 212-447-8152
Emergency: 800-222-1222
(English)   212-340-4494
    212-POISONS
    (212-764-7667)

Emergency: 212-VENENOS
(Spanish)   (212-836-3667)
TDD: 212-689-9014

ROCHESTER

Finger Lakes Regional Poison and Drug Information Center (*) University of Rochester Medical Center

601 Elmwood Ave.
Box 321
Rochester, NY 14642
Business: 585-273-4155
Emergency: 800-222-1222
TTY: 585-273-3854

SYRACUSE

Central New York Poison Center (*) SUNY Upstate Medical University

750 East Adams St.
Syracuse, NY 13210
Business: 315-464-7078
Emergency: 800-222-1222
www.cnypoison.org

NORTH CAROLINA

CHARLOTTE

Carolinas Poison Center (*) Carolinas Medical Center

P.O. Box 32861
Charlotte, NC 28232
Business: 704-512-3795
Emergency: 800-222-1222
TDD: 800-735-8262
TTY: 800-735-2962
www.ncpoisoncenter.org

NORTH DAKOTA

(MINNEAPOLIS, MN)

Minnesota Poison Control System (*), Hennepin County Medical Center

701 Park Ave.
Mail Code 820
Minneapolis, MN 55415
Business: 612-873-3144
Emergency: 800-222-1222
www.ndpoison.org

OHIO

CINCINNATI

Cincinnati Drug and Poison Information Center (*) Regional Poison Control System

3333 Burnet Ave.
Vernon Place, 3rd Floor
Cincinnati, OH 45229
Business: 513-636-5111
Emergency: 800-222-1222
TDD/TTY: 800-253-7955
www.cincinnatichildrens.org/dpic

CLEVELAND

Greater Cleveland Poison Control Center

11100 Euclid Ave.
MP 6007
Cleveland, OH 44106-6007
Business: 216-844-1573
Emergency: 800-222-1222
    216-231-4455 (OH)

COLUMBUS

Central Ohio Poison Center (*)

700 Children's Dr.
Room L032
Columbus, OH 43205-2696
Business: 614-722-2635
Emergency: 800-222-1222
TTY: 614-228-2272
www.bepoisonsmart.com

OKLAHOMA

OKLAHOMA CITY

Oklahoma Poison Control Center (*) Children's Hospital at OU Medical Center

940 Northeast 13th St.
Room 3510
Oklahoma City, OK 73104
Business: 405-271-5062
Emergency: 800-222-1222
www.oklahomapoison.org

OREGON

PORTLAND

Oregon Poison Center (*) Oregon Health Sciences University

3181 S.W. Sam Jackson Park Rd.,
CB550
Portland, OR 97239
Business: 503-494-8968
Emergency: 800-222-1222
www.oregonpoison.com

POISON CONTROL CENTERS (cont.)

PENNSYLVANIA

PHILADELPHIA

The Poison Control Center (*)
Children's Hospital of
Philadelphia

34th Street & Civic Center Blvd.
Philadelphia, PA 19104-4399
Business: 215-590-2003
Emergency: 800-222-1222
215-386-2100 (PA)
TDD/TTY: 215-590-8789
www.poisoncontrol.chop.edu

PITTSBURGH

Pittsburgh Poison Center (*)
Children's Hospital of Pittsburgh

3705 Fifth Ave.
Pittsburgh, PA 15213
Business: 412-390-3300
Emergency: 800-222-1222
412-681-6669
www.chp.edu/clinical/03a_
poison.php

PUERTO RICO

SANTURCE

San Jorge Children's Hospital
Poison Center

268 San Jorge St.
Santurce, PR 00912
Business: 787-726-5660
Emergency: 800-222-1222
TTY: 787-641-1934
www.poisoncenter.net

RHODE ISLAND

(BOSTON, MA)

Regional Center for Poison
Control and Prevention (*)
(Serving Massachusetts and
Rhode Island)

300 Longwood Ave.
Boston, MA 02115
Business: 617-355-6609
Emergency: 800-222-1222
TDD/TTY: 888-244-5313
www.maripoisoncenter.com

SOUTH CAROLINA

COLUMBIA

Palmetto Poison Center (*)
College of Pharmacy
University of South Carolina

Columbia, SC 29208
Business: 803-777-7909
Drug Info: 800-777-7805
Emergency: 800-222-1222
803-922-1117 (SC)
www.pharm.sc.edu/PPS/pps.htm

SOUTH DAKOTA

(MINNEAPOLIS, MN)

Hennepin Regional Poison
Center (*), Hennepin County
Medical Center

701 Park Ave.
Minneapolis, MN 55415
Business: 612-873-3144
Emergency: 800-222-1222
www.mnpoison.org

SIOUX FALLS

Provides education only—Does
not manage exposure cases.

Sioux Valley Poison Control
Center (*)

1305 W. 18th St.
Box 5039
Sioux Falls, SD 57117-5039
Business: 605-328-6670
www.sdpoison.org

TENNESSEE

NASHVILLE

Tennessee Poison Center (*)

1161 21st Ave. South
501 Oxford House
Nashville, TN 37232-4632
Business: 615-936-0760
Emergency: 800-222-1222
www.poisonlifeline.org

TEXAS

AMARILLO

Texas Panhandle
Poison Center (*)
Northwest Texas Hospital

1501 S. Coulter Dr.
Amarillo, TX 79106
Business: 806-354-1630
Emergency: 800-222-1222
www.poisoncontrol.org

DALLAS

North Texas Poison Center (*)
Texas Poison Center Network
Parkland Health and Hospital
System

5201 Harry Hines Blvd.
Dallas, TX 75235
Business: 214-589-0911
Emergency: 800-222-1222
www.poisoncontrol.org

EL PASO

West Texas Regional
Poison Center (*)
Thomason Hospital

4815 Alameda Ave.
El Paso, TX 79905
Business 915-534-3800
Emergency: 800-222-1222
www.poisoncontrol.org

GALVESTON

Southeast Texas Poison Center (*)
The University of Texas
Medical Branch

3.112 Trauma Bldg.
301 University Ave.
Galveston, TX 77555-1175
Business: 409-766-4403
Emergency: 800-222-1222
www.poisoncontrol.org

SAN ANTONIO

South Texas
Poison Center (*)
The University of Texas Health
Science Center–San Antonio

7703 Floyd Curl Dr., MC 7849
San Antonio, TX 78229-3900
Business: 210-567-5762
Emergency: 800-222-1222
www.poisoncontrol.org

TEMPLE

Central Texas Poison Center (*)
Scott & White Memorial Hospital

2401 South 31st St.
Temple, TX 76508
Business: 254-724-7401
Emergency: 800-222-1222
www.poisoncontrol.org

UTAH

SALT LAKE CITY

Utah Poison Control Center (*)

585 Komas Dr.
Suite 200
Salt Lake City, UT 84108
Business: 801-587-0600
Emergency: 800-222-1222
801-587-0600 (UT)
http://uuhsc.utah.edu/poison

VERMONT

(PORTLAND, ME)

Northern New England
Poison Center

Maine Medical Center
22 Bramhall St.
Portland, ME 04102
Business: 207-662-7220
Emergency: 800-222-1222
www.nnepc.org

VIRGINIA

CHARLOTTESVILLE

Blue Ridge Poison Center (*)
University of Virginia
Health System

P.O. Box 800774
Charlottesville, VA 22908-0774
Business: 434-924-0347
Emergency: 800-222-1222
www.healthsystem.virginia.edu.
brpc

RICHMOND

Virginia Poison Center (*)
Virginia Commonwealth
University

P.O. Box 980522
Richmond, VA 23298-0522
Business: 804-828-4780
Emergency: 800-222-1222
804-828-9123
www.vcu.edu/mcved/vpc

WASHINGTON

SEATTLE

Washington Poison Center (*)

155 NE 100th St.
Suite 400
Seattle, WA 98125-8011
Business: 206-517-2350
Emergency: 800-222-1222
206-526-2121 (WA)
TDD: 800-572-0638 (WA)
www.wapc.org

WEST VIRGINIA

CHARLESTON

West Virginia
Poison Center (*)

3110 MacCorkle Ave. SE
Charleston, WV 25304
Business: 304-347-1212
Emergency: 800-222-1222
www.wvpoisoncenter.org

WISCONSIN

MILWAUKEE

Children's Hospital
of Wisconsin Statewide
Poison Center

9000 W. Wisconsin Ave.
P.O. Box 1997, Mail Station 677A
Milwaukee, WI 53226
Business: 414-266-2952
Emergency: 800-222-1222
TDD/TTY: 414-266-2542
www.chw.org

WYOMING

(OMAHA, NE)

The Poison Center (*)
Children's Hospital

8401 W. Dodge St., Suite 115
Omaha, NE 68114
Business: 402-955-5555
Emergency: 800-222-1222
www.nebraskapoison.com

DRUG INFORMATION CENTERS

ALABAMA

BIRMINGHAM

**Drug Information Service
University of Alabama
UAB Hospital Pharmacy**

Drug Information-JT1720
619 S. 19th St.
Birmingham, AL 35249-6860
Mon.-Fri. 8 AM-5 PM
  205-934-2162
www.health.uab.edu/pharmacy

**Global Drug Information Service
Samford University
McWhorter School of Pharmacy**

800 Lakeshore Dr.
Birmingham, AL 35229-7027
Mon.-Wed. 8 AM-9 PM
Thurs.-Fri. 8 AM-4:30 PM
  205-726-2519 or 2891
www.samford.edu/schools/
pharmacy/dic/index.html

HUNTSVILLE

**Huntsville Hospital Drug
Information Center**

101 Sivley Rd.
Huntsville, AL 35801
Mon.-Fri. 7 AM-3:30 PM
  256-265-8284

ARIZONA

TUCSON

**Arizona Poison and Drug
Information Center
Arizona Health Sciences Center
University Medical Center**

1501 N. Campbell Ave.
Room 1156
Tucson, AZ 85724
7 days/week, 24 hours
  520-626-6016
  800-222-1222 **(Emergency)**
www.pharmacy.arizona.edu

ARKANSAS

LITTLE ROCK

**Arkansas Drug Information
Center**

4301 W. Markham St.
Slot 522-2
Little Rock, AR 72205
Mon.-Fri. 8:30 AM-5 PM
  501-686-5072
(Little Rock area only - **for health-
care professionals only**)
  800-228-1233
(AR only - **for healthcare
professionals only**)

CALIFORNIA

LOS ANGELES

**Los Angeles Regional
Drug Information Center
LAC & USC Medical Center**

1200 N. State St.
Trailer 25
Los Angeles, CA 90033
Mon.-Fri. 8 AM-4 PM
Closed 12 PM to 1 PM
  323-226-7741

SAN DIEGO

**Drug Information Service
University of California
San Diego Medical Center**

200 West Arbor Dr.
MC 8925
San Diego, CA 92103-8925
Mon.-Fri. 9 AM-5 PM
  619-543-6971
**(for healthcare professionals
only)**

SAN FRANCISCO

**Drug Information Analysis
Service
University of California,
San Francisco**

533 Parnassus Ave.
Room U12
San Francisco, CA 94143-0622
Mon.-Fri. 8:30 AM-4:30 PM
  415-502-9540
(for healthcare professionals only)

STANFORD

**Drug Information Center
University of California
Stanford Hospital and Clinics**

300 Pasteur Dr.
Room H-0301
Stanford, CA 94305
Mon.-Fri. 8 AM-4 PM
  650-723-6422

COLORADO

DENVER

**Rocky Mountain Poison
and Drug Center**

990 Bannock St.
(Physical address)
777 Bannock St.
(Mailing address)
Denver, CO 80264
  303-739-1123
  800-222-1222 **(Emergency)**
www.rmpdc.org

CONNECTICUT

FARMINGTON

**Drug Information Service
University of Connecticut
Health Center**

263 Farmington Ave.
Farmington, CT 06030
Mon.-Fri. 7:30 AM-4 PM
  860-679-2783

HARTFORD

**Drug Information Center
Hartford Hospital**

P.O. Box 5037
80 Seymour St.
Hartford, CT 06102
Mon.-Fri. 8:30 AM-5 PM
  860-545-2221
  860-545-2961(After 5 PM)
www.hartfordhospital.org

NEW HAVEN

**Drug Information Center
Yale-New Haven Hospital**

20 York St.
New Haven, CT 06540-3202
Mon.-Fri. 8:30 AM-5 PM
  203-688-2248
www.ynhh.org

DISTRICT OF COLUMBIA

**Drug Information Service
Howard University Hospital**

Room BB06
2041 Georgia Ave. NW
Washington, DC 20060
Mon.-Fri. 8:30 AM-4 PM
  202-865-1325
  800-222-1222 **(Emergency)**
www.huhosp.org/patientpublic/
pharmacy.htm

FLORIDA

FT. LAUDERDALE

**Nova Southeastern University
College of Pharmacy
Drug Information Center**

3200 S. University Dr.
Ft. Lauderdale, FL 33328
Mon.-Fri. 9 AM-5 PM
  954-262-3103
http://pharmacy.nova.edu

GAINESVILLE

**Drug Information &
Pharmacy Resource Center
Shands Hospital at
University of Florida**

P.O. Box 100316
Gainesville, FL 32610-0316
Mon.-Fri. 9 AM-5 PM
  352-265-0408
(for healthcare professionals only)
http://shands.org/professional/
drugs

JACKSONVILLE

**Drug Information Service
Shands Jacksonville**

655 W. 8th St.
Jacksonville, FL 32209
Mon.-Fri. 8:30 AM-5 PM
  904-244-4185
(for healthcare professionals only)
  904-244-4700
**(for consumers,
Mon.-Fri. 9:30 AM-4 PM)**

ORLANDO

**Orlando Regional Drug
Information Service
Orlando Regional
Healthcare System**

1414 Kuhl Ave., MP 192
Orlando, FL 32806
Mon.-Fri. 8 AM-4 PM
  321-841-8717

TALLAHASSEE

**Drug Information
Education Center
Florida Agricultural and
Mechanical University
College of Pharmacy and
Pharmaceutical Sciences**

Tallahassee, FL 32307
Mon.-Fri. 9 AM-5 PM
  850-488-5239

WEST PALM BEACH

**Drug Information Center
Nova Southeastern University,
West Palm Beach**

3970 RCA Blvd., Suite 7006A
Palm Beach Gardens, FL 33410
Mon.-Fri. 9 AM-5 PM
  561-622-0658
(for healthcare professionals only)

DRUG INFORMATION CENTERS (cont.)

GEORGIA

ATLANTA

Emory University Hospital Dept. of Pharmaceutical Services-Drug Information

1364 Clifton Rd. NE
Atlanta, GA 30322
Mon.-Fri. 8 AM-1 PM
   404-712-4644
(for healthcare professionals only)

Drug Information Service Northside Hospital

1000 Johnson Ferry Rd. NE
Atlanta, GA 30342
Mon.-Fri. 9 AM-5 PM
   404-851-8676 (GA only)

AUGUSTA

Drug Information Center Medical College of Georgia Hospital and Clinic

BI2101
1120 15th St.
Augusta, GA 30912
Mon.-Fri. 8:30 AM-5 PM
   706-721-2887

COLUMBUS

Columbus Regional Drug Information Center

710 Center St.
Columbus, GA 31902
Mon.-Fri. 8 AM-5 PM
   706-571-1934
(for healthcare professionals only)

IDAHO

POCATELLO

Drug Information Center Idaho State University School of Pharmacy

970 S. 5th St.
Campus Box 8092
Pocatello, ID 83209
Mon.-Thur. 8:30 AM-5 PM
Fri. 8:30 AM-3 PM
   208-282-4689
   800-334-7139 **(ID only)**
http://pharmacy.isu.edu

ILLINOIS

CHICAGO

Drug Information Center Northwestern Memorial Hospital

Feinberg Pavilion, LC 700
251 E. Huron St.
Chicago, IL 60611
Mon.-Fri. 8:30 AM-5 PM
   312-926-7573

Drug Information Services University of Chicago Hospitals

5841 S. Maryland Ave.
MC 0010
Chicago, IL 60637-1470
Mon.-Fri. 9 AM-5 PM
   773-702-1388

Drug Information Center University of Illinois at Chicago

833 S. Wood St.
MC 886
Chicago, IL 60612-7231
Mon.-Fri. 8 AM-4 PM
   312-996-5332
(for healthcare professionals only)
   312-996-3682
(for consumers, Mon.-Fri. 9 AM-12 PM)
www.uic.edu/pharmacy/
services/di/index.html

HARVEY

Drug Information Center Ingalls Memorial Hospital

1 Ingalls Dr.
Harvey, IL 60426
Mon.-Fri. 8 AM-4:30 PM
   708-333-2300

HINES

Drug Information Service Hines Veterans Administration Hospital

2100 S. 5th Ave.
Pharmacy Services
MC119
P.O. Box 5000
Hines, IL 60141-5000
Mon.-Fri. 8 AM-4:30 PM
   708-202-8387,
   ext. 23780

PARK RIDGE

Drug Information Center Advocate Lutheran General Hospital

1775 Dempster St.
Park Ridge, IL 60068
Mon.-Fri. 7:30 AM-4 PM
   847-723-8128
(for healthcare professionals only)

INDIANA

INDIANAPOLIS

Drug Information Center St. Vincent Hospital and Health Services

2001 W. 86th St.
Indianapolis, IN 46260
Mon.-Fri. 8 AM-4 PM
   317-338-3200
(for healthcare professionals only)

Drug Information Service Clarian Health Partners

Pharmacy Department I-65
at 21st St.
Room CG04
Indianapolis, IN 46202
Mon.-Fri. 8 AM-4:30 PM
   317-962-1750

MUNCIE

Drug Information Center Ball Memorial Hospital

2401 University Ave.
Muncie, IN 47303
Mon.-Fri. 8 AM-4:30 PM
   765-747-3035

IOWA

DES MOINES

Regional Drug Information Center Mercy Medical Center-Des Moines

1111 Sixth Ave.
Des Moines, IA 50314
Mon.-Fri. 8 AM-4:30 PM
(regional service; in-house service answered 7 days/week, 24 hours)
   515-247-3286

IOWA CITY

Drug Information Center University of Iowa Hospitals and Clinics

200 Hawkins Dr.
Iowa City, IA 52242
Mon.-Fri. 8 AM-4:30 PM
   319-356-2600

KANSAS

KANSAS CITY

Drug Information Center University of Kansas Medical Center

3901 Rainbow Blvd.
Kansas City, KS 66160
Mon.-Fri. 8:30 AM-4:30 PM
   913-588-2328
(for healthcare professionals only)

KENTUCKY

LEXINGTON

University of Kentucky Central Pharmacy Chandler Medical Center

800 Rose St., C-114
Lexington, KY 40536-0293
7 days/week, 24 hours
   859-323-5642

LOUISIANA

MONROE

Louisiana Drug and Poison Information Center University of Louisiana at Monroe College of Pharmacy

Sugar Hall
Monroe, LA 71209-6430
Mon.-Fri. 8 AM-4:30 PM
   318-342-1710

NEW ORLEANS

Xavier University Drug Information Center Tulane University Hospital and Clinic

1440 Canal St.
Suite 808
New Orleans, LA 70112
Mon.-Fri. 9 AM-5 PM
   504-588-5670

MARYLAND

ANDREWS AFB

Drug Information Services

79 MDSS/SGQP
1050 W. Perimeter Rd.
Suite D1-119
Andrews AFB, MD 20762-6660
Mon.-Fri. 7:30 AM-5 PM
   240-857-4565

BALTIMORE

Drug Information Service Johns Hopkins Hospital

600 N. Wolfe St.
Carnegie 180
Baltimore, MD 21287-6180
Mon.-Fri. 8:30 AM-5 PM
   410-955-6348

DRUG INFORMATION CENTERS (cont.)

**Drug Information Service
University of Maryland
School of Pharmacy**

Pharmacy Hall Room 760
20 North Pine St.
Baltimore, MD 21201
Mon.-Fri. 8:30 AM-5 PM
  410-706-7568
(for consumers only)
  410-706-0898
(for healthcare professionals only)
www.pharmacy.umaryland.edu/
umdi

EASTON
**Drug Information Pharmacy Dept.
Memorial Hospital**

219 S. Washington St.
Easton, MD 21601
7 days/week, 7 AM-5:30 PM
  410-822-1000, ext. 5645

MASSACHUSETTS
BOSTON
**Drug Information Services
Brigham and Women's Hospital**

75 Francis St.
Boston, MA 02115
Mon.-Fri. 7 AM-3 PM
  617-732-7166

WORCESTER
**Drug Information Pharmacy
UMass Memorial Medical Center
Healthcare Hospital**

55 Lake Ave. North
Worcester, MA 01655
Mon.-Fri. 8:30 AM-5 PM
  508-856-3456
  508-856-2775 (24-hour)

MICHIGAN
ANN ARBOR
**Drug Information Service
Dept. of Pharmacy Services
University of Michigan
Health System**

1500 East Medical Center Dr.
UH B2D301
Box 0008
Ann Arbor, MI 48109-0008
Mon.-Fri. 8 AM-5 PM
  734-936-8200

DETROIT
**Drug Information Center
Department of Pharmacy
Services
Detroit Receiving Hospital and
University Health Center**

4201 St. Antoine Blvd.
Detroit, MI 48201
Mon.-Fri. 9 AM-5 PM
  313-745-4556
www.dmcpharmacy.org

LANSING
**Drug Information Services
Sparrow Hospital**

1215 East Michigan Ave.
Lansing, MI 48912
7 days/week, 24 hours
  517-364-2444

PONTIAC
**Drug Information Center
St. Joseph Mercy Oakland**

44405 Woodward Ave.
Pontiac, MI 48341
Mon.-Fri. 8 AM-4:30 PM
  248-858-3055

ROYAL OAK
**Drug Information Services
William Beaumont Hospital**

3601 West 13 Mile Rd.
Royal Oak, MI 48073-6769
Mon.-Fri. 8 AM-4:30 PM
  248-898-4077

SOUTHFIELD
**Drug Information Service
Providence Hospital**

16001 West 9 Mile Rd.
Southfield, MI 48075
Mon.-Fri. 8 AM-4 PM
  248-849-3125

MISSISSIPPI
JACKSON
**Drug Information Center
University of Mississippi
Medical Center**

2500 N. State St.
Jackson, MS 39216
Mon.-Fri. 8 AM-4:30 PM
  601-984-2060

MISSOURI
KANSAS CITY
**University of Missouri-
Kansas City
Drug Information Center**

2411 Holmes St., MG-200
Kansas City, MO 64108
Mon.-Fri. 9 AM-4 PM
  816-235-5490
http://druginfo.umkc.edu/

SPRINGFIELD
**Drug Information Center
St. John's Hospital**

1235 E. Cherokee St.
Springfield, MO 65804
Mon.-Fri. 8 AM-4:30 PM
  417-820-3488

ST. JOSEPH
**Regional Medical Center
Pharmacy**

5325 Faraon St.
St. Joseph, MO 64506
7 days/week, 24 hours
  816-271-6141

MONTANA
MISSOULA
**Drug Information Service
University of Montana
School of Pharmacy
and Allied Health Sciences**

32 Campus Dr.
1522 Skaggs Bldg.
Missoula, MT 59812-1522
Mon.-Fri. 8 AM-5 PM
  406-243-5254
  800-501-5491
www.umt.edu/druginfo

NEBRASKA
OMAHA
**Drug Informatics Service
School of Pharmacy
Creighton University**

2500 California Plaza
Health Science Library
Room 204
Omaha, NE 68178
Mon.-Fri. 8:30 AM-4:30 PM
  402-280-5101
http://druginfo.creighton.edu

NEW JERSEY
NEWARK
**New Jersey Poison Information
and Education System**

65 Bergen St.
Newark, NJ 07107
Mon.-Fri. 8 AM- 5 PM
  973-972-9280
  800-222-1222 **(Emergency)**
www.njpies.org

NEW BRUNSWICK
**Drug Information Service
Robert Wood Johnson
University Hospital**

Pharmacy Department
1 Robert Wood Johnson Pl.
New Brunswick, NJ 08901
Mon.-Fri. 8:30 AM-4:30 PM
  732-937-8842

NEW MEXICO
ALBUQUERQUE
**New Mexico Poison Center
University of New Mexico
Health Sciences Center**

MSC09 5080
1 University of New Mexico
Albuquerque, NM 87131
7 days/week, 24 hours
  505-272-4261
  800-222-1222 **(Emergency)**
http://hsc.unm.edu/pharmacy/
poison

NEW YORK
BROOKLYN
**International Drug
Information Center
Long Island University
Arnold & Marie Schwartz College
of Pharmacy & Health Sciences**

75 DeKalb Ave.
RM-HS509
Brooklyn, NY 11201
Mon.-Fri. 9 AM-5 PM
  718-488-1064
www.liu.edu

NEW HYDE PARK
**Drug Information Center
St. John's University at Long
Island Jewish Medical Center**

270-05 76th Ave.
New Hyde Park, NY 11040
Mon.-Fri. 8 AM-3 PM
  718-470-DRUG (3784)

DRUG INFORMATION CENTERS (cont.)

NEW YORK CITY
Drug Information Center
Memorial Sloan-Kettering
Cancer Center

1275 York Ave.
RM S-702
New York, NY 10021
Mon.-Fri. 9 AM-5 PM
212-639-7552

Drug Information Center
Mount Sinai Medical Center

1 Gustave Levy Pl.
New York, NY 10029
Mon.-Fri. 9 AM-5 PM
212-241-6619
(for in-house healthcare professionals only)

Drug Information Service
New York Presbyterian Hospital

Room K04
525 E. 68th St.
New York, NY 10021
Mon.-Fri. 9 AM-5 PM
212-746-0741

ROCHESTER
Finger Lakes
Poison and Drug
Information Center
University of Rochester

601 Elmwood Ave.
Rochester, NY 14642
Mon.-Fri. 8 AM-5 PM
585-275-3718

ROCKVILLE CENTER
Drug Information Center
Mercy Medical Center

1000 North Village Ave.
Rockville Center, NY 11571-9024
Mon.-Fri. 8 AM-4 PM
516-705-1053

NORTH CAROLINA
BUIES CREEK
Drug Information Center
School of Pharmacy
Campbell University

P.O. Box 1090
Buies Creek, NC 27506
Mon.-Fri. 8:30 AM-4:30 PM
910-893-1200, ext. 2701
800-760-9697 (Toll free)
ext. 2701
800-327-5467 **(NC only)**

CHAPEL HILL
University of North
Carolina Hospitals
Drug Information Center
Dept. of Pharmacy

101 Manning Dr.
Chapel Hill, NC 27514
Mon.-Fri. 8 AM-4:30 PM
919-966-2373

DURHAM
Drug Information Center
Duke University HealthSystems

DUMC Box 3089
Durham, NC 27710
Mon.-Fri. 8 AM-5 PM
919-684-5125

GREENVILLE
Eastern Carolina Drug
Information Center
Pitt County Memorial Hospital
Dept. of Pharmacy Service

P.O. Box 6028
2100 Stantonsburg Rd.
Greenville, NC 27835
Mon.-Fri. 8 AM-5 PM
252-847-4257

WINSTON-SALEM
Drug Information Service Center
Wake-Forest University
Baptist Medical Center

Medical Center Blvd.
Winston-Salem, NC 27157
Mon.-Fri. 8 AM-5 PM
336-716-2037
(for healthcare professionals only)

OHIO
ADA
Drug Information Center
Raabe College of Pharmacy
Ohio Northern University

Ada, OH 45810
Mon.-Thurs. 8:30 AM-5 PM,
7-10 PM
Fri. 8:30 AM- 4 PM;
Sun. 2 PM-10 PM
419-772-2307
www.onu.edu/pharmacy/druginfo

CINCINNATI
Drug and Poison
Information Center
Children's Hospital
Medical Center

3333 Burnet Ave. VP-3
Cincinnati, OH 45229
Mon.-Fri. 9 AM-5 PM
513-636-5054
(Administration)
513-636-5111
(7 days/week, 24 hours)

CLEVELAND
Drug Information Service
Cleveland Clinic Foundation

9500 Euclid Ave.
Cleveland, OH 44195
Mon.-Fri. 8:30 AM-4:30 PM
216-444-6456
(for healthcare professionals only)

COLUMBUS
Drug Information Center
Ohio State University Hospital
Dept. of Pharmacy

Doan Hall 368
410 W. 10th Ave.
Columbus, OH 43210-1228
7 days/week, 24 hours
614-293-8679
(for in-house healthcare professionals only)

Drug Information Center
Riverside Methodist Hospital

3535 Olentangy River Road
Columbus, OH 43214
7 days/week, 24 hours
614-566-5425

TOLEDO
Drug Information Services
St. Vincent Mercy Medical Center

2213 Cherry St.
Toledo, OH 43608-2691
Mon.-Fri. 7 AM-5 PM
419-251-4227
www.rx.medctr.ohio-state.edu

OKLAHOMA
OKLAHOMA CITY
Drug Information Service
Integris Health

3300 Northwest Expressway
Oklahoma City, OK 73112
Mon.-Fri. 8 AM-4:30 PM
405-949-3660

Drug Information Center
OU Medical Center
Presbyterian Tower

700 NE 13th St.
Oklahoma City, OK 73104
Mon.-Fri. 8 AM-4:30 PM
405-271-6226
Fax: 405-271-6281

TULSA
Drug Information Center
Saint Francis Hospital

6161 S. Yale Ave.
Tulsa, OK 74136
Mon.-Fri. 8 AM-4:30 PM
918-494-6339
(for healthcare professionals only)

PENNSYLVANIA
PHILADELPHIA
Drug Information Center
Temple University Hospital
Dept. of Pharmacy

3401 N. Broad St.
Philadelphia, PA 19140
Mon.-Fri. 8 AM-4:30 PM
215-707-4644

Drug Information Service
Tenet Health System
Hahnemann University Hospital
Department of Pharmacy

MS 451
Broad and Vine Streets
Philadelphia, PA 19102
Mon.-Fri. 8 AM-4 PM
215-762-DRUG (3784)
(for healthcare professionals only)

Drug Information Service
Dept. of Pharmacy
Thomas Jefferson
University Hospital

111 S. 11th St.
Philadelphia, PA 19107-5089
Mon.-Fri. 8 AM-5 PM
215-955-8877

University of Pennsylvania
Health System Drug
Information Service
Hospital of the University
of Pennsylvania
Department of Pharmacy

3400 Spruce St.
Philadelphia, PA 19104
Mon.-Fri. 8:30 AM-4 PM
215-662-2903

DRUG INFORMATION CENTERS (cont.)

PITTSBURGH

Pharmaceutical Information Center
Mylan School of Pharmacy
Duquesne University

431 Mellon Hall
Pittsburgh, PA 15282
Mon.-Fri. 8 AM-4 PM
  412-396-4600

Drug Information Center
University of Pittsburgh

302 Scaife Hall
200 Lothrop St.
Pittsburgh, PA 15213
Mon.-Fri. 8:30 AM-4:30 PM
  412-647-3784
(for healthcare professionals only)

UPLAND

Drug Information Center
Crozer-Chester Medical Center
Dept. of Pharmacy

1 Medical Center Blvd.
Upland, PA 19013
Mon.-Fri. 8 AM-4:30 PM
  610-447-2851
(for healthcare professionals only)

PUERTO RICO

PONCE

Centro Informacion
Medicamentos
Escuela de Medicina de Ponce

P.O. Box 7004
Ponce, PR 00732-7004
Mon.-Fri. 8 AM-4:30 PM
  787-840-2575

SAN JUAN

Centro de Informacion de
Medicamentos-CIM
Escuela de Farmacia-RCM

P.O. Box 365067
San Juan, PR 00936-5067
Mon.-Fri. 8 AM-5:30 PM
  787-758-2525, ext. 1516

SOUTH CAROLINA

CHARLESTON

Drug Information Service
Medical University
of South Carolina

150 Ashley Ave.
Rutledge Tower Annex
Room 604
P.O. Box 250584
Charleston, SC 29425-0810
Mon.-Fri. 9 AM-5:30 PM
  843-792-3896
  800-922-5250

COLUMBIA

Drug Information Service
University of South Carolina
College of Pharmacy

Columbia, SC 29208
Mon.-Fri. 8 AM-5 PM
  803-777-7804
www.pharm.sc.edu

SPARTANBURG

Drug Information Center
Spartanburg Regional
Healthcare System

101 E. Wood St.
Spartanburg, SC 29303
Mon.-Fri. 8 AM-4:30 PM
  864-560-6910

TENNESSEE

KNOXVILLE

Drug Information Center
University of Tennessee
Medical Center at Knoxville

1924 Alcoa Highway
Knoxville, TN 37920-6999
Mon.-Fri. 8 AM-4:30 PM
  865-544-9124

MEMPHIS

South East Regional
Drug Information Center
VA Medical Center

1030 Jefferson Ave.
Memphis, TN 38104
Mon.-Fri. 6:30 AM-4 PM
  901-523-8990, ext. 6720

Drug Information Center
University of Tennessee

875 Monroe Ave.
Suite 116
Memphis, TN 38163
Mon.-Fri. 8 AM-5 PM
  901-448-5556

TEXAS

AMARILLO

Drug Information Center
Texas Tech Health Sciences
Center
School of Pharmacy

1300 Coulter Rd.
Amarillo, TX 79106
Mon.-Fri. 8 AM-5 PM
  806-356-4008

GALVESTON

Drug Information Center
University of Texas
Medical Branch

301 University Blvd.
Galveston, TX 77555-0701
Mon.-Fri. 8 AM-5 PM
  409-772-2734

HOUSTON

Drug Information Center
Ben Taub General Hospital
Texas Southern University/HCHD

1504 Taub Loop
Houston, TX 77030
Mon.-Fri. 8:30 AM-5 PM
  713-873-3710

LACKLAND A.F.B.

Drug Information Center
Dept. of Pharmacy
Wilford Hall Medical Center

2200 Bergquist Dr.
Suite 1
Lackland A.F.B., TX 78236
7 days/week, 24 hours
  210-292-5414

LUBBOCK

Drug Information and
Consultation Service
Covenant Medical Center

3615 19th St.
Lubbock, TX 79410
Mon.-Fri. 8 AM-5 PM
  806-725-0408

SAN ANTONIO

Drug Information Service
University of Texas
Health Science Center
at San Antonio
Department of Pharmacology

7703 Floyd Curl Drive
San Antonio, TX 78229-3900
Mon.-Fri. 8 AM-4 PM
  210-567-4280

TEMPLE

Drug Information Center
Scott and White Memorial
Hospital

2401 S. 31st St.
Temple, TX 76508
Mon.-Fri. 8 AM-5 PM
  254-724-4636

UTAH

SALT LAKE CITY

Drug Information Service
University of Utah Hospital

421 Wakara Way
Suite 204
Salt Lake City, UT 84108
Mon.-Fri. 7 AM-5 PM
  801-581-2073

VIRGINIA

HAMPTON

Drug Information Center
Hampton University School
of Pharmacy

Hampton Harbors Annex
Hampton, VA 23668
Mon.-Fri. 9 AM-4 PM
  757-728-6693

WEST VIRGINIA

MORGANTOWN

West Virginia Center for
Drug and Health Information
West Virginia University
Robert C. Byrd
Health Sciences Center

1124 HSN, P.O. Box 9520
Morgantown, WV 26506
Mon.-Fri. 8:30 AM-5 PM
  304-293-6640
  800-352-2501 **(WV only)**
www.hsc.wvu.edu/SOP

WYOMING

LARAMIE

Drug Information Center
University of Wyoming

P.O. Box 3375
Laramie, WY 82071
Mon.-Fri. 8:30 AM-4:30 PM
  307-766-6988

Herb/Drug Interactions

Below is a selection of common herbal remedies known to interact with conventional medications. Following the name of each herb is a list of the specific pharmaceutical categories with which it may interact, together with a brief description of each interaction's results.

Please remember that this table is not all-inclusive. For further information on any herb of interest, consult the latest edition of *PDR® for Herbal Medicines,* a compendium of information on more than 700 medicinal herbs.

Aloe
(Aloe vera)
Antiarrhythmics Aloe-induced hypokalemia may affect cardiac rhythm
Antidiabetic Agents Increased risk of hypoglycemia
Cardiac Glycosides Increases effect of cardiac glycosides
Corticosteroids, Licorice, Thiazide Diuretics, Loop Diuretics Increased potassium loss

Alpine Cranberry
(Vaccinium vitis-idaea)
Medication and Food that Increase Uric Acid Levels Decreased effect of Alpine Cranberry

Arnica
(Arnica montana)
Anticoagulants, Antiplatelet Agents, Low Molecular Weight Heparins, Thrombolytic Agents Coumarin component in Arnica may increase anticoagulant effect

Astragalus (Huang-Qi)
(Astragalus species)
Anticoagulants, Antiplatelet Agents, Low Molecular Weight Heparins, Thrombolytic Agents Astragalus may potentiate anticoagulant effects
Immunosuppressants Decreased effectiveness of immunosuppressive effect due to immunostimulant effect of Astragalus

Belladonna
(Atropa belladonna)
Amantadine Hydrochloride, Quinidine, Tricyclic Antidepressants Increases anticholinergic effect of herb

Bilberry
(Vaccinium myrtillus)
Anticoagulants, Antiplatelet Agents, Low Molecular Weight Heparins, Thrombolytic Agents Bilberry may potentiate anticoagulant effects with concomitant use
Salicylates, Warfarin Sodium Increases prothrombin time; caution should be observed when used concurrently

Bladderwrack
(Fucus vesiculosus)
Anticoagulants, Antiplatelet Agents, Low Molecular Weight Heparins, Thrombolytic Agents Bladderwrack may potentiate anticoagulant effects with concomitant use
Hypoglycemic Drugs Herb may have an additive hypoglycemic effect when taken with other hypoglycemic drugs

Brewer's Yeast
(Saccharomyces cerevisiae)
MAO Inhibitors Increase in blood pressure

Buckthorn
(Rhamnus catharticus)
Antiarrhythmics Increased effect due to potassium loss with chronic use of herb
Cardiac Glycosides Increased effect due to potassium loss with chronic use of herb
Corticosteroids Increases hypokalemic effects
Digoxin Herb may cause hypokalemia, which may increase digoxin toxicity
Licorice Root Increases hypokalemic effects
Thiazide Diuretics Increases hypokalemic effects
Other Medications Resorption of other medications could be reduced, due to a laxative effect.

Cascara Sagrada
(Rhamnus purshiana)
Antiarrhythmics Potentiate arrhythmias with prolonged use of Cascara
Cardiac Glycosides Increased effect due to potassium loss with chronic use of herb
Corticosteroids Increase hypokalemic effect
Digoxin Herb may cause hypokalemia, which may increase digoxin toxicity
Indomethacin Decreases therapeutic effect of Cascara
Iron May result in adverse sequellae with concomitant use
Licorice, Thiazide Diuretics Increased risk of hypokalemic effect

Castor Oil Plant
(Ricinus communis)
Cardioactive Steroids Increased effect due to potassium loss with chronic use of herb

Cayenne
(Capsicum annuum)
Aspirin, Salicylic Acid Compounds Decreased bioavailability of aspirin with concomitant use
Barbiturates Further studies in humans needed for concomitant use
Theophylline Herb may increase absorption, resulting in toxicity; use cautiously and monitor for side effects

Chamomile (German)
(Matricaria recutita)
Alcohol May increase sedative effect
Anticoagulants German Chamomile may increase risk of bleeding with concomitant use
Benzodiazepines May increase sedative effect

Chaste Tree
(Vitex agnus-castus)
Dopamine Agonists May result in increased dopaminergic side effects
Dopamine-2 Antagonists May result in decreased dopaminergic effect of herb

Chinese Rhubarb (Da-Huang)
(Rheum palmatum)
Cardiac Glycosides Increased effect due to potassium loss with chronic use of herb
Digoxin Herb may cause hypokalemia, which may increase digoxin toxicity

Coffee
(Coffea arabica)
Drugs, unspecified Herb can hinder (or decrease) resorption of other drugs

Digitalis
(Digitalis purpurea)
Methylxanthines, Phosphodiesterase Inhibitors, Quinidine, Sympathomimetic Agents Increased risk of cardiac arrhythmias with concomitant use

Echinacea
(Echinacea angustifolia)
Corticosteroids Echinacea may interfere with the anticancer chemotherapeutic effect of corticosteroids
Immunosuppressants The immune-stimulating effect of Echinacea may interfere with drugs that have immunosuppressant effects

Herb/Drug Interactions (cont.)

Evening Primrose
(Oenothera biennis)

Anticoagulants, Antiplatelet Agents, Low Molecular Weight Heparins, Thrombolytic Agents Evening Primrose oil may potentiate anticoagulant effects with concomitant use

Anticonvulsants Evening Primrose oil may lower seizure threshold and decrease effectiveness of anticonvulsant medications

Phenothiazines Evening Primrose oil may reduce the seizure threshold with concomitant use

Fenugreek
(Trigonella foenum-graecum)

Hypoglycemic Drugs Herb may have an additive hypoglycemic effect when taken with other hypoglycemic drugs

Feverfew
(Tanacetum parthenium)

Anticoagulants, Antiplatelet Agents, Low Molecular Weight Heparins, Thrombolytic Agents Feverfew may potentiate drug effects

Flax
(Linum usitatissimum)

Drugs, unspecified Absorption of other drugs may be delayed when taken simultaneously

Ginkgo
(Ginkgo biloba)

Anticoagulants, Antiplatelets, Low Molecular Weight Heparins, Thrombolytics, NSAIDs Ginkgo may potentiate drug effects

Anticonvulsants Concomitant use may precipitate seizures in epileptic patients with concomitant use

Buspirone, Fluoxetine, SSRIs Concomitant use resulted in hypomanic episode in a case report

Insulin Ginkgo may alter insulin requirements

MAO Inhibitors Ginkgo may potentiate drug effects

Nicardipine Ginkgo extract may reduce hypotensive effects

Nifedipine Herb may increase mean plasma concentration of nifedipine

Papaverine Herb may increase incidence of adverse effects

Thiazide Diuretics Concomitant use may increase blood pressure

Ginseng
(Panax ginseng)

Estrogen (conjugated) May result in symptoms of estrogen excess or interference

Hypoglycemic Drugs Due to hypoglycemic effects of Ginseng, concomitant use may theoretically increase risk of hypoglycemia

Loop Diuretics Increases diuretic resistance

MAO Inhibitors Combination increases chance for agitation, depression, headache, insomnia, tremors, manic-type symptoms

Nifedipine Herb increases mean plasma concentration of nifedipine

Green Tea
(Camellia sinensis)

Alkaline Drugs Decreased absorption of alkaline drugs due to tannin component in tea

Guarana
(Paullinia cupana)

Cardiac Glycosides Increased effect due to potassium loss with chronic use of herb

Digoxin Herb may cause hypokalemia, which may increase digoxin toxicity

Licorice
(Glycyrrhiza glabra)

Antiarrhythmics Licorice-induced hypokalemia increases risk of arrhythmias

Anticoagulants, Antiplatelet Agents, Low Molecular Weight Heparins, Thrombolytic Agents Licorice may potentiate drug effects

Antidiabetic Agents Licorice may reduce drug effects, causing hyperglycemia

Antihypertensive Drugs Herb may reduce drug effectiveness

Combination contraceptives Concomitant use may cause elevated blood pressure and fluid retention

Corticosteroids Licorice may potentiate drug effects

Digitalis Glycoside Preparations Licorice-induced hypokalemia increases risk of digitalis toxicity

Glucocorticoids Licorice may potentiate drug effects

Insulin Concomitant use may synergistically cause hypokalemia and sodium retention

Laxatives Additive potassium loss with concurrent use

Loop Diuretics, Thiazide Diuretics Herb may potentiate drug effects, resulting in hypokalemia and hypertension

MAO Inhibitors Increased risk of toxicity associated with excessive inhibition of monoamine oxidase

Potassium Supplements Increased risk for developing hypokalemia

Testosterone Concomitant use may reduce endogenous testosterone levels in men as well as women being treated for polycystic ovary disease

Milk Thistle
(Silybum marianum)

Butyrophenones, Phenothiazines Silymarin in combination with butyrophenones or phenothiazines causes a decrease in lipid peroxidation

Phentolamine Mesylate Silymarin antagonizes the effect of phentolamine

Yohimbine Hydrochloride Silymarin antagonizes the effect of yohimbine

Papaya
(Carica papaya)

Warfarin Sodium Concomitant use may increase INR levels

Psyllium
(Plantago ovata)

Antidiabetic Agents Mean area-under-the-curve (AUC) for glucose and insulin was reduced when herb was administered with a glucose load

Carbamazepine Reduced bioavailability with concomitant use

Drugs, unspecified Absorption of other drugs may be decreased if taken simultaneously with herb

Insulin Effect unspecified; insulin dose should be decreased

Psyllium Seed
(Plantago afra)

Drugs, unspecified Absorption of other drugs may be delayed or decreased if taken simultaneously

Saw Palmetto
(Serenoa repens)

Alpha Adrenergic Blockers Concomitant use may result in additive alpha adrenergic blocking effect

Androgens Saw Palmetto antagonizes the effects of androgens

Hormones, Hormone-Like Drugs, or Adrenergic Drugs Herb interferes with therapy due to the possible estrogenic, androgenic, and alpha-adrenergic effects

Iron Saw Palmetto's tannin content may complex with concomitantly administered iron, resulting in nonabsorbable insoluble components, which may result in adverse sequelae on blood components

Warfarin Increased risk of bleeding with concurrent use

Herb/Drug Interactions (cont.)

Senna
(Cassia senna)

Antiarrhythmics Senna-induced hypokalemia may increase risk of arrhythmia

Digitalis Glycoside Preparations Senna-induced hypokalemia may increase toxicity of digitalis preparations

Estrogen Senna decreases estrogen levels when taken with estrogen supplements

Indomethacin Decreased therapeutic effect of Senna

Nifedipine Inhibits activity of Senna via calcium channel blockade

St. John's Wort
(Hypericum perforatum)

Note: The herb may interact with multiple drugs, including antianxiety drugs, anticoagulants, antidepressants, anti-HIV drugs, calcium channel blockers, cardiac glycosides, oral contraceptives, statins, sympathomimetics, and many others. For a comprehensive list of interactions, consult the latest edition of *PDR for Herbal Medicines.*

Uva-Ursi
(Arctostaphylos uva-ursi)

Iron Uva-Ursi's tannin content may complex with concomitantly administered iron, resulting in nonabsorbable insoluble components, which may result in adverse sequelae on blood components

Loop Diuretics, Thiazide Diuretics The sodium-sparing effect of Uva-Ursi may antagonize the diuretic effect of loop diuretics

Medication and Food that Increase Uric Acid Levels Decreases antibacterial effect of herb

Nonsteroidal Anti-Inflammatory Drugs Uva-Ursi may potentiate the gastrointestinal irritation caused by NSAIDs

Valerian
(Valeriana officinalis)

Alcohol Additive sedation and depressant effects when combined with Valerian

Anticoagulants, Antiplatelet Agents, Low Molecular Weight Heparins, Barbiturates, Benzodiazipines Concurrent use may increase central nervous system depression

Hepatotoxic Agents Concurrent use may result in elevated liver transaminases with or without concomitant hepatic damage

Iron Valerian's tannin content may complex with concomitantly administered iron, resulting in nonabsorbable insoluble components, which may result in adverse sequelae on blood components

Loperamide Concurrent use may result in delirium with symptoms of confusion, agitation, and disorientation

Opioid Analgesics Additive central nervous system depression when combined with Valerian

Thrombolytic Agents Concurrent use may potentiate anticoagulant effects

White Willow
(Salix species)

Alcohol, Barbiturates Enhances toxicity of salicylates

Antiplatelet Drugs, Medications That Prolong PT Time Risk of additive effect with salicylates

Carbonic Anhydrase Inhibitors Potentiates action of salicylates

Nonsteroidal Anti-Inflammatory Drugs Use with caution; salicylate component of herb may decrease serum concentration and clearance of NSAIDs

Wild Yam
(Dioscorea villosa)

Estrogen Concurrent use may result in additive effect

Indomethacin Wild Yam may decrease the anti-inflammatory effect of indomethacin

Yohimbe Bark
(Pausinystalia yohimbe)

Antihypertensive agents, unspecified May need to adjust antihypertensive medications due to hypertensive effect of Yohimbe

Carbamazepine, Lithium Herb may exacerbate bipolar disorder by precipitating manic episodes

Clomipramine Increased risk of hypertension with concurrent use

Clonidine Reduced effectiveness with concurrent use

Ethanol Increased intoxication and anxiogenic effects with concurrent use

Guanabenz, Guanadrel, Guanethidine, Guanfacine Herb counteracts the effect of these substances

Minoxidil Yohimbe may counteract antihypertensive effect

Morphine Herb may enhance and/or prolong the effects of morphine

Naloxone Concurrent use may increase cortisol levels as well as symptoms of nervousness, anxiety, tremors, palpitations, hot and cold flashes, and nausea

Naltrexone Yohimbe may increase side effects (anxiety or nervousness), which may decrease compliance with treatment

OTC stimulants Concurrent use may potentiate hypertensive effects

Overview of Commonly Used Herbs

The following is a quick reference guide to some of the most commonly used herbal supplements. The information is based mainly on the findings of the German Regulatory Authority's "Commission E". For a complete evidence-based review of more than 700 herbs, consult the latest edition of the *PDR® for Herbal Medicines*.

Aloe *(Aloe vera)*. The gel from the Aloe plant is an ancient remedy used externally for its antibacterial, antiviral, anti-inflammatory, and pain-relieving effects. It is used topically in skin moisturizers and to treat burns, wounds, psoriasis, and frostbite. While the internal use of Aloe is suggested as a treatment for several conditions including constipation, there is no evidence of its efficacy. In fact, internal use is not recommended because of the risk of serious adverse effects.

Warning: Aloe should not be used by pregnant or breastfeeding women, by children under 12 years of age, or by people with severe intestinal disorders. Aloe should not be taken with certain drugs associated with potassium loss—such as diuretics, corticosteroids, and antiarrhythmics and other heart medications—or with the herb Licorice. If taken with antidiabetic agents, Aloe may increase the risk of hypoglycemia.

Arnica *(Arnica montana)*. The Arnica plant is used externally for pain and inflammation due to injury, and as an anti-infectious agent. Arnica should be discontinued immediately in the event of an allergic reaction to external application. The herb should not be used on open skin wounds.

Warning: Although Europeans take Arnica internally to treat respiratory infections, internal use is not recommended due to the risk of serious cardiac adverse effects.

Astragalus *(Astragalus species)*. Astragalus, or Huang-Qi, is used to improve immune function and strengthen the cardiovascular system. Compounds in Astragalus may also have beneficial antiviral, antioxidant, memory-enhancing, and liver-protecting effects, although the nature of those effects on specific diseases has not been established.

Warning: The use of Astragalus must be carefully monitored by a physician due to its potentially dangerous adverse effects, particularly in people with immune disorders or those taking blood-thinning medications.

Barberry *(Berberis vulgaris)*. Both the fruit and root bark of the Barberry plant are used in folk medicine. The berry is a source of vitamin C, which stimulates the immune system, improves iron absorption, and protects against scurvy. The fruit's acid content has a mild diuretic effect that is thought to aid in urinary tract infections. Barberry root bark may reduce blood pressure, relieve constipation, and have some antibiotic effects.

Warning: Pregnant and nursing women should not use Barberry.

Bilberry *(Vaccinium myrtillus)*. The astringent effects of Bilberry fruit are used to treat inflammation of the mouth and throat, and both the fruit and leaves are used for diarrhea. Reports citing Bilberry as a treatment for diabetic retinopathy need further confirmation.

Warning: The herb should not be used with blood-thinning drugs, including aspirin. Pregnant and nursing women should not use Bilberry.

Black Cohosh *(Cimicifuga racemosa)*. The hormone-modulating effects of Black Cohosh theoretically make it useful for women with menopausal symptoms and premenstrual syndrome, but clinical trials are inconclusive.

Warning: Due to a risk of spontaneous abortion, Black Cohosh should not be used during pregnancy; it should also be avoided during breastfeeding. In addition, the herb should not be combined with antihypertensive drugs or iron supplements.

Butcher's Broom *(Ruscus aculeatus)*. This herb, native to the Mediterranean regions of Europe, Africa, and western Asia, is used medicinally as a diuretic, anti-inflammatory, and for its beneficial effects on circulation. Butcher's Broom is used to relieve the discomforts of hemorrhoids, such as itching and burning, and for the leg heaviness, pain, cramping, and swelling associated with chronic venous insufficiency.

Cat's Claw *(Uncaria tomentosa)*. The root of the South American Cat's Claw contains compounds that have immune-stimulating, anti-inflammatory, and anticancer effects. Although human studies have yet to be conducted, Cat's Claw is often used to treat cancer; arthritis and rheumatic disorders; and AIDS and other viral diseases. It has also been used to treat diarrhea, gastritis, asthma, menstrual irregularities, and wounds. Because of the herb's effects on estradiol and progesterone, Cat's Claw has sometimes been used as a contraceptive.

Warning: Cat's Claw should not be used by pregnant or breastfeeding women, or by people with autoimmune disorders, multiple sclerosis, or tuberculosis. Transplant recipients and children under 2 years of age should also not use this herb. Cat's Claw should not be combined with anticoagulant, antiplatelet, or thrombolytic agents.

Cayenne *(Capsicum annuum)*. Externally, Cayenne is used to relieve the pain of muscle tension and spasm, diabetic neuropathy, and rheumatism. Cayenne is sometimes taken internally to relieve gastrointestinal disorders, although human studies have yet to confirm such uses.

Warning: Topical Cayenne preparations should not be used for more than two consecutive days, with a two-week break between applications. It should never be used on broken skin or near the eyes. When used internally, Cayenne preparations should not be taken with aspirin or antifungal drugs. They should also be avoided by people who have stomach ulcers, stomach inflammation, chronic irritable bowel, gastrointestinal disease, renal disease, and by those who are undergoing inhalation therapy.

Chamomile (German) *(Matricaria recutita)*. Chamomile tea—which has anti-inflammatory, antispasmodic, and muscle-relaxing effects—is used to treat gastrointestinal disorders such as indigestion and gas. It is also used for menstrual complaints, nervousness, and general debility. It is used topically for inflammation of the mouth and throat, rhinitis, toothache, earache, headache, and influenza. The oil is used in mouthwashes.

Warning: Chamomile should not be used by pregnant women.

Comfrey *(Symphytum officinale)*. This herb is applied topically as an anti-inflammatory; it is used for bruises and sprains and to promote bone healing.

Warning: Because of possible toxic adverse effects, Comfrey should not be taken internally. The herb is contraindicated in pregnant and breastfeeding women. It should also not be used by people with a history of liver or kidney disease.

Dandelion *(Taraxacum officinale)*. Dandelion, commonly used as an addition to the salad bowl, is recommended as an effective remedy for digestive and liver complaints, urinary tract infection, and as an appetite stimulant.

Overview of Commonly Used Herbs (cont.)

Warning: Although the herb is sometimes used for gallbladder complaints, this should only be done under a doctor's supervision. People with bile duct obstruction or stomach ulcer should not use Dandelion.

Dong Quai *(Angelica sinensis)*. Dong Quai root is used in China as a women's health tonic. It is popularly used as a remedy for fibrocystic breast disease, premenstrual syndrome, painful periods, and menopausal symptoms. Dong Quai is also used in cardiovascular disease to treat high blood pressure and improve poor circulation. It is has also been used for rheumatism, ulcers, anemia, allergies, constipation, as a blood tonic, and to strengthen the uterus and aid patients in supportive functions before pregnancy. In Japan, the herb is used as an analgesic, sedative, and nutrient.

Warning: Dong Quai should not be used by pregnant or breastfeeding women. The herb can also cause photosensitivity. It is contraindicated in patients with hemorrhagic disease, hypermenorrhea, chronic diarrhea, abdominal bloating, or acute infections including colds and flu. It should not be used by people with bleeding disorders, or by those taking blood thinners.

Echinacea *(Echinacea purpurea)*. This species of Echinacea is a well-established immune-system stimulator; it is used to treat flu, fevers, coughs and colds, bronchitis, urinary tract infections, wounds and burns, and inflammation of the mouth and pharynx. It is also used to prevent infection.

Warning: Echinacea should not be used in patients who have autoimmune disorders such as multiple sclerosis, collagen disease, AIDS or HIV infection, leucosis, and tuberculosis. Parenteral administration should not be used in patients with diabetes or those prone to allergies, especially to members of the composite family *(Asteraceae)*. The herb is also contraindicated in pregnant or breastfeeding women. Echinacea should not be used with the following: anticancer agents, drugs used to prevent organ rejection, corticosteroids, immunosuppressants, or drugs metabolized by cytochrome P450 3A4 antibodies.

English Hawthorn *(Crataegus laevigata)*. Hawthorn contains several compounds that are considered beneficial to the heart. It is used for cardiac insufficiency, angina, congestive heart failure, and irregular heartbeat.

Warning: Hawthorn should not be used in children under 12, or in the first trimester of pregnancy. People taking Hawthorn must be carefully monitored by a physician, especially in cases where it is combined with cardiac glycosides, beta-blockers, calcium channel blockers, antiarrhythmics, or antiplatelet agents. Hawthorn should not be taken with cisapride. Overuse can lead to low blood pressure, irregular heartbeat, and excessive sleepiness.

Evening Primrose *(Oenothera biennis)*. The anti-inflammatory compounds in Evening Primrose oil have been extensively studied, but no definitive indication has been accepted. Some herbalists consider the oil useful for treating breast pain, premenstrual syndrome, menopausal symptoms, and cyclic mastalgia. Other common uses include hypertension, rheumatoid arthritis, thrombosis, and autoimmune disease (e.g., multiple sclerosis and Raynaud's phenomenon). Capsules containing at least 500 mg of the oil are approved in Germany as a remedy for eczema.

Warning: People with seizure disorder or schizophrenia should not take Evening Primrose oil. It should not be used by people with bleeding disorders or by those taking blood thinners.

Feverfew *(Tanacetum parthenium)*. Feverfew is used to treat migraine headaches, allergies, and arthritic and rheumatic diseases. It has also been used to treat tinnitus, vertigo, arthritis, fever, toothache, insect bites, and asthma.

Warning: Feverfew should not be used during pregnancy or breastfeeding. It is also contraindicated in people with bleeding disorders and those using anticoagulants, including aspirin. This herb should not be used in children under 2 years of age.

Flax *(Linum usitatissimum)*. Ground Flax (also known as Linseed) is used internally to relieve constipation. It is also used externally as a compress to relieve skin inflammation.

Warning: Flax should not be used internally by patients with bowel or esophageal obstruction or in the presence of gastrointestinal or esophageal inflammation. Flax may delay absorption of other drugs taken simultaneously.

Fo-Ti *(Polygonum multiflorum)*. The Asian herb Fo-Ti is used for constipation, atherosclerosis, fatigue, high cholesterol, and as an immune enhancer.

Warning: Because of its laxative action, the herb may cause diarrhea. Taking the unprocessed root may cause skin rash, and overdosage may cause numbness in the extremities.

Garlic *(Allium sativum)*. Garlic is used as a treatment for hardening of the arteries, high blood pressure, and for reducing cholesterol levels. It may also have antibacterial and antiviral effects. It is used internally as an adjuvant to dietetic measures for elevated lipid levels and the prevention of age-related vascular changes and arteriosclerosis. Recent studies, however, found garlic ineffective for reducing cholesterol.

Warning: Garlic can cause allergic skin and respiratory reactions. It should not be used by people with bleeding disorders, or by those using blood thinners (including aspirin) or NSAID therapy. Garlic significantly induces the metabolism of chlorzoxazone and should not be used with this drug. Starting or stopping Garlic intake while taking protease inhibitors should not be done without consulting a physician. Nursing women should also avoid Garlic.

Ginger *(Zingiber officinale)*. Ginger root is a treatment for motion sickness and loss of appetite. It is also indicated for dyspeptic complaints, for nausea and vomiting associated with chemotherapy, and for helping to control nausea and vomiting in postoperative patients.

Warning: Ginger should not be used for morning sickness associated with pregnancy, or by nursing mothers, without physician approval. People who have gallstones or bleeding disorders should not take Ginger. The herb is also contraindicated in those using blood thinners (including aspirin) or NSAID therapy.

Ginkgo *(Ginkgo biloba)*. Ginkgo may be helpful for treating dementia, Alzheimer's disease, peripheral arterial occlusive disease, vertigo, and tinnitus of vascular origin.

Warning: Ginkgo should not be used by people who have bleeding disorders or by those using blood thinners (including aspirin) or NSAID therapy. Patients with a history of seizures should use the herb with caution, since Ginkgo may lower the seizure threshold.

Ginseng *(Panax ginseng)*. The Ginseng root is used for alleviating fatigue and improving concentration and stamina. Ginseng may also have antiviral, antioxidant, and anticancer effects.

Warning: People with cardiovascular disease or diabetes should use the herb cautiously. People who are taking diabetes drugs, diuretics, blood thinners (including aspirin), MAO inhibitors, or NSAIDs should not take Ginseng. It should not be used during pregnancy or breastfeeding, or by those with bleeding disorders. Taking large amounts can result in Ginseng abuse syndrome, which is characterized by high blood pressure, insomnia, water

Overview of Commonly Used Herbs (cont.)

retention, skin eruptions, diarrhea, and muscle tension. Concomitant use of Ginseng with conjugated estrogens may result in symptoms of estrogen excess.

Goldenseal *(Hydrastis canadensis)*. Goldenseal contains the compound berberine, which is used for gastritis, gastric ulcer, gallbladder disease, and acute diarrhea. It is also used externally as an antiseptic for wounds and herpes labialis.

Berberine is also used as an adjunct treatment in various cancers and in neutropenia resulting from radiation and chemotherapy.

Warning: Goldenseal should not be used by pregnant or breastfeeding women, by women with a history of miscarriage, or by those with bleeding disorders. It should also not be combined with blood thinners (including aspirin) or NSAIDs. In addition, the herb should not be used in people with glucose-6-phosphate-dehydrogenase deficiency. Use of Goldenseal for extended periods can result in digestive disorders, constipation, excitement, hallucination or delirium, and decreased vitamin B absorption. Overdosage may result in convulsion, difficulty breathing, and paralysis.

Gotu Kola *(Centella asiatica)*. Gotu Kola is used internally for chronic venous insufficiency and venous hypertension. In animal and lab studies, Gotu Kola was also effective for ulcers and varicose veins. The herb is used externally to treat wounds; if a rash develops, discontinue topical use.

Warning: Gotu Kola should not be used during pregnancy.

Great Burnet *(Sanguisorba officinalis)*. Great Burnet may be used for its astringent, decongestant, and diuretic properties. It is used internally for dysentery, enteritis, hemorrhoids, phlebitis, menopausal symptoms, intestinal bladder problems, and venous disorders. It is also prepared for external use as a plaster for wounds and ulcers.

Green Tea *(Camellia sinensis)*. Green tea, which is rich in catechins and flavonoids, is used to help prevent cancer. The antibacterial effects of Green Tea mouthwash are useful in the prevention of dental cavities. Keep in mind that Green Tea contains caffeine and should be used sparingly by pregnant and breastfeeding women and by those who are caffeine-sensitive or have sensitive stomachs. Consuming too much Green Tea may result in hyperacidity, gastric irritation, reduction of appetite, and diarrhea; however, these symptoms can generally be avoided by the addition of milk. Green Tea should be used cautiously by those with weakened cardiovascular systems, renal disease, thyroid hyperfunction, elevated susceptibility to spasm, and anxiety disorders. The herb reacts with alkaline medication and may delay resorption.

Horse Chestnut *(Aesculus hippocastanum)*. Both the seed and leaf of Horse Chestnut are used medicinally. The seed is indicated for the symptoms of chronic venous insufficiency, including pain, cramping, swelling, sensations of heaviness, and night cramping. Horse Chestnut leaf is used for venous disorders such as varicose veins, hemorrhoids, and phlebitis.

Warning: People taking blood thinners (including aspirin) should not use Horse Chestnut.

Kava *(Piper methysticum)*. The active compounds in Kava are lactones, which have antispasmodic, muscle-relaxing, and anticonvulsive effects; Kava can also thin the blood. The herb is used for nervousness, insomnia, tension, stress, and agitation.

Warning: Kava has been associated with severe liver injury in a small number of patients in other countries. People who have liver problems or who take drugs that can affect the liver should consult a physician before using

Kava. The herb is also contraindicated in patients with depression, in those with neurologic disorders, and in pregnant or nursing women. Overuse of Kava can result in skin rash or weight loss. Kava use for more than three months should be supervised by a physician. The herb should not be combined with the following: alcohol, anti-anxiety or mood-altering drugs (including barbiturates), levodopa, drugs metabolized by P450 (CYP) enzymes, blood thinners, hepatotoxic drugs, and MAO inhibitors.

Licorice *(Glycyrrhiza glabra)*. The sweet root of the Licorice plant has a long history of use in traditional medicine. It contains various compounds with anti-inflammatory and other soothing effects that make it helpful as a treatment for ulcers and digestive disorders such as gastritis. It also acts as an expectorant for cough and bronchitis.

Warning: Licorice is contraindicated in pregnant women and in people with hepatitis and other liver disorders, kidney disease, diabetes, arrhythmias, high blood pressure, muscle cramping, and low potassium levels. Licorice should not be taken with digoxin, blood thinners, diuretics, or medications that lower blood pressure. It should also not be combined with laxatives, combination contraceptives, MAO inhibitors, potassium supplements, testosterone, or drugs metabolized by P450 (CYP) enzymes.

Ma Huang *(Ephedra sinica)*. Ma Huang contains compounds that alleviate bronchial constriction and is used in folk remedies as a treatment for coughs and bronchitis.

Warning: Because of the severe adverse effects linked to ephedrine alkaloids—including heart attack, stroke, and death—the FDA banned dietary supplements containing ephedra in February 2004. The risks of this herb outweigh any possible benefits, especially for pregnant or breastfeeding women, children and teenagers, and for people with the following: anxiety, depression, high blood pressure, glaucoma, brain tumors, seizure disorders, prostate disorders, stomach ulcers, pheochromocytoma, thyrotoxicosis, cerebral perfusions, adrenal tumors, cardiac arrhythmia, or thyroid disease. Ma-Huang should not be combined with caffeine, decongestants, diet medications containing sympathomimetics or caffeine, stimulants, glaucoma medication, MAO Inhibitors, anesthetics, or labor-inducing drugs. Overdosage may result in death.

Milk Thistle *(Silybum marianum)*. The compounds in Milk Thistle seed have protective and regenerative effects on the liver. It is used as a treatment for liver and gallbladder disorders such as jaundice, toxic liver damage, cirrhosis of the liver, and gallbladder pain. It is also used for dyspeptic complaints.

Warning: The herb should not be used with antipsychotic drugs, Yohimbe, or male hormones.

Pumpkin Seed *(Cucurbita pepo)*. Pumpkin seed has anti-inflammatory and antioxidant properties. It is used to treat irritable bladder and symptoms of benign prostatic hyperplasia (obstructed urinary flow). It does not, however, appear to relieve an enlarged prostate.

Warning: INR may increase when Pumpkin Seed is combined with blood thinners, saw palmetto, or Vitamin E.

Pygeum *(Pygeum africanum)*. Pygeum bark contains compounds that inhibit the inflammation and swelling associated with benign prostatic hyperplasia.

Warning: The herb should not be used by pregnant or breastfeeding women. People with stomach disorders should check with their physician before using Pygeum.

Overview of Commonly Used Herbs (cont.)

Saw Palmetto *(Serenoa repens)*. The anti-inflammatory and hormone-modulating effects of Saw Palmetto theoretically make it useful for treating symptoms of benign prostatic hyperplasia, but clinical trials are inconclusive. The herb has also been used for treating irritable bladder.

Warning: Saw Palmetto should not be used by pregnant or breastfeeding women. The herb should be avoided by those who have hormone-driven cancers or a family history of such cancers. People with stomach disorders and those taking hormones or hormone-like drugs should check with their physician before using Saw Palmetto.

St. John's Wort *(Hypericum perforatum)*. St. John's wort is one of the better studied herbs. Various compounds in St. John's wort have antidepressant, anti-inflammatory, and antibacterial effects. It is used internally for depression and anxiety, and externally for wounds, burns, skin inflammation, and blunt injuries.

Warning: St. John's wort can cause photosensitivity if taken for too long or at high doses. It can also cause gastrointestinal discomfort and headache. Combining St. John's wort with antidepressant medications such as MAO inhibitors, selective serotonin reuptake inhibitors (including fluoxetine, paroxetine, sertraline, fluvoxamine, or citalopram), or nefazodone could cause "serotonin syndrome"—a condition characterized by sweating, tremor, confusion, and agitation. The herb should also not be combined with the following: antibiotics that have photosensitizing effects, cyclosporine, indinavir, combination oral contraceptives, reserpine, barbiturates, theophylline, or digoxin. Taking St. John's wort with drugs that are metabolized by P450 liver enzymes may decrease their effectiveness.

Stinging Nettle *(Urtica dioica)*. Both the flowers and root of the Stinging Nettle plant contain beneficial compounds used in various conditions. The flower is used internally and externally for rheumatism. It is also used internally for urinary tract infections and kidney and bladder stones. The root is used for irritable bladder and to help relieve symptoms of benign prostatic hyperplasia (obstructed urinary flow), although it does not reduce prostate enlargement.

Warning: Stinging Nettle should not be used by people who suffer from fluid retention due to impaired cardiac or kidney function. The herb should not be used during pregnancy.

Uva-Ursi *(Arctostaphylos uva-ursi)*. Uva-ursi is used in the treatment of urinary tract infections because of its astringent and antibacterial effects.

Warning: The herb should not be used by pregnant or breastfeeding women; it should also not be used in children under 12 years of age, as it could cause liver damage. Uva-ursi should not be combined with diuretics, NSAIDs, or with substances (food or medication) that promote acidity in the urine, since this reduces its antibacterial effect. Individuals with kidney disorders, irritated digestive disorders, and acidic urine should not take Uva-ursi.

Valerian *(Valeriana officinalis)*. Valerian root contains sedative compounds that are useful in nervousness and insomnia. It is also used for many other unproven uses such as headache, anxiety disorders, premenstrual syndrome, and menopausal symptoms.

Warning: Patients should avoid operating motor vehicles for several hours after taking Valerian. The herb should not be used by pregnant or breastfeeding women. It should also not be used in children less than 14 years old without medical supervision. Valerian extract or bath oils should not be used by people suffering from skin disorders, fever, infectious disease, heart disease, or muscle tension. The herb should be avoided in patients with preexisting liver disease. Valerian should not be combined with the following: alcohol, barbiturates, benzodiazepines, blood thinners, hepatoxic agents, supplemental iron, loperamide, or opioid analgesics.

Vitex *(Vitex agnus-castus)*. Also known as Chaste Tree, Vitex is used as a treatment for premenstrual syndrome and menopausal symptoms, menstrual cycle irregularities, and mastalgia/mastodynia.

Warning: Because of its hormonal effects, Vitex should not be used by pregnant or breastfeeding women. Occasionally, rash can occur. The herb should not be used with drugs that affect dopamine levels.

Wild Yam *(Dioscorea villosa)*. Popular reports have led to the belief that Wild Yam is a "natural" source of the hormone progesterone. While Wild Yam is used as a constituent of artificial progesterone pharmaceutically, the body cannot complete the conversion process by itself. The herb may be useful in treating high cholesterol.

Warning: Because of possible hormonal effects, pregnant and nursing women should not use Wild Yam. The herb should not be taken with estrogen-containing drugs or indomethacin.

Yohimbe *(Pausinystalia yohimbe)*. Yohimbe is prepared pharmaceutically under the brand name Yocon and is used to treat erectile dysfunction. Compounds in Yohimbe stimulate norepinephrine, which improves blood flow to the penis. It is also used for debility and exhaustion. The risks, however, of unregulated ingestion of the herb are thought to outweigh the benefits. Therefore, it is recommended that Yohimbe be taken only under strict medical supervision.

Warning: Yohimbe should not be used by women, especially pregnant or breastfeeding women. Children under 12 years of age should not take the herb. It is also contraindicated in patients with liver or kidney disease, post-traumatic stress disorder, high blood pressure, panic disorder, or Parkinson's disease. The herb should not be combined with the following: alcohol, blood pressure medication, carbamazepine, clomipramine, clonidine, guanabenz, guanadrel, guanethidine, guanfacine, lithium, minoxidil, morphine, naloxone, naltrexone, OTC stimulants, reserpine, sibutramine, or valproic acid. Patients should check with their doctor before taking Yohimbe with any OTC product. It should also not be taken with tyramine-containing foods such as wine and aged cheese.

SECTION 6

PRODUCT IDENTIFICATION GUIDE

For quick identification, this section provides full-color reproductions of product packaging, as well as some actual-sized photographs of tablets and capsules. In all, the section contains more than 100 photos.

Products in this section are arranged alphabetically by manufacturer. In some instances, not all dosage forms and sizes are pictured. For more information on any of the products in this section,

please turn to the page indicated above the product's photo or check directly with the product's manufacturer.

While every effort has been made to guarantee faithful reproduction of the photos in this section, changes in size, color, and design are always a possibility. Be sure to confirm a product's identity with the manufacturer or your pharmacist.

MANUFACTURER'S INDEX

Adams Respiratory Therapeutics 502

Awareness Corporation. 502

Boehringer Ingelheim Consumer H.C..............503

Eniva Nutraceutics Corporation......................503

Mannatech, Inc. 503

Matrixx Initiatives, Inc. 503

Memory Secret 504

Novartis Consumer Health, Inc......................504

Procter & Gamble 507

Reese Pharmaceutical Company....................508

Schering-Plough HealthCare Products.............508

Tahitian Noni International 508

Topical Biomedics, Inc. 508

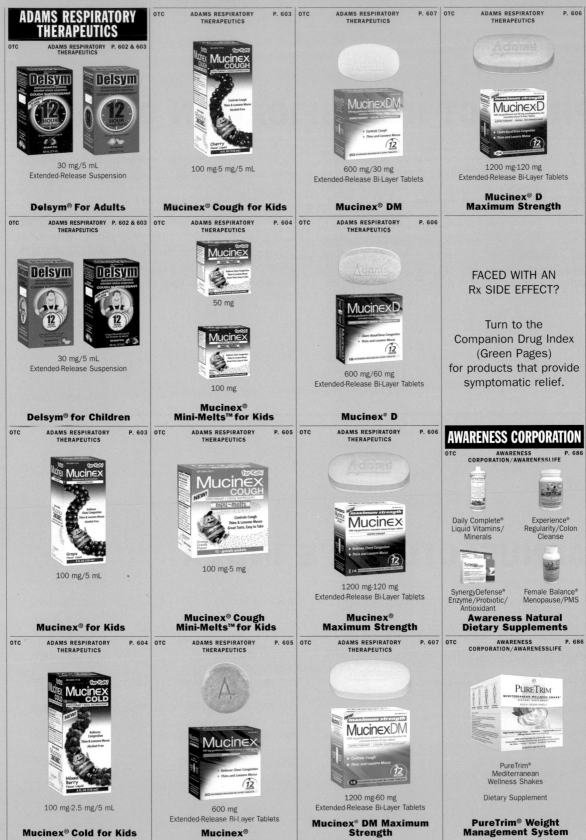

ADAMS RESPIRATORY THERAPEUTICS

OTC   ADAMS RESPIRATORY   P. 602 & 603
THERAPEUTICS

30 mg/5 mL
Extended-Release Suspension

Delsym® For Adults

OTC   ADAMS RESPIRATORY   P. 602 & 603
THERAPEUTICS

30 mg/5 mL
Extended-Release Suspension

Delsym® for Children

OTC   ADAMS RESPIRATORY   P. 603
THERAPEUTICS

100 mg/5 mL

Mucinex® for Kids

OTC   ADAMS RESPIRATORY   P. 604
THERAPEUTICS

100 mg-2.5 mg/5 mL

Mucinex® Cold for Kids

OTC   ADAMS RESPIRATORY   P. 603
THERAPEUTICS

100 mg-5 mg/5 mL

Mucinex® Cough for Kids

OTC   ADAMS RESPIRATORY   P. 604
THERAPEUTICS

50 mg

100 mg

**Mucinex®
Mini-Melts™ for Kids**

OTC   ADAMS RESPIRATORY   P. 605
THERAPEUTICS

100 mg-5 mg

**Mucinex® Cough
Mini-Melts™ for Kids**

OTC   ADAMS RESPIRATORY   P. 605
THERAPEUTICS

600 mg
Extended-Release Bi-Layer Tablets

Mucinex®

OTC   ADAMS RESPIRATORY   P. 607
THERAPEUTICS

600 mg/30 mg
Extended-Release Bi-Layer Tablets

Mucinex® DM

OTC   ADAMS RESPIRATORY   P. 606
THERAPEUTICS

600 mg/60 mg
Extended-Release Bi-Layer Tablets

Mucinex® D

OTC   ADAMS RESPIRATORY   P. 606
THERAPEUTICS

1200 mg-120 mg
Extended-Release Bi-Layer Tablets

**Mucinex®
Maximum Strength**

OTC   ADAMS RESPIRATORY   P. 607
THERAPEUTICS

1200 mg-60 mg
Extended-Release Bi-Layer Tablets

**Mucinex® DM Maximum
Strength**

OTC   ADAMS RESPIRATORY   P. 606
THERAPEUTICS

1200 mg-120 mg
Extended-Release Bi-Layer Tablets

**Mucinex® D
Maximum Strength**

FACED WITH AN
Rx SIDE EFFECT?

Turn to the
Companion Drug Index
(Green Pages)
for products that provide
symptomatic relief.

AWARENESS CORPORATION

OTC   AWARENESS   P. 686
CORPORATION/AWARENESSLIFE

Daily Complete®
Liquid Vitamins/
Minerals

Experience®
Regularity/Colon
Cleanse

SynergyDefense®
Enzyme/Probiotic/
Antioxidant

Female Balance®
Menopause/PMS

**Awareness Natural
Dietary Supplements**

OTC   AWARENESS   P. 686
CORPORATION/AWARENESSLIFE

PureTrim®
Mediterranean
Wellness Shakes

Dietary Supplement

**PureTrim® Weight
Management System**

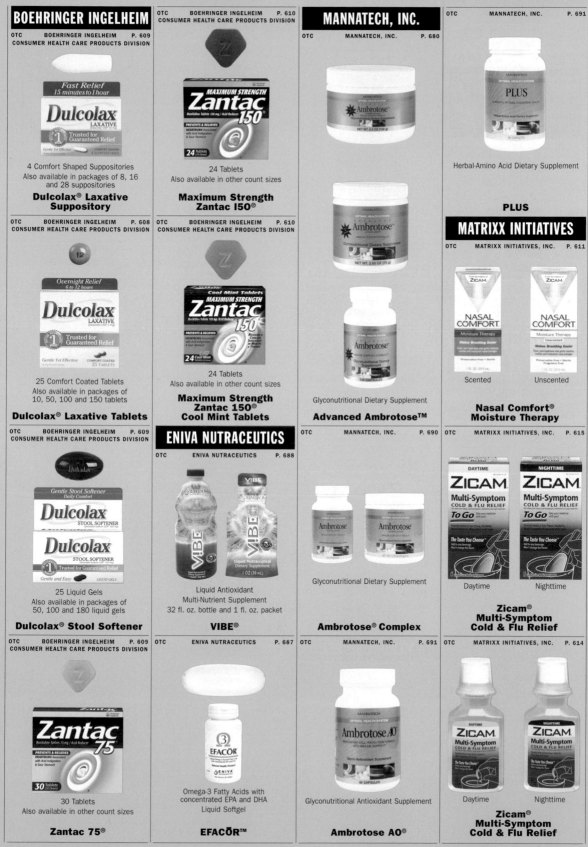

BOEHRINGER INGELHEIM

OTC   BOEHRINGER INGELHEIM   P. 609
CONSUMER HEALTH CARE PRODUCTS DIVISION

Fast Relief
15 minutes to 1 hour

Dulcolax LAXATIVE

4 Comfort Shaped Suppositories
Also available in packages of 8, 16
and 28 suppositories

**Dulcolax® Laxative
Suppository**

OTC   BOEHRINGER INGELHEIM   P. 608
CONSUMER HEALTH CARE PRODUCTS DIVISION

Overnight Relief
6 to 12 hours

Dulcolax LAXATIVE

25 Comfort Coated Tablets
Also available in packages of
10, 50, 100 and 150 tablets

Dulcolax® Laxative Tablets

OTC   BOEHRINGER INGELHEIM   P. 609
CONSUMER HEALTH CARE PRODUCTS DIVISION

Gentle Stool Softener
Daily Comfort

Dulcolax STOOL SOFTENER
Dulcolax STOOL SOFTENER

25 Liquid Gels
Also available in packages of
50, 100 and 180 liquid gels

Dulcolax® Stool Softener

OTC   BOEHRINGER INGELHEIM   P. 609
CONSUMER HEALTH CARE PRODUCTS DIVISION

Zantac 75

30 Tablets
Also available in other count sizes

Zantac 75®

OTC   BOEHRINGER INGELHEIM   P. 610
CONSUMER HEALTH CARE PRODUCTS DIVISION

MAXIMUM STRENGTH Zantac 150

24 Tablets
Also available in other count sizes

**Maximum Strength
Zantac 150®**

OTC   BOEHRINGER INGELHEIM   P. 610
CONSUMER HEALTH CARE PRODUCTS DIVISION

Cool Mint Tablets
MAXIMUM STRENGTH Zantac 150

24 Tablets
Also available in other count sizes

**Maximum Strength
Zantac 150®
Cool Mint Tablets**

ENIVA NUTRACEUTICS

OTC   ENIVA NUTRACEUTICS   P. 688

VIBE

Liquid Antioxidant
Multi-Nutrient Supplement
32 fl. oz. bottle and 1 fl. oz. packet

VIBE®

OTC   ENIVA NUTRACEUTICS   P. 687

EFACOR

Omega-3 Fatty Acids with
concentrated EPA and DHA
Liquid Softgel

EFACŌR™

MANNATECH, INC.

OTC   MANNATECH, INC.   P. 680

Ambrotose™

Ambrotose™

Glyconutritional Dietary Supplement

Advanced Ambrotose™

OTC   MANNATECH, INC.   P. 690

Glyconutritional Dietary Supplement

Ambrotose® Complex

OTC   MANNATECH, INC.   P. 691

Ambrotose AO

Glyconutritional Antioxidant Supplement

Ambrotose AO®

OTC   MANNATECH, INC.   P. 691

PLUS

Herbal-Amino Acid Dietary Supplement

PLUS

MATRIXX INITIATIVES

OTC   MATRIXX INITIATIVES, INC.   P. 611

NASAL COMFORT Moisture Therapy
NASAL COMFORT Moisture Therapy

Scented   Unscented

**Nasal Comfort®
Moisture Therapy**

OTC   MATRIXX INITIATIVES, INC.   P. 615

ZICAM Multi-Symptom COLD & FLU RELIEF To Go
ZICAM Multi-Symptom COLD & FLU RELIEF To Go

Daytime   Nighttime

**Zicam®
Multi-Symptom
Cold & Flu Relief**

OTC   MATRIXX INITIATIVES, INC.   P. 614

ZICAM Multi-Symptom COLD & FLU RELIEF
ZICAM Multi-Symptom COLD & FLU RELIEF

Daytime   Nighttime

**Zicam®
Multi-Symptom
Cold & Flu Relief**

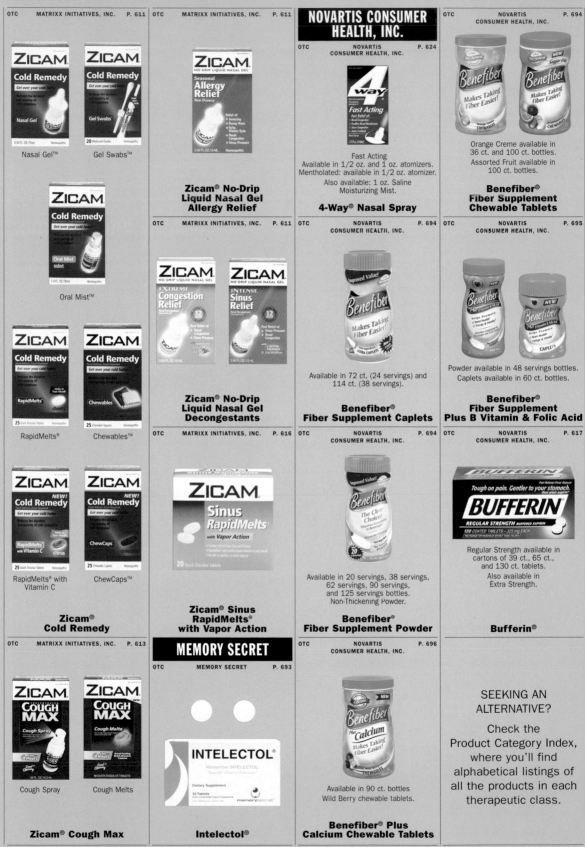

OTC   MATRIXX INITIATIVES, INC.   P. 611

Nasal Gel™

Gel Swabs™

Oral Mist™

RapidMelts®

Chewables™

RapidMelts® with Vitamin C

ChewCaps™

**Zicam®
Cold Remedy**

OTC   MATRIXX INITIATIVES, INC.   P. 613

Cough Spray

Cough Melts

Zicam® Cough Max

OTC   MATRIXX INITIATIVES, INC.   P. 611

**Zicam® No-Drip
Liquid Nasal Gel
Allergy Relief**

OTC   MATRIXX INITIATIVES, INC.   P. 611

**Zicam® No-Drip
Liquid Nasal Gel
Decongestants**

OTC   MATRIXX INITIATIVES, INC.   P. 616

**Zicam® Sinus
RapidMelts®
with Vapor Action**

MEMORY SECRET

OTC   MEMORY SECRET   P. 693

Intelectol®

NOVARTIS CONSUMER HEALTH, INC.

OTC   NOVARTIS   P. 624
CONSUMER HEALTH, INC.

Fast Acting
Available in 1/2 oz. and 1 oz. atomizers.
Mentholated: available in 1/2 oz. atomizer.
Also available: 1 oz. Saline
Moisturizing Mist.

4-Way® Nasal Spray

OTC   NOVARTIS   P. 694
CONSUMER HEALTH, INC.

Available in 72 ct. (24 servings) and
114 ct. (38 servings).

**Benefiber®
Fiber Supplement Caplets**

OTC   NOVARTIS   P. 694
CONSUMER HEALTH, INC.

Available in 20 servings, 38 servings,
62 servings, 90 servings,
and 125 servings bottles.
Non-Thickening Powder.

**Benefiber®
Fiber Supplement Powder**

OTC   NOVARTIS   P. 696
CONSUMER HEALTH, INC.

Available in 90 ct. bottles
Wild Berry chewable tablets.

**Benefiber® Plus
Calcium Chewable Tablets**

OTC   NOVARTIS   P. 694
CONSUMER HEALTH, INC.

Orange Creme available in
36 ct. and 100 ct. bottles.
Assorted Fruit available in
100 ct. bottles.

**Benefiber®
Fiber Supplement
Chewable Tablets**

OTC   NOVARTIS   P. 695
CONSUMER HEALTH, INC.

Powder available in 48 servings bottles.
Caplets available in 60 ct. bottles.

**Benefiber®
Fiber Supplement
Plus B Vitamin & Folic Acid**

OTC   NOVARTIS   P. 617
CONSUMER HEALTH, INC.

Regular Strength available in
cartons of 39 ct., 65 ct.,
and 130 ct. tablets.
Also available in
Extra Strength.

Bufferin®

SEEKING AN ALTERNATIVE?

Check the
Product Category Index,
where you'll find
alphabetical listings of
all the products in each
therapeutic class.

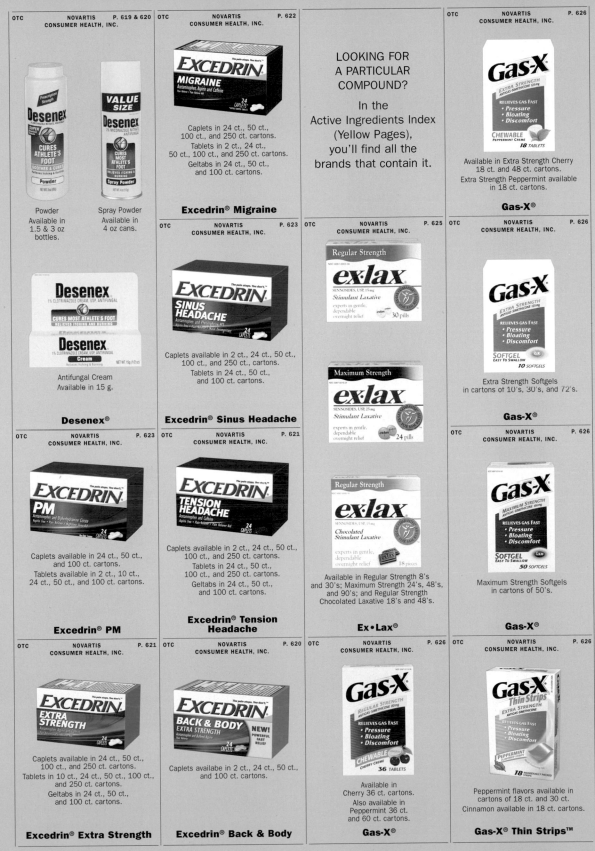

OTC NOVARTIS P. 619 & 620
CONSUMER HEALTH, INC.

Powder
Available in
1.5 & 3 oz
bottles.

Spray Powder
Available in
4 oz cans.

OTC NOVARTIS P. 622
CONSUMER HEALTH, INC.

Caplets in 24 ct., 50 ct.,
100 ct., and 250 ct. cartons.
Tablets in 2 ct., 24 ct.,
50 ct., 100 ct., and 250 ct. cartons.
Geltabs in 24 ct., 50 ct.,
and 100 ct. cartons.

Excedrin® Migraine

LOOKING FOR
A PARTICULAR
COMPOUND?

In the
Active Ingredients Index
(Yellow Pages),
you'll find all the
brands that contain it.

OTC NOVARTIS P. 626
CONSUMER HEALTH, INC.

Available in Extra Strength Cherry
18 ct. and 48 ct. cartons.
Extra Strength Peppermint available
in 18 ct. cartons.

Gas-X®

OTC NOVARTIS P. 623
CONSUMER HEALTH, INC.

Antifungal Cream
Available in 15 g.

Desenex®

OTC NOVARTIS P. 623
CONSUMER HEALTH, INC.

Caplets available in 2 ct., 24 ct., 50 ct.,
100 ct., and 250 ct., cartons.
Tablets in 24 ct., 50 ct.,
and 100 ct. cartons.

Excedrin® Sinus Headache

OTC NOVARTIS P. 625
CONSUMER HEALTH, INC.

Available in Regular Strength 8's
and 30's; Maximum Strength 24's, 48's,
and 90's; and Regular Strength
Chocolated Laxative 18's and 48's.

Ex•Lax®

OTC NOVARTIS P. 626
CONSUMER HEALTH, INC.

Extra Strength Softgels
in cartons of 10's, 30's, and 72's.

Gas-X®

OTC NOVARTIS P. 623
CONSUMER HEALTH, INC.

Caplets available in 24 ct., 50 ct.,
and 100 ct. cartons.
Tablets available in 2 ct., 10 ct.,
24 ct., 50 ct., and 100 ct. cartons.

Excedrin® PM

OTC NOVARTIS P. 621
CONSUMER HEALTH, INC.

Caplets available in 2 ct., 24 ct., 50 ct.,
100 ct., and 250 ct. cartons.
Tablets in 24 ct., 50 ct.,
100 ct., and 250 ct. cartons.
Geltabs in 24 ct., 50 ct.,
and 100 ct. cartons.

**Excedrin® Tension
Headache**

OTC NOVARTIS P. 626
CONSUMER HEALTH, INC.

Maximum Strength Softgels
in cartons of 50's.

Gas-X®

OTC NOVARTIS P. 621
CONSUMER HEALTH, INC.

Caplets available in 24 ct., 50 ct.,
100 ct., and 250 ct. cartons.
Tablets in 10 ct., 24 ct., 50 ct., 100 ct.,
and 250 ct. cartons.
Geltabs in 24 ct., 50 ct.,
and 100 ct. cartons.

Excedrin® Extra Strength

OTC NOVARTIS P. 620
CONSUMER HEALTH, INC.

Caplets availabe in 2 ct., 24 ct., 50 ct.,
and 100 ct. cartons.

Excedrin® Back & Body

OTC NOVARTIS P. 626
CONSUMER HEALTH, INC.

Available in
Cherry 36 ct. cartons.
Also available in
Peppermint 36 ct.
and 60 ct. cartons.

Gas-X®

OTC NOVARTIS P. 626
CONSUMER HEALTH, INC.

Peppermint flavors available in
cartons of 18 ct. and 30 ct.
Cinnamon available in 18 ct. cartons.

Gas-X® Thin Strips™

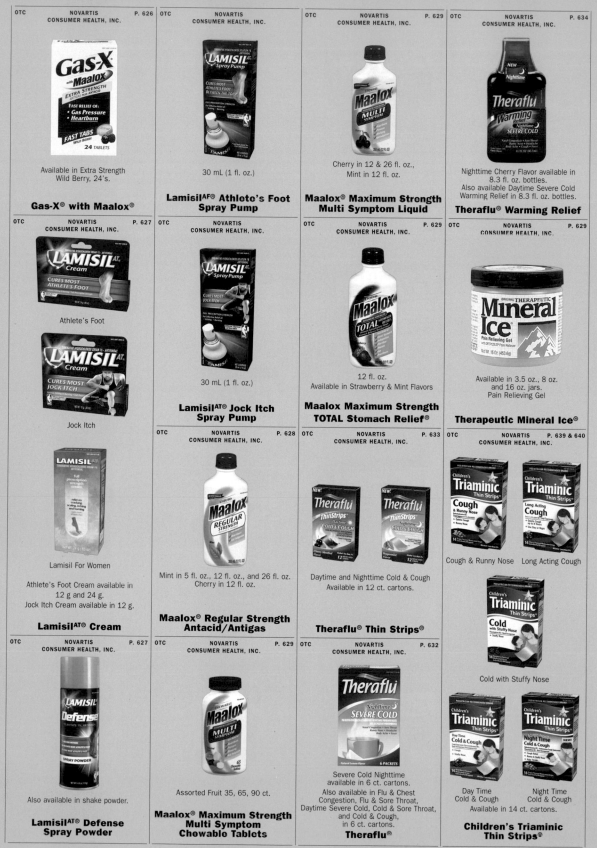

OTC   NOVARTIS CONSUMER HEALTH, INC.   P. 626

Available in Extra Strength
Wild Berry, 24's.

Gas-X® with Maalox®

OTC   NOVARTIS CONSUMER HEALTH, INC.   P. 627

Athlete's Foot

Jock Itch

Lamisil For Women

Athlete's Foot Cream available in
12 g and 24 g.
Jock Itch Cream available in 12 g.

Lamisil^AT® Cream

OTC   NOVARTIS CONSUMER HEALTH, INC.   P. 627

Also available in shake powder.

Lamisil^AT® Defense
Spray Powder

OTC   NOVARTIS CONSUMER HEALTH, INC.   P. 626

30 mL (1 fl. oz.)

Lamisil^AF® Athlote's Foot
Spray Pump

OTC   NOVARTIS CONSUMER HEALTH, INC.

30 mL (1 fl. oz.)

Lamisil^AT® Jock Itch
Spray Pump

OTC   NOVARTIS CONSUMER HEALTH, INC.   P. 628

Mint in 5 fl. oz., 12 fl. oz., and 26 fl. oz.
Cherry in 12 fl. oz.

Maalox® Regular Strength
Antacid/Antigas

OTC   NOVARTIS CONSUMER HEALTH, INC.   P. 629

Assorted Fruit 35, 65, 90 ct.

Maalox® Maximum Strength
Multi Symptom
Chewable Tablets

OTC   NOVARTIS CONSUMER HEALTH, INC.   P. 629

Cherry in 12 & 26 fl. oz.,
Mint in 12 fl. oz.

Maalox® Maximum Strength
Multi Symptom Liquid

OTC   NOVARTIS CONSUMER HEALTH, INC.   P. 629

12 fl. oz.
Available in Strawberry & Mint Flavors

Maalox Maximum Strength
TOTAL Stomach Relief®

OTC   NOVARTIS CONSUMER HEALTH, INC.   P. 633

Daytime and Nighttime Cold & Cough
Available in 12 ct. cartons.

Theraflu® Thin Strips®

OTC   NOVARTIS CONSUMER HEALTH, INC.   P. 632

Severe Cold Nighttime
available in 6 ct. cartons.
Also available in Flu & Chest
Congestion, Flu & Sore Throat,
Daytime Severe Cold, Cold & Sore Throat,
and Cold & Cough,
in 6 ct. cartons.

Theraflu®

OTC   NOVARTIS CONSUMER HEALTH, INC.   P. 634

Nighttime Cherry Flavor available in
8.3 fl. oz. bottles.
Also available Daytime Severe Cold
Warming Relief in 8.3 fl. oz. bottles.

Theraflu® Warming Relief

OTC   NOVARTIS CONSUMER HEALTH, INC.   P. 629

Available in 3.5 oz., 8 oz.
and 16 oz. jars.
Pain Relieving Gel

Therapeutic Mineral Ice®

OTC   NOVARTIS CONSUMER HEALTH, INC.   P. 639 & 640

Cough & Runny Nose   Long Acting Cough

Cold with Stuffy Nose

Day Time   Night Time
Cold & Cough   Cold & Cough
Available in 14 ct. cartons.

Children's Triaminic
Thin Strips®

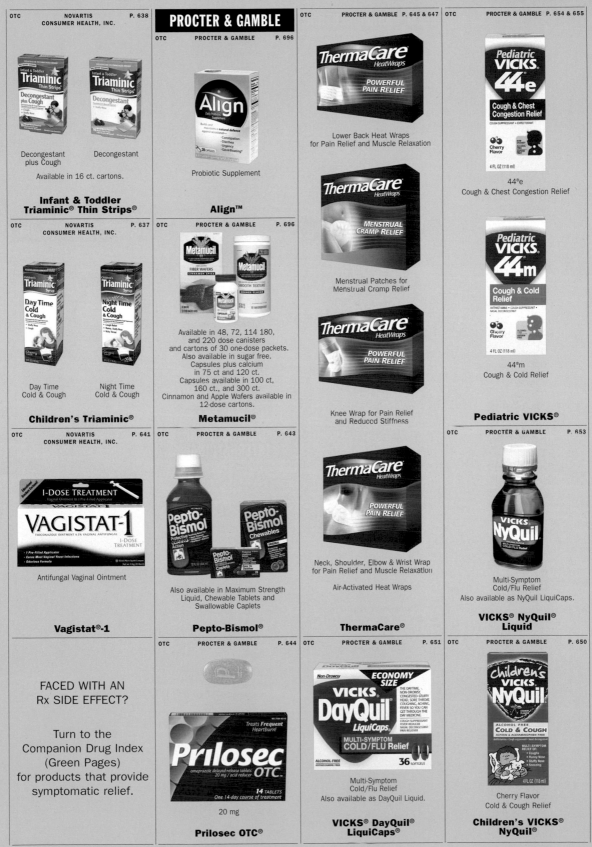

OTC   NOVARTIS   P. 638
CONSUMER HEALTH, INC.

Decongestant plus Cough   Decongestant

Available in 16 ct. cartons.

Infant & Toddler Triaminic® Thin Strips®

OTC   NOVARTIS   P. 637
CONSUMER HEALTH, INC.

Day Time Cold & Cough   Night Time Cold & Cough

Children's Triaminic®

OTC   NOVARTIS   P. 641
CONSUMER HEALTH, INC.

Antifungal Vaginal Ointment

Vagistat®-1

FACED WITH AN
Rx SIDE EFFECT?

Turn to the
Companion Drug Index
(Green Pages)
for products that provide
symptomatic relief.

PROCTER & GAMBLE

OTC   PROCTER & GAMBLE   P. 696

Probiotic Supplement

Align™

OTC   PROCTER & GAMBLE   P. 696

Available in 48, 72, 114 180,
and 220 dose canisters
and cartons of 30 one-dose packets.
Also available in sugar free.
Capsules plus calcium
in 75 ct and 120 ct.
Capsules available in 100 ct,
160 ct., and 300 ct.
Cinnamon and Apple Wafers available in
12-dose cartons.

Metamucil®

OTC   PROCTER & GAMBLE   P. 643

Also available in Maximum Strength
Liquid, Chewable Tablets and
Swallowable Caplets

Pepto-Bismol®

OTC   PROCTER & GAMBLE   P. 644

Treats Frequent Heartburn!

20 mg

Prilosec OTC®

OTC   PROCTER & GAMBLE   P. 645 & 647

Lower Back Heat Wraps
for Pain Relief and Muscle Relaxation

Menstrual Patches for
Menstrual Cramp Relief

Knee Wrap for Pain Relief
and Reduced Stiffness

Neck, Shoulder, Elbow & Wrist Wrap
for Pain Relief and Muscle Relaxation

Air-Activated Heat Wraps

ThermaCare®

OTC   PROCTER & GAMBLE   P. 651

Multi-Symptom
Cold/Flu Relief
Also available as DayQuil Liquid.

**VICKS® DayQuil®
LiquiCaps®**

OTC   PROCTER & GAMBLE   P. 654 & 655

44®e
Cough & Chest Congestion Relief

44®m
Cough & Cold Relief

Pediatric VICKS®

OTC   PROCTER & GAMBLE   P. 653

Multi-Symptom
Cold/Flu Relief
Also available as NyQuil LiquiCaps.

**VICKS® NyQuil®
Liquid**

OTC   PROCTER & GAMBLE   P. 650

Cherry Flavor
Cold & Cough Relief

**Children's VICKS®
NyQuil®**

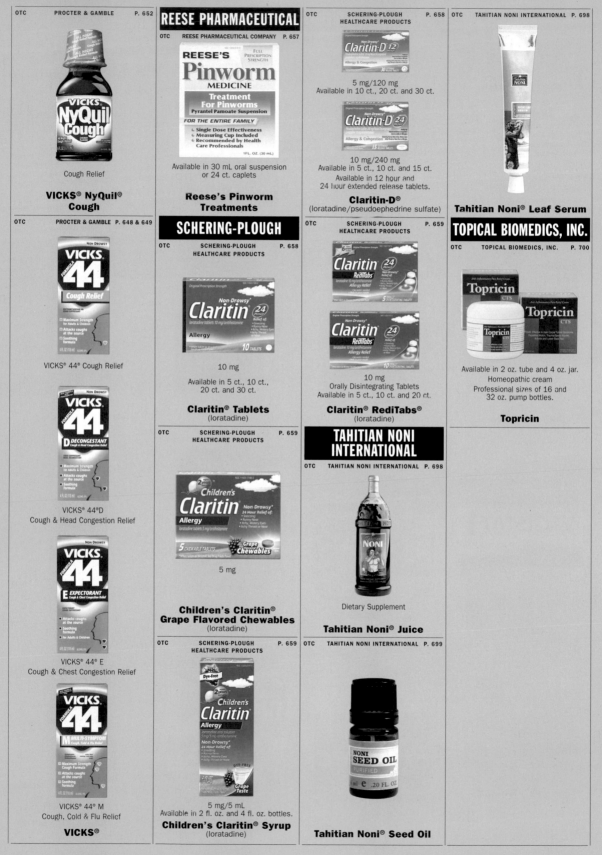

OTC   PROCTER & GAMBLE   P. 652

Cough Relief

VICKS® NyQuil® Cough

OTC   PROCTER & GAMBLE   P. 648 & 649

VICKS® 44® Cough Relief

VICKS® 44®D
Cough & Head Congestion Relief

VICKS® 44® E
Cough & Chest Congestion Relief

VICKS® 44® M
Cough, Cold & Flu Relief

VICKS®

OTC   REESE PHARMACEUTICAL COMPANY   P. 657

REESE PHARMACEUTICAL

Available in 30 mL oral suspension
or 24 ct. caplets

Reese's Pinworm Treatments

SCHERING-PLOUGH

OTC   SCHERING-PLOUGH
HEALTHCARE PRODUCTS   P. 658

10 mg
Available in 5 ct., 10 ct.,
20 ct. and 30 ct.

Claritin® Tablets
(loratadine)

OTC   SCHERING-PLOUGH
HEALTHCARE PRODUCTS   P. 659

5 mg

**Children's Claritin®
Grape Flavored Chewables**
(loratadine)

OTC   SCHERING-PLOUGH
HEALTHCARE PRODUCTS   P. 659

5 mg/5 mL
Available in 2 fl. oz. and 4 fl. oz. bottles.

Children's Claritin® Syrup
(loratadine)

OTC   SCHERING-PLOUGH
HEALTHCARE PRODUCTS   P. 658

5 mg/120 mg
Available in 10 ct., 20 ct. and 30 ct.

10 mg/240 mg
Available in 5 ct., 10 ct. and 15 ct.
Available in 12 hour and
24 hour extended release tablets.

Claritin-D®
(loratadine/pseudoephedrine sulfate)

OTC   SCHERING-PLOUGH
HEALTHCARE PRODUCTS   P. 659

10 mg
Orally Disintegrating Tablets
Available in 5 ct., 10 ct. and 20 ct.

Claritin® RediTabs®
(loratadine)

**TAHITIAN NONI
INTERNATIONAL**

OTC   TAHITIAN NONI INTERNATIONAL   P. 698

Dietary Supplement

Tahitian Noni® Juice

OTC   TAHITIAN NONI INTERNATIONAL   P. 699

Tahitian Noni® Seed Oil

OTC   TAHITIAN NONI INTERNATIONAL   P. 698

Tahitian Noni® Leaf Serum

TOPICAL BIOMEDICS, INC.

OTC   TOPICAL BIOMEDICS, INC.   P. 700

Available in 2 oz. tube and 4 oz. jar.
Homeopathic cream
Professional sizes of 16 and
32 oz. pump bottles.

Topricin

NONPRESCRIPTION DRUG INFORMATION

This section presents information on nonprescription drugs, self-testing kits, and other medical products marketed for home use by consumers. It is made possible through the courtesy of the manufacturers whose products appear on the following pages. The information concerning each product has been prepared, edited, and approved by the manufacturer's professional staff.

Pharmaceutical product descriptions in this section must be in compliance with the Code of Federal Regulations' labeling requirements for over-the-counter drugs. The descriptions are designed to provide all information necessary for informed use, including, when applicable, active ingredients, inactive ingredients, Indications, actions, warnings, cautions, drug interactions, symptoms and treatment of oral overdosage, dosage and directions for use, professional labeling, and how supplied. In some cases, additional information has been supplied to complement the standard labeling.

In compiling this section, the publisher has emphasized the necessity of describing products comprehensively. The descriptions seen here include all information made available by the manufacturer. The publisher does not warrant or guarantee any product described here, and does not perform any independent analysis of the information provided. Inclusion of a product in this book does not represent an endorsement, and the publisher does not necessarily advocate the use of any product listed.

Actavis, Inc.
7205 WINDSOR BOULEVARD
BALTIMORE, MD 21244

Direct Inquiries to:
Customer Service
(800) 432-8534

PERMETHRIN LOTION 1%
(Actavis, Inc.)
Lice Treatment

Description:
EACH FLUID OUNCE CONTAINS: Active Ingredient: Permethrin 280 mg (1%). Inactive Ingredients: Balsam fir canada, cetyl alcohol, citric acid, FD&C Yellow No. 6, fragrance, hydrolyzed animal protein, hydroxyethylcellulose, polyoxyethylene 10 cetyl ether, propylene glycol, stearalkonium chloride, water, isopropyl alcohol 5.6 g (20%), methylparaben 56 mg (0.2%), and propylparaben 22 mg (0.08%).
Permethrin Lotion 1% kills lice and their unhatched eggs with usually only one application. Permethrin Lotion 1% protects against head lice reinfestation for 14 days. The creme rinse formula leaves hair manageable and easy to comb.

Indications: For the treatment of head lice. For prophylactic use during head lice epidemics.

Warnings: For external use only. Keep out of eyes when rinsing hair. Adults and children: Close eyes and do not open eyes until product is rinsed out. If product gets into the eyes, immediately flush with water. Do not use near the eyes or permit contact with mucous membranes, such as inside the nose, mouth, or vagina, as irritation may occur. Children: Also protect children's eyes with a washcloth, towel or other suitable material or method. This product should not be used on pediatric patients less than 2 months of age. Itching, redness, or swelling of the scalp may occur. If skin irritation persists or infection is present or develops, discontinue use and consult a doctor. Consult a doctor if infestation of eyebrows or eyelashes occurs. This product may cause breathing difficulty or an asthmatic episode in susceptible persons. As with any drug, if you are pregnant or nursing a baby, seek the advice of a health professional before using this product. Keep this and all drugs out of the reach of children. In case of accidental ingestion, seek professional assistance or contact a Poison Control Center immediately.

Dosage and Administration:
Treatment: Permethrin Lotion 1% should be used after hair has been washed with patient's regular shampoo, rinsed with water and towel dried. A sufficient amount should be applied to saturate hair and scalp (especially behind the ears and on the nape of the neck). Leave on hair for 10 minutes but not longer. Rinse with water. A single application is usually sufficient. If live lice are observed seven days or more after the first application of this product, a second treatment should be given. For proper head lice management, remove nits with the nit comb provided. Head lice live on the scalp and lay small white eggs (nits) on the hair shaft close to the scalp. The nits are most easily found on the nape of the neck or behind the ears. All personal headgear, scarfs, coats, and bed linen should be disinfected by machine washing in hot water and drying, using the hot cycle of a dryer for at least 20 minutes. Personal articles of clothing or bedding that cannot be washed may be dry-cleaned, sealed in a plastic bag for a period of about 2 weeks, or sprayed with a product specifically designed for this purpose. Personal combs and brushes may be disinfected by soaking in hot water (above 130°F) for 5 to 10 minutes. Thorough vacuuming of rooms inhabited by infected patients is recommended.
Prophylaxis: Prophylactic use of Permethrin Lotion 1% is only recommended for individuals exposed to head lice epidemics in which at least 20% of the population at an institution are infested and for immediate household members of infested individuals. Casual use is strongly discouraged.
The method of application of Permethrin Lotion 1% for prophylaxis is identical to that described above for treatment of a lice infestation except nit removal is not required.

Directions For Use: One application of Permethrin Lotion 1% has been shown to protect greater than 95% of patients against reinfestation for at least two weeks. In epidemic settings, a second prophylactic application is recommended two weeks after the first because the life cycle of a head louse is approximately four weeks.

How Supplied: Bottles of 2 fl. oz. (59 mL) with nit removal comb and Family Pack of 2 bottles, 2 fl. oz. (59 mL) each, with 2 nit removal combs.
Store at 15° to 25°C (59° to 77°F).
Manufactured by
Alpharma USPD Inc.
Baltimore, MD 21244
FORM NO. 5242   Rev. 9/99
              VC1587

Adams Respiratory Therapeutics
14841 SOVEREIGN ROAD
FORT WORTH, TX 76155

Direct Inquiries to:
Phone: 817-786-1200
Fax: 817-786-1150
866-MUCINEX

DELSYM® LIQUID
(Adams Respiratory Therapeutics)
Dextromethorphan polistirex
equivalent to 30 mg
dextromethorphan hydrobromide
Cough suppressant
Grape Flavor

Drug Facts
**Active ingredient
(in each 5 mL teaspoonful)**   **Purpose**
Dextromethorphan polistirex
equivalent to 30 mg
dextromethorphan
hydrobromide .... Cough suppressant

Use: temporarily relieves cough due to minor throat and bronchial irritation as may occur with the common cold or inhaled irritants

Warnings:
Do not use
- if you are now taking a prescription monoamine oxidase inhibitor (MAOI) (certain drugs for depression, psychiatric or emotional conditions, or Parkinson's disease), or for 2 weeks after stopping the MAOI drug. If you do not know if your prescription drug contains an MAOI, ask a doctor or pharmacist before taking this product.

Ask a doctor before use if you have
- chronic cough that lasts as occurs with smoking, asthma or emphysema
- cough that occurs with too much phlegm (mucus)

Stop use and ask a doctor if
- cough lasts more than 7 days, cough comes back, or occurs with fever, rash or headache that lasts. These could be signs of a serious condition.

If pregnant or breast-feeding, ask a health professional before use.
Keep out of reach of children. In case of overdose, get medical help or contact a Poison Control Center right away.

Directions:
- shake bottle well before use
- dose as follows or as directed by a doctor

adults and children 12 years of age and over	2 teaspoonfuls every 12 hours, not to exceed 4 teaspoonfuls in 24 hours
children 6 to under 12 years of age	1 teaspoonful every 12 hours, not to exceed 2 teaspoonfuls in 24 hours
children 2 to under 6 years of age	1/2 teaspoonful every 12 hours, not to exceed 1 teaspoonful in 24 hours
children under 2 years of age	consult a doctor

Other information:
- **each 5 mL teaspoonful contains:** sodium 6 mg
- store at 20°-25°C (68°-77°F)

Inactive ingredients: citric acid anhydrous, D&C Red #33, edetate disodium, ethylcellulose, FD&C Blue #1, flavor, high fructose corn syrup, methylparaben, polyethylene glycol 3350, polysorbate 80, propylene glycol, propylparaben, purified water, sucrose, tragacanth, vegetable oil, xanthan gum

How Supplied: Grape flavored liquid in bottles of 89 mL (3 fl oz)
(adult NDC 63824-171-63) (children's NDC 63824-172-63)

Shown in Product Identification Guide, page 502

DELSYM® LIQUID
(Adams Respiratory Therapeutics)
**Dextromethorphan polistirex
equivalent to 30 mg
dextromethorphan hydrobromide
Cough suppressant
Orange Flavor**

Drug Facts
**Active Ingredient
(in each 5 mL teaspoonful)   Purpose**
Dextromethorphan polistirex equivalent to 30 mg dextromethorphan hydrobromide .... Cough suppressant

Use: temporarily relieves cough due to minor throat and bronchial irritation as may occur with the common cold or inhaled irritants

Warnings:
Do not use
• if you are now taking a prescription monoamine oxidase inhibitor (MAOI) (certain drugs for depression, psychiatric or emotional conditions, or Parkinson's disease), or for 2 weeks after stopping the MAOI drug. If you do not know if your prescription drug contains an MAOI, ask a doctor or pharmacist before taking this product.
Ask a doctor before use if you have
• chronic cough that lasts as occurs with smoking, asthma or emphysema
• cough that occurs with too much phlegm (mucus)
Stop use and ask a doctor if
• cough lasts more than 7 days, cough comes back, or occurs with fever, rash or headache that lasts. These could be signs of a serious condition.
If pregnant or breast-feeding, ask a health professional before use.
Keep out of reach of children. In case of overdose, get medical help or contact a Poison Control Center right away.

Directions:
• **shake bottle well before use**
• dose as follows or as directed by a doctor

adults and children 12 years of age and over	2 teaspoonfuls every 12 hours, not to exceed 4 teaspoonfuls in 24 hours
children 6 to under 12 years of age	1 teaspoonful every 12 hours, not to exceed 2 teaspoonfuls in 24 hours
children 2 to under 6 years of age	1/2 teaspoonful every 12 hours, not to exceed 1 teaspoonful in 24 hours
children under 2 years of age	consult a doctor

Other information:
• **each 5 mL teaspoonful contains:** sodium 6 mg
• store at 20°-25°C (68°-77°F)

Inactive ingredients: citric acid, edetate disodium, ethylcellulose, FD&C Yellow No. 6, flavor, high fructose corn syrup, methylparaben, polyethylene glycol 3350, polysorbate 80, propylene glycol, propylparaben, purified water, sucrose, tragacanth, vegetable oil, xanthan gum

How Supplied: Orange flavored liquid in bottles of 89 mL (3 fl oz) (adult NDC 63824-175-63) (children's NDC 63824-176-63) and bottles of 148 mL (5 fl oz) (adult NDC 63824-175-65) (children's NDC 63824-176-65).

Shown in Product Identification Guide, page 502

MUCINEX® COUGH LIQUID
(Adams Respiratory Therapeutics)
**5 mg dextromethorphan HBr
and 100 mg guaifenesin
Cough suppressant and expectorant
Cherry Flavor**

Drug Facts
**Active ingredients
(in each 5 mL tsp)   Purpose**
Dextromethorphan HBr 5 mg .... Cough suppressant
Guaifenesin 100 mg .... Expectorant

Uses:
• helps loosen phlegm (mucus) and thin bronchial secretions to rid the bronchial passageways of bothersome mucus and make coughs more productive
• temporarily relieves:
• cough due to minor throat and bronchial irritation as may occur with the common cold or inhaled irritants
• the intensity of coughing
• the impulse to cough to help your child get to sleep

Warnings:
Do not use
• in a child who is taking a prescription monoamine oxidase inhibitor (MAOI) (certain drugs for depression, psychiatric, or emotional conditions, or Parkinson's disease), or for 2 weeks after stopping the MAOI drug. If you do not know if your child's prescription drug contains an MAOI, ask a doctor or pharmacist before giving this product.
Ask a doctor before use if the child has
• cough that occurs with too much phlegm (mucus)

• persistent or chronic cough such as occurs with asthma

Stop use and ask a doctor if cough lasts more than 7 days, comes back, or occurs with fever, rash, or persistent headache. These could be signs of a serious illness.
Keep out of reach of children. In case of overdose, get medical help or contact a Poison Control Center right away.

Directions:
• do not take more than 6 doses in any 24-hour period

Age	Dose
children 6 years to under 12 years	1-2 teaspoonfuls every 4 hours
children 2 years to under 6 years	1/2-1 teaspoonful every 4 hours
children under 2 years	ask a doctor

Other information:
• **each teaspoonful contains:** sodium 3.0 mg
• tamper evident: do not use if seal under bottle cap printed "SEALED for YOUR PROTECTION" is torn or missing.
• store between 20-25°C (68-77°F)
• dosage cup provided

Inactive ingredients: citric acid anhydrous, dextrose, D&C red #33, FD&C red #40, flavors, glycerin, methylparaben, potassium sorbate, propylene glycol, propylparaben, purified water, saccharin sodium, sodium hydroxide, sucralose, xanthan gum

How Supplied: Bottles of 4 fl oz (118 mL) (NDC 63824-174-64).

Shown in Product Identification Guide, page 502

MUCINEX® LIQUID
(Adams Respiratory Therapeutics)
**100 mg guaifenesin
Expectorant
Grape Flavor**

Drug Facts
**Active ingredient
(in each 5 mL tsp)   Purpose**
Guaifenesin 100 mg .... Expectorant

Uses: helps loosen phlegm (mucus) and thin bronchial secretions to rid the bronchial passageways of bothersome mucus and make coughs more productive

Warnings:
Ask a doctor before use if the child has
• cough that occurs with too much phlegm (mucus)
• persistent or chronic cough such as occurs with asthma

Stop use and ask a doctor if
• cough lasts more than 7 days, comes back, or occurs with fever, rash, or persistent headache. These could be signs of a serious illness.

Continued on next page

Mucinex Liquid—Cont.

Keep out of reach of children. In case of overdose, get medical help or contact a Poison Control Center right away.

Directions:
- do not take more than 6 doses in any 24-hour period

Age	Dose
children 6 years to under 12 years	1-2 teaspoonfuls every 4 hours
children 2 years to under 6 years	1/2-1 teaspoonful every 4 hours
children under 2 years	ask a doctor

Other information:
- **each teaspoonful contains:** sodium 3.0 mg
- tamper evident: do not use if seal under bottle cap printed "SEALED for YOUR PROTECTION" is torn or missing.
- store between 20-25°C (68-77°F)
- dosage cup provided

Inactive ingredients: citric acid anhydrous, dextrose, FD&C blue #1, FD&C red #40, flavor, glycerin, methylparaben, potassium sorbate, propylene glycol, propylparaben, purified water, saccharin sodium, sodium hydroxide, sucralose, xanthan gum

How Supplied: Bottles of 4 fl oz (118 mL) (NDC 63824-173-64).

Shown in Product Identification Guide, page 502

MUCINEX® COLD LIQUID

(Adams Respiratory Therapeutics)
100 mg guaifenesin and
2.5 mg Phenylephrine HCl
Expectorant
Nasal Decongestant
Mixed Berry Flavor

Drug Facts
Active ingredients
(in each 5 mL tsp)   **Purpose**
Guaifenesin 100 mg .... Expectorant
Phenylephrine
HCl 2.5 mg .... Nasal decongestant

Uses:
- helps loosen phlegm (mucus) and thin bronchial secretions to rid the bronchial passageways of bothersome mucus and make coughs more productive
- temporarily relieves:
  - nasal congestion due to a cold
  - stuffy nose

Warnings:
Do not use
- in a child who is taking a prescription monoamine oxidase inhibitor (MAOI) (certain drugs for depression, psychiatric, or emotional conditions, or Parkinson's disease), or for 2 weeks after stopping the MAOI drug. If you do not know if your child's prescription drug contains an MAOI, ask a doctor or pharmacist before giving this product.

Ask a doctor before use if the child has
- heart disease
- high blood pressure
- thyroid disease
- diabetes
- cough that occurs with too much phlegm (mucus)
- persistent or chronic cough such as occurs with asthma

When using this product
- **do not use more than directed**

Stop use and ask a doctor if
- you get nervous, dizzy or sleepless
- symptoms do not get better within 7 days or occur with fever
- cough lasts more than 7 days, comes back, or occurs with fever, rash, or persistent headache. These could be signs of a serious illness.

Keep out of reach of children. In case of overdose, get medical help or contact a Poison Control Center right away.

Directions:
- do not take more than 6 doses in any 24-hour period

Age	Dose
children 6 years to under 12 years	2 teaspoonfuls every 4 hours
children 2 years to under 6 years	1 teaspoonful every 4 hours
children under 2 years	ask a doctor

Other information:
- **each teaspoonful contains:** sodium 5.0 mg
- tamper evident: do not use if seal under bottle cap printed "SEALED for YOUR PROTECTION" is torn or missing.
- store between 20-25°C (68-77°F)
- dosage cup provided

Inactive ingredients: citric acid anhydrous, dextrose, D&C red #33, FD&C blue #1, FD&C red#40, flavors, glycerin, methylparaben, potassium sorbate, propyl gallate, propylene glycol, propylparaben, purified water, saccharin sodium, sodium hydroxide, sorbitol solution, sucralose, xanthan gum

How Supplied: Bottles of 4 fl oz (118 mL) (NDC 63824-177-64).

Shown in Product Identification Guide, page 502

MUCINEX® MINI-MELTS™

(Adams Respiratory Therapeutics)
100 mg guaifenesin
Expectorant
Bubble Gum Flavor

Drug Facts
Active ingredient
(in each packet)   **Purpose**
Guaifenesin, USP 100 mg ... Expectorant

Uses: helps loosen phlegm (mucus) and thin bronchial secretions to rid the bronchial passageways of bothersome mucus and make coughs more productive

Warnings:
Ask a doctor before use if you have
- persistent or chronic cough such as occurs with smoking, asthma, chronic bronchitis, or emphysema
- cough that occurs with too much phlegm (mucus)

Stop use and ask a doctor if
- cough lasts more than 7 days, comes back, or occurs with fever, rash, or persistent headache. These could be signs of a serious illness.

If pregnant or breastfeeding, ask a health professional before use.
Keep out of reach of children. In case of overdose, get medical help or contact a Poison Control Center right away.

Directions:
- empty entire contents of packet onto tongue and swallow
- for best taste, do not chew granules
- do not take more than 6 doses in any 24-hour period

Age	Dose
adults and children 12 years and over	2 to 4 packets every 4 hours
children 6 years to under 12 years	1 to 2 packets every 4 hours
children 2 years to under 6 years	1 packet every 4 hours
children under 2 years	ask a doctor

Other information:
- **phenylketonurics:** contains phenylalanine 1.0 mg per packet
- **each packet contains:** magnesium 10.0 mg and sodium 2.0 mg
- store between 15-25°C (59-77°F)
- tamper evident: do not use if carton is open or if packets are torn or open

Inactive ingredients: aspartame, banana flavor, butylated methacrylate copolymer, carbomer, carboxymethylcellulose, sodium, magnesium stearate, microcrystalline cellulose, povidone, sodium bicarbonate, sorbitol, stearic acid, talc, triethyl citrate, tutti-frutti flavor

How Supplied: Cartons of 12 packets of 100 mg guaifenesin granules (NDC 63824-154-12)

Shown in Product Identification Guide, page 502

MUCINEX® MINI-MELTS™

(Adams Respiratory Therapeutics)
50 mg guaifenesin
Expectorant
Grape Flavor

Drug Facts
Active ingredient
(in each packet)   **Purpose**
Guaifenesin, USP 50 mg .... Expectorant

Uses:
helps loosen phlegm (mucus) and thin bronchial secretions to rid the bronchial

passageways of bothersome mucus and make coughs more productive

Warnings:

Ask a doctor before use if the child has

- persistent or chronic cough such as occurs with asthma or chronic bronchitis
- cough that occurs with too much phlegm (mucus)

Stop use and ask a doctor if

- cough lasts more than 7 days, comes back, or occurs with fever, rash, or persistent headache. These could be signs of a serious illness.

Keep out of reach of children. In case of overdose, get medical help or contact a Poison Control Center right away.

Directions:

- empty entire contents of packet onto tongue and swallow
- for best taste, do not chew granules
- do not take more than 6 doses in any 24-hour period

Age	Dose
children 6 years to under 12 years	2 to 4 packets every 4 hours
children 2 years to under 6 years	1 to 2 packets every 4 hours
children under 2 years	ask a doctor

Other information:

- phenylketonurics: contains phenylalanine 0.6 mg per packet
- each packet contains: magnesium 10.0 mg and sodium 2.0 mg
- store between 15-25°C (59-77°F)
- tamper evident: do not use if carton is open or if packets are torn or open

Inactive ingredients: aspartame, butylated methacrylate copolymer, carbomer, carboxymethylcellulose sodium, grape flavor, magnesium stearate, microcrystalline cellulose, povidone, raspberry flavor, sodium bicarbonate, sorbitol, stearic acid, talc, triethyl citrate

How Supplied: Cartons of 12 packets of 50 mg guaifenesin granules (NDC 63824-153-12)

Shown in Product Identification Guide, page 502

MUCINEX® COUGH MINI-MELTS™
(Adams Respiratory Therapeutics)
100 mg guaifenesin and
5 mg dextromethorphan HBr
Expectorant
Cough suppressant
Orange Creme Flavor

Drug Facts

Active ingredients
(in each packet) .... **Purpose**
Dextromethorphan
HBr 5 mg .... Cough suppressant
Guaifenesin 100 mg .... Expectorant

Uses:

- helps loosen phlegm (mucus) and thin bronchial secretions to rid the bronchial passageways of bothersome mucus and make coughs more productive
- temporarily relieves:
  - cough due to minor throat and bronchial irritation as may occur with the common cold or inhaled irritants
  - the intensity of coughing
  - the impulse to cough to help you get to sleep

Warnings:

Do not use

- if you are now taking a prescription monoamine oxidase inhibitor (MAOI) (certain drugs for depression, psychiatric, or emotional conditions, or Parkinson's disease), or for 2 weeks after stopping the MAOI drug. If you do not know if your prescription drug contains a MAOI, ask a doctor or pharmacist before taking this product.

Ask a doctor before use if you have

- persistent or chronic cough such as occurs with smoking, asthma, chronic bronchitis, or emphysema
- cough that occurs with too much phlegm (mucus)

Stop use and ask a doctor if

- cough lasts more than 7 days, comes back, or occurs with fever, rash, or persistent headache. These could be signs of a serious illness.

If pregnant or breast-feeding, ask a healthcare professional before use.

Keep out of reach of children. In case of overdose, get medical help or contact a Poison Control Center right away.

Directions:

- empty entire contents of packet onto tongue and swallow
- for best taste, do not chew granules
- do not take more than 6 doses in any 24-hour period

Age	Dose
adults and children 12 years and over	2 to 4 packets every 4 hours
children 6 years to under 12 years	1 to 2 packets every 4 hours
children 2 years to under 6 years	1 packet every 4 hours
children under 2 years	ask a doctor

Other information:

- **each packet contains:** magnesium 6.0 mg and sodium 2.0 mg
- **phenylketonurics:** contains phenylalanine 2.0 mg per packet
- store between 15-25°C (59-77°F)
- tamper evident: do not use if carton is open or if packets are torn or open

Inactive ingredients: aspartame, butylated methacrylate copolymer, carbomer homopolymer, creme flavor, magnesium stearate, microcrystalline cellulose, orange flavor, povidone, sodium bicarbonate, sodium carboxymethylcellulose, sorbitol, stearic acid, talc, triethyl citrate

How Supplied: Cartons of 12 packets of 100 mg guaifenesin and 5 mg dextromethorphan HBr granules (NDC 63824-156-12)

Shown in Product Identification Guide, page 502

MUCINEX®
(Adams Respiratory Therapeutics)
600 mg Guaifenesin
Extended-Release Bi-Layer Tablets
Expectorant

Drug Facts

Active Ingredient: **Purpose:**
(in each extended-release bi-layer tablet)
Guaifenesin 600 mg .... Expectorant

Uses: helps loosen phlegm (mucus) and thin bronchial secretions to rid the bronchial passageways of bothersome mucus and make coughs more productive

Warnings:

Do not use

- for children under 12 years of age

Ask a doctor before use if you have

- persistent or chronic cough such as occurs with smoking, asthma, chronic bronchitis, or emphysema
- cough accompanied by too much phlegm (mucus)

Stop use and ask a doctor if

- cough lasts more than 7 days, comes back, or occurs with fever, rash, or persistent headache. These could be signs of a serious illness.

If pregnant or breast-feeding, ask a health professional before use.

Keep out of reach of children. In case of overdose, get medical help or contact a Poison Control Center right away.

Directions:

- do not crush, chew, or break tablet
- take with a full glass of water
- this product can be administered without regard for the timing of meals
- adults and children 12 years of age and over: one or two tablets every 12 hours. Do not exceed 4 tablets in 24 hours.
- children under 12 years of age: do not use

Other Information:

- tamper evident: do not use if seal on bottle printed "SEALED for YOUR PROTECTION" is broken or missing
- store between 20–25°C (68–77°F)

Inactive Ingredients: carbomer 934P, NF; FD&C blue #1 aluminum lake; hypromellose, USP; magnesium stearate, NF; microcrystalline cellulose, NF; sodium starch glycolate, NF

How Supplied:
Bottles of 20 tablets (NDC 63824-008-20), 40 tablets (NDC 63824-008-40), 60 tablets (NDC 63824-008-60), 100 tablets (NDC 63824-008-10) and 500 tablets (NDC 63824-008-50). A round bi-layer tablet de-

Continued on next page

Mucinex—Cont.

bossed with "A" on the light blue, marbled layer and "600" on the white layer. Each tablet provides 600 mg guaifenesin. US Patent Nos. 6,372,252 B1 and 6,955,821 B2

Shown in Product Identification Guide, page 502

MUCINEX®
(Adams Respiratory Therapeutics)
1200 mg guaifenesin
Extended-Release Bi-Layer Tablets
Expectorant

Drug Facts

Active ingredient	Purpose

(in each extended-release bi-layer tablet)
Guaifenesin 1200 mg .... Expectorant

Uses: helps loosen phlegm (mucus) and thin bronchial secretions to rid the bronchial passageways of bothersome mucus and make coughs more productive

Warnings:
Do not use
• for children under 12 years of age

Ask a doctor before use if you have
• persistent or chronic cough such as occurs with smoking, asthma, chronic bronchitis, or emphysema
• cough accompanied by too much phlegm (mucus)

Stop use and ask a doctor if
• cough lasts more than 7 days, comes back, or occurs with fever, rash, or persistent headache. These could be signs of a serious illness.

If pregnant or breast-feeding, ask a health professional before use.
Keep out of reach of children. In case of overdose, get medical help or contact a Poison Control Center right away.

Directions:
• do not crush, chew, or break tablet
• take with a full glass of water
• this product can be administered without regard for the timing of meals
• adults and children 12 years of age and over: 1 tablet every 12 hours. Do not exceed 2 tablets in 24 hours.
• children under 12 years of age: do not use

Other information:
• tamper evident: do not use if carton is open or if seal on bottle printed "SEALED for YOUR PROTECTION" is broken or missing
• store between 20-25°C (68-77°F)

Inactive ingredients: carbomer 934P, NF; FD&C blue #1 aluminum lake; hypromellose, USP; magnesium stearate, NF; microcrystalline cellulose, NF; sodium starch glycolate, NF

How Supplied: Boxes of 14 tablets (NDC 63824-023-14) and 28 tablets (NDC 63824-023-28). A modified oval bi-layer tablet debossed with "Adams" on the blue layer and "1200" on the white layer. Each tablet provides 1200 mg guaifenesin. US Patent Nos. 6,372,252 B1 and 6,955,821 B2

Shown in Product Identification Guide, page 502

MUCINEX® D
(Adams Respiratory Therapeutics)
600 mg Guaifenesin and 60 mg Pseudoephedrine HCl
Extended-Release Bi-Layer Tablets
Expectorant and Nasal Decongestant

Drug Facts

Active Ingredients:	Purpose:

(in each extended-release bi-layer tablet)
Guaifenesin 600 mg .... Expectorant
Pseudoephedrine HCl 60 mg .... Nasal Decongestant

Uses:
• helps loosen phlegm (mucus) and thin bronchial secretions to rid the bronchial passageways of bothersome mucus and make coughs more productive
• temporarily relieves nasal congestion due to:
  • common cold
  • hay fever
  • upper respiratory allergies
• temporarily restores freer breathing through the nose
• promotes nasal and/or sinus drainage
• temporarily relieves sinus congestion and pressure

Warnings:
Do not use if you are now taking a prescription monoamine oxidase inhibitor (MAOI) (certain drugs for depression, psychiatric or emotional conditions, or Parkinson's disease), or for 2 weeks after stopping the MAOI drug. If you do not know if your prescription drug contains a MAOI, ask a doctor or pharmacist before taking this product.

Ask a doctor before use if you have
• heart disease
• high blood pressure
• thyroid disease
• diabetes
• trouble urinating due to an enlarged prostate gland
• persistent or chronic cough such as occurs with smoking, asthma, chronic bronchitis, or emphysema
• cough accompanied by too much phlegm (mucus)

When using this product
• do not use more than directed

Stop use and ask a doctor if
• you get nervous, dizzy, or sleepless
• symptoms do not get better within 7 days, come back or occur with a fever,

rash, or persistent headache. These could be signs of a serious illness.

If pregnant or breast-feeding, ask a health professional before use.

Keep out of reach of children. In case of overdose, get medical help or contact a Poison Control Center right away.

Directions:
• do not crush, chew, or break tablet
• take with a full glass of water
• this product can be administered without regard for timing of meals
• adults and children 12 years and older: two tablets every 12 hours; not more than 4 tablets in 24 hours
• children under 12 years of age: do not use

Other Information:
• tamper evident: do not use if printed seal on blister is broken or missing
• store at 20-25°C (68-77°F)

Inactive Ingredients: carbomer 934P, NF; FD&C yellow #6 aluminum lake; hypromellose, USP; magnesium stearate, NF; microcrystalline cellulose, NF; sodium starch glycolate, NF

How Supplied: Boxes of 18 tablets (in blisters of 6) (NDC 63824-057-18), 36 tablets (in blisters of 6) (NDC 63824-057-36). A modified oval bi-layer tablet debossed with "Adams" on the orange layer and "600" on the white layer. Each tablet provides 600 mg guaifenesin and 60 mg pseudoephedrine HCl. US Patent Nos. 6,372,252 B1 and 6,955,821 B2

Shown in Product Identification Guide, page 502

MUCINEX® D
(Adams Respiratory Therapeutics)
1200 mg guaifenesin and
120 mg Pseudoephedrine HCl
Extended-Release Bi-Layer Tablets
Expectorant
Nasal Decongestant

Drug Facts

Active ingredients	Purpose

(in each extended-release bi-layer tablet)
Guaifenesin 1200 mg .... Expectorant
Pseudoephedrine HCl 120 mg .... Nasal Decongestant

Uses:
• helps loosen phlegm (mucus) and thin bronchial secretions to rid the bronchial passageways of bothersome mucus and make coughs more productive
• temporarily relieves nasal congestion due to:
  • common cold • hay fever
  • upper respiratory allergies
• temporarily restores freer breathing through the nose
• promotes nasal and/or sinus drainage
• temporarily relieves sinus congestion and pressure

Warnings:

Do not use

- if you are now taking a prescription monoamine oxidase inhibitor (MAOI) (certain drugs for depression, psychiatric or emotional conditions, or Parkinson's disease), or for 2 weeks after stopping the MAOI drug. If you do not know if your prescription drug contains a MAOI, ask a doctor or pharmacist before taking this product.

Ask a doctor before use if you have

- heart disease
- high blood pressure
- thyroid disease   • diabetes
- trouble urinating due to an enlarged prostate gland
- persistent or chronic cough such as occurs with smoking, asthma, chronic bronchitis, or emphysema
- cough accompanied by too much phlegm (mucus)

When using this product

- **do not use more than directed**

Stop use and ask a doctor if

- you get nervous, dizzy, or sleepless
- symptoms do not get better within 7 days, come back or occur with a fever, rash, or persistent headache. These could be signs of a serious illness.

If pregnant or breast-feeding, ask a health professional before use.
Keep out of reach of children. In case of overdose, get medical help or contact a Poison Control Center right away.

Directions:

- do not crush, chew, or break tablet
- take with a full glass of water
- this product can be administered without regard for timing of meals
- adults and children 12 years and older: 1 tablet every 12 hours; not more than 2 tablets in 24 hours
- children under 12 years of age: do not use

Other information:

- tamper evident: do not use if printed seal on blister is broken or missing
- store at 20-25°C (68-77°F)

Inactive ingredients: carbomer 934P, NF; FD&C yellow #6 aluminum lake; hypromellose, USP; magnesium stearate, NF; microcrystalline cellulose, NF; sodium starch glycolate, NF

How Supplied: Boxes of 24 tablets (in blisters of 6) (NDC 63824-041-24). A modified oval bi-layer tablet debossed with "Adams" on the peach layer and "1200" on the white layer. Each tablet provides 1200 mg guaifenesin and 120 mg pseudoephedrine HCl. US Patent Nos. 6,372,252 B1 and 6,955,821 B2
Shown in Product Identification Guide, page 502

MUCINEX® DM
(Adams Respiratory Therapeutics)
600 mg Guaifenesin and 30 mg
Dextromethorphan HBr
Extended-Release Bi-Layer Tablets
Expectorant and Cough Suppressant

Drug Facts

Active Ingredients:　　　　　**Purpose:**
(in each extended-release bi-layer tablet)
Dextromethorphan HBr
30 mg .... Cough suppressant
Guaifenesin 600 mg .... Expectorant

Uses:

- helps loosen phlegm (mucus) and thin bronchial secretions to rid the bronchial passageways of bothersome mucus and make coughs more productive
- temporarily relieves:
cough due to minor throat and bronchial irritation as may occur with the common cold or inhaled irritants
- the intensity of coughing
- the impulse to cough to help you get to sleep

Warnings:

Do not use

- for children under 12 years of age
- if you are now taking a prescription monoamine oxidase inhibitor (MAOI) (certain drugs for depression, psychiatric or emotional conditions, or Parkinson's disease), or for 2 weeks after stopping the MAOI drug. If you do not know if your prescription drug contains a MAOI, ask a doctor or pharmacist before taking this product.

Ask a doctor before use if you have

- persistent or chronic cough such as occurs with smoking, asthma, chronic bronchitis, or emphysema
- cough accompanied by too much phlegm (mucus)

When using this product

- do not use more than directed

Stop use and ask a doctor if

- cough lasts more than 7 days, comes back, or occurs with fever, rash, or persistent headache. These could be signs of a serious illness.

If pregnant or breast-feeding, ask a health professional before use.
Keep out of reach of children. In case of overdose, get medical help or contact a Poison Control Center right away.

Directions:

- do not crush, chew, or break tablet
- take with a full glass of water
- this product can be administered without regard for timing of meals
- adults and children 12 years and older: one or two tablets every 12 hours; not more than 4 tablets in 24 hours
- children under 12 years of age: do not use

Other Information:

- tamper evident: do not use if seal on bottle printed "SEALED for YOUR PROTECTION" is broken or missing
- store at 20–25°C (68–77°F)

Inactive Ingredients: carbomer 934P, NF; D&C yellow #10 aluminum lake; hypromellose, USP; magnesium stearate, NF; microcrystalline cellulose, NF; sodium starch glycolate, NF

How Supplied:

Bottles of 20 tablets (NDC 63824-056-20), 40 tablets (NDC 63824-056-40) and 54 tablets (NDC 63824-056-54).
A modified oval bi-layer tablet debossed with "Adams" on the yellow layer and "600" on the white layer. Each tablet provides 600 mg guaifenesin and 30 mg dextromethorphan HBr. US Patent Nos. 6,372,252 B1 and 6,955,821 B2
Shown in Product Identification Guide, page 502

MUCINEX® DM
(Adams Respiratory Therapeutics)
1200 mg guaifenesin and
60 mg Dextromethorphan HBr
Extended-Release Bi-Layer Tablets
Expectorant
Cough Suppressant

Drug Facts

Active ingredients　　　　　　**Purpose**
(in each extended-release bi-layer tablet)
Dextromethorphan HBr
60 mg .... Cough suppressant
Guaifenesin 1200 mg .... Expectorant

Uses:

- helps loosen phlegm (mucus) and thin bronchial secretions to rid the bronchial passageways of bothersome mucus and make coughs more productive
- temporarily relieves:
- cough due to minor throat and bronchial irritation as may occur with the common cold or inhaled irritants
- the intensity of coughing
- the impulse to cough to help you get to sleep

Warnings:

Do not use

- for children under 12 years of age
- if you are now taking a prescription monoamine oxidase inhibitor (MAOI) (certain drugs for depression, psychiatric or emotional conditions, or Parkinson's disease), or for 2 weeks after stopping the MAOI drug. If you do not know if your prescription drug contains a MAOI, ask a doctor or pharmacist before taking this product.

Ask a doctor before use if you have

- persistent or chronic cough such as occurs with smoking, asthma, chronic bronchitis, or emphysema
- cough accompanied by too much phlegm (mucus)

When using this product

- do not use more than directed

Continued on next page

Mucinex DM—Cont.

Stop use and ask a doctor if

- cough lasts more than 7 days, comes back, or occurs with fever, rash, or persistent headache. These could be signs of a serious illness.

If pregnant or breast-feeding, ask a health professional before use.

Keep out of reach of children. In case of overdose, get medical help or contact a Poison Control Center right away.

Directions:

- do not crush, chew, or break tablet
- take with a full glass of water
- this product can be administered without regard for timing of meals
- adults and children 12 years and older: 1 tablet every 12 hours; not more than 2 tablets in 24 hours
- children under 12 years of age: do not use

Other information:

- tamper evident: do not use if carton is open or if seal on bottle printed "SEALED for YOUR PROTECTION" is broken or missing
- store at 20-25°C (68-77°F)

Inactive ingredients: carbomer 934P, NF; D&C yellow #10 aluminum lake; hypromellose, USP; magnesium stearate, NF; microcrystalline cellulose, NF; sodium starch glycolate, NF

How Supplied: Boxes of 14 tablets (NDC 63824-072-14) and 28 tablets (NDC 63824-072-28). A modified oval bi-layer tablet debossed with "Adams" on the yellow layer and "1200" on the white layer. Each tablet provides 1200 mg guaifenesin and 60 mg Dextromethorphan HBr. US Patent Nos. 6,372,252 B1 and 6,955,821 B2

Shown in Product Identification Guide, page 502

Beutlich LP, Pharmaceuticals

1541 SHIELDS DRIVE
WAUKEGAN, IL 60085-8304

Direct Inquiries to:
(847) 473-1100
(800) 238-8542 in the U.S. and Canada
M-Th: 7:30 a.m. - 4:00 p.m. CT
FAX: (847) 473-1122
http://www.beutlich.com
E-mail: beutlich@beutich.com

HURRICAINE® Topical Anesthetic
20% Benzocaine Oral Anesthetic
(Beutlich LP)

Formats available: Gel, Liquid, Snap-n-Go™ Swabs and Spray

Uses: for the temporary relief of occasional minor irritation and pain, associated with

- Canker sores
- Sore mouth and throat
- Minor dental procedures
- Minor injury of the mouth and gums
- Minor irritation of the mouth and gums dentures or orthodontic appliances

Works fast – within 20 seconds
Safe – available OTC
Tastes good – great flavors
No artificial colors

Packaging Available

GEL

1 oz. jar Wild Cherry - NDC #0283-0871-31
1 oz. jar Pina Colada - NDC #0283-0886-31
1 oz. jar Watermelon - NDC #0283-0293-31
1 oz. jar Fresh Mint - NDC #0283-0998-31
5.25 g. tube - Wild Cherry - NDC #0283-0871-75

LIQUID

1 fl. oz. jar Wild Cherry - NDC #0283-0569-31
1 fl. oz. jar Pina Colada - NDC #0283-1886-31
Snap-n-Go Swabs - 72 each per box NDC #0283-0569-72
Snap-n-Go Swabs - 8 each per travel pack - NDC #0283-0569-08

SPRAY

2 oz. Aerosol Wild Cherry with 1 extension tube NDC #0283-0679-02

SPRAY KIT

2 oz. Aerosol Wild Cherry with 200 extension tubes NDC #0283-0679-60

Boehringer Ingelheim Consumer Health Care Products Division

DIVISION OF BOEHRINGER INGELHEIM PHARMACEUTICALS, INC.
900 RIDGEBURY ROAD
P.O. BOX 368
RIDGEFIELD, CT 06877

Direct Inquiries to:
(888) 285-9159

DULCOLAX® LAXATIVE TABLETS
(Boehringer Ingelheim Consumer Health Care Products Division)
[*dul cō-lax*]
brand of bisacodyl USP
Tablets of 5 mg laxative

Drug Facts
Active Ingredient:
(in each tablet) **Purpose:**
Bisacodyl USP, 5 mg .... Laxative

Uses:

- relieves occasional constipation and irregularity
- this product usually causes bowel movement in 6 to 12 hours

Warnings:

Do not use if you cannot swallow without chewing

Ask a doctor before use if you have

- stomach pain, nausea or vomiting
- a sudden change in bowel habits that lasts more than 2 weeks

When using this product

- do not chew or crush tablet
- do not use within 1 hour after taking an antacid or milk
- you may have stomach discomfort, faintness or cramps

Stop use and ask a doctor if

- rectal bleeding or failure to have a bowel movement occurs after use of a laxative. These could be signs of a serious condition.
- you need to use a laxative for more than 1 week

If pregnant or breast-feeding, ask a doctor before use.

Keep out of reach of children. In case of overdose, get medical help or contact a Poison Control Center right away.

Directions:

adults and children 12 years and over	take 1 to 3 tablets (usually 2) daily
children 6 to under 12 years	take 1 tablet daily
children under 6 years	ask a doctor

Other Information:

- store at 20-25°C (68-77°F)
- avoid excessive humidity

Inactive Ingredients: acacia, acetylated monoglyceride, carnauba wax, cellulose acetate phthalate, corn starch, dibutyl phthalate, docusate sodium, gelatin, glycerin, iron oxides, kaolin, lactose, magnesium stearate, methylparaben, pharmaceutical glaze, polyethylene glycol, povidone, propylparaben, Red No. 30 lake, sodium benzoate, sorbitan monooleate, sucrose, talc, titanium dioxide, white wax, Yellow No. 10 lake.

How Supplied: Boxes of 10, 25, 50, 100 and 150 comfort coated tablets

Questions about DULCOLAX?
Call toll-free **1-888-285-9159**
Or visit **www.Dulcolax.com**
Se habla Español.
Boehringer Ingelheim Consumer Health Care Products Division
Division of Boehringer Ingelheim Pharmaceuticals, Inc., Ridgefield, CT 06877
Made in Mexico

Shown in Product Identification Guide, page 503

DULCOLAX® LAXATIVE SUPPOSITORIES
(Boehringer Ingelheim Consumer Health Care Products Division)
[*dul cō-lax*]
brand of bisacodyl USP
Suppositories of 10 mg laxative

Drug Facts
Active Ingredient:
(in each suppository)   Purpose:
Bisacodyl USP, 10 mg .... Laxative

Uses:
- relieves occasional constipation and irregularity
- this product usually causes bowel movement in 15 minutes to 1 hour

Warnings:
For rectal use only
Do not use when abdominal pain, nausea or vomiting are present

Ask a doctor before use if you have
- stomach pain, nausea or vomiting
- a sudden change in bowel habits that lasts more than 2 weeks

When using this product you may have abdominal discomfort, faintness, rectal burning and mild cramps

Stop use and ask a doctor if
- rectal bleeding or failure to have a bowel movement occurs after use of a laxative. These could be signs of a serious condition.
- you need to use a laxative for more than 1 week

If pregnant or breast-feeding, ask a doctor before use.
Keep out of reach of children. If swallowed, get medical help or contact a Poison Control Center right away.

Directions:

adults and children 12 years and over	1 suppository once daily. Remove foil. Insert suppository well into rectum, pointed end first. Retain about 15 to 20 minutes.
children 6 to under 12 years	½ suppository once daily
children under 6 years	ask a doctor

Other Information:
- store at controlled room temperature 20-25°C (68-77°F)

Inactive Ingredients: hydrogenated vegetable oil

How Supplied: Boxes of 4, 8, 16 and 28 comfort shaped suppositories

Questions about DULCOLAX?
Call toll-free **1-888-285-9159**
Or visit www.Dulcolax.com
Se habla Español.
Boehringer Ingelheim Consumer Health Care Products Division
Division of Boehringer Ingelheim Pharmaceuticals, Inc., Ridgefield, CT 06877
Made in Italy
Shown in Product Identification Guide, page 503

DULCOLAX® STOOL SOFTENER
(Boehringer Ingelheim Consumer Health Care Products Division)
[*dul cō-lax*]
brand of docusate sodium USP
Liquid gel of 100 mg stool softener

Drug Facts
Active Ingredient:
(in each liquid gel)   Purpose:
Docusate sodium, 100 mg .... Stool softener

Uses:
- temporary relief of occasional constipation
- this product generally produces bowel movement within 12 to 72 hours

Warnings:
Do not use if abdominal pain, nausea or vomiting are present

Ask a doctor before use if you
- have noticed a sudden change in bowel habits that persists over a period of 2 weeks
- are presently taking mineral oil

Stop use and ask a doctor if
- rectal bleeding or failure to have a bowel movement occur after use, which may indicate a serious condition
- you need to use a laxative for more than 1 week

If pregnant or breast-feeding, ask a health professional before use.
Keep out of reach of children. In case of overdose, get medical help or contact a Poison Control Center immediately.

Directions:

adults and children 12 years and over	take 1 to 3 liquid gels daily
children 2 to under 12 years	take 1 liquid gel daily
children under 2 years	ask a doctor

Other Information:
- each liquid gel contains: sodium 5 mg

- store at 15-30°C (59-86°F)
- protect from excessive moisture

Inactive Ingredients: FD&C Red #40, FD&C Yellow #6, gelatin, glycerin, polyethylene glycol, propylene glycol, purified water, sorbitol special.

How Supplied: Bottles of 25, 50, 100 and 180 Liquid Gels

Questions about DULCOLAX?
Call toll-free **1-888-285-9159**
Or visit www.Dulcolax.com
Se habla Español.
Boehringer Ingelheim Consumer Health Care Products Division
Division of Boehringer Ingelheim Pharmaceuticals, Inc., Ridgefield, CT 06877
Shown in Product Identification Guide, page 503

ZANTAC 75®
(Boehringer Ingelheim Consumer Health Care Products Division)
brand of ranitidine USP
Tablet of 75 mg acid reducer

Drug Facts
Active ingredient
(in each tablet)   Purpose
Ranitidine 75 mg (as ranitidine hydrochloride 84 mg) .... Acid reducer

Uses
- relieves heartburn associated with acid indigestion and sour stomach
- prevents heartburn associated with acid indigestion and sour stomach brought on by certain foods and beverages

Warnings
Allergy alert: Do not use if you are allergic to ranitidine or other acid reducers

Do not use
- if you have trouble or pain swallowing food, vomiting with blood, or bloody or black stools. These may be signs of a serious condition. See your doctor.
- with other acid reducers

Ask a doctor before use if you have
- frequent **chest pain**
- frequent wheezing, particularly with heartburn
- unexplained weight loss
- nausea or vomiting
- stomach pain
- had heartburn over 3 months. This may be a sign of a more serious condition
- heartburn with **lightheadedness, sweating or dizziness**
- chest pain or shoulder pain with shortness of breath; sweating; pain spreading to arms, neck or shoulders; or lightheadedness

Stop use and ask a doctor if
- your heartburn continues or worsens

Continued on next page

Zantac 75—Cont.

- you need to take this product for more than 14 days

If pregnant or breast-feeding, ask a health professional before use.

Keep out of reach of children. In case of overdose, get medical help or contact a Poison Control Center right away.

Directions

- adults and children 12 years and over:
  - to **relieve** symptoms, swallow 1 tablet with a glass of water
  - to **prevent** symptoms, swallow 1 tablet with a glass of water **30 to 60 minutes before** eating food or drinking beverages that cause heartburn
  - can be used up to twice daily (do not take more than 2 tablets in 24 hours)
- children under 12 years: ask a doctor

Other information

- do not use if printed foil under bottle cap is open or torn
- store at 20°-25°C (68°-77°F)
- avoid excessive heat or humidity
- this product is sodium and sugar free

Inactive ingredients

Hypromellose, magnesium stearate, microcrystalline cellulose, synthetic red iron oxide, titanium dioxide, triacetin

Read the directions, consumer information leaflet and warnings before use. Keep the carton. It contains important information.

Questions about ZANTAC?

Call toll-free **1-888-285-9159**

Or visit **www.zantacotc.com**

Boehringer Ingelheim Consumer Health Care Products Division

Division of Boehringer Ingelheim Pharmaceuticals, Inc., Ridgefield, CT 06877

Copyright © 2007, Boehringer Ingelheim Pharmaceuticals, Inc. All rights reserved.

Shown in Product Identification Guide, page 503

MAXIMUM STRENGTH
ZANTAC 150®
(Boehringer Ingelheim Consumer Health Care Products Division) brand of ranitidine USP Tablet of 150 mg acid reducer

Drug Facts

Active ingredient (in each tablet)   **Purpose**

Ranitidine 150 mg (as ranitidine hydrochloride 168 mg) .... Acid reducer

Uses

- relieves heartburn associated with acid indigestion and sour stomach
- prevents heartburn associated with acid indigestion and sour stomach brought on by certain foods and beverages

Warnings

Allergy alert: Do not use if you are allergic to ranitidine or other acid reducers

Do not use

- if you have trouble or pain swallowing food, vomiting with blood, or bloody or black stools. These may be signs of a serious condition. See your doctor.
- with other acid reducers
- if you have kidney disease, except under the advice and supervision of a doctor

Ask a doctor before use if you have

- frequent **chest pain**
- frequent wheezing, particularly with heartburn
- unexplained weight loss
- nausea or vomiting
- stomach pain
- had heartburn over 3 months. This may be a sign of a more serious condition.
- heartburn with **lightheadedness, sweating or dizziness**
- chest pain or shoulder pain with shortness of breath; sweating; pain spreading to arms, neck or shoulders; or lightheadedness

Stop use and ask a doctor if

- your heartburn continues or worsens
- you need to take this product for more than 14 days

If pregnant or breast-feeding, ask a health professional before use.

Keep out of reach of children. In case of overdose, get medical help or contact a Poison Control Center right away.

Directions

- adults and children 12 years and over:
  - to **relieve** symptoms, swallow 1 tablet with a glass of water
  - to **prevent** symptoms, swallow 1 tablet with a glass of water **30 to 60 minutes before** eating food or drinking beverages that cause heartburn
  - can be used up to twice daily (do not take more than 2 tablets in 24 hours)
- children under 12 years: ask a doctor

Other information

- do not use if printed foil under bottle cap is open or torn
- store at 20°-25°C (68°-77°F)
- avoid excessive heat or humidity
- this product is sodium and sugar free

Inactive ingredients

Hypromellose, magnesium stearate, microcrystalline cellulose, synthetic red iron oxide, titanium dioxide, triacetin

Read the directions, consumer information leaflet and warnings before use. Keep the carton. It contains important information.

Questions about ZANTAC?

Call toll-free **1-888-285-9159**

Or visit **www.zantacotc.com**

Boehringer Ingelheim Consumer Health Care Products Division

Division of Boehringer Ingelheim Pharmaceuticals, Inc., Ridgefield, CT 06877

Copyright © 2007, Boehringer Ingelheim Pharmaceuticals, Inc. All rights reserved.

Shown in Product Identification Guide, page 503

MAXIMUM STRENGTH
ZANTAC 150®
COOL MINT TABLETS
(Boehringer Ingelheim Consumer Health Care Products Division) brand of ranitidine USP Cool Mint Tablet of 150 mg acid reducer

Drug Facts

Active ingredient (in each tablet)   **Purpose**

Ranitidine 150 mg (as ranitidine hydrochloride 168 mg) .... Acid reducer

Uses

- relieves heartburn associated with acid indigestion and sour stomach
- prevents heartburn associated with acid indigestion and sour stomach brought on by eating or drinking certain foods and beverages

Warnings

Allergy alert: Do not use if you are allergic to ranitidine or other acid reducers

Do not use

- with other acid reducers
- if you have kidney disease, except under the advice and supervision of a doctor
- if you have trouble or pain swallowing food, vomiting with blood, or bloody or black stools. These may be signs of a serious condition. See your doctor.

Ask a doctor before use if you have

- nausea or vomiting
- stomach pain
- unexplained weight loss
- frequent **chest pain**
- frequent wheezing, particularly with heartburn
- had heartburn over 3 months. This may be a sign of a more serious condition.
- heartburn with **lightheadedness, sweating or dizziness**
- chest pain or shoulder pain with shortness of breath; sweating; pain spreading to arms, neck or shoulders; or lightheadedness

Stop use and ask a doctor if

- your heartburn continues or worsens
- you need to take this product for more than 14 days

If pregnant or breast-feeding, ask a health professional before use.

Keep out of reach of children. In case of overdose, get medical help or contact a Poison Control Center right away.

Directions

- adults and children 12 years and over:
  - to **relieve** symptoms, swallow 1 tablet with a glass of water

- to **prevent** symptoms, swallow 1 tablet with a glass of water **30 to 60 minutes before** eating food or drinking beverages that cause heartburn
- can be used up to twice daily (up to 2 tablets in 24 hours)
- do not chew tablet
- children under 12 years: ask a doctor

Other information
- do not use if individual unit is open or torn
- store at 20°-25°C (68°-77°F)
- avoid excessive heat or humidity
- this product is sodium and sugar free

Inactive ingredients

Carrageenan, FD&C blue no.1, flavors, hypromellose, magnesium stearate, microcrystalline cellulose, polyethylene glycol, polysorbate, sucralose, and titanium dioxide

Read the directions, consumer information leaflet and warnings before use. Keep the carton. It contains important information.

Questions about ZANTAC?

Call toll-free **1-888-285-9159**
Or visit **www.zantacotc.com**
Boehringer Ingelheim Consumer Health Care Products Division
Division of Boehringer Ingelheim Pharmaceuticals, Inc., Ridgefield, CT 06877
Copyright © 2007, Boehringer Ingelheim Pharmaceuticals, Inc. All rights reserved.
Shown in Product Identification Guide, page 503

Matrixx Initiatives, Inc.
4742 NORTH 24TH STREET
SUITE 455
PHOENIX, AZ 85016

Direct Inquiries to:
Phone - (602) 385-8888
Fax - (602) 385-8850
http://www.zicam.com

NASAL COMFORT™
(Matrixx)
Moisture Therapy

Scented:
Ingredients: Purified water, high purity sodium chloride, spearmint oil (no preservatives).

Unscented:
Ingredients: Purified water, high purity sodium chloride, aloe vera (no preservatives).

Description:
Makes Breathing Easier

Dry heated rooms, air conditioning, allergens, colds, certain medications and environmental pollutants all contribute to the irritation and dehydration of nasal passages. Nasal Comfort™ Moisture Therapy not only soothes and moisturizes sensitive nasal membranes, but also helps your nose cleanse and filter the air you

breathe. Used twice a day, our pure hypertonic formula provides refreshing relief from dryness, irritation and conditions that can lead to congestion.
- Safe to use with all medications
- Non-habit forming
- *Preservative Free* and so pure you can use it as often as you need it
- Spearmint oil is light, refreshing and soothes nasal passages
- Patented *Micro-Filtration Sprayer* prevents product contamination and is easy to use

Discover easier, more comfortable breathing. Make Nasal Comfort™ Moisture Therapy part of your daily routine.

Instructions: Shake well before every use. Before first use, prime sprayer until the fine mist is delivered. Use twice daily (before bed and in the morning), or as often as needed. One spray per nostril. Wipe nozzle clean after each use. For more information, see enclosed insert. 1 oz bottle lasts 45 days when used twice daily.

Other Information:
Do not share sprayer with others as this may spread germs.
Keep out of reach of children.

How Supplied: 1 FL. OZ.
Shown in Product Identification Guide, page 503

ZICAM® Allergy Relief
(Matrixx)
[zĭ'kăm]

Drug Facts:

Active Ingredients: **Purpose:**
Luffa operculata 4x, 12x, 30x
Galphimia glauca 12x, 30x
Histanium hydrochloricum 12x, 30x, 200x
Sulphur 12x,
    30x, 200x .... Upper respiratory allergy symptom relief

Uses:
- Relieves symptoms of hay fever and other upper respiratory allergies such as: *sinus pressure *runny nose *sneezing *itchy eyes *watery eyes *nasal congestion

Warnings: For nasal use only. Ask a doctor before use if you have ear, nose or throat sensitivity or if you are susceptible to nose bleeds. **When using this product** avoid contact with eyes. In case of accidental contact with eyes, flush with water and immediately seek professional help. The use of this container by more than one person may spread infection. **Stop use and ask a doctor** if symptoms persist. **If pregnant or breast-feeding,** ask a health professional before use. **Keep out of reach of children.** If swallowed, get medical help or contact a Poison Control Center right away.

Directions:
- Adults and children 6 years of age and older (with adult supervision):
  - Remove cap and safety clip.

- Hold with thumb at bottom of bottle and nozzle between your fingers.
- Before using the first time, prime pump by depressing several times.
- Place tip of nozzle just past nasal opening (approximately 1/8").
- While inside nasal opening, slightly angle nozzle outward.
- Pump once into each nostril.
- After application, press lightly on outside of each nostril for about 5 seconds.
- Wait at least 30 seconds before blowing nose.
- Use once every 4 hours.
- Optimal results may not be seen for 1-2 weeks. After 1-2 weeks, may need to use only 1-2 times daily. For best results, use up to one week before contact with known causes of your allergies.
- Children under 6 years of age: Consult a doctor before use.

Inactive Ingredients: benzalkonium chloride, benzyl alcohol, edetate disodium, glycerine, hydroxyethylcellulose, potassium chloride, potassium phosphate, purified water, sodium chloride, sodium phosphate

How Supplied: *ZICAM®* Allergy Relief nasal pump: 0.5 FL OZ (15 mL) pump bottle
Shown in Product Identification Guide, page 504

ZICAM® Cold Remedy Nasal Gel™
(Matrixx)
[zĭ-kăm]

ZICAM® Cold Remedy Gel Swabs™

ZICAM® Cold Remedy RapidMelts®

ZICAM® Cold Remedy RapidMelts®
with Vitamin C

ZICAM® Cold Remedy Oral Mist™

ZICAM® Cold Remedy Chewables™

ZICAM® Cold Remedy ChewCaps

Drug Facts:
ZICAM® Cold Remedy Nasal Gel™, ZICAM® Cold Remedy Gel Swabs™ only:

Active Ingredient: **Purpose:**
Zincum
Gluconicum 2x .... Reduces duration and severity of the common cold
ZICAM® Cold Remedy RapidMelts®, ZICAM® Cold Remedy RapidMelts® with Vitamin C, ZICAM® Cold Remedy Oral Mist™, ZICAM® Cold Remedy Chewables™, ZICAM® Cold Remedy ChewCaps only:

Active Ingredient: **Purpose:**
Zincum
Aceticum 2x .... Reduces duration and severity of the common cold
Zincum Gluconicum 1x

Continued on next page

Zicam Cold Remedy—Cont.

Uses:
- Reduces the duration of the common cold
- Reduces severity of cold symptoms:
  - sore throat • stuffy nose • sneezing • coughing • congestion

Warnings:
ZICAM® Cold Remedy Nasal Gel™, ZICAM® Cold Remedy Gel Swabs™ only: **For nasal use only.** Ask doctor before use if you have ear, nose of throat sensitivity or if you are susceptible to nose bleeds. **When using this product** avoid contact with eyes. In case of accidental contact with eyes, flush with water and immediately seek professional help. Temporary discomfort such as burning, stinging, sneezing or increased nasal discharge may result. To help avoid possible irritation, do not sniff up gel. Use of this container by more than one person may spread infection. **Stop use and ask a doctor** if symptoms persist or are accompanied by fever. ZICAM® Cold Remedy was formulated to shorten the duration of the common cold and may not be effective for flu or allergies. **If pregnant or breast feeding,** ask a health professional before use. **Keep out of reach of children.** If swallowed, get medical help or contact a Poison Control Center right away.

ZICAM® Cold Remedy RapidMelts®, ZICAM® Cold Remedy RapidMelts® with Vitamin C, ZICAM® Cold Remedy Oral Mist™, ZICAM® Cold Remedy Chewables™, ZICAM® Cold Remedy ChewCaps only:
For oral use only. Stop use and ask a doctor if symptoms persist or are accompanied by fever. ZICAM® Cold Remedy was formulated to shorten the duration of the common cold and may not be effective for flu or allergies. **If pregnant or breast feeding,** ask a health professional before use. **Keep out of reach of children.**

ZICAM® Cold Remedy Oral Mist™ only: **When using this product** avoid contact with eyes. In case of accidental contact with eyes, flush with water and immediately seek professional help.

Directions:
ZICAM® Cold Remedy Nasal Gel™:
- For best results, use at the first sign of a cold and continue to use for an additional 48 hours after symptoms subside.
- Adults and children 3 years of age and older (with adult supervison):
- Remove cap and safety clip
- Hold with thumb at the bottom of the bottle and nozzle between your fingers.
- Prior to initial use, prime pump by holding it upright and depressing several times (into a tissue) until the gel is dispensed.
- Place tip of nozzle just past nasal opening (approximately 1/8″).
- While inside nasal opening, slightly angle nozzle outward.
- Pump once into each nostril. To help avoid possible irritation, do not sniff up gel. This product helps put gel in the lower part of the nose.
- After application, press lightly on the outside of each nostril for about 5 seconds.
- Wait at least 30 seconds before blowing nose.
- Use once every 4 hours.
- Children under 3 years of age, consult doctor before use.

ZICAM® Cold Remedy Gel Swabs™:
- For best results, use at the first sign of a cold and continue to use for an additional 48 hours after symptoms subside.
- Adults and children 3 years of age and older (with adult supervison):
- Open tube (also see illustrations on side of carton & insert):
- With thumb and index finger, pinch the tube on both yellow dots.
- With other hand, gently bend base of handle back and forth until seal is broken.
- Pull out swab.
- Apply medication just inside first nostril. Press lightly on the outside of first nostril for about 5 seconds. Re-dip swab in tube. Apply medication to second nostril. Press lightly on the outside of second nostril for about 5 seconds. Do not insert swab more than ¼″ past nasal opening.
- Discard swab after use.
- Wait at least 30 seconds before blowing nose.
- Use one tube every 4 hours.
- Children under 3 years of age: Consult a doctor before use.

ZICAM® Cold Remedy RapidMelts®
ZICAM® Cold Remedy RapidMelts® with Vitamin C:
- For best results, use at the first sign of a cold and continue to use for an additional 48 hours after symptoms subside.
- Adults and children 3 years of age and older (with adult supervison):
- Dissolve entire tablet in mouth. Do not chew. Do not swallow whole.
- Take one tablet at the onset of symptoms.
- Repeat every three hours until symptoms are gone.
- To avoid minor stomach upset, do not take on an empty stomach.
- Do not eat or drink for 15 minutes after use. Do not eat or drink citrus fruits or juices for 30 minutes before or after use. Otherwise, drink plenty of fluids.
- Children under 3 years of age, consult doctor before use.

ZICAM® Cold Remedy Chewables™
ZICAM® Cold Remedy ChewCaps:
- For best results, use at the first sign of a cold and continue to use for an additional 48 hours after symptoms subside.
- Adults and children 6 years of age and older (with adult supervison):
- Take one Chewable™ or ChewCap at the onset of symptoms. Chew thoroughly before swallowing.
- Repeat every three hours until symptoms are gone.
- To avoid minor stomach upset, do not take on an empty stomach.
- Do not eat or drink for 15 minutes after use. Do not eat or drink citrus fruits or juices for 30 minutes before or after use. Otherwise, drink plenty of water.
- These products are not recommended for children under the age of 6 due to the hazard of choking.

ZICAM® Cold Remedy Oral Mist™:
- For best results, use at the first sign of a cold and continue to use for an additional 48 hours after symptoms subside.
- Adults and children 3 years of age and older (with adult supervision):
- Spray four times in mouth at the onset of symptoms. Spray on inside of cheeks, roof of mouth and gums. Retain for 15 seconds. Swallow.
- Repeat every three hours until symptoms are gone.
- To avoid minor stomach upset, do not take on an empty stomach.
- Do not eat or drink for 15 minutes after use. Do not eat or drink citrus fruits or juices for 30 minutes before or after use. Otherwise, drink plenty of water.
- Children under 3 years of age, consult doctor before use.

Inactive Ingredients:
ZICAM® Cold Remedy Nasal Gel™, ZICAM® Cold Remedy Gel Swabs™ only: benzalkonium chloride, glycerin, hydroxyethylcellulose, purified water, sodium chloride, sodium hydroxide

ZICAM® Cold Remedy RapidMelts® only: crospovidone, magnesium stearate, mannitol, microcrystalline cellulose, natural & artificial cherry flavor, polysorbate 80, polyvinyl pyrolidone, purified talc, silicon dioxide, sodium lauryl sulphate, sodium starch glycolate, sorbitan monostearate, sucralose

ZICAM® Cold Remedy RapidMelts® with Vitamin C only: ascorbic acid, carnauba wax, crospovidone, ethylcellulose, FD&C yellow #6, magnesium stearate, mannitol, microcrystalline cellulose, mono and diglycerides, natural orange flavor, polyethylene glycol, polysorbate 80, polyvinyl pyrolidone, purified talc, silicon dioxide, sodium lauryl sulphate, sodium starch glycolate, sorbitan monostearate, sucralose.

ZICAM® Cold Remedy Chewables™ only: FD&C red #40, glycerin, HPMC, lecithin, malitol syrup, maltodextrin, mono and diglycerides, natural and artifical strawberry flavor, partially hydrogenated cotton seed and soy oil, sugar.

ZICAM® Cold Remedy ChewCaps only: acetylated mono-diglycerides, confectioner's glaze, dextrose monohydrate, FD&C red #40 and #28, FD&C yellow #6, HPMC, lecithin, magnesium stearate, maltitol syrup, maltodextrin, mono and di-glycerides, natural and artifical cinnamon flavor, opaglos red #2, partially hydrogenated cotton seed and soy oil, polyethylene glycol, purified talc, silicon dioxide, sodium carboxymethylcellulose, sucralose, sugar, titanium dioxide.

ZICAM® Cold Remedy Oral Mist™ only: benzalkonium chloride, glycerin, peppermint flavor, purified water, sucralose.

ZICAM® Cold Remedy Nasal Gel™: 0.5 FL OZ (15mL) pump bottle; ZICAM® Cold Remedy Gel Swabs™ and 20 medicated swabs; ZICAM® Cold Remedy RapidMelts® and ZICAM® Cold Remedy RapidMelts® with Vitamin C: 25 quick dissolve tablets; ZICAM® Cold Remedy Chewables™: 25 chewable squares; ZICAM® Cold Remedy ChewCaps: 25 chewable caplets; ZICAM® Cold Remedy Oral Mist™: 1.0 FL OZ (30mL)

Shown in Product Identification Guide, page 504

ZICAM® Extreme Congestion Relief (Matrixx)
ZICAM® Intense Sinus Relief (Matrixx)

[zī 'kăm]

Drug Facts:

Active Ingredient:	Purpose:
Oxymetazoline HCl 0.05%	Nasal decongestant

Uses:
- Temporarily relieves nasal congestion due to:
  *common cold *sinusitis *hay fever *upper respiratory allergies
- Helps clear nasal passages
- Shrink swollen membranes
- Temporarily relieves sinus congestion and pressure

Warnings: For nasal use only. Ask a doctor before use if you have heart disease, high blood pressure, thyroid disease, diabetes, trouble urinating due to enlarged prostrate gland. **When using this product do not use more than directed.** Do not use for more than 3 days. Use only as directed. Frequent or prolonged use may cause nasal congestion to recur or worsen. Temporary discomfort such as burning, stinging, sneezing, or an increase in nasal discharge may result. Use of this container by more than one person may spread infection. **Stop use and ask a doctor** if symptoms persist. **If pregnant or breast-feeding,** ask a health professional before use. **Keep out of reach of children. If swallowed,** get medical help or contact a Poison Control Center right away.

Directions: Adults and children 6 to under 12 years of age (with adult supervision): Pump 2 or 3 times in each nostril without tilting your head, not more often than once every 10 to 12 hours. Sniff deeply. Do not exceed 2 doses in any 24-hour period. Wipe nozzle clean after use. Children under 6 years of age: Consult a doctor.
To use pump:
Remove cap and safety clip.
Hold with thumb at bottom of bottle and nozzle between fingers.
Before using the first time, prime pump by depressing several times.

ZICAM® Extreme Congestion Relief only

Inactive Ingredients: alkoxylated diester, aloe barbadensis gel, benzalkonium chloride, benzyl alcohol, disodium EDTA, disodium phosphate, glycerin, hydroxyethylcellulose, hydroxylated lecithin, monosodium phosphate, purified water

ZICAM® Intense Sinus Relief only

Inactive Ingredients: alkoxylated diester, aloe barbadensis gel, benzalkonium chloride, benzyl alcohol, disodium EDTA, disodium phosphate, di-alpha tocopherol, eucalyptol, glycerin, hydroxyethylcellulose, hydroxylated lecithin, menthol, monosodium phosphate, polysorbate 80, purified water

How Supplied: *ZICAM®* Extreme Congestion Relief and ZICAM® Intense Sinus Relief nasal pump: 0.5 FL OZ (15 mL) pump bottle

---

ZICAM® Cough Max Cough Spray
ZICAM® Cough Max Cough Melts

Active Ingredients:	Purpose:
Cough Max: (in each 0.25 mL spray)	
Dextromethorphan HBr 6.0 mg	Cough Suppressant
Cough Max Cough Melts: (in each tablet)	
Dextromethorphan HBr 30 mg	Cough Suppressant

Cough Max/Cough Max Melts

Uses: temporarily relieves cough due to minor throat and bronchial irritation associated with a cold.

Warnings:

Cough Max/Cough Max Cough Melts:

Do not use if you are now taking a prescription monoamine oxidase inhibitor (MAOI) (certain drugs for depression, psychiatric, or emotional conditions, or Parkinson's disease), or for 2 weeks after stopping the MAOI drug. If you do not know if your prescription drug contains an MAOI, ask a doctor or pharmacist before taking this product.

Cough Max/Cough Max Melts:
Ask a doctor before use if you have
- cough accompanied by excessive phlegm (mucus).
- persistent or chronic cough such as occurs with smoking, asthma, or emphysema.

Stop use and ask a doctor if
- cough lasts more than 7 days, comes back, or occurs with fever, rash, or headache that lasts. These could be signs of a serious condition.

If pregnant or breast-feeding, ask a health professional before use.

Keep out of reach of children. In case of overdose, get medical help or contact a Poison Control Center right away.

Directions:
Cough Max:
- Remove safety cap.
- Prime pump by spraying into a tissue.
- Hold close to mouth and depress sprayer fully. Swallow.

12 yrs & older	5 sprays (30.0 mg Dextromethorphan HBr)
Under 12 yrs	consult a doctor

- Repeat every 6-8 hours, not to exceed 4 doses per day.
- May be followed by water or liquids if desired.

Cough Max Melts:
- Adults and children 12 years of age and older:
  - Dissolve entire tablet in mouth. Do not swallow whole.
  - Repeat every 6-8 hours, do not exceed 4 doses per day.
  - To avoid minor stomach upset, do not take on an empty stomach.
- Under 12 years of age, consult a doctor.

Inactive Ingredients:

Cough Max Cough Melts:

Inactive Ingredients: Acetylated mono-diglycerides, crospovidone, dextrose monohydrate, FD&C Red #40, magnesium stearate, mannitol, microcrystalline cellulose, natural & cherry flavor, polysorbate 80, purified talc, silicon dioxide, styrene and divinyl benzene resin, sucralose

Cough Max:

Inactive Ingredients: citric acid, glycerin, hydroxylated lecithin, menthol, natural flavors, polyethylene glycol, polysorbate 60, potassium sorbate, purified water, sucralose

Other Information:
Store at room temperature 15°C-29°C (59°F-84°F)

Questions?
Comments?
call 877-942-2626
toll-free or visit us on the web at www.zicam.com

Shown in Product Identification Guide, page 504

ZICAM® MULTI-SYMPTOM LIQUID DAYTIME

Drug Facts
Active ingredients:

(in each 15mL = 1 tablespoon)	*Purpose*
Acetaminophen 325 mg	Pain reliever/fever reducer
Dextromethorphan HBr 10 mg	Cough suppressant
Guaifenesin 200 mg	Expectorant

Uses: Temporarily relieves common cold and flu symptoms:
- helps loosen phlegm (mucus) and thin

Continued on next page

Zicam Liquid Daytime—Cont.

bronchial secretions to rid the bronchial passage ways of bothersome mucus
- cough due to minor throat and bronchial irritation
- minor aches and pains
- sore throat
- muscular aches
- headache
- fever

Warnings:

Liver warning: This product contains acetaminophen. Severe liver damage may occur if you take:
- more than 12 tablespoons in any 24 hour period
- with any other drugs containing acetaminophen
- 3 or more alcoholic drinks everyday while using this product

Sore throat warning: If sore throat is severe, persists for more than two days, is accompanied by or followed by fever, headache, rash, nausea, or vomiting, consult a doctor promptly.

Do not use

- **with any other medicines containing acetaminophen** (prescription or non prescription). Ask a doctor or pharmacist before using with other drugs if you are not sure.
- if you are now taking a prescription monoamine oxidase inhibitor (MAOI) (certain drugs for depression, psychiatric or emotional conditions, or Parkinson's disease), or for 2 weeks after stopping the MAOI drug. If you do not know if your prescription drug contains an MAOI, ask a doctor or pharmacist before taking this product.

Ask a doctor before use if you have:

- liver disease
- cough that occurs with too much phlegm (mucus)
- persistent or chronic cough as occurs with smoking, asthma, chronic bronchitis or emphysema
- a sodium restricted diet

Stop use and ask a doctor if:

- redness or swelling is present
- fever gets worse or lasts for more than 3 days
- pain or cough get worse or do not get better within 7 days or are accompanied by a fever
- cough comes back or occurs with rash, fever, or headache that lasts
- new symptoms occur

These could be signs of a serious condition

If pregnant or breast feeding, ask a health professional before use. **Keep out of reach of children.**

Overdose warning: taking more than the recommended dose can cause serious health problems. In case of overdose, get medical help or contact a poison control center right away. Quick medical attention is critical for adults as well as

children even if you do not notice any signs or symptoms.

Directions:

- Take only as directed – see overdose warning
- Only use enclosed measuring cup designed for use with this product
- Adults and children 12 years and over
  - Take 2 tablespoons (Tbsp) or 30mL
  - May be added to 6-8 ounces of hot or cold beverage (tea, juice, soda)
  - Take every 4 hours as needed
  - Do not exceed 12 tablespoons in any 24 hour period
- Children under 12 years of age, consult a doctor

Other information:

- store at room temperature 15°-29°C (59°-84°F)
- do not use if plastic neck wrap or foil inner seal is broken or missing
- contains 10 mg potassium per dosage unit
- contains 30 mg sodium per dosage unit

Inactive ingredients: acesulfame potassium, disodium EDTA, glycerin, hydroxyethylcellulose, polyethylene glycol, potassium sorbate, purified water, sodium chloride, sucralose.

Questions? Comments?

call 877-942-2626 toll-free or visit us on the web at www.zicam.com
Shown in Product Identification Guide, page 503

ZICAM MULTISYMPTOM COLD & FLU NIGHTIME LIQUID

Drug Facts
Active ingredients:
(in each
15mL = 1 tablespoon)   Purpose
Acetaminophen
325 mg .... Pain reliever/fever reducer
Dextromethorphan HBr
10 mg .... Cough suppressant
Doxylamine Succinate
6.25 mg .... Antihistamine

Uses: temporarily relieves common cold and flu symptoms:
- cough due to minor throat and bronchial irritation
- minor aches and pains
- sore throat
- muscular aches
- headache
- fever
- runny nose
- watery eyes
- sneezing

Warnings:

Liver warning: This product contains acetaminophen. Severe liver damage may occur if you take:
- more than 12 tablespoons in any 24 hour period
- with any other drugs containing acetaminophen

- 3 or more alcoholic drinks everyday while using this product

Sore throat warning: If sore throat is severe, persists for more than two days, is accompanied by or followed by fever, headache, rash, nausea, or vomiting, consult a doctor promptly.

Do not use

- **with any other medicines containing acetaminophen** (prescription or non prescription). Ask a doctor or pharmacist before using with other drugs if you are not sure.
- if you are now taking a prescription monoamine oxidase inhibitor (MAOI) (certain drugs for depression, psychiatric or emotional conditions, or Parkinson's disease), or for 2 weeks after stopping the MAOI drug. If you do not know if your prescription drug contains an MAOI, ask a doctor or pharmacist before taking this product.

Ask a doctor before use if you have:

- liver disease
- glaucoma
- difficulty in urination due to enlarged prostate
- a breathing problem such as emphysema or chronic bronchitis
- cough that occurs with too much phlegm (mucus)
- persistent or chronic cough as occurs with smoking, asthma or emphysema
- a sodium restricted diet

Ask a doctor or pharmacist before use if you are taking sedatives or tranquilizers

When using this product:

- may cause excitability especially in children
- be careful when driving a motor vehicle or operating machinery
- may cause marked drowsiness
- alcohol, sedatives, and tranquilizers may intensify drowsiness effect
- avoid alcoholic beverages

Stop use and ask a doctor if:

- redness or swelling is present
- fever gets worse or lasts for more than 3 days
- pain or cough get worse or do not get better within 7 days or are accompanied by a fever
- cough comes back or occurs with rash, fever, or headache that lasts
- new symptoms occur

These could be signs of a serious condition

If pregnant or breast feeding, ask a health professional before use. **Keep out of reach of children.**

Overdose warning: taking more than the recommended dose can cause serious health problems. In case of overdose, get medical help or contact a poison control center right away. Quick medical attention is critical for adults as well as children even if you do not notice any signs or symptoms.

Directions:
- Take only as directed – see overdose warning
- Only use enclosed measuring cup designed for use with this product
- Adults and children 12 years and over
  - Take 2 tablespoons (Tbsp) or 30mL
  - May be added to 6-8 ounces of hot or cold beverage (tea, juice, soda)
  - Take every 4 hours as needed
  - Do not exceed 12 tablespoons in any 24 hour period
- Children under 12 years of age, consult a doctor

Other information
- store at room temperature 15°-29°C (59°-84°F)
- do not use if plastic neck wrap or foil inner seal is broken or missing
- contains 10 mg potassium per dosage unit
- contains 30 mg sodium per dosage unit

Inactive ingredients: acesulfame potassium, disodium EDTA, glycerin, hydroxyethylcellulose, polyethylene glycol, potassium sorbate, purified water, sodium chloride, sucralose.

Questions? Comments?

call 877-942-2626 toll-free or visit us on the web at www.zicam.com

Shown in Product Identification Guide, page 503

ZICAM® MULTISYMPTOM COLD & FLU DAYTIME TO GO

Drug Facts
Active ingredient:
(on each spoon)   *Purpose*
Acetaminophen
650 mg ...... Pain Reliever/Fever Reducer
Chlorpheniramine maleate
4 mg .... Antihistamine
Dextromethorphan
HBr 20 mg .... Cough Suppressant
Phenylephrine
HCl 10 mg .... Nasal Decongestant

Uses: temporarily relieves common cold and flu symptoms:
- nasal and sinus congestion • cough due to minor throat and bronchial irritation • minor aches & pains • runny nose • sore throat • muscular aches • watery eyes • sneezing • headache • fever

Warnings:

Liver warning: This product contains acetaminophen. Severe liver damage may occur if you take more than 6 single doses in any 24 hour period.

Sore Throat Warning: If sore throat is severe, persists for more than two days, is accompanied by or followed by fever, headache, rash, nausea, or vomiting, consult a doctor promptly.

Do not use
- **with any other medicines containing acetaminophen** (prescription or non prescription). Ask a doctor or pharmacist before using with other drugs if you are not sure.
- if you are now taking a prescription monoamine oxidase inhibitor (MAOI) (certain drugs for depression, psychiatric or emotional conditions, or Parkinson's disease), or for 2 weeks after stopping the MAOI drug. If you do not know if your prescription drug contains an MAOI, ask a doctor or pharmacist before taking this product.

Ask a doctor before use if you have
- liver disease
- heart disease
- thyroid disease
- diabetes
- high blood pressure
- glaucoma
- difficulty in urination due to enlarged prostate
- a breathing problem such as emphysema or chronic bronchitis
- cough that occurs with too much phlegm (mucus)
- persistent or chronic cough as occurs with smoking, asthma, or emphysema

Ask a doctor or pharmacist before use if you are taking sedatives or tranquilizers

When using this product
- **do not use more than directed**
- may cause excitability especially in children
- be careful when driving a motor vehicle or operating machinery
- alcohol, sedatives, and tranquilizers may increase drowsiness
- may cause drowsiness
- avoid alcoholic beverages

Stop use and ask a doctor if
- redness or swelling is present
- fever gets worse and lasts more than 3 days
- pain, nasal congestion, or cough gets worse or does not get better within 7 days or are accompanied by a fever
- cough comes back or occurs with rash or headache that lasts
- you get nervous, dizzy or sleepless
- new symptoms occur

These could be signs of a serious condition.

If pregnant or breast feeding, ask a health professional before use. **Keep out of reach of children.**

Overdose Warning: Taking more than the recommended dose can cause serious health problems.
In case of overdose, get medical help or contact a Poison Control Center right away. Quick medical attention is critical for adults as well as for children even if you do not notice any signs or symptoms.

Directions
- Take only as directed – see overdose warning.
- Remove spoon from protective wrapper.
- Peel back lid completely from spoon.
- Stir spoon in 4 to 8 ounces of hot or cold beverage (tea, juice, soda).
- Mix for 30 seconds or until uniform.
- Lick remaining medicine off spoon. Use caution when placing spoon in mouth.
- Discard protective wrapper, lid and spoon.
- Take one dose [or spoon] every 4 hours as needed.
- Adults and children 12 years and over, one dose every 4 hours.
- Do not exceed 6 doses in any 24 hour period.
- Children under 12 years of age: consult a doctor.

Inactive ingredients: citric acid, glycerin, hydroxyethylcellulose, polyethylene glycol, potassium chloride, propylene glycol, purified water, sodium carboxymethylcellulose, sodium citrate, sucralose

Shown in Product Identification Guide, page 503

ZICAM® MULTISYMPTOM COLD & FLU NIGHTIME TO GO

Drug Facts
Active ingredient:
(on each spoon)   *Purpose*
Acetaminophen
650 mg ...... Pain Reliever/Fever Reducer
Dextromethorphan
HBr 20 mg .... Cough Suppressant
Doxylamine
succinate 12.5 mg .... Antihistamine
Phenylephrine
HCl 10 mg .... Nasal Decongestant

Uses: temporarily relieves common cold and flu symptoms:
- nasal and sinus congestion • cough due to minor throat and bronchial irritation • minor aches & pains • runny nose • sore throat • muscular aches • watery eyes • sneezing • headache • fever

Warnings:

Liver warning: This product contains acetaminophen. Severe liver damage may occur if you take more than 6 single doses in any 24 hour period.

Sore Throat Warning: If sore throat is severe, persists for more than two days, is accompanied by or followed by fever, headache, rash, nausea, or vomiting, consult a doctor promptly.

Do not use
- **with any other medicines containing acetaminophen** (prescription or non prescription). Ask a doctor or pharmacist before using with other drugs if you are not sure.
- if you are now taking a prescription monoamine oxidase inhibitor (MAOI) (certain drugs for depression, psychiatric or emotional conditions, or Parkinson's disease), or for 2 weeks after

Continued on next page

Zicam Cold & Flu Nightime—Cont.

stopping the MAOI drug. If you do not know if your prescription drug contains an MAOI, ask a doctor or pharmacist before taking this product.

Ask a doctor before use if you have
- liver disease
- heart disease
- thyroid disease
- diabetes
- high blood pressure
- glaucoma
- difficulty in urination due to enlarged prostate
- a breathing problem such as emphysema or chronic bronchitis
- cough that occurs with too much phlegm (mucus)
- persistent or chronic cough as occurs with smoking, asthma, or emphysema

Ask a doctor or pharmacist before use if you are taking sedatives or tranquilizers

When using this product
- **do not use more than directed**
- may cause excitability especially in children
- be careful when driving a motor vehicle or operating machinery
- alcohol, sedatives, and tranquilizers may increase drowsiness
- may cause marked drowsiness
- avoid alcoholic beverages

Stop use and ask a doctor if
- redness or swelling is present
- fever gets worse and lasts more than 3 days
- pain, nasal congestion, or cough gets worse or does not get better within 7 days or are accompanied by a fever
- cough comes back or occurs with rash or headache that lasts
- you get nervous, dizzy or sleepless
- new symptoms occur

These could be signs of a serious condition.

If pregnant or breast feeding, ask a health professional before use. **Keep out of reach of children.**

Overdose Warning: Taking more than the recommended dose can cause serious health problems. In case of overdose, get medical help or contact a Poison Control Center right away. Quick medical attention is critical for adults as well as for children even if you do not notice any signs or symptoms.

Directions
- Take only as directed – see overdose warning.
- Remove spoon from protective wrapper.
- Peel back lid completely from spoon.
- Stir spoon in 4 to 8 ounces of hot or cold beverage (tea, juice, soda).
- Mix for 30 seconds or until uniform.
- Lick remaining medicine off spoon. Use caution when placing spoon in mouth.
- Discard protective wrapper, lid and spoon.

- Take one dose [or spoon] every 4 hours as needed.
- Adults and children 12 years and over, one dose every 4 hours.
- Do not exceed 6 doses in any 24 hour period.
- Children under 12 years of age: consult a doctor.

Inactive ingredients: citric acid, glycerin, hydroxyethylcellulose, polyethylene glycol, potassium chloride, propylene glycol, purified water, sodium carboxymethylcellulose, sodium citrate, sucralose

Shown in Product Identification Guide, page 503

ZICAM® SINUS MELTS

Drug Facts

Active ingredients:
(in each tablet)   **Purpose**
Acetaminophen
325 mg .... Pain reliever
Phenylephrine
HCl 5 mg .... Nasal decongestant

Uses: temporarily relieves sinus symptoms: • Sinus pain • Headache • Nasal and sinus congestion

Warnings:

Alcohol warning: If you consume 3 or more alcoholic drinks per day, ask your doctor whether you should take acetaminophen or other pain relievers/fever reducers. Acetaminophen may cause liver damage. **Taking more than the recommended dose (overdose) may cause serious liver damage.**

Do not use:
- With other medicines containing acetaminophen
- If you are now taking a prescription monoamine oxidase inhibitor (MAOI) (certain drugs for depression, psychiatric or emotional conditions, or Parkinson's disease), or for 2 weeks after stopping the MAOI drug. If you do not know if your prescription drug contains an MAOI, ask a doctor or pharmacist before taking this product.

Ask a doctor before use if you have
- Heart disease • Thyroid disease • Diabetes • High blood pressure • Difficulty in urination due to enlarged prostate

When using this product, do not use more than directed

Stop use and ask a doctor if
- Redness or swelling is present • You get nervous, dizzy or sleepless • Fever gets worse and lasts for more than 3 days
- New symptoms occur • Symptoms do not get better within 7 days or are accompanied by a fever

These could be signs of a serious condition

If pregnant or breast feeding, ask a health professional before use. **Keep out of reach of children**

Overdose warning: taking more than the recommended dose can cause serious health problems. In case of overdose, get medical help or contact a Poison Control Center right away. Quick medical attention is critical for adults as well as children even if you do not notice any signs or symptoms

Directions:
- Take only as directed – see overdose warning
- Do not exceed 6 doses per 24 hours
- Adults and children 12 years and over
  - Dissolve 2 entire tablets in mouth. Do not swallow whole.
  - One dose every 4 hours as needed
  - Do not exceed 6 doses every 24 hours
- Children under 12 years
  - Do not use this adult product in children under 12 years of age; this will provide more than the recommended dose (overdose) and may cause liver damage.

Inactive ingredients: acetylated monoglyceride, crospovidone, dextrose monohydrate, ethylcellulose, green color*, magnesium stearate, microcrystalline cellulose, polacrilin potassium, polyethylene glycol, polysorbate 80, silicon dioxide, sodium lauryl sulfate, sucralose, talc, triethyl citrate, natural & artificial flavors

Other Information:
- Store at room temperature 15°-29°C (59°-84°F)
- Do not use if foil seal is torn or broken
  Shown in Product Identification Guide, page 504

Mission Pharmacal Company
10999 IH 10 WEST, SUITE 1000
SAN ANTONIO, TX 78230-1355

Direct Inquiries to:
P.O. Box 786099
San Antonio TX 78278-6099
(800) 292-7364

THERA-GESIC® Maximum Strength Analgesic Pain Relieving Creme (Mission Pharmacal)
pain relieving crème

Drug Facts

Active Ingredients: **Purpose:**
Menthol 1% .... Analgesic
Methyl Salicylate 15% .. Counterirritant

Use:
temporary relief of minor aches and pains of muscles and joints associated with:
- arthritis • simple backaches • strains
- bruises • sprains

Warnings:

For external use only. Use only as directed. Avoid contact with eyes or mucous membranes.

Do not bandage tightly, wrap or cover until after washing the areas where THERA-GESIC® has been applied.

Do not use
- immediately after shower or bath
- if skin is sensitive to oil of wintergreen (methyl salicylate)
- on wounds or damaged skin

Ask a doctor before use
- for children under 2 and to 12 years of age
- if prone or sensitive to allergic reactions from aspirin or salicylate

When using this product
- discontinue use if skin irritation develops, or redness is present
- do not swallow
- do not use a heating pad after application of THERA-GESIC®

Stop use and ask a doctor if condition worsens, or if symptoms persist for more than 7 days or clear up and occur again within a few days.

If pregnant or breast-feeding, ask a health professional before use.

Keep out of reach of children to avoid accidental poisoning. If swallowed, get medical help or contact a Poison Control Center right away.

Directions:

Adults and children 12 or more years of age: Apply thin layers of creme into and around the sore or painful area, not more than 3 to 4 times daily. The number of thin layers controls the intensity of the action of THERA-GESIC®. One thin layer provides a mild effect, two thin layers provide a strong effect and three thin layers provide a very strong effect. SEE WARNINGS. Wash hands thoroughly after application.

Other Information:

Once THERA-GESIC® has penetrated the skin, the area may be washed, leaving it dry, clean and fragrance-free without decreasing the effectiveness of the product. Avoid contact with clothing or other surfaces. Store at 20–25°C (68–77°F).

Inactive Ingredients:

Carbomer 934, Dimethicone, Glycerine, Methylparaben, Propylparaben, Sodium Lauryl Sulfate, Trolamine, Water.

Questions?
(210) 696–8400 (M-F 8:30–5:00 CST)

How Supplied: Net wt. 3 oz., NDC 0178-0320-03; Net wt. 5 oz., NDC 0178-0320-05.

FACED WITH AN Rx SIDE EFFECT?
Turn to the
Companion Drug Index
for products that
provide symptomatic
relief.

Novartis Consumer Health, Inc.

**200 KIMBALL DRIVE
PARSIPPANY, NJ 07054-0622**

Direct Inquiries to:
Consumer & Professional Affairs
(800) 452-0051
Fax: (800) 635-2801

Or write to the above address

**BUFFERIN®
(Novartis Consumer Health, Inc.)
Regular/Extra Strength
Pain Reliever/Fever Reducer**

Drug Facts
Regular Strength

Active Ingredients: (in each tablet)	Purpose:
Buffered aspirin equal to 325 mg aspirin	Pain reliever/fever reducer

(buffered with calcium carbonate, magnesium oxide and magnesium carbonate)

Extra Strength

Active Ingredients: (in each tablet)	Purpose:
Buffered aspirin equal to 500 mg aspirin	Pain reliever/fever reducer

(buffered with calcium carbonate, magnesium oxide and magnesium carbonate)

Uses:
- for the temporary relief of minor aches and pains associated with:
  - headache
  - cold
  - muscular aches
  - arthritis
  - toothache
  - premenstrual & menstrual cramps
- temporarily reduces fever

Warnings:

Reye's syndrome: Children and teenagers who have or are recovering from chicken pox or flu-like symptoms should not use this product. When using this product, if changes in behavior with nausea and vomiting occur, consult a doctor because these symptoms could be an early sign of Reye's syndrome, a rare but serious illness.

Allergy alert: Aspirin may cause a severe allergic reaction, which may include:
- hives
- facial swelling
- asthma (wheezing)
- shock

Alcohol warning: If you consume 3 or more alcoholic drinks every day, ask your doctor whether you should take aspirin or other pain relievers/fever reducers. Aspirin may cause stomach bleeding.

Do not use if you have ever had an allergic reaction to any other pain reliever/fever reducer.

Ask a doctor before use if you have
- kidney disease
- a magnesium-restricted diet
- asthma • bleeding problems • ulcers

- stomach problems that last or come back, such as heartburn, upset stomach, or pain

Ask a doctor or pharmacist before use if you are

taking a prescription drug for:
- anticoagulation (thinning the blood)
- diabetes • gout • arthritis

Stop use and ask a doctor if
- allergic reaction occurs. Seek medical help right away.
- pain gets worse or lasts for more than 10 days
- new symptoms occur
- fever gets worse or lasts for more than 3 days
- painful area is red or swollen
- ringing in the ears or loss of hearing occurs

If pregnant or breast-feeding, ask a health professional before use.

It is especially important not to use aspirin during the last 3 months of pregnancy unless definitely directed to do so by a doctor because it may cause problems in the unborn child or complications during delivery.

Keep out of reach of children. In case of overdose, get medical help or contact a Poison Control Center right away.

Directions:
Regular Strength
Drink a full glass of water with each dose.
- adults and children 12 years and over: take 2 tablets every 4 hours; not more than 12 tablets in 24 hours
- children under 12 years: ask a doctor

Extra Strength
Drink a full glass of water with each dose.
- adults and children 12 years and over: take 2 tablets every 6 hours; not more than 8 tablets in 24 hours
- children under 12 years: ask a doctor

Other Information:
Regular Strength
- **each tablet contains:** calcium 65 mg and magnesium 50 mg
- store at room temperature
- read all product information before using.

Extra Strength
- **each tablet contains:** calcium 90 mg and magnesium 70 mg
- store at room temperature
- read all product information before using.

Inactive Ingredients: benzoic acid, carnauba wax, citric acid, corn starch, FD&C blue #1, hypromellose, magnesium stearate, mineral oil, polysorbate 20, povidone, propylene glycol, simethicone emulsion, sodium phosphate, sorbitan monolaurate, titanium dioxide, zinc stearate

Questions or comments?
1-800-468-7746

How Supplied:
Regular Strength and Extra Strength are available in 39 ct., 65 ct., and 130 ct. cartons.

Shown in Product Identification Guide, page 504

BUCKLEY'S® CHEST CONGESTION MIXTURE
(Novartis Consumer Health, Inc.)
Guaifenesin/Expectorant

Drug Facts
Active ingredient:
(in each 5 mL,
1 teaspoon)   **Purpose**
Guaifenesin 100 mg .... Expectorant

Uses:
• helps loosen phlegm (mucus) and thin bronchial secretions to drain bronchial tubes and make coughs more productive

Warnings:
Ask a doctor before use if you have
• cough that occurs with too much phlegm (mucus)
• cough that lasts or is chronic such as occurs with smoking, asthma, chronic bronchitis, or emphysema
Stop use and ask a doctor if
• cough lasts more than 7 days, comes back, or is accompanied by fever, rash, or persistent headache. These could be signs of a serious condition.
If pregnant or breast-feeding, ask a health professional before use
Keep out of reach of children, in case of overdose get medical help or contact a Poison Control Center right away

Directions:
• shake well before taking
• adults and children 12 years of age and over: 2 to 4 teaspoons every 4 hours not to exceed 6 doses in 24 hours
• children 6 to 12 years of age: 1 teaspoonful every 4 hours not to exceed 6 doses in 24 hours
• children under 6 years of age: ask a doctor

Other information:
• store at controlled room temperature 20-25°C (68-77°F)
• protect from freezing

Inactive Ingredients: acesulfame potassium, ammonium carbonate, butylparaben, camphor, Canadian fir balsam gum, carrageenan, glycerin, menthol, pine needle oil, propylene glycol, propylparaben, purified water, tincture of capsicum

Questions? Call **1-800-452-0051** 24 hours a day, 7 days a week.

How Supplied: Available in 4 fl. oz. bottles.

BUCKLEY'S® COUGH MIXTURE
(Novartis Consumer Health, Inc.)
Dextromethorphan HBr/ Cough Suppressant

Drug Facts
Active ingredient:
(in each 5 mL,
1 teaspoon)   **Purpose**
Dextromethorphan HBr
12.5 mg .... Cough suppressant

Uses:
• temporarily relieves cough due to minor throat and bronchial irritation associated with a cold

Warnings:
Do not use if you are now taking a prescription monoamine oxidase inhibitor (MAOI) (certain drugs for depression, psychiatric, or emotional conditions, or Parkinson's disease) or for 2 weeks after stopping the MAOI drug. If you do not know if your prescription drug contains an MAOI, ask a doctor or pharmacist before taking this product.
Ask a doctor before use if you have
• a cough that occurs with too much phlegm (mucus)
• a cough that lasts or is chronic such as occurs with smoking, asthma, chronic bronchitis, or emphysema
Stop use and ask a doctor if
• cough gets worse or lasts for more than 7 days
• cough comes back or occurs with fever, rash or headache that lasts. These could be signs of a serious condition.
If pregnant or breast-feeding, ask a health professional before use
Keep out of reach of children, in case of overdose get medical help or contact a Poison Control Center right away

Directions:
• shake well before taking
• adults and children 12 years of age and over: 1 teaspoon every 4 hours not to exceed 6 doses in 24 hours
• children under 12 years of age: ask a doctor

Other information:
Store at 15°C-30°C (59°F-86°F)

Inactive Ingredients: ammonium carbonate, butylparaben, camphor, Canadian fir balsam gum, carrageenan viscarin, glycerin, menthol, pine needle oil, propylparaben sodium, purified water, sodium saccharin, tincture of capsicum

Questions? Call **1-800-452-0051** 24 hours a day, 7 days a week.

How Supplied: Available in 4 fl. oz. bottles.

COMTREX® Maximum Strength Day/Night Cold & Cough
(Novartis Consumer Health, Inc.)
Pain Reliever/Fever Reducer

Drug Facts
Active Ingredients: **Purpose:**
(in each caplet)
Acetaminophen
325 mg .... Pain reliever/fever reducer
Chlorpheniramine maleate
2 mg* .... Antihistamine*
Dextromethorphan HBr
10 mg .... Cough suppressant
Phenylephrine HCl
5 mg .... Nasal decongestant

*antihistamine in nighttime dose only

Uses:
• **daytime** (orange caplets) – for temporary relief of the following symptoms:
  • nasal congestion
  • sore throat pain   • cough
  • minor aches and pains
  • reduction of fever • headache
• **nighttime** (blue caplets) – provides the same relief as the daytime caplets plus temporarily relieves:
  • runny nose • sneezing

Warnings:
• **Alcohol warning:** If you consume 3 or more alcoholic drinks every day, ask your doctor whether you should take acetaminophen or other pain relievers/ fever reducers. Acetaminophen may cause liver damage.
• **Sore throat warning:** Severe or persistent sore throat or sore throat accompanied by high fever, headache, nausea, and vomiting may be serious. Ask a doctor right away. Do not use for more than 2 days or give to children under 3 years of age unless directed by a doctor.

Do not use
• for more than 7 days
• if you are now taking a prescription monoamine oxidase inhibitor (MAOI) (certain drugs for depression, psychiatric or emotional conditions, or Parkinson's disease), or for 2 weeks after stopping the MAOI drug. If you do not know if your prescription drug contains an MAOI, ask a doctor or pharmacist before taking this product.
• with any other products containing acetaminophen. Taking more than directed may cause liver damage.

Ask a doctor before use if you have
• glaucoma • heart disease
• high blood pressure • diabetes
• thyroid disease
• trouble urinating due to an enlarged prostate gland
• cough that occurs with too much phlegm (mucus)
• chronic cough that lasts or as occurs with smoking, asthma or emphysema
• a breathing problem such as emphysema or chronic bronchitis

Ask a doctor or pharmacist before use if you are taking sedatives or tranquilizers

When using this product
• **do not use more than directed**
• when using nighttime product:
  • excitability may occur, especially in children
  • may cause marked drowsiness
  • alcohol, sedatives and tranquilizers may increase drowsiness
  • avoid alcoholic drinks
  • be careful when driving a motor vehicle or operating machinery

Stop use and ask a doctor if
• new symptoms occur
• you get nervous, dizzy, or sleepless
• redness or swelling is present
• fever gets worse or lasts more than 3 days

- pain, cough or nasal congestion gets worse or lasts for more than 7 days
- cough comes back, or occurs with rash, or headache that lasts. These could be signs of a serious condition.

If pregnant or breast-feeding ask a health professional before use.

Keep out of reach of children.

Overdose warning: Taking more than the recommended dose can cause serious health problems. In case of overdose, get medical help or contact a Poison Control Center right away. Quick medical attention is critical for adults as well as for children even if you do not notice any signs or symptoms.

Directions:

do not use more than directed **(see Overdose warning)**
- children under 12 years of age: ask a doctor
- adults and children 12 years of age and over:
  - **daytime** – take 2 orange caplets every 4 hours, while symptoms persist, not to exceed 8 daytime caplets in 24 hours, or as directed by your doctor
  - **nighttime** – take 2 blue caplets, if needed, to be taken no sooner than 4 hours after the last daytime caplets, not to exceed 4 nighttime caplets in 24 hours, or as directed by your doctor.

Other Information:
- store at room temperature

Inactive Ingredients:
- **daytime caplet** – benzoic acid, carnauba wax, corn starch, D&C yellow no. 10 lake, FD&C red no. 40 lake, hypromellose, magnesium stearate, microcrystalline cellulose, polyethylene glycol, polysorbate 80, stearic acid, titanium dioxide
- **nighttime caplet** – benzoic acid, carnauba wax, corn starch, D&C yellow no. 10 lake, FD&C blue no. 1 lake, hypromellose, magnesium stearate, microcrystalline cellulose, polyethylene glycol, stearic acid, titanium dioxide

Questions or comments?
1-800-468-7746

How Supplied: Available in 20 ct. carton.

COMTREX® Maximum Strength Non-Drowsy Cold & Cough
(Novartis Consumer Health, Inc.)
Pain Reliever/Fever Reducer, Cough Suppressant, Nasal Decongestant
Acetaminophen, Dextromethorphan HBr, Phenylephrine HCl

Fast Relief of:
- Nasal Congestion • headache
- Sore Throat Pain • coughing

Drug Facts
Active Ingredients
(in each caplet): **Purposes:**

Acetaminophen
325 mg ..... Pain reliever/fever reducer

Dextromethorphan HBr
10 mg .... Cough suppressant
Phenylephrine HCl
5 mg .... Nasal decongestant

Uses:
- for temporary relief of the following symptoms:
  - headache • sore throat pain
  - cough • minor aches and pains
  - nasal congestion
- temporarily reduces fever

Warnings:

Alcohol warning: If you consume 3 or more alcoholic drinks every day, ask your doctor whether you should take acetaminophen or other pain relievers/fever reducers. Acetaminophen may cause liver damage.

Sore throat warning: Severe or persistent sore throat or sore throat accompanied by high fever, headache, nausea, and vomiting may be serious. Ask a doctor right away. Do not use for more than 2 days or give to children under 3 years of age unless directed by a doctor.

Do not use
- for more than 7 days
- if you are now taking a prescription monoamine oxidase inhibitor (MAOI) (certain drugs for depression, psychiatric or emotional conditions, or Parkinson's disease), or for 2 weeks after stopping the MAOI drug. If you do not know if your prescription drug contains an MAOI, ask a doctor or pharmacist before taking this product.
- with any other products containing acetaminophen. Taking more than directed may cause liver damage.

Ask a doctor before use if you have
- heart disease • high blood pressure
- diabetes • thyroid disease
- cough that occurs with too much phlegm (mucus)
- chronic cough that lasts or as occurs with smoking, asthma, or emphysema
- trouble urinating due to an enlarged prostate gland

When using this product • do not use more than directed

Stop use and ask a doctor if
- you get nervous, dizzy, or sleepless
- new symptoms occur
- redness or swelling is present
- fever gets worse or lasts more than 3 days
- pain, cough or nasal congestion gets worse or lasts more than 7 days
- cough comes back, or occurs with rash, or headache that lasts. These could be signs of a serious condition.

If pregnant or breast-feeding, ask a health professional before use.

Keep out of reach of children.

Overdose warning: Taking more than the recommended dose can cause serious health problems. In case of overdose, get medical help or contact a Poison Control Center right away. Quick medical attention is critical for adults as well as for children even if you do not notice any signs or symptoms.

Directions:
- do not use more than directed (see overdose warning
- adults and children 12 years of age and over: take 2 caplets every 4 hours, while symptoms persist
- do not use more than 12 caplets in 24 hours
- children under 12 years of age: consult a doctor

Other Information:
- store at room temperature

Inactive Ingredients: benzoic acid, carnauba wax, corn starch, D&C yellow no. 10 lake, FD&C red no. 40 lake, hypromellose, magnesium stearate, microcrystalline cellulose, polyethylene glycol, polysorbate 80, stearic acid, titanium dioxide

Questions or comments?
1-800-468-7746

How Supplied:
Available in cartons of 10 and 20 ct.

DESENEX® ANTIFUNGALS
(Novartis Consumer Health, Inc.)
All products are Prescription Strength
Shake Powder
Liquid Spray
Spray Powder
Jock Itch Spray Powder

Drug Facts

Active Ingredient: **Purpose:**
Miconazole nitrate 2% .... Antifungal

Uses: *Shake Powder, Liquid Spray, and Spray Powder*
- cures most athlete's foot (tinea pedis) and ringworm (tinea corporis) • relieves itching, scaling, burning, and discomfort that can accompany athlete's foot
Jock Itch Spray Powder
- cures most jock itch (tinea cruris) • relieves itching, scaling, burning and discomfort that can accompany jock itch

Warnings:
For external use only
Flammability Warning: Contents under pressure. Do not puncture or incinerate. Flammable mixture; do not use near fire or flame, or expose to heat or temperatures above 49°C (120°F). Use only as directed. Intentional misuse by deliberately concentrating and inhaling the contents can be harmful or fatal.
Do not use
- in or near the mouth or the eyes
- for nail or scalp infections
When using this product
- do not get into the eyes or mouth
Stop use and ask a doctor if
- irritation occurs or gets worse
- no improvement within 4 weeks for athlete's foot and ringworm, or no improvement within 2 weeks for jock itch.

Continued on next page

Desenex Antifungals—Cont.

Keep out of reach of children. If swallowed, get medical help or contact a poison control center right away.

Directions:
- adults and children 2 years and older
- wash the affected area with soap and water and dry completely before applying

Shake Powder
- apply a thin layer over affected area twice a day (morning and night) or as directed by a doctor
- pay special attention to the spaces between the toes. Wear well-fitting, ventilated shoes and change shoes and socks at least once a day.
- use every day for 4 weeks
- supervise children in the use of this product
- children under 2 years of age: ask a doctor

Liquid Spray and Spray Powder
- shake can well, hold 4″ to 6″ from skin
- spray a thin layer over affected area twice a day (morning and night) or as directed by a doctor
- for athlete's foot pay special attention to the spaces between the toes. Wear well-fitting, ventilated shoes and change shoes and socks at least once a day.
- use daily for 4 weeks
- supervise children in the use of this product
- children under 2 years of age: ask a doctor

Jock Itch Spray Powder
- shake can well, hold 4″ to 6″ from skin
- spray a thin layer over affected area twice a day (morning and night) or as directed by a doctor
- use daily for 2 weeks
- supervise children in the use of this product
- children under 2 years of age: ask a doctor

Other Information: • store at controlled room temperature 20-25°C (68-77°F)
- see bottom of can for lot number and expiration date

For Spray Powders and Liquid Spray
- if clogging occurs, remove button and clean nozzle with a pin

Inactive Ingredients: *Shake Powder—* corn starch, corn starch/acrylamide/sodium acrylate polymer, fragrance, talc
*Liquid Spray—*polyethylene glycol 300, polysorbate 20, SD alcohol 40-B (15%w/w) Propellant: dimethyl ether
Spray Powder, Jock Itch Spray Powder— aloe vera gel, aluminum starch octenyl succinate, isopropyl myristate, propylene carbonate, SD alcohol 40-B (10% w/w), sorbitan monooleate, stearalkonium hectorite Propellant: isobutane/propane

How Supplied: *Shake Powder*-1.5 oz, 3 oz, plastic bottles. *Spray Powder*-4 oz cans. *Liquid Spray*-4.6 oz cans. *Jock Itch Spray Powder*-4 oz cans

Shown in Product Identification Guide, page 505

DESENEX® CREAM
(Novartis Consumer Health, Inc.)
1% clotrimazole cream, USP, antifungal

Drug Facts
Active Ingredient: **Purpose:**
Clotrimazole USP, 1% .... Antifungal

Uses:
- cures most athlete's foot (tinea pedis), most jock itch (tinea cruris), and ringworm (tinea corporis)
- relieves itching, burning, cracking, and discomfort which accompany these conditions

Warnings:
For external use only

Do not use
- in or near the mouth or the eyes
- for vaginal yeast infections
- on nail or scalp

Stop use and ask a doctor if
- irritation occurs or gets worse
- there is no improvement within 4 weeks for athlete's foot or ringworm or within 2 weeks for jock itch

Keep out of reach of children. If swallowed, get medical help or contact a poison control center right away.

Directions:
- Adults and children 2 years of age and older.
- use tip of cap to break the seal and open the tube
- wash the affected skin with soap and water and dry completely before applying
- for athelete's foot and ringworm, apply a thin layer over affected area morning and evening for 4 weeks or as directed by a doctor
- for athlete's foot, pay special attention to the spaces between the toes. Wear well-fitting, ventilated shoes and change shoes and socks at least once a day.
- for jock itch, apply a thin layer over affected area morning and evening for 2 weeks or as directed by a doctor
- Children under 2 years: ask a doctor

Other Information:
- store between 2°-30°C (36°-86°F)
- do not use if seal on tube is broken or is not visible

Inactive Ingredients: benzyl alcohol (1%), cetostearyl alcohol, cetyl esters wax, 2-octyldodecanol, polysorbate 60, purified water, sorbitan monostearate

Questions? call **1-800-452-0051** 24 hours a day, 7 days a week.

How Supplied: ½ oz cartons.
Shown in Product Identification Guide, page 505

EXCEDRIN® BACK & BODY
(Novartis Consumer Health, Inc.)

Drug Facts
Active Ingredients *Purposes*
(in each caplet)
Acetaminophen 250 mg   Pain reliever
Buffered aspirin equal to   Pain reliever
250 mg aspirin (buffered
with calcium carbonate)

Uses:
- for the temporary relief of:
  - minor pain of arthritis • backache
  - muscular aches

Warnings:

Reye's syndrome: Children and teenagers who have or are recovering from chicken pox or flu-like symptoms should not use this product. When using this product, if changes in behavior with nausea and vomiting occur, consult a doctor because these symptoms could be an early sign of Reye's syndrome, a rare but serious illness.

Allergy alert: Aspirin may cause a severe allergic reaction which may include:
- hives   • facial swelling
- asthma (wheezing) • shock

Alcohol warning: If you consume 3 or more alcoholic drinks every day, ask your doctor whether you should take acetaminophen and aspirin or other pain relievers/fever reducers. Acetaminophen and aspirin may cause liver damage and stomach bleeding.

Do not use
- if you have ever had an allergic reaction to any other pain reliever/fever reducer
- with any other products containing acetaminophen. **(see Overdose Warning)**

Ask a doctor before use if you have
- asthma • ulcers • bleeding problems
- stomach problems that last or come back, such as heartburn, upset stomach, or stomach pain

Ask a doctor or pharmacist before use if you are taking a prescription drug for:
- anticoagulation (thinning of the blood)
- diabetes • gout • arthritis

Stop use and ask a doctor if • an allergic reaction occurs. Seek medical help right away.
- new symptoms occur
- symptoms do not get better or worsen
- ringing in the ears or loss of hearing occurs
- painful area is red or swollen
- pain gets worse or lasts for more than 10 days
- fever gets worse or lasts for more than 3 days

If pregnant or breast-feeding, ask a health professional before use. It is especially important not to use aspirin during the last 3 months of pregnancy unless definitely directed to by a doctor because it may cause problems in the unborn child or complications during delivery.

Keep out of reach of children.

Overdose warning: Taking more than the recommended does can cause serious health problems, including serious liver damage. In case of overdose, get medical help or contact a Poison Control Center right away. Quick medical attention is critical for adults as well as for children even if you do not notice any signs or symptoms.

Directions:
- do not use more than directed **(see Overdose Warning)**
- drink a full glass of water with each dose
- adults and children 12 years and over: take 2 caplets every 6 hours; not more than 8 caplets in 24 hours
- children under 12 years: ask a doctor

Other Information:
- **each caplet contains:** calcium 80 mg
- store at controlled room temperature 20°-25° C (68°-77° F)
- read all product information before using. Keep this box for important information

Inactive Ingredients: benzoic acid, corn starch, croscarmellose sodium, D&C yellow #10 lake, FD&C blue #1 lake, FD&C blue #2 lake, hydroxypropylcellulose, hypromellose, microcrystalline cellulose, mineral oil, polysorbate 20, povidone, propylene glycol, silicone dioxide, simethicone emulsion, sorbitan monolaurate, stearic acid, zinc stearate

Questions or comments?
1-800-468-7746

How Supplied: Caplets available in 24 ct., 50 ct. and 100 ct. cartons.

Shown in Product Identification Guide, page 505

EXCEDRIN® TENSION HEADACHE
(Novartis Consumer Health, Inc.)
PAIN RELIEVER

Drug Facts
Active Ingredients   **Purpose:**
(in each geltab/tablets/caplets):
Acetaminophen
   500 mg .... Pain reliever
(formulated with 65 mg caffeine)

Uses:
- temporarily relieves minor aches and pains due to:
  - headache • muscular aches

Warnings:
Alcohol warning: If you consume 3 or more alcoholic drinks every day, ask your doctor whether you should take acetaminophen or other pain relievers/fever reducers. Acetaminophen may cause liver damage.

Caffeine warning: The recommended dose of this product contains about as much caffeine as a cup of coffee. Limit the use of caffeine-containing medications, foods, or beverages while taking this product because too much caffeine may cause nervousness, irritability, sleeplessness, and, occasionally, rapid heartbeat.

Do not use
- with any other products containing acetaminophen. **(see Overdose Warning)**

Stop use and ask a doctor if
- new symptoms occur
- symptoms do not get better or worsen
- painful area is red or swollen
- pain gets worse or lasts for more than 10 days
- fever gets worse or lasts for more than 3 days

If pregnant or breast-feeding, ask a health professional before use.

Keep out of reach of children.

Overdose warning: Taking more than the recommended dose can cause serious health problems, including serious liver damage. In case of overdose, get medical help or contact a Poison Control Center right away. Quick medical attention is critical for adults as well as for children even if you do not notice any signs or symptoms.

Directions:
- do not use more than directed **(see overdose warning)**
- adults and children 12 years of age and over: take 2 geltabs, tablets or caplets every 6 hours; not more than 8 geltabs, tablets or caplets in 24 hours
- children under 12 years of age: ask a doctor

Other Information:
- store at room temperature

Inactive Ingredients:
Tablets/Caplets
benzoic acid, corn starch, croscarmellose sodium*, FD&C blue #1, FD&C red #40, FD&C yellow #6, gelatin, glycerin, hypromellose, magnesium stearate, methylparaben*, microcrystalline cellulose, mineral oil, polysorbate 20, povidone, pregelatinized starch, propylene glycol, propylparaben*, simethicone emulsion, sorbitan monolaurate, stearic acid, titanium dioxide
Geltabs
benzoic acid, corn starch, croscarmellose sodium*, FD&C blue #1, FD&C red #40, FD&C yellow #6, gelatin, glycerin, hypromellose, magnesium stearate, methylparaben*, microcrystalline cellulose, mineral oil, polysorbate 20, povidone, pregelatinized starch, propylene glycol, propylparaben*, simethicone emulsion, sorbitan monolaurate, stearic acid, titanium dioxide

---

*may contain these ingredients

Questions or comments?
1-800-468-7746

How Supplied: Tablets in 24 ct., 50 ct., 100 ct. and 250 ct. cartons. Caplets in 24 ct., 50 ct., 100 ct. and 250 ct. cartons. Geltabs in 24 ct., 50 ct., and 100 ct. cartons.

Shown in Product Identification Guide, page 505

EXCEDRIN® EXTRA STRENGTH
(Novartis Consumer Health, Inc.)
PAIN RELIEVER

Drug Facts
Active Ingredients: **Purpose:**
(in each caplet/tablet/geltab)
Acetaminophen 250 mg ..... Pain reliever
Aspirin 250 mg .... Pain reliever
Caffeine 65 mg .... Pain reliever aid

Uses:
- temporarily relieves minor aches and pains due to:
  - headache
  - a cold • arthritis • muscular aches
  - sinusitis • toothache
  - premenstrual & menstrual cramps

Warnings:
Reye's syndrome: Children and teenagers who have or are recovering from chicken pox or flu-like symptoms should not use this product. When using this product, if changes in behavior with nausea and vomiting occur, consult a doctor because these symptoms could be an early sign of Reye's syndrome, a rare but serious illness.

Allergy alert: Aspirin may cause a severe allergic reaction, which may include:
- hives • facial swelling
- asthma (wheezing) • shock

Alcohol warning: If you consume 3 or more alcoholic drinks every day, ask your doctor whether you should take acetaminophen and aspirin or other pain relievers/fever reducers. Acetaminophen and aspirin may cause liver damage and stomach bleeding.

Caffeine warning: The recommended dose of this product contains about as much caffeine as a cup of coffee. Limit the use of caffeine-containing medications, foods, or beverages while taking this product because too much caffeine may cause nervousness, irritability, sleeplessness, and, occasionally, rapid heart beat.

Do not use
- if you have ever had an allergic reaction to any other pain reliever/fever reducer
- with any other products containing acetaminophen. **(see Overdose Warning)**

Ask a doctor before use if you have
- asthma
- ulcers
- bleeding problems
- stomach problems such as heartburn, upset stomach, or stomach pain that do not go away or return

Ask a doctor or pharmacist before use if you are taking a prescription drug for:
- anticoagulation (thinning of the blood)
- diabetes • gout • arthritis

Stop use and ask a doctor if
- an allergic reaction occurs. Seek medical help right away.
- new symptoms occur

Continued on next page

Excedrin Extra Strength—Cont.

- symptoms do not get better or worsen
- ringing in the ears or loss of hearing occurs
- painful area is red or swollen
- pain gets worse or lasts for more than 10 days
- fever gets worse or lasts for more than 3 days

If pregnant or breast-feeding, ask a health professional before use. It is especially important not to use aspirin during the last 3 months of pregnancy unless definitely directed to do so by a doctor because it may cause problems in the unborn child or complications during delivery.

Keep out of reach of children.

Overdose warning: Taking more than the recommended dose can cause serious health problems, including serious liver damage. In case of overdose, get medical help or contact a Poison Control Center right away. Quick medical attention is critical for adults as well as for children even if you do not notice any signs or symptoms.

Directions:
- do not use more than directed **(see overdose warning)**
- drink a full glass of water with each dose
- adults and children 12 years and over: take 2 caplets, tablets, or geltabs every 6 hours; not more than 8 caplets, tablets, or geltabs in 24 hours
- children under 12 years: ask a doctor

Other Information:
- store at room temperature
- read all product information before using.

Inactive Ingredients:
Tablets/Caplets
benzoic acid, carnauba wax, FD&C blue #1*, hydroxypropyl cellulose, hypromellose, microcrystalline cellulose, mineral oil, polysorbate 20, povidone, propylene glycol, simethicone emulsion, sorbitan monolaurate, stearic acid, titanium dioxide*

* may also contain these ingredients.

Inactive Ingredients:
Geltabs
benzoic acid, D&C yellow #10 lake, disodium EDTA, FD&C blue #1 lake, FD&C red #40 lake, ferric oxide, gelatin, glycerin, hydroxypropyl cellulose, hypromellose, maltitol solution, microcrystalline cellulose, mineral oil, pepsin, polysorbate 20, povidone, propylene glycol, propyl gallate, simethicone emulsion, sorbitan monolaurate, stearic acid, titanium dioxide

Questions or comments?
1-800-468-7746

How Supplied: Caplets available in 24 ct., 50 ct., 100 ct., and 250 ct. cartons. Tablets available in 2 ct., 10 ct., 24 ct., 50 ct., 100 ct. and 250 ct. cartons. Geltabs available in 24 ct., 50 ct. and 100 ct. cartons.

Shown in Product Identification Guide, page 505

EXCEDRIN® MIGRAINE PAIN RELIEVER/PAIN RELIEVER AID
(Novartis Consumer Health, Inc.)

Drug Facts
Active Ingredients   **Purposes:**
(in each caplet/tablet/geltab):
Acetaminophen 250 mg ..... Pain reliever
Aspirin 250 mg .... Pain reliever
Caffeine 65 mg .... Pain reliever aid

Use:
- treats migraine

Warnings:
Reye's syndrome: Children and teenagers who have or are recovering from chicken pox or flu-like symptoms should not use this product. When using this product, if changes in behavior with nausea and vomiting occur, consult a doctor because these symptoms could be an early sign of Reye's syndrome, a rare but serious illness.

Allergy alert: Aspirin may cause a severe allergic reaction, which may include:
- hives • facial swelling
- asthma (wheezing) • shock

Alcohol warning: If you consume 3 or more alcoholic drinks every day, ask your doctor whether you should take acetaminophen and aspirin or other pain relievers/fever reducers. Acetaminophen and aspirin may cause liver damage and stomach bleeding.

Caffeine warning: The recommended dose of this product contains about as much caffeine as a cup of coffee. Limit the use of caffeine-containing medications, foods, or beverages while taking this product because too much caffeine may cause nervousness, irritability, sleeplessness, and, occasionally, rapid heartbeat.

Do not use
- if you have ever had an allergic reaction to any other pain reliever/fever reducer
- with any other products containing acetaminophen. **(see Overdose Warning)**

Ask a doctor before use if you have
- never had migraines diagnosed by a health professional
- a headache that is different from your usual migraines
- the worst headache of your life
- fever and stiff neck
- headaches beginning after or caused by head injury, exertion, coughing or bending
- experienced your first headache after the age of 50
- daily headaches
- a migraine so severe as to require bed rest

- asthma • bleeding problems
- ulcers
- stomach problems such as heartburn, upset stomach, or stomach pain that do not go away or recur
- problems or serious side effects from taking pain relievers or fever reducers
- vomiting with your migraine headache

Ask a doctor or pharmacist before use if you are
- taking a prescription drug for:
  - anticoagulation (thinning of the blood)
  - diabetes • gout • arthritis
- under a doctor's care for any serious condition
- taking any other drug
- taking any other product that contains aspirin, acetaminophen, or any other pain reliever/fever reducer

Stop use and ask a doctor if
- an allergic reaction occurs. Seek medical help right away.
- your migraine is not relieved or worsens after first dose
- new or unexpected symptoms occur
- stomach pain or upset gets worse or lasts
- ringing in the ears or loss of hearing occurs

If pregnant or breast-feeding, ask a health professional before use. It is especially important not to use aspirin during the last 3 months of pregnancy unless definitely directed to do so by a doctor because it may cause problems in the unborn child or complications during delivery.

Keep out of reach of children.

Overdose warning: Taking more than the recommended dose can cause serious health problems, including serious liver damage. In case of overdose, get medical help or contact a Poison Control Center right away. Quick medical attention is critical for adults as well as for children even if you do not notice any signs or symptoms.

Directions:
- do not use more than directed **(see Overdose Warning)**
- adults: take 2 tablets, caplets or geltabs with a glass of water
- if symptoms persist or worsen, ask your doctor
- do not take more than 2 tablets, caplets or geltabs in 24 hours, unless directed by a doctor
- under 18 years of age: ask a doctor

Other Information:
- store at 20°-25°C (68°-77F)
- read all product information before using. Keep the box for important information.

Inactive Ingredients:
Tablets/Caplets
benzoic acid, carnauba wax, FD&C blue #1*, hydroxypropylcellulose, hypromellose, microcrystalline cellulose, mineral oil, polysorbate 20, povidone, propylene

glycol, simethicone emulsion, sorbitan monolaurate, stearic acid, titanium dioxide*

———

*may contain these ingredients

Geltabs

benzoic acid, D&C yellow #10 lake, disodium EDTA, FD&C blue #1 lake, FD&C red #40 lake, ferric oxide, gelatin, glycerin, hydroxypropylcellulose, hypromellose, maltitol solution, microcrystalline cellulose, mineral oil, pepsin, polysorbate 20, povidone, propylene glycol, propyl gallate, simethicone emulsion, sorbitan monolaurate, stearic acid, titanium dioxide

Questions or comments?
1-800-468-7746

How Supplied: Tablets in 2 ct., 24 ct., 50 ct., 100 ct. and 250 ct. cartons. Caplets in 24 ct., 50 ct., 100 ct. and 250 ct. cartons. Geltabs in 24 ct., 50 ct., and 100 ct. cartons.

Shown in Product Identification Guide, page 505

———

EXCEDRIN PM®
(Novartis Consumer Health, Inc.)
PAIN RELIEVER/NIGHTTIME SLEEP AID

Drug Facts

Active Ingredients: **Purpose:**
(in each caplets/tablets)
Acetaminophen 500 mg ..... Pain reliever
Diphenhydramine
citrate 38 mg .... Nighttime sleep aid

Uses: for the temporary relief of occasional headaches and minor aches and pains with accompanying sleeplessness.

Warnings:

Alcohol warning: If you consume 3 or more alcoholic drinks every day, ask your doctor whether you should take acetaminophen or other pain relievers/fever reducers. Acetaminophen may cause liver damage.

Do not use
- in children under 12 years of age
- with any other product containing diphenhydramine, even one used on skin
- with any other products containing acetaminophen. **(see Overdose Warning)**

Ask a doctor before use if you have
- glaucoma
- a breathing problem such as emphysema or chronic bronchitis
- trouble urinating due to an enlarged prostate gland

Ask a doctor or pharmacist before use if you are taking sedatives or tranquilizers.

When using this product
- avoid alcoholic drinks
- drowsiness may occur
- be careful when driving a motor vehicle or operating machinery

Stop use and ask a doctor if
- new symptoms occur
- sleeplessness lasts continuously for more than 2 weeks. Insomnia may be a symptom of serious underlying medical illness.
- pain gets worse or lasts for more than 10 days
- painful area is red or swollen
- fever gets worse or lasts for more than 3 days

If pregnant or breast-feeding, ask a health professional before use.

Keep out of reach of children.

Overdose warning: Taking more than the recommended dose can cause serious health problems, including serious liver damage. In case of overdose, get medical help or contact a Poison Control Center right away. Quick medical attention is critical for adults as well as for children even if you do not notice any signs or symptoms.

Directions:
- do not use more than directed **(see overdose warning)**
- children under 12 years of age: consult a doctor
- adults and children 12 years and over: take 2 caplets or tablets at bedtime, if needed, or as directed by a doctor

Other Information:
- store at room temperature
- read all product information before using.

Inactive Ingredients: benzoic acid, carnauba wax, croscarmellose sodium*, crospovidone*, D&C yellow #10 lake, FD&C blue #1 lake, hypromellose, magnesium stearate, methylparaben*, microcrystalline cellulose, mineral oil, polysorbate 20, povidone, pregelatinized starch, propylene glycol, propylparaben*, simethicone emulsion, sodium citrate, sorbitan monolaurate, stearic acid, titanium dioxide

———

*may contain these ingredients

Questions or comments?
1-800-468-7746

How Supplied: Caplets available in 24 ct., 50 ct. and 100 ct. cartons. Tablets available in 2 ct., 10 ct., 24 ct., 50 ct. and 100 ct. cartons.

Shown in Product Identification Guide, page 505

———

EXCEDRIN® SINUS HEADACHE
(Novartis Consumer Health, Inc.)
Acetaminophen and Phenylephrine HCl

Drug Facts

Active Ingredients:
(in each caplet/tablet)   **Purposes:**
Acetaminophen
    325 mg .... Pain reliever
Phenylephrine HCl
    5 mg .... Nasal decongestant

Uses:
- temporarily relieves:
  - headache • minor aches and pains
  - nasal congestion • sinus congestion and pressure
- helps clear nasal passages; shrinks swollen membranes

Warnings:

Alcohol warning: If you consume 3 or more alcoholic drinks every day, ask your doctor whether you should take acetaminophen or other pain relievers/fever reducers. Acetaminophen may cause liver damage.

Do not use
- with any other products containing acetaminophen. **(see Overdose Warning)**
- if you are now taking a prescription monoamine oxidase inhibitor (MAOI) (certain drugs for depression, psychiatric or emotional conditions, or Parkinson's disease), or for 2 weeks after stopping the MAOI drug. If you do not know if your prescription drug contains an MAOI, ask a doctor or pharmacist before taking this product.

Ask a doctor before use if you have
- trouble urinating due to an enlarged prostate gland
- heart disease • high blood pressure
- thyroid disease • diabetes

When using this product
- do not use more than directed

Stop use and ask a doctor if
- new symptoms occur
- you get nervous, dizzy, or sleepless
- redness or swelling is present
- pain or nasal congestion gets worse or lasts more than 7 days
- fever gets worse or lasts more than 3 days

If pregnant or breast-feeding, ask a health professional before use.

Keep out of reach of children.

Overdose warning:

Taking more than the recommended dose can cause serious health problems, including serious liver damage. In case of overdose, get medical help or contact a Poison Control Center right away. Quick medical attention is critical for adults as well as for children even if you do not notice any signs or symptoms.

Directions:
- do not use more than directed **(see Overdose Warning)**
- children under 12 years of age: ask a doctor
- adults and children 12 years of age and over: take 2 caplets or tablets, every 4 hours
- do not take more than 12 caplets or tablets in 24 hours

Other Information:
- store at room temperature
- read all product information before using.

Continued on next page

Excedrin Sinus Headache—Cont.

Inactive Ingredients: benzoic acid, carnauba wax, corn starch, FD&C blue # 1, hypromellose, magnesium stearate, microcrystalline cellulose, mineral oil, polysorbate 20, povidone, propylene glycol, simethicone emulsion, sorbitan monolaurate, stearic acid, titanium dioxide

Questions or comments?
1–800–468–7746

How Supplied:
Caplets available in 2 ct., 24 ct., 50 ct., 100 ct. & 250 ct. cartons.
Tablets available in 24 ct., 50 ct. & 100 ct. cartons.

Shown in Product Identification Guide, page 505

4-WAY® MENTHOL
(Novartis Consumer Health, Inc.)
Nasal Decongestant

Drug Facts
Active Ingredient: **Purpose:**
Phenylephrine hydrochloride
   1% .... Nasal decongestant

Uses:
temporarily relieves nasal congestion due to:
   • common cold • hay fever
   • upper respiratory allergies

Warnings:
Ask a doctor before use if you have
• heart disease • high blood pressure
• thyroid disease • diabetes
• trouble urinating due to an enlarged prostate gland
When using this product
• **do not use more than directed**
• do not use more than 3 days
• use only as directed
• frequent or prolonged use may cause nasal congestion to recur or worsen
• temporary discomfort such as burning, stinging, sneezing, or an increase in nasal discharge may occur
• infection may spread if this container is used by more than one person
Stop use and ask a doctor if symptoms persist
If pregnant or breast-feeding, ask a health professional before use.
Keep out of reach of children. If swallowed, get medical help or contact a Poison Control Center right away.

Directions:
• adults and children 12 years and older: 2 or 3 sprays in each nostril not more than every 4 hours.
• children under 12 years: ask a doctor. Use instructions: with head in a normal, upright position, put atomizer tip into nostril. Squeeze bottle with firm, quick pressure while inhaling. Wipe nozzle clean after each use.

Other Information:
• store at room temperature
• container is filled to proper level for best spray action

Inactive Ingredients: benzalkonium chloride, boric acid, camphor, eucalyptol, menthol, polysorbate 80, sodium borate, water

Questions or comments?
1-800-468-7746

How Supplied:
Available in 0.5 and 1.0 fl oz cartons.

4-WAY® MOISTURIZING RELIEF
(Novartis Consumer Health, Inc.)
Nasal Decongestant
Xylometazoline Hydrochloride 0.1%

Drug Facts
Active ingredient: *Purpose*
Xylometazoline   Nasal decongestant
hydrochloride 0.1%

Uses:
• temporarily relieves nasal congestion due to:
   • a cold • hay fever
   • upper respiratory allergies
• soothes nasal discomfort caused by dryness

Warnings:
Ask a doctor before use if you have
• heart disease   • high blood pressure
• thyroid disease   • diabetes
• trouble urinating due to an enlarged prostate gland
When using this product
• **do not use more than directed**
• do not use more than 3 days
• use only as directed
• frequent or prolonged use may cause nasal congestion to recur or worsen
• temporary discomfort such as burning, stinging, sneezing, or an increase in nasal discharge may occur
• infection may spread if this container is used by more than one person
Stop use and ask a doctor if symptoms persist
If pregnant or breast-feeding, ask a health professional before use.
Keep out of reach of children. If swallowed, get medical help or contact a Poison Control Center right away.

Directions:
• adults and children 12 years of age and over: 2 or 3 sprays in each nostril not more often than every 8 to 10 hours
• do not use more than 3 doses in 24 hours
• children under 12 years: ask a doctor
Use instructions: with head in a normal, upright position, put atomizer tip into nostril. Squeeze bottle with firm, quick pressure while inhaling. Wipe nozzle clean after each use.

Other information
• store at room temperature
• container is filled to proper level for best spray action
• non-USP for assay

Inactive ingredients: benzalkonium chloride, dibasic sodium phosphate, edetate disodium, hypromellose, monobasic sodium phosphate, purified water, sodium chloride, sorbitol solution

Questions or comments? 1-800-452-0051

How Supplied: Available in 0.5 and 1.0 oz sizes.

4-WAY® Fast Acting Nasal Spray
(Novartis Consumer Health, Inc.)
Phenylephrine hydrochloride 1%, nasal decongestant

Active Ingredient: **Purpose:**
Phenylephrine hydrochloride
   1% .... Nasal decongestant

Uses:
temporarily relieves nasal congestion due to:
   • common cold
   • hay fever
   • upper respiratory allergies

Warnings:
Ask a doctor before use if you have
• heart disease
• high blood pressure
• thyroid disease
• diabetes
• trouble urinating due to an enlarged prostate gland
When using this product
• **do not use more than directed**
• do not use more than 3 days
• use only as directed
• frequent or prolonged use may cause nasal congestion to recur or worsen
• temporary discomfort such as burning, stinging, sneezing, or an increase in nasal discharge may occur
• infection may spread if this container is used by more than one person
Stop use and ask a doctor if symptoms persist
If pregnant or breast-feeding, ask a health professional before use.
Keep out of reach of children. If swallowed, get medical help or contact a Poison Control Center right away.

Directions:
• adults and children 12 years and older: 2 or 3 sprays in each nostril not more than every 4 hours.
• children under 12 years: ask a doctor.
Use instructions: with head in a normal, upright position, put atomizer tip into nostril. Squeeze bottle with firm, quick pressure while inhaling. Wipe nozzle clean after each use.

Other Information:
• store at room temperature
• container is filled to proper level for best spray action

Inactive Ingredients: benzalkonium chloride, boric acid, sodium borate, water

Questions or comments?
1-800-468-7746

How Supplied:
Available in 0.5 and 1.0 fl oz cartons.
Shown in Product Identification Guide, page 504

4-WAY® SALINE
(Novartis Consumer Health, Inc.)
Moisturizing Mist

Uses:
Helps make nasal passages feel clear and more comfortable by providing gentle, soothing, moisture to dry, irritated nasal passages due to colds, allergies, air pollution, smoke, air travel, overuse of decongestant sprays/drops and dry air (low humidity).

Directions:

Adults and children 2 years of age and over:	2 to 3 sprays in each nostril as often as needed or as directed by your doctor.
Children under 2 years of age:	Use only as directed by your doctor.

Use Instructions: With head in a normal, upright position, put atomizer tip into nostril. Squeeze bottle with firm, quick pressure while inhaling. Wipe nozzle clean after each use.

Cautions: Keep out of reach of children. The use of this dispenser by more than one person may spread infections.

Ingredients: Water, Boric Acid, Glycerin, Sodium Chloride, Sodium Borate, Eucalyptol, Menthol, Polysorbate 80, Benzalkonium Chloride

Note: Container is filled to proper level for best spray action. Store at room temperature.

Questions or comments?
1-800-468-7746

How Supplied:
Available in 1.0 fl oz cartons.

EX•LAX® CHOCOLATED STIMULANT
(Novartis Consumer Health, Inc.)
LAXATIVE
Sennosides, USP, 15mg

Drug Facts
Active Ingredient   Purpose:
(in each piece):
Sennosides, USP,
   15 mg .... Stimulant laxative

Uses:
• relieves occasional constipation (irregularity)
• generally produces bowel movement in 6 to 12 hours

Warnings:
Do not use laxative products when abdominal pain, nausea, or vomiting are present unless directed by a doctor

Ask a doctor before use if you have
• noticed a sudden change in bowel habits that persists over a period of 2 weeks

Ask a doctor or pharmacist before use if you
• are taking a prescription drug. Laxatives may affect how other drugs work. Take this product 2 or more hours before or after other drugs.

When using this product
• do not use for a period longer than 1 week

Stop use and ask a doctor if
• rectal bleeding or failure to have a bowel movement occur after use of a laxative. These may be signs of a serious condition.

If pregnant or breast-feeding, ask a health professional before use.

Keep out of reach of children. In case of overdose, get medical help or contact a Poison Control Center right away.

Directions:

adults and children 12 years of age and older	chew 2 chocolated pieces once or twice daily
children 6 to under 12 years of age	chew 1 chocolated piece once or twice daily
children under 6 years of age	ask a doctor

Other Information:
• each piece contains: **potassium 10mg**
• store at controlled room temperature 20-25°C (68-77°F)

Inactive Ingredients: cocoa, confectioners sugar, hydrogenated palm kernel oil, lecithin, non-fat dry milk, vanillin

Questions? call **1-800-452-0051**
24 hours a day, 7 days a week.

How Supplied: Cartons of 18 ct. pieces.
Shown in Product Identification Guide, page 505

EX•LAX® Laxative Pills
(Novartis Consumer Health, Inc.)
Regular Strength
Maximum Strength
Laxative Pills
Senosides, USP, 15mg
Senosides, USP, 25mg

Active Ingredients: Regular Strength: Sennosides, USP, 15 mg.
Maximum Strength: Sennosides, USP, 25 mg.

Purpose: Stimulant Laxative

Uses:
• relieves occasional constipation (irregularity)
• generally produces bowel movement in 6 to 12 hours

Warnings:
Do not use laxative products when abdominal pain, nausea, or vomiting are present unless directed by a doctor

Ask a doctor before use if you have
• noticed a sudden change in bowel habits that persists over a period of 2 weeks

Ask a doctor or pharmacist before use if you
• are taking a prescription drug. Laxatives may affect how other drugs work. Take this product 2 or more hours before or after other drugs.

When using this product
• do not use for a period longer than 1 week

Stop use and ask a doctor if
• rectal bleeding or failure to have a bowel movement occur after use of a laxative. These may be signs of a serious condition.

If pregnant or breast-feeding, ask a health professional before use.

Keep out of reach of children. In case of overdose, get medical help or contact a Poison Control Center right away.

Directions:
• swallow pill(s) with a glass of water
• swallow pill(s) whole, do not crush, break or chew

adults and children 12 years of age and older	2 pills once or twice daily
children 6 to under 12 years of age	1 pill once or twice daily
children under 6 years of age	ask a doctor

Other Information:
• each pill contains: **calcium 50mg**
• store at controlled room temperature 20-25°C (68-77°F)

Continued on next page

Ex·Lax Laxative Pills—Cont.

Inactive Ingredients:

Regular Strength:

acacia, alginic acid, carnauba wax, colloidal silicon dioxide, dibasic calcium phosphate, iron oxides, magnesium stearate, microcrystalline cellulose, sodium benzoate, sodium lauryl sulfate, starch, stearic acid, sucrose, talc, titanium dioxide

Maximum Strength:

acacia, alginic acid, carnauba wax, colloidal silicon dioxide, dibasic calcium phosphate, FD&C blue no. 1 aluminium lake, magnesium stearate, microcrystalline cellulose, sodium benzoate, sodium lauryl sulfate, starch, stearic acid, sucrose, talc, titanium dioxide

Questions? call **1-800-452-0051**
24 hours a day, 7 days a week.

How Supplied: Available in Regular Strength 8 and 30 ct, Maximum Strength 24, 48 and 90 cts cartons.

Shown in Product Identification Guide, page 505

GAS-X® REGULAR STRENGTH Antigas Chewable Tablets
GAS-X® EXTRA STRENGTH Antigas Softgels and Chewable Tablets
GAS-X® MAXIMUM STRENGTH Antigas Softgels
GAS-X® WITH MAALOX® EXTRA STRENGTH Antigas/Antacid Chewable Tablets
(Novartis Consumer Health, Inc.)

Active Ingredients: Purpose

Regular Strength Tablets
   Simethicone 80 mg .... Antigas
Extra Strength Softgels and Tablets
   Simethicone 125 mg .... Antigas
Maximum Strength Softgels
   Simethicone 166 mg .... Antigas
Gas-X with Maalox Fast tabs
   Calcium carbonate 500 mg ..... Antigas
   Simethicone 125 mg .... Antigas

Inactive Ingredients:

Regular Strength Tablets
Cherry Creme:
calcium carbonate, D&C Red 30 aluminum lake, dextrose, flavors, maltodextrin, propylene glycol, soy protein isolate
Peppermint Creme:
calcium carbonate, dextrose, flavors, maltodextrin, starch
Extra Strength
Softgels:
D&C Yellow 10, FD&C Blue 1, FD&C Red 40, gelatin, glycerin, peppermint oil, purified water, sorbitol, titanium dioxide

Cherry Creme Tablets:
calcium phosphate tribasic, colloidal silicon dioxide, D&C Red 30 aluminum lake, dextrose, flavors, maltodextrin, propylene glycol soy protein isolate
Peppermint Creme Tablets:
calcium phosphate tribasic, colloidal silicon dioxide, D&C Red 30 aluminum lake, D&C Yellow 10 aluminum lake, dextrose, flavors, maltodextrin, starch
Maximum Strength Softgels
FD&C Blue 1, FD&C Red 40, gelatin, glycerin, peppermint oil, purified water, sorbitol
GAS-X with Maalox Fast tabs
Wild Berry:
colloidal silicon dioxide, D&C Red 30, dextrose, flavors, maltodextrin, mannitol, pregelatinized starch, talc, tribasic calcium phosphate

Use:
GAS-X
For the relief of
• pressure and bloating commonly referred to as gas
GAS-X with Maalox
For the relief of
• pressure and bloating commonly referred to as gas
• acid indigestion
• heartburn
• sour stomach
• upset stomach associated with these symptoms

Warnings:
GAS-X
Keep out of reach of children.
GAS-X with Maalox
Ask a doctor or pharmacist before use if you are
• now taking a prescription drug. Antacids may interact with certain prescription drugs.
Keep out of reach of children.

Directions:
Regular Strength Tablets
• adults: chew 1 or 2 tablets as needed after meals and at bedtime
• do not exceed 6 tablets in 24 hours except under the advice and supervision of a physician
Extra Strength
Tablets
• adults: chew 1 or 2 tablets at needed after meals and at bedtime
• do not exceed 4 tablets in 24 hours except under the advice and supervision of a physician
Softgels
• adults: swallow with water one or two Softgels as needed after meals and at bedtime
• do not exceed 4 Softgels in 24 hours except under the advice and supervision of a physician
Maximum Strength Tablets
• adults: chew 1 or 2 tablets as needed after meals and at bedtime
• do not exceed 6 tablets in 24 hours except under the advice and supervision of a physician

Gas-X with Maalox Fast tabs
• chew 1 to 2 tablets as symptoms occur or as directed by a physician
• do not take more than 4 tablets in a 24-hour period or use the maximum dosage for more than 2 weeks except under the advice and supervision of a physician

Other Information:
Regular Strength Tablets
• each tablet contains: **calcium 30mg**
• store at controlled room temperature 20-25°C (68-77°F)
• protect from moisture
Extra Strength
Tablets
• each tablet contains: **calcium 45mg**
• store at controlled room temperature 20-25°C (68-77°F)
• protect from moisture
Softgels
• store at controlled room temperature 20-25°C (68-77°F)
• protect from heat and moisture
Gas-X with Maalox Tablets
• each tablet contains: **calcium 45mg**
• store at controlled room temperature 20-25°C (68-77°F)
• protect from moisture

Questions?
Call **1-800-452-0051** 24 hours a day, 7 days a week.

How Supplied:
Regular Strength Chewable tablets are available in peppermint creme 36 and 60 cts., and cherry creme 36 ct. carton.
Extra Strength Chewable tablets are available in peppermint creme and cherry creme 18 ct. carton.
Extra Strength Softgels are available in 10, 30 and 72 ct. cartons.
Maximum Strength Softgels are available in 50 ct. cartons.
Gas-X® With Maalox® Tablets are available in wild berry 24 ct. cartons.

Shown in Product Identification Guide, page 505 and 506

GAS-X® THIN STRIPS™
(Novartis Consumer Health, Inc.)
Extra Strength
Anti-Gas Simethicone 62.5 mg
Alcohol: less than 0.5%

Description:
Extra Strength Gas-X® Thin Strips™ offers fast, effective, and convenient relief of pressure and bloating. They melt on your tongue so you can discreetly take them anywhere. And they provide a great mouth freshening feel too!

Drug Facts
Active Ingredient (per strip):   Purpose:
Simethicone 62.5 mg .... Antigas

Use:
For the relief of
• Pressure, bloating, and fullness commonly referred to as gas

Warnings:

Keep out of reach of children

Directions:

- Adults: allow 2 to 4 strips to dissolve on tongue as needed after meals and at bedtime
- Do not exceed 8 strips in 24 hours except under the advice and supervision of a physician

Other Information:

- Store at a controlled room temperature 20-25°C (68-77°F)
- Protect from moisture

Inactive Ingredients:

Cinnamon flavor:

corn starch modified, ethyl alcohol, FD&C Red #40, flavor, hypromellose, maltodextrin, polyethylene glycol, sorbitol, sucralose, titanium dioxide, water

Peppermint flavor:

corn starch modified, ethyl alcohol, FD&C Blue #1, flavor, hypromellose, maltodextrin, menthol, polyethylene glycol, sorbitol, sucralose, titanium dioxide, water

Questions?

Call **1-800-452-0051** 24 hours a day, 7 days a week.

How Supplied:

Available in Cinnamon and Peppermint flavors, 18 ct. Individually packed strips.
Shown in Product Identification Guide, page 505

LAMISIL^{AT}® CREAM
(Novartis Consumer Health, Inc.)

Drug Facts

Active Ingredient:	Purpose:

Terbinafine hydrochloride 1% .... Antifungal

Uses:

- **cures most athlete's foot (tinea pedis)**
- **cures most jock itch (tinea cruris) and ringworm (tinea corporis)**
- **relieves itching, burning, cracking and scaling which accompany these conditions**

Warnings:

For external use only
Do not use • on nails or scalp
- in or near the mouth or the eyes
- for vaginal yeast infections
When using this product do not get into the eyes. If eye contact occurs, rinse thoroughly with water.
Stop use and ask a doctor if too much irritation occurs or gets worse.
Keep out of reach of children. If swallowed, get medical help or contact a poison control center right away.

Directions:

- adults and children 12 years and over
  - use the tip of the cap to break the seal and open the tube
  - wash the affected skin with soap and water and dry completely before applying

- **for athlete's foot** wear well-fitting, ventilated shoes. Change shoes and socks at least once daily
  - **between the toes only:** apply twice a day (morning and night) for **1 week** or as directed by a doctor.

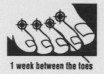

1 week between the toes

- **on the bottom or sides of the foot:** apply twice a day (morning and night) for **2 weeks** or as directed by a doctor.

2 weeks on the bottom or sides of the foot

- **for jock itch and ringworm:** apply once a day (morning **or** night) for **1 week** or as directed by a doctor.
- wash hands after each use
- children under 12 years: ask a doctor

Other Information:

- do not use if seal on tube is broken or is not visible
- store at controlled room temperature 20–25°C (68–77°F)

Inactive Ingredients: benzyl alcohol, cetyl alcohol, cetyl palmitate, isopropyl myristate, polysorbate 60, purified water, sodium hydroxide, sorbitan monostearate, stearyl alcohol.

How Supplied: Athlete's Foot — Net wt. 12g (.42 oz.) tube and 24g (.85 oz.) tube and 30g tube, Jock Itch — Net wt. 12g (.42 oz.) tube.
Questions? call **1-800-452-0051** 24 hours a day, 7 days a week.
Shown in Product Identification Guide, page 506

LAMISIL^{AF} DEFENSE™
(Novartis Consumer Health, Inc.)
TOLNAFTATE 1%, ANTIFUNGAL
Shake Powder
Spray Powder

Drug Facts

Active Ingredient:	Purpose:

Tolnaftate 1% .... Antifungal

Uses:

- Proven clinically effective in the treatment of most athlete's foot (tinea pedis) and ringworm (tinea corporis)
- Helps prevent most athlete's foot with daily use
- For effective relief of itching, burning and cracking

Warnings:

For external use only
Flammability Warning: (for Spray Powder only): Contents under pressure. Do not puncture or incinerate. Flammable mixture; do not use near fire or flame, or expose to heat or temperatures above 49°C (120°F). Use only as directed. Intentional misuse by deliberately concentrating and inhaling contents can be harmful or fatal.

Do not use
- in or near the mouth or eyes
- on nails or scalp

When using this product
- avoid contact with eyes

Stop use and ask a doctor if
- irritation occurs or gets worse
- no improvement within 4 weeks

Keep out of reach of children. If swallowed, get medical help or contact a poison control center right away.

Directions:

Shake Powder:

- adults and children 2 years and older
  - Wash affected area and dry thoroughly
  - Apply a thin layer over affected area twice daily (morning and night) or as directed by a doctor
  - For athlete's foot: pay special attention to spaces between the toes; wear well-fitting, ventilated shoes and change shoes and socks at least once daily
  - Use daily for 4 weeks; if condition persists longer, ask a doctor.
  - To prevent athlete's foot, apply once or twice daily (morning and/or night)
  - Supervise children in the use of this product
- Children under 2 years of age: ask a doctor

Spray Powder:

- adults and children 2 years and older
  - Wash affected area and dry thoroughly
  - Shake can well, hold 4″ to 6″ from skin
  - Spray a thin layer over affected area twice a day (morning and night) or as directed by a doctor
  - For athlete's foot: pay special attention to spaces between the toes; wear well-fitting, ventilated shoes and change shoes and socks at least once daily
  - Use daily for 4 weeks; if condition persists longer, ask a doctor
  - To prevent athlete's foot, apply once or twice daily (morning and/or night)
  - Supervise children in the use of this product
- Children under 2 years of age: ask a doctor

Other Information:

Shake Powder:

- store between 15°C to 25°C (59°F to 77°F)

Continued on next page

Lamisil Defense—Cont.

- see container bottom for lot number and expiration date

Spray Powder:

- store between 20°C to 25°C (68°F to 77°F)
- see container bottom for lot number and expiration date
- In case of clogging, remove button and clean nozzle with a pin

Inactive Ingredients:

Shake Powder: corn starch, fragrance, talc

Spray Powder: aluminum starch octenyl succinate, fragrance, isopropyl myristate, propylene carbonate, SD alcohol 40-B (11% w/w), sorbitan oleate, stearalkonium hectorite, talc.
Propellant: isobutane/propane
Tamper-evident aerosol can for your protection.
Questions call **1-800-452-0051** 24 hours a day, 7 days a week.

How Supplied:
Shake Powder available in 4 oz bottles.
Spray Powder available in 4.6 oz cans.
Shown in Product Identification Guide, page 506

MAALOX® MAXIMUM STRENGTH MULTI SYMPTOM ANTACID/ ANTIGAS LIQUID
(Novartis Consumer Health, Inc.)
Oral Suspension Antacid/Anti-Gas

- Cherry
- Mint

Drug Facts:

Active Ingredients	Maximum Strength Maalox® Max® Antacid/ AntiGas Per Tsp. (5 mL)	Purpose
Aluminum Hydroxide	400 mg	antacid
(equivalent to dried gel, USP)		
Magnesium Hydroxide	400 mg	antacid
Simethicone	40 mg	antigas

Uses: For the relief of
- acid indigestion • heartburn
- sour stomach
- upset stomach associated with these symptoms
- bloating and pressure commonly referred to as gas

Warnings:
Ask a doctor before use if you have kidney disease or • a magnesium-restricted diet.

Ask a doctor or pharmacist before use if you are taking a prescription drug. Antacids may interact with certain prescription drugs.
Stop use and ask a doctor if symptoms last for more than 2 weeks
Keep out of reach of children.

Directions:
- shake well before using
- Adults/children 12 years and older: take 2 to 4 teaspoonsful four times a day or as directed by a physician
- do not take more than 12 teaspoonsful in 24 hours or use the maximum dosage for more than 2 weeks.
- Children under 12 years: consult a physician
To aid in establishing proper dosage schedules, the following information is provided:

MAALOX® Maximum Strength Multi Symptom Antacid/AntiGas	
	Per 2 Tsp. (10 mL) (Minimum Recommended Dosage)
Acid neutralizing capacity	38.8 mEq

Inactive Ingredients: butylparaben, carboxymethylcellulose sodium, flavor, glycerin, hypromellose, microcrystalline cellulose, potassium citrate, propylene glycol, propylparaben, purified water, saccharin sodium, sorbitol.

PROFESSIONAL LABELING
Indications:
As an antacid for symptomatic relief of hyperacidity associated with the diagnosis of peptic ulcer, gastritis, peptic esophagitis, gastric hyperacidity, or hiatal hernia. As an antiflatulent to alleviate the symptoms of gas, including postoperative gas pain.

Warnings:
Prolonged use of aluminum-containing antacids in patients with renal failure may result in or worsen dialysis osteomalacia. Elevated tissue aluminum levels contribute to the development of the dialysis encephalopathy and osteomalacia syndromes. Small amounts of aluminum are absorbed from the gastrointestinal tract and renal excretion of aluminum is impaired in renal failure. Aluminum is not well removed by dialysis because it is bound to albumin and transferrin, which do not cross dialysis membranes. As a result, aluminum is deposited in bone, and dialysis osteomalacia may develop when large amounts of aluminum are ingested orally by patients with impaired renal function.
Aluminum forms insoluble complexes with phosphate in the gastrointestinal tract, thus decreasing phosphate absorption. Prolonged use of aluminum-containing antacids by normophosphatemic patients may result in hypophosphatemia if phosphate intake is not adequate. In its more severe forms, hypophosphatemia can lead to anorexia, malaise, muscle weakness, and osteomalacia.

Advantages: In addition to the fast acting antacid ingredients, Aluminum Hydroxide and Magnesium Hydroxide, MAALOX® Maximum Strength Multi Symptom Antacid/Antigas contains the powerful antigas ingredient, simethicone, to provide concurrent fast relief from discomfort associated with gas.

Questions? call **1-800-452-0051** 24 hours a day, 7 days a week.

How Supplied:
Cherry is available in plastic bottles of 12 fl. oz. (355 mL) and 26 fl. oz. (769 mL).
Mint is available in plastic bottles of 12 fl. oz. (355 mL) and 26 fl. oz. (769 mL).

MAALOX® REGULAR STRENGTH
(Novartis Consumer Health, Inc.)
Liquid Antacid & Antigas

Active ingredients:
(in each 5 mL = 1 teaspoonful)   *Purpose*
Aluminum hydroxide (equiv. to dried gel, USP) 200 mg .... Antacid
Magnesium hydroxide 200 mg .... Antacid
Simethicone 20 mg .... Antigas

Uses: for the relief of:
- acid indigestion • heartburn
- sour stomach
- upset stomach associated with these symptoms
- pressure and bloating commonly referred to as gas

Warnings:
Ask a doctor before use if you have
- kidney disease
- a magnesium-restricted diet

Ask a doctor or pharmacist before use if you are taking a prescription drug. Antacids may interact with certain prescription drugs.

Stop use and ask a doctor if symptoms last for more than 2 weeks
Keep out of reach of children.

Directions:
- shake well before using
- Adults/children 12 years and older: take 2 to 4 teaspoonsful four times a day or as directed by a physician
- do not take more than 16 teaspoonsful in 24 hours or use the maximum dosage for more than 2 weeks
- Children under 12 years: consult a physician

Other information:
- each teaspoonful contains: **magnesium 85 mg**
- store at controlled room temperature 20-25°C (68-77°F)
- protect from freezing

Inactive ingredients:

butylparaben, carboxymethylcellulose sodium, flavor, glycerin, hypromellose, microcrystalline cellulose, propylene glycol, propylparaben, purified water, saccharin sodium, sorbitol

Questions?

call **1-800-452-0051** 24 hours a day, 7 days a week.

How Supplied: Mint available in 5 fl. oz. (148 mL), 12 fl. oz. (355 mL) and 26 fl. oz. (769 mL) bottles. Cherry available in 12 fl. oz. (355 mL) bottles.

Shown in Product Identification Guide, page 506

MAALOX TOTAL STOMACH RELIEF®
(Novartis Consumer Health, Inc.)
Peppermint
Strawberry

Drug Facts:

Active ingredient
(in each 15 mL*)   **Purpose**
Bismuth
subsalicylate 525 mg .... Upset stomach reliever/Antidiarrheal

---

*15 mL = 1 tablespoon

Uses:
- upset stomach
- indigestion
- nausea
- diarrhea
- gas
- heartburn

Warnings:

Do not use
- if you have bloody or black stool
- an ulcer
- a bleeding problem

Reye's syndrome: Children and teenagers who have or are recovering from chicken pox or flu-like symptoms should not use this product. When using this product, if changes in behavior with nausea and vomiting occur, consult a doctor because these symptoms could be an early sign of Reye's syndrome, a rare but serious illness.

Allergy alert: Do not take this product if you are
- allergic to salicylates (including aspirin)
- taking other salicylate-containing products (such as aspirin)

Ask a doctor or pharmacist before use if you
- are taking a prescription drug for anticoagulation (blood thinning), diabetes, gout, or arthritis
- have fever
- have mucus in the stool

When using this product a temporary, but harmless, darkening of the stool and/or tongue may occur

Stop use and ask a doctor if
- symptoms get worse
- ringing in the ears or a loss of hearing occurs
- diarrhea or symptoms last more than 2 days

If pregnant or breast-feeding, ask a health care professional before use.

Keep out of reach of children. In case of overdose, get medical help or contact a poison control center right away.

Directions:
- shake well before using
- adults and children 12 years of age and older: 2 tablespoons (30 mL) every 1/2 hour to 1 hour, as required, not to exceed 8 tablespoons (120 mL) in 24 hours
- use until diarrhea stops but not more than 2 days
- children under 12 years of age: ask a doctor
- drink plenty of clear liquids to prevent dehydration caused by diarrhea

Other Information:
- each tablespoon contains: **sodium 6 mg**
- each tablespoon contains: **salicylate 232 mg**
- store at controlled room temperature 20-25°C (68-77°F)
- keep tightly closed and avoid freezing

Peppermint flavor:

Inactive Ingredients: carboxymethylcellulose sodium, ethyl alcohol, flavor, methylparaben, microcrystalline cellulose, propylene glycol, propylparaben, purified water, salicylic acid, sodium salicylate, sorbitol, sucralose, xanthan gum

Stawberry flavor:

Inactive ingredients: carboxymethylcellulose sodium, flavor, methylparaben, microcrystalline cellulose, propylene glycol, propylparaben, purified water, salicylic acid, sodium salicylate, sorbitol, sucralose, xanthan gum

Questions? call **1-800-452-0051** 24 hours a day, 7 days a week.
Made in Canada
www.maaloxus.com

How Supplied: Plastic bottles of 12 fl. oz. (355 mL).

Shown in Product Identification Guide, page 506

MAALOX® MAXIMUM STRENGTH MULTI SYMPTOM
(Novartis Consumer Health, Inc.)
ANTACID/ANTIGAS CHEWABLE TABLETS

Drug Facts:

Active Ingredients:
(in each tablet)   **Purpose:**
Calcium carbonate
  1000 mg .... Antacid
Simethicone 60 mg .... Antigas

Uses:
For the relief of
- acid indigestion • heartburn
- sour stomach
- upset stomach associated with these symptoms
- bloating and pressure commonly referred to as gas

Warnings:

Ask a doctor before use if you have:
- kidney stones • a calcium-restricted diet

Ask a doctor or pharmacist before use if you are: presently taking a prescription drug. Antacids may interact with certain prescription drugs.

Stop use and ask a doctor if:
symptoms last for more than 2 weeks.
Keep out of reach of children.

Directions:
- Chew 1 to 2 tablets as symptoms occur or as directed by a physician
- do not take more than 8 tablets in a 24-hour period or use the maximum dosage for more than 2 weeks except under the advice and supervision of a physician

Other Information:
- each tablet contains: **calcium 400 mg**
- store at controlled room temperature 20–25°C (68–77°F)
- keep tightly closed and dry

Inactive Ingredients: acesulfame K, colloidal silicon dioxide, croscarmellose sodium, D&C Red #30 aluminum lake, D&C Yellow #10 aluminum lake, dextrose, FD&C Red #40 aluminum lake, FD&C Yellow #6 aluminum lake, flavors, magnesium stearate, maltodextrin, mannitol, pregelatinized starch.

Questions? call **1-800-452-0051** 24 hours a day, 7 days a week.

How Supplied:

Assorted Fruit — Plastic Bottles of 35, 65 and 90 tablets.

Shown in Product Identification Guide, page 506

MINERAL ICE®
(Novartis Consumer Health, Inc.)
Pain Reliever

Drug Facts

Active Ingredient: **Purpose:**
Menthol 2% .... Topical analgesic

Uses:
- temporarily relieves minor aches and pains of muscles and joints associated with:
  - arthritis • simple backache • strains
  - bruises • sport injuries • sprains
- provides cooling penetrating relief

Continued on next page

Mineral Ice—Cont.

Warnings:

For external use only

Do not use
• with other topical pain relievers
• with heating pads or heating devices

When using this product
• do not use in or near the eyes
• do not apply to wounds or damaged skin
• do not bandage tightly

Stop use and ask a doctor if
• condition worsens
• symptoms last more that 7 days or clear up and occur again within a few days
• redness or irritation develops

If pregnant or breast-feeding, ask a health professional before use.

Keep out of reach of children. If swallowed, get medical help or contact a Poison Control Center right away.

Directions:
• clean affected area before applying product
• adults and children 2 years of age and older: apply to affected area not more than 3 to 4 times daily
• children under 2 years of age: ask a doctor

Other Information:
• store in a cool place
• keep lid tightly closed
• do not use, pour, spill or store near heat or open flame

Inactive Ingredients: ammonium hydroxide, carbomer, cupric sulfate, FD&C blue no. 1, isopropyl alcohol, magnesium sulfate, sodium hydroxide, thymol, water

Questions or comments?

1-800-468-7746

How Supplied:

Available in 3.5 oz, 8.0 oz & 16.0 oz jars.
Shown in Product Identification Guide, page 506

THERAFLU® Cold & Cough

(Novartis Consumer Health, Inc.)
Cough Suppressant
(Dextromethorphan HBr)
Antihistamine (Pheniramine maleate)
Nasal Decongestant
(Phenylephrine HCl)

Drug Facts

Active Ingredients: **Purpose:**
(in each packet)
Dextromethorphan hydrobromide
20 mg .... Cough suppressant
Pheniramine maleate
20 mg .... Antihistamine
Phenylephrine hydrochloride
10 mg .... Nasal decongestant

Uses:
• temporarily relieves these symptoms due to a cold:
  • nasal and sinus congestion
  • cough due to minor throat and bronchial irritation

• temporarily relieves these symptoms due to hay fever or other upper respiratory allergies:
  • runny nose • sneezing • itchy nose and throat
  • itchy, watery eyes

Warnings:

Do not use • if you are now taking a prescription monoamine oxidase inhibitor (MAOI) (certain drugs for depression, psychiatric, or emotional conditions, or Parkinson's disease), or for 2 weeks after stopping the MAOI drug. If you do not know if your prescription drug contains an MAOI, ask a doctor or pharmacist before taking this product.

Ask a doctor before use if you have
• heart disease • high blood pressure
• thyroid disease • diabetes • glaucoma
• a breathing problem such as emphysema, asthma, or chronic bronchitis
• trouble urinating due to an enlarged prostate gland • cough that occurs with smoking, too much phlegm (mucus) or chronic cough that lasts
• a sodium-restricted diet

Ask a doctor or pharmacist before use if you are taking sedatives or tranquilizers.

When using this product • do not exceed recommended dosage • avoid alcoholic drinks • may cause marked drowsiness • alcohol, sedatives, and tranquilizers may increase drowsiness • be careful when driving a motor vehicle or operating machinery • excitability may occur, especially in children

Stop use and ask a doctor if
• nervousness, dizziness, or sleeplessness occur
• symptoms do not improve within 7 days or occur with a fever
• cough persists for more than 7 days, comes back or occurs with a fever, rash, or persistent headache. These could be signs of a serious condition.

If pregnant or breast-feeding, ask a health care professional before use.

Keep out of reach of children. In case of overdose, get medical help or contact a poison control center right away.

Directions:
• take every 4 hours; not to exceed 6 packets in 24 hours or as directed by a doctor.
• adults and children 12 years of age and over: dissolve contents of one packet in 8 oz. hot water; sip while hot. Consume entire drink within 10–15 minutes.
• children under 12 years of age: consult a doctor.
• If using a microwave, add contents of one packet to 8 oz. of cool water; stir briskly before and after heating. Do not overheat.

Other Information:
• each packet contains: **sodium 46 mg**
• store at controlled room temperature 20-25°C (68-77°F)

How Supplied: 6 packets in a carton.

Inactive Ingredients: acesulfame K, citric acid, D&C yellow 10, FD&C Yellow 6, lecithin, magnesium stearate, malto-dextrin, natural flavors, silicon dioxide, sodium citrate, sucrose, tribasic calcium phosphate

Questions? call **1-800-452-0051**
24 hours a day, 7 days a week.

THERAFLU® Cold & Sore Throat

(Novartis Consumer Health, Inc.)
Pain Reliever-Fever Reducer
(Acetaminophen)
Antihistamine (Pheniramine maleate)
Nasal Decongestant
(Phenylephrine HCl)

Drug Facts

Active Ingredients: **Purpose:**
(in each packet)
Acetaminophen
325 mg .... Pain reliever/
                                        Fever reducer
Pheniramine maleate
20 mg .... Antihistamine
Phenylephrine hydrochloride
10 mg .... Nasal decongestant

Uses:
• temporarily relieves these symptoms due to a cold:
  • minor aches and pains • headache
  • minor sore throat pain • nasal congestion • temporarily reduces fever
• temporarily relieves these symptoms due to hay fever or other upper respiratory allergies:
  • runny nose • sneezing • itchy nose and throat • itchy, watery eyes

Warnings:

Alcohol Warning: If you consume 3 or more alcoholic drinks every day, ask your doctor whether you should take acetaminophen or other pain relievers/fever reducers. Acetaminophen may cause liver damage.

Do not use • if you are now taking a prescription monoamine oxidase inhibitor (MAOI) (certain drugs for depression, psychiatric, or emotional conditions, or Parkinson's disease), or for 2 weeks after stopping the MAOI drug. If you do not know if your prescription drug contains an MAOI, ask a doctor or pharmacist before taking this product.
• with any other product containing acetaminophen **(see Overdose Warning)**

Ask a doctor before use if you have
• heart disease • high blood pressure
• thyroid disease • diabetes • glaucoma
• a breathing problem such as emphysema or chronic bronchitis
• trouble urinating due to an enlarged prostate gland
• a sodium-restricted diet

Ask a doctor or pharmacist before use if you are taking sedatives or tranquilizers.

When using this product • do not exceed recommended dosage • avoid alcoholic drinks • may cause drowsiness • alcohol, sedatives, and tranquilizers may increase drowsiness • be careful when driving a motor vehicle or operating machinery • excitability may occur, especially in children

Stop use and ask a doctor if • nervousness, dizziness, or sleeplessness occur
• pain or nasal congestion gets worse or lasts more than 7 days
• fever gets worse or lasts more than 3 days
• redness or swelling is present
• new symptoms occur
• sore throat is severe, persists for more than 2 days, is accompanied or followed by fever, headache, rash, nausea, or vomiting. These could be signs of a serious condition.

If pregnant or breast-feeding, ask a health care professional before use.

Keep out of reach of children.

Overdose Warning: Taking more than the recommended dose can cause serious health problems, including serious liver damage. In case of overdose, get medical help or contact a poison control center right away. Prompt medical attention is critical for adults as well as for children even if you do not notice any signs or symptoms.

Directions:
• do not use more than directed **(see Overdose Warning)**
• take every 4 hours; not to exceed 6 packets in 24 hours or as directed by a doctor.
• adults and children 12 years of age and over: dissolve contents of one packet into 8 oz. hot water; sip while hot. Consume entire drink within 10–15 minutes.
• children under 12 years of age: consult a doctor.
• If using a microwave, add contents of one packet to 8 oz. of cool water; stir briskly before and after heating. Do not overheat.

Other Information:
• each packet contains: **sodium 44 mg**
• store at controlled room temperature 20-25°C (68-77°F)

How Supplied: 6 packets in a carton.

Inactive Ingredients: acesulfame K, citric acid, D&C Yellow 10, FD&C Yellow 6, lecithin, magnesium stearate, maltodextrin, natural flavors, silicon dioxide, sodium citrate, sucrose, tribasic calcium phosphate
Questions? call **1-800-452-0051**
24 hours a day, 7 days a week.

**THERAFLU® Flu & Chest Congestion
(Novartis Consumer Health, Inc.)
Pain Reliever-Fever Reducer
(Acetaminophen)
Expectorant (Guaifenesin)**

Drug Facts

Active Ingredients: **Purpose:**
(in each packet):
Acetaminophen
1000 mg .... Pain reliever/
                                       Fever reducer
Guaifenesin
400 mg .... Expectorant

Uses: • temporarily relieves these symptoms due to a cold:
• minor aches and pains • headache
• minor sore throat pain
• helps loosen phlegm (mucus) and thin bronchial secretions to drain bronchial tubes and make coughs more productive
• temporarily reduces fever

Warnings: Alcohol Warning: If you consume 3 or more alcoholic drinks every day, ask your doctor whether you should take acetaminophen or other pain relievers/fever reducers. Acetaminophen may cause liver damage.

Do not use • with any other product containing acetaminophen **(see Overdose Warning)**

Ask a doctor before use if you have
• a breathing problem such as emphysema, asthma, or chronic bronchitis
• cough that occurs with smoking, too much phlegm (mucus) or chronic cough that lasts

Stop use and ask a doctor if
• pain or cough gets worse or lasts more than 7 days
• fever gets worse or lasts more than 3 days
• redness or swelling is present
• new symptoms occur
• cough comes back or occurs with rash or headache that lasts. These could be signs of a serious condition.
• sore throat is severe, persists for more than 2 days, is accompanied or followed by fever, headache, rash, nausea, or vomiting

If pregnant or breast-feeding, ask a health care professional before use.

Keep out of reach of children.

Overdose Warning: Taking more than the recommended dose can cause serious health problems, including serious liver damage. In case of overdose, get medical help or contact a poison control center right away. Prompt medical attention is critical for adults as well as for children even if you do not notice any signs or symptoms.

Directions:
• do not use more than directed **(see Overdose Warning)**
• take every 6 hours; not to exceed 4 packets in 24 hours or as directed by a doctor.
• adults and children 12 years of age and over: dissolve contents of one packet into 8 oz. hot water; sip while hot. Consume entire drink within 10–15 minutes.
• children under 12 years of age: consult a doctor.
• If using a microwave, add contents of one packet to 8 oz. of cool water; stir briskly before and after heating. Do not overheat.

Other Information:
• Phenylketonurics: Contains Phenylalanine 24 mg per packet
• each packet contains: **sodium 15 mg**
• each packet contains: **potassium 10 mg**

• store at controlled room temperature 20-25°C (68-77°F)

How Supplied: 6 packets in a carton.

Inactive Ingredients: acesulfame K, aspartame, citric acid, D&C Yellow 10, FD&C Red 40, maltodextrin, natural flavors, silicon dioxide, sodium citrate, sucrose, tribasic calcium phosphate
Questions? call **1-800-452-0051**
24 hours a day, 7 days a week.

**THERAFLU® Flu & Sore Throat
(Novartis Consumer Health, Inc.)
Pain Reliever-Fever Reducer
(Acetaminophen)
Antihistamine (Pheniramine maleate)
Nasal Decongestant
(Phenylephrine HCl)**

Drug Facts

Active Ingredients: **Purpose:**
(in each packet)
Acetaminophen
650 mg .... Pain reliever/
                                       Fever reducer
Pheniramine maleate
20 mg .... Antihistamine
Phenylephrine hydrochloride
10 mg .... Nasal decongestant

Uses:
• temporarily relieves these symptoms due to a cold:
• minor aches and pains • headache
• minor sore throat pain • nasal congestion • temporarily reduces fever
• temporarily relieves these symptoms due to hay fever or other upper respiratory allergies:
• runny nose • sneezing • itchy nose and throat • itchy, watery eyes

Warnings:

Alcohol Warning: If you consume 3 or more alcoholic drinks every day, ask your doctor whether you should take acetaminophen or other pain relievers/fever reducers. Acetaminophen may cause liver damage.

Do not use • if you are now taking a prescription monoamine oxidase inhibitor (MAOI) (certain drugs for depression, psychiatric, or emotional conditions, or Parkinson's disease), or for 2 weeks after stopping the MAOI drug. If you do not know if your prescription drug contains an MAOI, ask a doctor or pharmacist before taking this product.
• with any other product containing acetaminophen **(see Overdose Warning)**

Ask a doctor before use if you have
• heart disease • high blood pressure
• thyroid disease • diabetes • glaucoma
• a breathing problem such as emphysema, asthma or chronic bronchitis
• trouble urinating due to an enlarged prostate gland
• a sodium-restricted diet

Continued on next page

Theraflu Flu & Sore Th.—Cont.

Ask a doctor or pharmacist before use if you are taking sedatives or tranquilizers.
When using this product • do not exceed recommended dosage • avoid alcoholic drinks • may cause drowsiness • alcohol, sedatives, and tranquilizers may increase drowsiness • be careful when driving a motor vehicle or operating machinery • excitability may occur, especially in children
Stop use and ask a doctor if • nervousness, dizziness, or sleeplessness occur
• pain or nasal congestion gets worse or lasts more than 7 days
• fever gets worse or lasts more than 3 days
• redness or swelling is present
• new symptoms occur
• sore throat is severe, persists for more than 2 days, is accompanied or followed by fever, headache, rash, nausea, or vomiting. These could be signs of a serious condition.
If pregnant or breast-feeding, ask a health care professional before use.
Keep out of reach of children.
Overdose Warning: Taking more than the recommended dose can cause serious health problems, including serious liver damage. In case of overdose, get medical help or contact a poison control center right away. Prompt medical attention is critical for adults as well as for children even if you do not notice any signs or symptoms.

Directions:

• do not use more than directed **(see Overdose Warning)**
• take every 4 hours; not to exceed 6 packets in 24 hours or as directed by a doctor.
• adults and children 12 years of age and over: dissolve contents of one packet in 8 oz. hot water; sip while hot. Consume entire drink within 10–15 minutes.
• children under 12 years of age: consult a doctor.
• If using a microwave, add contents of one packet to 8 oz. of cool water; stir briskly before and after heating. Do not overheat.

Other Information:

• each packet contains: **sodium 51 mg**
• each packet contains: **potassium 10 mg**
• store at controlled room temperature 20-25°C (68-77°F)

How Supplied: 6 packets in a carton.

Inactive Ingredients: acesulfame K, citric acid, D&C Yellow 10, FD&C Blue 1, FD&C Red 40, lecithin, maltodextrin, medium chain triglycerides, natural flavors, silicon dioxide, sodium chloride, sodium citrate, sucrose, triacetin, tribasic calcium phosphate
Questions? call **1-800-452-0051**
24 hours a day, 7 days a week.

THERAFLU® Nighttime Severe Cold
(Novartis Consumer Health, Inc.)
Pain Reliever-Fever Reducer (Acetaminophen)
Antihistamine (Pheniramine maleate)
Nasal Decongestant (Phenylephrine HCl)

Drug Facts

Active Ingredients:　　　　　　**Purpose:**
(in each packet)
Acetaminophen
　650 mg .... Pain reliever/
　　　　　　　　　　　　　　　Fever reducer
Pheniramine maleate
　20 mg .... Antihistamine
Phenylephrine hydrochloride
　10 mg .... Nasal decongestant
Uses:
• temporarily relieves these symptoms due to a cold:
　• minor aches and pains • headache
　• minor sore throat pain • nasal congestion • temporarily reduces fever
• temporarily relieves these symptoms due to hay fever or other upper respiratory allergies:
　• runny nose • sneezing • itchy nose and throat • itchy, watery eyes

Warnings:

Alcohol Warning: If you consume 3 or more alcoholic drinks every day, ask your doctor whether you should take acetaminophen or other pain relievers/fever reducers. Acetaminophen may cause liver damage.
Do not use • if you are now taking a prescription monoamine oxidase inhibitor (MAOI) (certain drugs for depression, psychiatric, or emotional conditions, or Parkinson's disease), or for 2 weeks after stopping the MAOI drug. If you do not know if your prescription drug contains an MAOI, ask a doctor or pharmacist before taking this product.
• with any other product containing acetaminophen **(see Overdose Warning)**
Ask a doctor before use if you have
• heart disease • high blood pressure
• thyroid disease • diabetes • glaucoma
• a breathing problem such as emphysema, asthma, or chronic bronchitis
• trouble urinating due to an enlarged prostate gland
• a sodium-restricted diet
Ask a doctor or pharmacist before use if you are taking sedatives or tranquilizers.
When using this product • do not exceed recommended dosage • avoid alcoholic drinks
• may cause drowsiness • alcohol, sedatives, and tranquilizers may increase drowsiness
• be careful when driving a motor vehicle or operating machinery
• excitability may occur, especially in children
Stop use and ask a doctor if • nervousness, dizziness, or sleeplessness occur
• pain or nasal congestion gets worse or lasts more than 7 days

• fever gets worse or lasts more than 3 days
• redness or swelling is present
• new symptoms occur
• sore throat is severe, persists for more than 2 days, is accompanied or followed by fever, headache, rash, nausea, or vomiting. These could be signs of a serious condition.
If pregnant or breast-feeding, ask a health care professional before use.
Keep out of reach of children.
Overdose Warning: Taking more than the recommended dose can cause serious health problems, including serious liver damage. In case of overdose, get medical help or contact a poison control center right away. Prompt medical attention is critical for adults as well as for children even if you do not notice any signs or symptoms.

Directions:

• do not use more than directed (see **Overdose Warning**)
• take every 4 hours; not to exceed 6 packets in 24 hours or as directed by a doctor
• adults and children 12 years of age and over: dissolve contents of one packet into 8 oz. hot water; sip while hot. Consume entire drink within 10–15 minutes.
• children under 12 years of age: consult a doctor.
• If using a microwave, add contents of one packet to 8 oz. of cool water; stir briskly before and after heating. Do not overheat.

Other Information:
• each packet contains: **sodium 44 mg**
• store at controlled room temperature 20-25°C (68-77°F)

How Supplied: 6 packets in a carton

Inactive Ingredients: acesulfame K, citric acid, D&C Yellow 10, FD&C Yellow 6, lecithin, maltodextrin, natural flavors, silicon dioxide, sodium citrate, sucrose, tribasic calcium phosphate
Questions? call **1-800-452-0051**
24 hours a day, 7 days a week.
Shown in Product Identification Guide, page 506

THERAFLU® Daytime Severe Cold
(Novartis Consumer Health, Inc.)
Pain Reliever-Fever Reducer (Acetaminophen)
Nasal Decongestant (Phenylephrine HCl)

Drug Facts

Active Ingredients:　　　　　　**Purpose:**
(in each packet)
Acetaminophen
　650 mg .... Pain reliever/
　　　　　　　　　　　　　　　Fever reducer
Phenylephrine hydrochloride
　10 mg .... Nasal decongestant

Uses: • temporarily relieves these symptoms due to a cold:
• headache
• minor aches and pains
• minor sore throat pain
• nasal and sinus congestion
• temporarily reduces fever

Warnings:

Alcohol Warning: If you consume 3 or more alcoholic drinks every day, ask your doctor whether you should take acetaminophen or other pain relievers/fever reducers. Acetaminophen may cause liver damage.

Do not use • if you are now taking a prescription monoamine oxidase inhibitor (MAOI) (certain drugs for depression, psychiatric, or emotional conditions, or Parkinson's disease), or for 2 weeks after stopping the MAOI drug. If you do not know if your prescription drug contains an MAOI, ask a doctor or pharmacist before taking this product.
• with any other product containing acetaminophen (**see Overdose Warning**)

Ask a doctor before use if you have
• heart disease • high blood pressure
• thyroid disease • diabetes
• trouble urinating due to an enlarged prostate gland
• a sodium-restricted diet

When using this product • do not exceed recommended dosage

Stop use and ask a doctor if • nervousness, dizziness, or sleeplessness occur
• pain or nasal congestion gets worse or lasts more than 7 days
• fever gets worse or lasts more than 3 days
• redness or swelling is present
• new symptoms occur
• sore throat is severe, persists for more than 2 days, is accompanied or followed by fever, headache, rash, nausea, or vomiting. These could be signs of a serious condition.

If pregnant or breast-feeding, ask a health care professional before use.

Keep out of reach of children.

Overdose Warning: Taking more than the recommended dose can cause serious health problems, including serious liver damage. In case of overdose, get medical help or contact a poison control center right away. Prompt medical attention is critical for adults as well as for children even if you do not notice any signs or symptoms.

Directions:
• do not use more than directed (**see Overdose Warning**)
• take every 4 hours; not to exceed 6 packets in 24 hours or as directed by a doctor
• adults and children 12 years of age and over: dissolve contents of one packet in 8 oz. hot water; sip while hot. Consume entire drink within 10–15 minutes.
• children under 12 years of age: consult a doctor.
• If using a microwave, add contents of one packet to 8 oz. of cool water; stir

briskly before and after heating. Do not overheat.

Other Information:
• each packet contains: **sodium 44 mg**
• store at controlled room temperature 20-25°C (68-77°F)

How Supplied: 6 packets in a carton.

Inactive Ingredients: acesulfame K, citric acid, D&C Yellow 10, FD&C Yellow 6, lecithin, maltodextrin, natural flavors, silicon dioxide, sodium citrate, sucrose, tribasic calcium phosphate
Questions? call **1-800-452-0051**
24 hours a day, 7 days a week.

THERAFLU® THINSTRIPS®
DAYTIME COLD & COUGH

Drug Facts
Active ingredient
(in each strip)   *Purposes*
Dextromethorphan 14.8 mg
(equivalent to 20 mg dextromethrophan HBr) .... Cough suppressant
Phenylephrine HCl
10 mg .... Nasal decongestant

Uses • temporarily relieves
• nasal congestion
• cough due to minor throat and bronchial irritation associated with a cold

Warnings:

Do not use • if you are now taking a prescription monoamine oxidase inhibitor (MAOI) (certain drugs for depression, psychiatric or emotional conditions, or Parkinson's disease), or for 2 weeks after stopping the MAOI drug. If you do not know if your prescription drug contains an MAOI, ask a doctor or pharmacist before giving this product.

Ask a doctor before use if you have
• heart disease • high blood pressure
• thyroid disease • diabetes
• trouble urinating due to an enlarged prostate gland
• cough that occurs with too much phlegm (mucus)
• cough that lasts or is chronic such as occurs with smoking, asthma or emphysema

When using this product • do not take more than directed

Stop use and ask a doctor if
• nervousness, dizziness or sleeplessness occurs
• symptoms do not improve within 7 days or occur with a fever
• new symptoms occur
• cough persists for more than 7 days, or occurs with rash, or headache that last. These could be signs of a serious condition.

If pregnant or breast-feeding, ask a health care professional before use.

Keep out of reach of children. In case of overdose, get medical help or contact a Poison Control Center right away.

Directions:
• adults and children 12 years of age and over: allow 1 strip to dissolve on tongue every 4 hours as needed
• do not exceed 6 strips in 24 hours or as directed by a doctor
• children under 12 years of age: ask a doctor

Other information:
• store at controlled room temperature 20-25°C (68-77°F)

Inactive ingredients:
acetone, alcohol, FD&C Red 40, flavor, hypromellose, mannitol, polacrilin, polyethylene glycol, polyethylene oxide, sodium polystyrene sulfonate, sucralose, water

Questions? call **1-800-452-0051** 24 hours a day, 7 days a week.

How Supplied: 12 Cherry Menthol Flavored medicated strips in a carton.
Shown in Product Identification Guide, page 506

THERAFLU® THINSTRIPS®
NIGHTTIME COLD & COUGH

Drug Facts
Active ingredient
(in each strip)   *Purposes*
Diphenhydramine HCl,
25 mg .... Antihistamine/Cough
                             suppressant
Phenylephrine HCl,
10 mg .... Nasal decongestant

Uses • temporarily relieves
• runny nose • sneezing • itchy nose or throat
• itchy, watery eyes due to hay fever
• nasal congestion
• cough due to minor throat and bronchial irritation associated with a cold

Warnings:

Do not use • if you are now taking a prescription monoamine oxidase inhibitor (MAOI) (certain drugs for depression, psychiatric or emotional conditions, or Parkinson's disease), or for 2 weeks after stopping the MAOI drug. If you do not know if your prescription drug contains an MAOI, ask a doctor or pharmacist before giving this product.

Do not use • with any other product containing diphenhydramine, even one used on skin

Ask a doctor before use if you have
• heart disease • high blood pressure
• thyroid disease
• diabetes • glaucoma
• cough that occurs with too much phlegm (mucous)
• chronic cough that lasts or as occurs with smoking, asthma or emphysema
• a breathing problem such as asthma or chronic bronchitis

Continued on next page

Theraflu ThinStrips—Cont.

- trouble urinating due to an enlarged prostate gland

Ask a doctor or pharmacist before use if you are

- taking sedatives or tranquilizers

When using this product • do not take more than directed

- marked drowsiness may occur • avoid alcoholic drinks
- alcohol, sedatives, and tranquilizers may increase the drowsiness
- excitability may occur, especially in children
- be careful when driving a motor vehicle or operating machinery

Stop use and ask a doctor if

- symptoms do not improve within 7 days or occur with a fever
- new symptoms occur
- nervousness, dizziness or sleeplessness occurs
- cough persists for more than 7 days, or occurs with rash, or headache that last. These could be signs of a serious condition.

If pregnant or breastfeeding, ask a health care professional before use.

Keep out of reach of children. In case of overdose, get medical help or contact a Poison Control Center right away.

Directions:

- adults and children 12 years of age and over: allow 1 strip to dissolve on tongue every 4 hours as needed
- do not exceed 6 strips in 24 hours or as directed by a doctor
- children under 12 years of age: ask a doctor

Other information:

- store at controlled room temperature 20-25°C (68-77°F)

Inactive ingredients:

acetone, alcohol, FD&C Blue # 1, flavor, hypromellose, mannitol, polyethylene glycol, polyethylene oxide, sodium polystyrene sulfonate, sucralose, water

Questions? call **1-800-452-0051** 24 hours a day, 7 days a week.

How Supplied: 12 Peppermint Flavored medicated strips in a carton.
Shown in Product Identification Guide, page 506

THERAFLU® CAPLETS DAYTIME SEVERE COLD
(Novartis Consumer Health, Inc.)

Drug Facts
Active ingredients
(in each caplet) **Purpose**
Acetaminophen
USP 325 mg .... Pain reliever/fever reducer
Dextromethorphan hydrobromide
USP 15 mg .... Cough suppressant

Phenylephrine hydrochloride
USP 5 mg .... Nasal decongestant

Uses • temporarily relieves
 • minor aches and pains • headache
 • minor sore throat pain • nasal and sinus congestion • cough due to minor throat and bronchial irritation
 • temporarily reduces fever

Warnings:

Alcohol Warning: If you consume 3 or more alcoholic drinks every day, ask your doctor whether you should take acetaminophen or other pain relievers/fever reducers. Acetaminophen may cause liver damage.

Do not use

- if you are now taking a prescription monoamine oxidase inhibitor (MAOI) (certain drugs for depression, psychiatric, or emotional conditions, or Parkinson's disease), or for 2 weeks after stopping the MAOI drug. If you do not know if your prescription drug contains an MAOI, ask a doctor or pharmacist before taking this product.
- with any other product containing acetaminophen **(see Overdose Warning)**

Ask a doctor before use if you have

- heart disease • high blood pressure
- thyroid disease • diabetes
- cough that occurs with too much phlegm(mucus) • trouble urinating due to an enlarged prostate gland • cough that lasts or is chronic such as occurs with smoking, asthma or emphysema

When using this product

- do not exceed recommended dosage

Stop use and ask a doctor if

- nervousness, dizziness, or sleeplessness occurs • redness or swelling is present • fever gets worse or lasts more than 3 days • new symptoms occur • pain, cough or nasal congestion gets worse or lasts more than 7 days
- sore throat is severe, persists for more than 2 days, is accompanied or followed by fever, headache, rash, nausea, or vomiting
- cough comes back or occurs with fever, rash or headache that lasts.
These could be signs of a serious condition.

If pregnant or breast-feeding, ask a health care professional before use.
Keep out of reach of children.

Overdose Warning: Taking more than the recommended dose can cause serious health problems, including serious liver damage. In case of overdose, get medical help or contact a poison control center right away. Prompt medical attention is critical for adults as well as for children even if you do not notice any signs or symptoms.

Directions:

- do not use more than directed **(see Overdose Warning)**
- take every 6 hours; not more than 8 caplets in 24 hours

- adults and children 12 years of age and over: take 2 caplets every 6 hours
- children under 12 years of age: consult a doctor

Other information • store at controlled room temperature 20–25° C (68–77° F)

Inactive ingredients acesulfame potassium, flavor, magnesium stearate, microcrystalline cellulose, polyethylene glycol, polyvinyl alcohol, povidone, sodium starch glycolate, starch, stearic acid, silicon dioxide, talc, titanium dioxide

Questions? Call **1-800-452-0051** 24 hours a day, 7 days a week

How Supplied: 24 coated caplets.

THERAFLU® WARMING RELIEF DAYTIME SEVERE COLD
(Novartis Consumer Health, Inc.)
Pain Reliever/Fever Reducer/Cough Suppressant/Nasal Decongestant

Drug Facts
Active Ingredients: **Purpose:**
(in each 15 mL tablespoonful)
Acetaminophen
325 mg .... Pain reliever/fever reducer
Dextromethorphan HBr
10 mg .... Cough suppressant
Phenylephrine HCl
5 mg .... Nasal decongestant

Uses:

- temporarily relieves
 • minor aches and pains • headache
 • minor sore throat pain
 • nasal congestion
 • cough due to minor throat and bronchial irritation
- temporarily reduces fever

Warnings:

Alcohol Warning: If you consume 3 or more alcoholic drinks every day, ask your doctor whether you should take acetaminophen or other pain relievers/fever reducers. Acetaminophen may cause liver damage.

Do not use

- if you are now taking a prescription monoamine oxidase inhibitor (MAOI) (certain drugs for depression, psychiatric, or emotional conditions, or Parkinson's disease), or for 2 weeks after stopping the MAOI drug. If you do not know if your prescription drug contains an MAOI, ask a doctor or pharmacist before taking this product.
- with any other product containing acetaminophen **(see Overdose Warning)**

Ask a doctor before use if you have

- heart disease • high blood pressure
- thyroid disease • diabetes
- cough that occurs with too much phlegm(mucus)
- trouble urinating due to an enlarged prostate gland
- cough that lasts or is chronic such as occurs with smoking, asthma or emphysema

When using this product
- **do not exceed recommended dosage**

Stop use and ask a doctor if
- nervousness, dizziness, or sleeplessness occurs
- pain, cough or nasal congestion gets worse or lasts more than 7 days
- fever gets worse or lasts more than 3 days
- redness or swelling is present
- new symptoms occur
- sore throat is severe, persists for more than 2 days, is accompanied or followed by fever, headache, rash, nausea, or vomiting.
- cough comes back or occurs with rash or headache that lasts. These could be signs of a serious condition.

If pregnant or breast-feeding, ask a health care professional before use.

Keep out of reach of children.

Overdose Warning: Taking more than the recommended dose can cause serious health problems, including serious liver damage. In case of overdose, get medical help or contact a poison control center right away. Prompt medical attention is critical for adults as well as for children even if you do not notice any signs or symptoms.

Directions:
- do not use more than directed **(see Overdose Warning)**
- adults and children 12 years of age and over: take 2 tablespoons (30 mL) in dose cup provided, every 4 hours as needed
- do not take more than 6 doses (12 tablespoons) in 24 hours
- Consult a physician for use in children under 12 years of age

Other Information:
- each tablespoon contains: **sodium 8 mg**
- store at controlled room temperature 20-25°C (68-77°F)

Inactive Ingredients: acesulfame potassium, alcohol, citric acid, edetate disodium, FD&C blue 1, FD&C red 40, flavors, glycerin, maltitol solution, propylene glycol, purified water, sodium benzoate, sodium citrate
Alcohol content: 10%

Questions? call **1-800-452-0051** 24 hours a day, 7 days a week.

How Supplied:
Available in 8.3 fl oz bottles. Cherry Flavor.
Shown in Product Identification Guide, page 506

THERAFLU® WARMING RELIEF NIGHTTIME SEVERE COLD
(Novartis Consumer Health, Inc.)
Cough Suppressant/Antihistamine/Pain Reliever/Fever Reducer/Nasal Decongestant

Drug Facts

Active Ingredients: **(in each 15 mL tablespoonful)**	**Purpose:**
Acetaminophen 325 mg	Pain reliever/fever reducer
Diphenhydramine HCl 12.5 mg	Antihistamine/ Cough suppressant
Phenylephrine HCl 5 mg	Nasal decongestant

Uses:
- temporarily relieves
  - minor aches and pains • headache
  - runny nose • sneezing
  - itchy nose or throat
  - itchy, watery eyes
  - minor sore throat pain
  - nasal and sinus congestion
  - cough due to minor throat and bronchial irritation
- temporarily reduces fever

Warnings:

Alcohol Warning: If you consume 3 or more alcoholic drinks every day, ask your doctor whether you should take acetaminophen or other pain relievers/fever reducers. Acetaminophen may cause liver damage.

Do not use
- if you are now taking a prescription monoamine oxidase inhibitor (MAOI) (certain drugs for depression, psychiatric, or emotional conditions, or Parkinson's disease), or for 2 weeks after stopping the MAOI drug. If you do not know if your prescription drug contains an MAOI, ask a doctor or pharmacist before taking this product.
- with any other product containing diphenhydramine, even one used on skin
- with any other product containing acetaminophen **(see Overdose Warning)**

Ask a doctor before use if you have
- heart disease • high blood pressure
- thyroid disease • diabetes • glaucoma
- a breathing problem such as emphysema or chronic bronchitis
- trouble urinating due to an enlarged prostate gland
- cough that occurs with too much phlegm (mucus)
- cough that lasts or is chronic such as occurs with smoking, asthma or emphysema

Ask a doctor or pharmacist before use if you are taking sedatives or tranquilizers.

When using this product
- **do not exceed recommended dosage**
- avoid alcoholic drinks
- may cause marked drowsiness
- alcohol, sedatives, and tranquilizers may increase drowsiness
- be careful when driving a motor vehicle or operating machinery
- excitability may occur, especially in children

Stop use and ask a doctor if
- nervousness, dizziness, or sleeplessness occurs
- pain, cough or nasal congestion gets worse or lasts more than 7 days
- fever gets worse or lasts more than 3 days

- redness or swelling is present
- new symptoms occur
- sore throat is severe, persists for more than 2 days, is accompanied or followed by fever, headache, rash, nausea, or vomiting
- cough comes back or occurs with rash or headache that lasts. These could be signs of a serious condition.

If pregnant or breast-feeding, ask a health care professional before use.

Keep out of reach of children.

Overdose Warning: Taking more than the recommended dose can cause serious health problems, including serious liver damage. In case of overdose, get medical help or contact a poison control center right away. Prompt medical attention is critical for adults as well as for children even if you do not notice any signs or symptoms.

Directions:
- do not use more than directed **(see Overdose Warning)**
- adults and children 12 years of age and over: take 2 tablespoons (30 mL) in dose cup provided, every 4 hours as needed
- do not take more than 6 doses (12 tablespoons) in 24 hours
- Consult a physician for use in children under 12 years of age

Other information:
- each tablespoon contains: **sodium 7 mg**
- each tablespoon contains: **potassium 5 mg**
- store at controlled room temperature 20-25°C (68-77°F)

Inactive Ingredients: acesulfame potassium, alcohol, citric acid, edetate disodium, FD&C blue 1, FD&C red 40, flavors, glycerin, maltitol solution, propylene glycol, purified water, sodium benzoate, sodium citrate
Alcohol content: 10%

Questions? call **1-800-452-0051** 24 hours a day, 7 days a week.

How Supplied:
Available in 8.3 fl oz bottles. Cherry Flavor.

THERAFLU® CAPLETS NIGHTTIME SEVERE COLD
(Novartis Consumer Health, Inc.)

Drug Facts

Active ingredients **(in each caplet)**	**Purpose**
Acetaminophen USP 325 mg	Pain reliever/fever reducer
Chlorpheniramine maleate USP 2 mg	Antihistamine
Dextromethorphan hydrobromide USP 10 mg	Cough suppressant
Phenylephrine hydrochloride USP 5 mg	Nasal decongestant

Continued on next page

Theraflu Caplets—Cont.

Uses • temporarily relieves • minor aches and pains • itchy nose or throat • minor sore throat pain • sneezing • runny nose • cough due to minor throat and bronchial irritation • nasal and sinus congestion • headache • temporarily reduces fever

Warnings:

Alcohol Warning: If you consume 3 or more alcoholic drinks every day, ask your doctor whether you should take acetaminophen or other pain relievers/fever reducers. Acetaminophen may cause liver damage.

Do not use • with any other product containing acetaminophen **(see Overdose Warning)**
• if you are now taking a prescription monoamine oxidase inhibitor (MAOI) (certain drugs for depression, psychiatric, or emotional conditions, or Parkinson's disease), or for 2 weeks after stopping the MAOI drug. If you do not know if your prescription drug contains an MAOI, ask a doctor or pharmacist before taking this product.

Ask a doctor before use if you have • a breathing problem such as emphysema or chronic bronchitis • heart disease • thyroid disease • diabetes • high blood pressure • glaucoma • cough that occurs with too much phlegm(mucus) • trouble urinating due to an enlarged prostate gland • cough that lasts or is chronic such as occurs with smoking, asthma or emphysema

Ask a doctor or pharmacist before use if you are taking sedatives or tranquilizers

When using this product • do not exceed recommended dosage • may cause marked drowsiness • be careful when driving a motor vehicle or operating machinery • avoid alcoholic drinks
• alcohol, sedatives and tranquilizers may increase drowsiness
• excitability may occur, especially in children

Stop use and ask a doctor if • nervousness, dizziness, or sleeplessness occurs • fever gets worse or lasts more than 3 days • redness or swelling is present • new symptoms occur • pain, cough or nasal congestion gets worse or lasts more than 7 days
• sore throat is severe, persists for more than 2 days, is accompanied or followed by fever, headache, rash, nausea, or vomiting
• cough comes back or occurs with fever, rash or headache that lasts. These could be signs of a serious condition.

If pregnant or breast-feeding, ask a health care professional before use.
Keep out of reach of children.

Overdose Warning: Taking more than the recommended dose can cause serious health problems, including serious liver damage. In case of overdose, get medical help or contact a poison control center right away. Prompt medical attention is critical for adults as well as for children even if you do not notice any signs or symptoms.

Directions

• do not use more than directed **(see Overdose Warning)**
• adults and children 12 years of age and older: take 2 caplets every 4 hours
• do not take more than 12 caplets in 24 hours • children under 12 years of age: consult a doctor

Other information

• store at controlled room temperature 20-25° C (68-77° F)

Inactive ingredients

acesulfame potassium, FD&C blue no. 1 lake, flavor, magnesium stearate, microcrystalline cellulose, polyethylene glycol, polyvinyl alcohol, povidone, purified water, sodium starch glycolate, starch, stearic acid, talc, titanium dioxide

Questions? Call **1-800-452-0051** 24 hours a day, 7 days a week

How Supplied: 29 coated caplets.

TRIAMINIC®
Chest & Nasal Congestion
(Novartis Consumer Health, Inc.)
Expectorant, Nasal Decongestant

Drug Facts

Active Ingredients:	**Purpose:**
(in each 5 mL, 1 teaspoon)	
Guaifenesin, USP, 50 mg	Expectorant
Phenylephrine HCl, USP, 2.5 mg	Nasal decongestant

Uses:

temporarily relieves
• chest congestion by loosening phlegm (mucus) to help clear bronchial passageways
• nasal and sinus congestion

Warnings:

Do not use

• in a child who is taking a prescription monoamine oxidase inhibitor (MAOI) (certain drugs for depression, psychiatric or emotional conditions, or Parkinson's disease), or for 2 weeks after stopping the MAOI drug. If you do not know if the child's prescription drug contains an MAOI, ask a doctor or pharmacist before giving this product.

Ask a doctor before use if the child has

• heart disease • high blood pressure
• thyroid disease • diabetes
• cough that occurs with too much phlegm (mucus)
• chronic cough that lasts or as occurs with asthma

When using this product

• do not exceed recommended dosage

Stop use and ask a doctor if

• nervousness, dizziness, or sleeplessness occurs
• symptoms do not improve within 7 days or occur with a fever
• cough persists for more than 7 days, comes back or occurs with a fever, rash, or persistent headache. These could be signs of a serious condition.

Keep out of reach of children. In case of overdose, get medical help or contact a poison control center right away.

Directions:

• take every 4 hours; not to exceed 6 doses in 24 hours or as directed by a doctor

children 6 to under 12 years of age	2 teaspoons
children 2 to under 6 years of age	1 teaspoon
children under 2 years of age	ask a doctor

Other Information:

• each teaspoon contains: **sodium 3 mg**
• contains no aspirin
• store at controlled room temperature 20-25°C (68-77°F)

Inactive Ingredients: acesulfame K, benzoic acid, citric acid, D&C Yellow 10, edetate disodium, FD&C Yellow 6, flavors, maltitol solution, propylene glycol, purified water, sodium citrate

Questions? call **1-800-452-0051** 24 hours a day, 7 days a week.

How Supplied: Available in cartons of 4 fl oz bottles. Tropical Flavor.

TRIAMINIC®
Cold & Allergy
(Novartis Consumer Health, Inc.)
Antihistamine, Nasal Decongestant
Orange Flavor

Drug Facts

Active Ingredients:	**Purpose:**
Chlorpheniramine maleate, USP, 1 mg	Antihistamine
Phenylephrine HCl, USP, 2.5 mg	Nasal decongestant

Uses:

temporarily relieves
• itchy, watery eyes • runny nose
• itchy nose or throat • sneezing
• nasal and sinus congestion

Warnings:

Do not use • in a child who is taking a prescription monoamine oxidase inhibitor (MAOI) (certain drugs for depression, psychiatric or emotional conditions, or Parkinson's disease), or for 2 weeks after stopping the MAOI drug. If you do not know if the child's prescription drug contains an MAOI, ask a doctor or pharmacist before giving this product.

Ask a doctor before use if the child has
- heart disease • high blood pressure
- thyroid disease • diabetes • glaucoma
- a breathing problem such as asthma or chronic bronchitis

Ask a doctor or pharmacist before use if the child is taking sedatives or tranquilizers

When using this product
- **do not exceed recommended dosage**
- may cause drowsiness
- sedatives and tranquilizers may increase drowsiness
- excitability may occur, especially in children

Stop use and ask a doctor if
- nervousness, dizziness or sleeplessness occurs
- symptoms do not improve within 7 days or occur with a fever. These could be signs of a serious condition.

Keep out of reach of children. In case of overdose, get medical help or contact a poison control center right away.

Directions: take every 4 hours; not to exceed 6 doses in 24 hours or as directed by a doctor

children 6 to under 12 years of age	2 teaspoons
children under 6 years of age	ask a doctor

Other Information:
- each teaspoon contains: **sodium 3 mg**
- contains no aspirin
- store at controlled room temperature 20-25°C (68-77°F)

Inactive Ingredients: acesulfame K, benzoic acid, citric acid, edetate disodium, FD&C Yellow 6, flavors, maltitol solution, purified water, sodium citrate

Questions? call **1-800-452-0051** 24 hours a day, 7 days a week.

How Supplied: 4 fl oz bottle in a carton.

TRIAMINIC®
Day Time Cold & Cough
(Novartis Consumer Health, Inc.)
Cough Suppressant,
Nasal Decongestant
Cherry Flavor

Drug Facts

Active Ingredients: **Purpose:**
(in each 5 mL, 1 teaspoon)
Dextromethorphan HBr,
  USP, 5 mg .... Cough suppressant
Phenylephrine HCl,
  USP, 2.5 mg .... Nasal decongestant

Uses:
temporarily relieves
- nasal and sinus congestion
- cough due to minor throat and bronchial irritation

Warnings:
Do not use
- in a child who is taking a prescription monoamine oxidase inhibitor (MAOI) (certain drugs for depression, psychiatric or emotional conditions, or Parkinson's disease), or for 2 weeks after stopping the MAOI drug. If you do not know if the child's prescription drug contains an MAOI, ask a doctor or pharmacist before giving this product.

Ask a doctor before use if the child has
- heart disease • high blood pressure
- thyroid disease • diabetes
- a breathing problem such as asthma or chronic bronchitis
- cough that occurs with too much phlegm (mucus) or chronic cough that lasts

When using this product
- **do not exceed recommended dosage**

Stop use and ask a doctor if
- nervousness, dizziness or sleeplessness occurs
- symptoms do not improve within 7 days or occur with a fever
- cough persists for more than 7 days, comes back or occurs with a fever, rash or persistent headache. These could be signs of a serious condition.

Keep out of reach of children. In case of overdose, get medical help or contact a poison control center right away.

Directions:
- take every 4 hours not to exceed 6 doses in 24 hours or as directed by a doctor

children 6 to under 12 years of age	2 teaspoons
children 2 to under 6 years of age	1 teaspoon
children under 2 years of age	ask a doctor

Other Information:
- each teaspoon contains: **sodium 2 mg**
- contains no aspirin
- store at controlled room temperature 20–25°C (68–77°F)

Inactive Ingredients: acesulfame K, benzoic acid, citric acid, edetate disodium, FD&C Red 40, flavors, maltitol solution, propylene glycol, purified water, sodium citrate

Questions? call **1-800-452-0051** 24 hours a day, 7 days a week.

How Supplied: Available in cartons of 4 fl oz and 8 fl oz bottles.
Shown in Product Identification Guide, page 507

TRIAMINIC®
Night Time Cold & Cough
(Novartis Consumer Health, Inc.)
Antihistamine/Cough Suppressant,
Nasal Decongestant
Grape Flavor

Drug Facts
Active Ingredients: **Purpose:**
(in each 5 mL, 1 teaspoon)
Diphenhydramine HCl,
USP, 6.25 mg .... Antihistamine/Cough
                                           suppressant
Phenylephrine HCl,
USP, 2.5 mg .... Nasal decongestant

Uses:
temporarily relieves
- sneezing
- itchy nose or throat
- runny nose
- itchy, watery eyes due to hay fever
- nasal and sinus congestion
- cough due to minor throat and bronchial irritation

Warnings:
Do not use
- in a child who is taking a prescription monoamine oxidase inhibitor (MAOI) (certain drugs for depression, psychiatric or emotional conditions, or Parkinson's disease), or for 2 weeks after stopping the MAOI drug. If you do not know if the child's prescription drug contains an MAOI, ask a doctor or pharmacist before giving this product.
- with any other product containing diphenhydramine, even one used on skin

Ask a doctor before use if the child has
- heart disease • high blood pressure
- thyroid disease • diabetes • glaucoma
- a breathing problem such as asthma or chronic bronchitis
- cough that occurs with too much phlegm (mucus) or chronic cough that lasts

Ask a doctor or pharmacist before use if the child is taking sedatives or tranquilizers

When using this product
- **do not exceed recommended dosage**
- may cause marked drowsiness
- sedatives and tranquilizers may increase drowsiness
- excitability may occur, especially in children

Stop use and ask a doctor if
- nervousness, dizziness or sleeplessness occurs
- symptoms do not improve within 7 days or occur with a fever
- cough persists for more than 7 days, comes back or occurs with a fever, rash, or persistent headache. These could be signs of a serious condition

Keep out of reach of children. In case of overdose, get medical help or contact a poison control center right away

Continued on next page

Triaminic Night Time—Cont.

Directions:
- take every 4 hours; not to exceed 6 doses in 24 hours or as directed by a doctor

children 6 to under 12 years of age	2 teaspoons
children under 6 years of age	ask a doctor

Other Information:
- each teaspoon contains **sodium 6 mg**
- contains no aspirin
- store at controlled room temperature 20–25°C (68–77°F)

Inactive Ingredients: acesulfame K, benzoic acid, citric acid, edetate disodium, FD&C Blue 1, FD&C Red 40, flavor, maltitol solution, propylene glycol, purified water, sodium citrate

Questions? call **1-800-452-0051** 24 hours a day, 7 days a week.

How Supplied:
Available in cartons of 4 fl oz and 8 fl oz bottles.

Shown in Product Identification Guide, page 507

TRIAMINIC®
Cough & Sore Throat
(Novartis Consumer Health, Inc.)
Pain Reliever/Fever Reducer/ Cough Suppressant

Drug Facts
Active Ingredients: **Purpose:**
(in each 5 mL, 1 teaspoon)
Acetaminophen, USP, 160 mg .... Pain reliever/ Fever reducer
Dextromethorphan HBr, USP, 5 mg .... Cough suppressant

Uses:
temporarily relieves
- minor aches and pains
- headache
- minor sore throat pain
- cough due to minor throat and bronchial irritation
- temporarily reduces fever

Warnings:
Do not use • in a child who is taking a prescription monoamine oxidase inhibitor (MAOI) (certain drugs for depression, psychiatric or emotional conditions, or Parkinson's disease), or for 2 weeks after stopping the MAOI drug. If you do not know if the child's prescription drug contains an MAOI, ask a doctor or pharmacist before giving this product.
- with any other product containing acetaminophen **(see Overdose Warning)**

Ask a doctor before use if the child has
- cough that occurs with too much phlegm (mucus)
- chronic cough that lasts, or as occurs with asthma

Stop use and ask a doctor if
- pain or cough gets worse or lasts more than 5 days
- fever gets worse or lasts more than 3 days
- redness or swelling is present
- new symptoms occur
- sore throat is severe, persists for more than 2 days or occurs with fever, headache, rash, nausea or vomiting
- cough comes back or occurs with a fever, rash or persistent headache. These could be signs of a serious condition.

Keep out of reach of children.

Overdose Warning: Taking more than the recommended dose can cause serious health problems, including serious liver damage. In case of overdose, get medical help or contact a poison control center right away. Prompt medical attention is critical for adults as well as for children even if you do not notice any signs or symptoms.

Directions:
- do not use more than directed (**see Overdose Warning**)
- take every 4 hours; not to exceed 5 doses in 24 hours or as directed by a doctor

children 6 to under 12 years of age	2 teaspoons
children 2 to under 6 years of age	1 teaspoon
children under 2 years of age	ask a doctor

Other Information:
- each teaspoon contains: **sodium 5 mg**
- contains no aspirin
- store at controlled room temperature 20-25°C (68-77°F)

Inactive Ingredients: citric acid, edetate disodium, FD&C Blue 1, FD&C Red 40, flavor, glycerin, polyethylene glycol, purified water, sodium benzoate, sodium citrate, sorbitol, sucrose

Questions? call **1-800-452-0051** 24 hours a day, 7 days a week.

How Supplied: Available in 4 fl oz cartons, Grape Flavor.

UNKNOWN DRUG?
Consult the
Product Identification Guide
(Gray Pages)
for full-color photos of
leading over-the-counter
medications.

INFANT & TODDLER TRIAMINIC THIN STRIPS®
(Novartis Consumer Health, Inc.)
Decongestant
Nasal Decongestant

Decongestant Plus Cough
Nasal Decongestant, Cough Suppressant

Drug Facts
Decongestant:
Active Ingredients: **Purpose:**
(in each strip)
Phenylephrine HCl 1.25 mg .... Nasal decongestant

Decongestant plus Cough:
Active Ingredients: **Purpose:**
(in each strip)
Dextromethorphan 1.83 mg (equivalent to 2.5 mg dextromethorphan HBr) .... Cough suppressant
Phenylephrine HCl 1.25 mg .... Nasal decongestant

Uses:
Decongestant:
temporarily relieves
- nasal and sinus congestion due to a cold

Decongestant plus Cough:
temporarily relieves
- nasal and sinus congestion due to a cold
- cough due to minor throat and bronchial irritation

Warnings:
Do not use
- in a child who is taking a prescription monoamine oxidase inhibitor (MAOI) (certain drugs for depression, psychiatric, or emotional conditions, or Parkinson's disease), or for 2 weeks after stopping the MAOI drug. If you do not know if the child's prescription drug contains an MAOI, ask a doctor or pharmacist before giving this product.

Ask a doctor before use if the child has
- heart disease • high blood pressure
- thyroid disease • diabetes

Decongestant plus Cough:
- chronic cough that lasts, or as occurs with asthma
- cough that occurs with too much phlegm (mucus)

When using this product
- do not exceed recommended dosage

Stop use and ask a doctor if
- nervousness, dizziness or sleeplessness occurs
- symptoms do not improve within 7 days or occur with a fever

Decongestant plus Cough:
- cough persists for more than 7 days, comes back or occurs with a fever, rash or persistent headache. These could be signs of a serious condition.

Keep out of reach of children. In case of overdose, get medical help or contact a poison control center right away.

Directions:
- take every 4 hours; not to exceed 6 doses in 24 hours or as directed by a doctor

| children 2 to 3 years of age | allow 2 strips to dissolve on tongue |
| children under 2 years of age | ask a doctor |

Other Information:
- contains no aspirin
- store at controlled room temperature 20-25°C (68-77°F)

Decongestant:

Inactive Ingredients: acetone, alcohol, FD&C Blue 1, FD&C Red 40, flavor, hypromellose, maltodextrin, microcrystalline cellulose, polyethylene glycol, propylene glycol, purified water, sodium polystyrene sulfonate, sucralose, titanium dioxide

Decongestant plus Cough:

Inactive Ingredients: acetone, alcohol, FD&C Blue 1, FD&C Red 40, flavor, hypromellose, microcrystalline cellulose, polacrilin, polyethylene glycol, propylene glycol, purified water, sodium polystyrene sulfonate, sucralose, titanium dioxide

Questions? call **1-800-452-0051** 24 hours a day, 7 days a week

Alcohol: less than 0.5%

How Supplied: 16 Mixed Berry Medicated Strips in a carton.
Shown in Product Identification Guide, page 507

TRIAMINIC® SOFTCHEWS®
Cough & Runny Nose
(Novartis Consumer Health, Inc.)
Antihistamine, Cough Suppressant
Cherry Flavor

Drug Facts

Active Ingredients: **Purpose:**
(in each tablet)
Chlorpheniramine maleate, USP, 1 mg .... Antihistamine
Dextromethorphan HBr, USP, 5 mg .... Cough Suppressant

Uses:
temporarily relieves
- sneezing
- itchy nose or throat
- runny nose
- itchy, watery eyes due to hay fever
- cough due to minor throat and bronchial irritation

Warnings:
Do not use • in a child who is taking a prescription monoamine oxidase inhibitor (MAOI) (certain drugs for depression, psychiatric, or emotional conditions, or Parkinson's disease), or for 2 weeks after stopping the MAOI drug. If you do not know if the child's prescription drug contains an MAOI, ask a doctor or pharmacist before giving this product.

Ask a doctor before use if the child has
- glaucoma
- a breathing problem such as asthma or chronic bronchitis
- cough that occurs with too much phlegm (mucus) or chronic cough that lasts

Ask a doctor or pharmacist before use if the child is taking sedatives or tranquilizers.

When using this product • do not use more than directed • may cause marked drowsiness • sedatives and tranquilizers may increase drowsiness • excitability may occur, especially in children

Stop use and ask a doctor if • symptoms do not improve within 7 days or occurs with a fever • cough persists for more than 7 days, comes back or occurs with a fever, rash, or persistent headache. These could be signs of a serious condition.

Keep out of reach of children. In case of overdose, get medical help or contact a poison control center right away.

Directions: • Let Softchews® tablet dissolve in mouth or chew Softchews® tablet before swallowing, whichever is preferred • take every 4 to 6 hours; not to exceed 6 doses in 24 hours or as directed by a doctor

| children 6 to under 12 years of age | 2 tablets |
| children under 6 years of age | ask a doctor |

Other Information:
- each Softchews® tablet contains: **sodium 5 mg**
- Phenylketonurics: Contains **Phenylalanine, 17.6 mg** per Softchews® tablet
- contains no aspirin • store at controlled room temperature 20–25°C (68–77°F)
- protect from light.

Inactive Ingredients: aspartame, carnauba wax, citric acid, crospovidone, D&C Red 27 aluminum lake, D&C Red 30 aluminum lake, ethylcellulose, FD&C Blue 2 aluminum lake, flavors, fractionated coconut oil, gum arabic, hypromellose, magnesium stearate, maltodextrin, mannitol, microcrystalline cellulose, mono- and di-glycerides, oleic acid, povidone, silicon dioxide, sodium bicarbonate, sodium chloride, sorbitol, starch, sucrose, triethyl citrate

Questions? call **1-800-452-0051** 24 hours a day, 7 days a week.

How Supplied: 18 Softchews® Tablets in a carton.

TRIAMINIC THIN STRIPS®
Cold with Stuffy Nose
(Novartis Consumer Health, Inc.)
Nasal Decongestant

Drug Facts
Active Ingredient: **Purpose:**
(in each strip)
Phenylephrine HCl, 2.5 mg .... Nasal decongestant

Uses:
temporarily relieves
- nasal and sinus congestion due to a cold

Warnings:

Do not use • in a child who is taking a prescription monoamine oxidase inhibitor (MAOI) (certain drugs for depression, psychiatric, or emotional conditions, or Parkinson's disease), or for 2 weeks after stopping the MAOI drug. If you do not know if the child's prescription drug contains an MAOI, ask a doctor or pharmacist before giving this product.

Ask a doctor before use if the child has
- heart disease • thyroid disease
- high blood pressure • diabetes

When using this product
- **do not exceed recommended dosage**

Stop use and ask a doctor if
- nervousness, dizziness, or sleeplessness occur
- symptoms do not improve within 7 days or occur with a fever. These could be signs of a serious condition.

Keep out of reach of children.

In case of overdose, get medical help or contact a poison control center right away.

Directions:
- take every 4 hours; not to exceed 6 doses in 24 hours or as directed by a doctor

children 6 to under 12 years of age:	allow 2 strips to dissolve on tongue
children 2 to under 6 years of age:	allow 1 strip to dissolve on tongue
children under 2 years of age	ask a doctor

Other Information:
- contains no aspirin
- store at controlled room temperature 20-25°C (68-77°F)

Inactive Ingredients: acetone, FD&C Blue 1, FD&C Red 40, flavors, hypromellose, maltodextrin, microcrystalline cellulose, polyethylene glycol, purified water, sodium polystyrene sulfonate, sucralose, titanium dioxide

Questions? call **1-800-452-0051** 24 hours a day, 7 days a week.

How Supplied: 14 Raspberry Flavored Medicated Strips in a carton.
Shown in Product Identification Guide, page 506

TRIAMINIC THIN STRIPS®
Cough & Runny Nose
(Novartis Consumer Health, Inc.)

Drug Facts

Active ingredient:	Purpose:
(in each strip)	

Diphenhydramine HCl
12.5 mg .... Cough suppressant/
Antihistamine

Uses:

temporarily relieves
• runny nose • sneezing
• itchy nose or throat
• itchy, watery eyes due to hay fever
• cough due to minor throat and bronchial irritation occurring with a cold

Warnings:

Do not use
• with any other product containing diphenhydramine, even one used on skin

Ask a doctor before use if the child has
• glaucoma
• cough that occurs with too much phlegm (mucus)
• cough that lasts or is chronic such as occurs with asthma or chronic bronchitis

Ask a doctor or pharmacist before use if the child is
• taking sedatives or tranquilizers

When using this product
• do not use more than directed
• marked drowsiness may occur. Sedatives and tranquilizers may increase the drowsiness effect.
• excitability may occur, especially in children

Stop use and ask a doctor if
• cough lasts more than 7 days, comes back, or is accompanied by fever, rash, or persistent headache. These could be signs of a serious condition.

Keep out of reach of children. In case of overdose, get medical help or contact a Poison Control Center right away.

Directions:
• children 6 to under 12 years of age: allow 1 strip to dissolve on tongue. May be taken every 4 hours.
• do not exceed 6 strips in 24 hours, or as directed by a doctor
• children under 6 years of age: ask a doctor

Other Information:
• store at controlled room temperature 20-25°C (68-77°F)

Inactive Ingredients: acetone, alcohol, FD&C Blue 1, FD&C Red 40, flavors, hydroxypropyl cellulose, hypromellose, maltodextrin, microcrystalline cellulose, polyethylene glycol, pregelatinized starch, propylene glycol, purified water, sodium polystyrene sulfonate, sorbitol, sucralose, titanium dioxide
Alcohol: less than 5%

Questions? call **1-800-452-0051**
24 hours a day, 7 days a week.

How Supplied:
14 Grape Flavored medicated strips in a carton.
Shown in Product Identification Guide, page 506

TRIAMINIC THIN STRIPS®
Day Time Cold & Cough
(Novartis Consumer Health, Inc.)
Cough Suppressant,
Nasal Decongestant

Drug Facts

Active Ingredients:	Purpose:
(in each strip)	

Dextromethorphan, 3.67 mg (equivalent to 5 mg dextromethorphan HBr) .... Cough suppressant
Phenylephrine HCl,
2.5 mg .... Nasal decongestant

Uses:

temporarily relieves
• nasal and sinus congestion due to a cold
• cough due to minor throat and bronchial irritation

Warnings:

Do not use
• in a child who is taking a prescription monoamine oxidase inhibitor (MAOI) (certain drugs for depression, psychiatric, or emotional conditions, or Parkinson's disease), or for 2 weeks after stopping the MAOI drug. If you do not know if the child's prescription drug contains an MAOI, ask a doctor or pharmacist before giving this product.

Ask a doctor before use if the child has
• heart disease • high blood pressure
• thyroid disease • diabetes • glaucoma
• cough that lasts or is chronic such as occurs with asthma
• cough that occurs with too much phlegm (mucus)

When using this product
• **do not exceed recommended dosage**

Stop use and ask a doctor if
• nervousness, dizziness, or sleeplessness occur
• symptoms do not improve within 7 days or occur with a fever
• cough persists for more than 7 days, comes back or occurs with a fever, rash or persistent headache. These could be signs of a serious condition.

Keep out of reach of children. In case of overdose, get medical help or contact a poison control center right away.

Directions:
• take every 4 hours; not to exceed 6 doses in 24 hours or as directed by a doctor

children 6 to under 12 years of age:	allow 2 strips to dissolve on tongue
children 2 to under 6 years of age:	allow 1 strip to dissolve on tongue
children under 2 years of age:	ask a doctor

Other Information:
• contains no aspirin
• store at controlled room temperature 20-25°C (68-77°F)

Inactive Ingredients: acetone, alcohol, FD&C Blue 1, FD&C Red 40, flavors, hypromellose, microcrystalline cellulose, polacrilin, polyethylene glycol, purified water, sodium polystyrene sulfonate, sucralose, titanium dioxide

Questions? call **1-800-452-0051**
24 hours a day, 7 days a week.

Alcohol: less than 0.5%

How Supplied: 14 Wild Berry Flavored Medicated Strips in a carton.
Shown in Product Identification Guide, page 506

TRIAMINIC® THIN STRIPS®
Night Time Cold & Cough
(Novartis Consumer Health, Inc.)

Drug Facts
Active ingredients   **Purposes**
(in each strip)
Diphenhydramine HCl,
12.5 mg .... Antihistamine/
Cough suppressant
Phenylephrine HCl,
5 mg .... Nasal decongestant

Uses • temporarily relieves
• cough due to minor sore throat and bronchial irritation
• nasal and sinus congestion • sneezing
• itchy nose or throat • runny nose
• itchy, watery eyes due to hay fever

Warnings:

Do not use • in a child who is taking a prescription monoamine oxidase inhibitor (MAOI) (certain drugs for depression, psychiatric or emotional conditions, or Parkinson's disease), or for 2 weeks after stopping the MAOI drug. If you do not know if the child's prescription drug contains an MAOI, ask a doctor or pharmacist before giving this product.
• with any other product containing diphenhydramine, even one used on skin

Ask a doctor before use if the child has
• heart disease • high blood pressure
• thyroid disease • diabetes • glaucoma
• cough that occurs with too much phlegm (mucus) or chronic cough that lasts
• a breathing problem such as asthma or chronic bronchitis

Ask a doctor or pharmacist before use if the child is taking sedatives or tranquilizers

When using this product
• **do not exceed recommended dosage**
• marked drowsiness may occur
• sedatives and tranquillizers may increase the drowsiness
• excitability may occur, especially in children

Stop use and ask a doctor if
• nervousness, dizziness, or sleeplessness occurs

• symptoms do not improve within 7 days or occur with a fever
• cough persists for more than 7 days, comes back or occurs with a fever, rash or persistent headache. These could be signs of a serious condition.

Keep out of reach of children. In case of overdose, get medical help or contact a Poison Control Center right away.

Directions:
• children 6 to under 12 years of age: allow 1 strip to dissolve on tongue. May be taken every 4 hours.
• do not exceed 6 strips in 24 hours, or as directed by a doctor
• children under 6 years of age: ask a doctor

Other information:
• store at controlled room temperature 20-25°C (68-77°F)

Inactive ingredients: acetone, FD&C Blue #1, FD&C Red #40, flavors, hypromellose, maltodextrin, mannitol, polyethylene glycol, sodium polystyrene sulfonate, sucralose, water

Questions? call **1-800-452-0051** 24 hours a day, 7 days a week

How Supplied: 14 Grape Flavored Medicated Strips in a carton.

Shown in Product Identification Guide, page 506

VAGISTAT®-1
Tioconazole Ointment 6.5%
Vaginal antifungal
(Novartis Consumer Health, Inc.)

Drug Facts
Active Ingredient: **Purpose:**
(in each applicator)
Tioconazole 300 mg (6.5%) .... Vaginal antifungal

Use:
• treats vaginal yeast infections

Warnings:
For vaginal use only
Do not use if you have never had a vaginal yeast infection diagnosed by a doctor
Ask a doctor before use if you have
• **vaginal itching and discomfort for the first time**
• **lower abdominal, back or shoulder pain, fever, chills, nausea, vomiting, or foul-smelling vaginal discharge. You may have a more serious condition.**
• vaginal yeast infections often (such as once a month or 3 in 6 months). You could be pregnant or have a serious underlying medical cause for your symptoms, including diabetes or a weakened immune system.
• been exposed to the human immunodeficiency virus (HIV) that causes AIDS
When using this product
• do not use tampons, douches, spermicides, or other vaginal products. Con-

doms and diaphragms may be damaged and fail to prevent pregnancy or sexually transmitted disease (STDs).
• do not have vaginal intercourse
• mild increase in vaginal burning, itching, or irritation may occur
Stop use and ask a doctor if
• **symptoms do not get better after 3 days**
• **symptoms last more than 7 days**
• **you get a rash or hives, abdominal pain, fever, chills, nausea, vomiting, or foul-smelling vaginal discharge**
If pregnant or breast-feeding, ask a health professional before use.
Keep out of reach of children. If swallowed, get medical help or contact a Poison Control Center right away.

Directions:
• before using this product read the enclosed brochure and instructions on foil packet for complete directions and information
• adults and children 12 years of age and over:
    • open the foil packet just before use and remove blue cap
    • insert entire contents of applicator into the vagina at bedtime. Throw applicator away after use.
• children under 12 years of age: ask a doctor

Other Information:
• this product is a 1-dose treatment, most women do not experience complete relief of their symptoms in just one day. Most women experience some relief within one day and complete relief of symptoms within 7 days.
• if you have questions about vaginal yeast infections, consult your doctor
• store at 15°-30°C (59°-86°F)
• see end flap of carton for lot number and expiration date

Inactive Ingredients: butylated hydroxyanisole, magnesium aluminum silicate, white petrolatum
Questions or comments?
1-888-824-4782

How Supplied: VAGISTAT-1 is supplied in a ready-to-use prefilled single close vaginal applicator. Each applicatorful will deliver approximately 4.6 grams of VAGISTAT-1 containing 6.5% of tioconazole per gram of ointment.

Shown in Product Identification Guide, page 507

Procter & Gamble
P.O. BOX 559
CINCINNATI, OH 45201

Direct Inquiries to:
Consumer Relations
(800) 832-3064

CHILDREN'S PEPTO
(Procter & Gamble)
Calcium carbonate/antacid

Drug Facts
Active Ingredient:
(in each tablet)   **Purpose:**
Calcium carbonate
    400 mg .... Antacid

Uses:
• relieves:
    • heartburn
    • sour stomach
    • acid indigestion
    • upset stomach due to these symptoms or overindulgence in food and drink

Warnings:
Ask a doctor or pharmacist before use if the child is • presently taking a prescription drug.
Antacids may interact with certain prescription drugs.
Stop use and ask a doctor if symptoms last more than two weeks.
Keep this and all drugs out of the reach of children.

Directions:
• find the right dose on chart below based on weight (preferred), otherwise use age
• repeat dose as needed
• do not take more than 3 tablets (ages 2–5) or 6 tablets (ages 6–11) in a 24-hour period, or use the maximum dosage for more than two weeks, except under the advice and supervision of a doctor.

Dosing Chart		
Weight (lbs.)	Age	Dose
under 24	under 2 yrs	ask a doctor
24–47	2–5 yrs	1 tablet
48–95	6–11 yrs	2 tablets

Other Information:
• each tablet contains: calcium 161 mg
• very low sodium
• store at room temperature, avoid excessive humidity

Inactive Ingredients: [Editor's note: "flavor" is applicable to both BUBBLEGUM AND WATERMELON] flavor, magnesium stearate, mannitol, povidone, red 27 aluminum lake, sorbitol, sugar, talc

Questions? 1-800-717-3786

How Supplied: Available in 24ct

HEAD & SHOULDERS INTENSIVE SOLUTIONS
(Procter & Gamble)
Dandruff Shampoo for Normal Hair

Head & Shoulders Intensive Solutions Dandruff Shampoo offers effective control of persistent dandruff, seborrheic dermatitis of the scalp, and other symptoms associated with dandruff. Double-

Continued on next page

Head & Shoulders—Cont.

blind and expert graded testing have proven that Intensive Solutions Dandruff Shampoo reduces persistent dandruff. It is also gentle enough to use everyday for clean, manageable hair. The formula ingredients below are for the Normal Hair version. Head & Shoulders Intensive Solutions is also available in versions for Oily Hair and Dry Damaged Hair. A 2-in-1 for Normal Hair version is available for increased manageability and prevention of hair damage.

Drug Facts

Active Ingredient: 2% Pyrithione zinc suspended in a mild surfactant base. Shampoo also includes mild conditioning agents.

Purpose: Anti-dandruff

Uses: Helps prevent recurrence of flaking and itching associated with persistent dandruff.

Warnings:

For external use only. When using this product
• Avoid contact with eyes. If contact occurs, rinse eyes thoroughly with water

Stop use and ask a doctor if
• Condition worsens or does not improve after regular use of this product as directed

Keep this and all drugs out of reach of children. If swallowed, get medical help or contact a Poison Control Center right away.

Directions:

• For maximum dandruff control, use every time you shampoo
• Wet hair, massage onto scalp, rinse, repeat if desired
• For best results use at least twice a week or as directed by a doctor

Inactive Ingredients:

Water, Sodium Laureth Sulfate, Sodium Lauryl Sulfate, Cocamide MEA, Zinc Carbonate, Glycol Distearate, Dimethicone, Fragrance, Cetyl Alcohol, Guar Hydroxypropyltrimonium Chloride, Magnesium Sulfate, Sodium Benzoate, Ammonium Laureth Sulfate, Magnesium Carbonate Hydroxide, Benzyl Alcohol, Sodium Chloride, Methylchloroisothiazolinone, Methylisothiazolinone, Sodium Xylenesulfonate, Red 4, blue 1.

How Supplied: All versions available in an 8.5 fl. oz. (251 mL) unbreakable plastic bottle.

Questions [*or comments*]*?*
1-800-723-9569

METAMUCIL® FIBER LAXATIVE
(Procter & Gamble)
[*met uh-mü sil*]
(psyllium husk)
Also see Metamucil Dietary Fiber Supplement in PDR for Nonprescription Drugs

Description: Metamucil contains psyllium husk (from the plant *Plantago ovata*), a bulk forming, natural therapeutic fiber for restoring and maintaining regularity when recommended by a physician. Metamucil contains no chemical stimulants and does not disrupt normal bowel function. Each dose of Metamucil powder and Metamucil Fiber Wafers contains approximately 3.4 grams of psyllium husk (or 2.4 grams of soluble fiber). Each dose of Metamucil capsules fiber laxative (5 capsules) contains approximately 2.6 grams of psyllium husk (or 2.0 grams of soluble fiber). Inactive ingredients, sodium, calcium, potassium, calories, carbohydrate, dietary fiber, and phenylalanine content are shown in the following table for all versions and flavors. Metamucil Smooth Texture Sugar-Free Unflavored and Metamucil capsules contains no sugar and no artificial sweeteners; Metamucil Smooth Texture Sugar-Free Orange Flavor contains aspartame (phenylalanine content per dose is 25 mg). Metamucil powdered products and Metamucil capsules are gluten-free. Metamucil Fiber Wafers contain gluten: Apple contains 0.7g/dose, Cinnamon contains 0.5g/dose. Each two-wafer dose contains 5 grams of fat.

Actions: The active ingredient in Metamucil is psyllium husk, a natural fiber which promotes elimination due to its bulking effect in the colon. This bulking effect is due to both the water-holding capacity of undigested fiber and the increased bacterial mass following partial fiber digestion. These actions result in enlargement of the lumen of the colon, and softer stool, thereby decreasing intraluminal pressure and straining, and speeding colonic transit in constipated patients.

Indications: Metamucil is indicated for the treatment of occasional constipation, and when recommended by a physician, for chronic constipation and constipation associated with irritable bowel syndrome, diverticulosis, hemorrhoids, convalescence, senility and pregnancy. Pregnancy: Category B. If considering use of Metamucil as part of a cholesterol-lowering program, see **Metamucil Dietary Fiber Supplement** in Dietary Supplement Section.

Drug Facts

Active Ingredient: **Purpose:**
(in each DOSE)
Psyllium husk
  approximately 3.4 g .... Fiber therapy
                              for regularity

For Metamucil capsules each dose of 5 capsules contains approximately 2.6 gm of psyllium husk.

Uses:
• effective in treating occasional constipation and restoring regularity

Warnings:
Choking: Taking this product without adequate fluid may cause it to swell and block your throat or esophagus and may cause choking. Do not take this product if you have difficulty in swallowing. If you experience chest pain, vomiting, or difficulty in swallowing or breathing after taking this product, seek immediate medical attention.

Allergy alert: This product may cause allergic reaction in people sensitive to inhaled or ingested psyllium.

Ask a doctor before use if you have:
• a sudden change in bowel habits persisting for 2 weeks
• abdominal pain, nausea or vomiting

Stop use and ask a doctor if:
• constipation lasts more than 7 days
• rectal bleeding occurs
These may be signs of a serious condition.

Keep out of reach of children. In case of overdose, get medical help or contact a Poison Control Center right away.

Directions: For Powders: Put one dose into an empty glass. Fill glass with at least 8 oz of water or your favorite beverage. Stir briskly and drink promptly. If mixture thickens, add more liquid and stir. Mix this product (child or adult dose) with at least 8 ounces (a full glass) of water or other fluid. **For Capsules:** Take product with 8 oz of liquid (swallow 1 capsule at a time) up to 3 times daily. Take this product with at least 8 oz (a full glass) of liquid. **For Wafers:** Take this product (child or adult dose) with at least 8 ounces (a full glass) of liquid. Taking these products without enough liquid may cause choking. See choking warning.

Adults 12 yrs. & older	Powders: 1 dose in 8 oz of liquid. Capsules: 5 capsules with 8 oz of liquid (swallow one capsule at a time). Wafers: 1 dose with 8 oz of liquid. Take at the first sign of irregularity; can be taken up to 3 times daily. Generally produces effect in 12 – 72 hours.
6 – 11 yrs.	Powders: ½ adult dose in 8 oz of liquid. Wafers: 1 wafer with 8 oz of liquid. Can be taken up to 3 times daily. Capsules: consider use of powder or wafer products
Under 6 yrs.	consult a doctor

Laxatives, including bulk fibers, may affect how well other medicines work. If you are taking a prescription medicine by mouth, take this product at least 2 hours before or 2 hours after the prescribed medicine. As your body adjusts to increased fiber intake, you may experience changes in bowel habits or minor bloating. **New Users:** Start with 1 dose per day; gradually increase to 3 doses per day as necessary.

Other Information:
• **Each product contains:** Potassium; sodium (See table for amount/dose)

Metamucil Fiber Laxative/Dietary Fiber Supplement

Versions/Flavors	Ingredients (alphabetical order)	Sodium mg/ dose	Calcium mg/ dose	Potassium mg/ dose	Calories kcal/ dose	Total Carbohydrate g/dose	Dietary Fiber/ (Soluble) g/dose	Dosage (Weight in gms)	How Supplied
Smooth Texture Orange Flavor Metamucil Powder	Citric Acid, FD&C Yellow #6, Natural and Artificial Flavor, Psyllium Husk, Sucrose	5	7	30	45	12	3 (2.4)	1 rounded tablespoon ~12g	Canisters: Doses: 48, 72, 114, 188; Cartons: 30 single-dose packets.
Smooth Texture Sugar-Free Orange Flavor Metamucil Powder	Aspartame, Citric Acid, FD&C Yellow #6, Maltodextrin, Natural and Artificial Flavor, Psyllium Husk	5	7	30	20	5	3 (2.4)	1 rounded teaspoon ~5.8g	Canisters: Doses: 30, 48, 72, 114, 180, 220; Cartons: 30 single-dose packets.
Smooth Texture Sugar-Free Unflavored Metamucil Powder	Citric Acid, Maltodextrin, Psyllium Husk	4	7	30	20	5	3 (2.4)	1 rounded teaspoon ~5.4g	Canisters: Doses: 48, 72 114.
Coarse Milled Unflavored Metamucil Powder	Psyllium Husk, Sucrose	3	6	30	25	7	3 (2.4)	1 rounded teaspoon ~7g	Canisters: Doses: 48, 72 114.
Coarse Milled Orange Flavor Metamucil Powder	Citric Acid, FD&C Yellow #6, Natural and Artificial Flavor, Psyllium Husk, Sucrose	5	6	30	40	11	3 (2.4)	1 rounded tablespoon ~11g	Canisters: Doses: 48,72 114.
Metamucil Capsules	Caramel color, FD&C Blue No. 1 Aluminum Lake, FD&C Red No. 40 Aluminum Lake, FD&C Yellow No. 6 Aluminum Lake, gelatin, polysorbate 80, psyllium husk	0	5	30	10	3	3 (2.4)	6 capsules 3.2g	Bottles: 100 ct, 160 ct, 300 ct
Fiber Laxative Wafers									
Apple Metamucil Wafers	(1)	20	14	60	120	17	6	2 wafers 24 g	Cartons: 12 doses
Cinnamon Metamucil Wafers	(2)	20	14	60	120	17	6	2 wafers 24 g	Cartons: 12 doses

(1) ascorbic acid, brown sugar, cinnamon, corn oil, corn starch, fructose, lecithin, molasses, natural and artificial flavors, oat hull fiber, psyllium husk, sodium bicarbonate, sucrose, water, wheat flour
(2) ascorbic acid, cinnamon, corn oil, corn starch, fructose, lecithin, molasses, natural and artificial flavors, nutmeg, oat hull fiber, oats, psyllium husk, sodium bicarbonate, sucrose, water, wheat flour

• **PHENYLKETONURICS:** Smooth Texture Sugar Free Orange product **contains phenylalanine** 25 mg per dose
• Each product contains a 100% natural, therapeutic fiber

Inactive Ingredients: See table Notice to Health Care Professionals: To minimize the potential for allergic reaction, health care professionals who frequently dispense powdered psyllium products should avoid inhaling airborne dust while dispensing these products. Handling and Dispensing: To minimize generating airborne dust, spoon product from the canister into a glass according to label directions.

How Supplied: Powder: canisters and cartons of single-dose packets. Capsules: 100, 160 and 300 count bottles. Wafers:

cartons of single dose packets. (See table) [See table above]
Questions? 1-800-983-4237
Shown in Product Identification Guide, page 507

PEPTO-BISMOL®
(Procter & Gamble)
ORIGINAL LIQUID,
MAXIMUM STRENGTH LIQUID,
ORIGINAL AND CHERRY FLAVOR
CHEWABLE TABLETS
AND EASY-TO-SWALLOW CAPLETS
For upset stomach, indigestion, heartburn, nausea and diarrhea.

Multi-symptom Pepto-Bismol® contains bismuth subsalicylate and is the only

leading OTC stomach remedy clinically proven effective for both upper and lower GI symptoms. It has been clinically proven in double-blind placebo-controlled trials for relief of upset stomach symptoms and diarrhea.

Active Ingredient:

(per tablespoon/per tablet/per caplet)
Original Liquid/Tablets/Caplets
Bismuth subsalicylate 262 mg
Maximum Strength Liquid
Bismuth subsalicylate 525 mg

Inactive Ingredients:
[**Original Liquid**] benzoic acid, flavor, magnesium aluminum silicate, methylcel-

Continued on next page

Pepto-Bismol—Cont.

lulose, red 22, red 28, saccharin sodium, salicylic acid, sodium salicylate, sorbic acid, water

[Maximum Strength Liquid] benzoic acid, flavor, magnesium aluminum silicate, methylcellulose, red 22, red 28, saccharin sodium, salicylic acid, sodium salicylate, sorbic acid, water

[Original Tablets] calcium carbonate, flavor, magnesium stearate, mannitol, povidone, red 27 aluminum lake, saccharin sodium, talc

[Cherry Tablets] adipic acid, calcium carbonate, flavor, magnesium stearate, mannitol, povidone, red 27 aluminum lake, red 40 aluminum lake, saccharin sodium, talc

[Caplets] calcium carbonate, magnesium stearate, mannitol, microcrystalline cellulose, polysorbate 80, povidone, red 27 aluminum lake, silicon dioxide, sodium starch glycolate.

Other Information:
Sodium Content
Original Liquid—each Tbsp contains: sodium 6 mg • low sodium
Maximum Strength Liquid—each Tbsp contains: sodium 6 mg • low sodium
Chewable Tablets—each Original or Cherry Flavor Tablet contains: calcium 140 mg, sodium less than 1 mg • very low sodium
Caplets—each Caplet contains: calcium 27 mg, sodium 3 mg • low sodium
Salicylate Content
Original Liquid—each Tbsp contains: salicylate 130 mg
Maximum Strength Liquid—each Tbsp contains: salicylate 236 mg
Chewable Tablets—each tablet contains:
[original] salicylate 102 mg
[cherry] salicylate 99 mg
Caplets—each caplet contains: salicylate 99 mg
All Forms are sugar free.

Indications:
• relieves upset stomach symptoms (i.e., indigestion, heartburn, nausea and fullness caused by over-indulgence in food and drink) without constipating; and,
• controls diarrhea.

Actions: For upset stomach symptoms, the active ingredient is believed to work via a topical effect on the stomach mucosa. For diarrhea, it is believed to work by several mechanisms in the gastrointestinal tract, including: 1) normalizing fluid movement via an antisecretory merchanism, 2) binding bacterial toxins and 3) antimicrobial activity.

Warnings:
Reye's syndrome: Children and teenagers who have or are recovering from chicken pox or flu-like symptoms should not use this product. When using this product, if changes in behavior with nausea and vomiting occur, consult a doctor because these symptoms could be an early sign of Reye's syndrome, a rare but serious illness.

Allergy alert: Contains salicylate. Do not take if you are
• allergic to salicylates (including aspirin)
• taking other salicylate products
Do not use if you have
• an ulcer
• a bleeding problem
• bloody or black stool
Ask a doctor before use if you have
• fever
• mucus in the stool
Ask a doctor or pharmacist before use if you are taking any drug for
• anticoagulation (thinning the blood)
• diabetes
• gout
• arthritis
When using this product a temporary, but harmless, darkening of the stool and/or tongue may occur
Stop use and ask a doctor if
• symptoms get worse
• ringing in the ears or loss of hearing occurs
• diarrhea lasts more than 2 days
If pregnant or breast feeding, ask a health professional before use.
Keep out of reach of children. In case of overdose, get medical help or contact a Poison Control Center right away.
Notes: May cause a temporary and harmless darkening of the tongue or stool. Stool darkening should not be confused with melena.
While no lead is intentionally added to Pepto-Bismol, this product contains certain ingredients that are mined from the ground and thus contain small amounts of naturally occurring lead. For example, bismuth, contained in the active ingredient of Pepto-Bismol, is mined and therefore contains some naturally occurring lead. The small amounts of naturally occurring lead in Pepto-Bismol are low in comparison to average daily lead exposure; this is for the information of healthcare professionals. Pepto-Bismol is indicated for treatment of acute upset stomach symptoms and diarrhea. It is not intended for chronic use.

Overdosage: In case of overdose, patients are advised to contact a physician or Poison Control Center. Emesis induced by ipecac syrup is indicated in large ingestions provided ipecac can be administered within one hour of ingestion. Activated charcoal should be administered after gastric emptying. Patients should be evaluated for signs and symptoms of salicylate toxicity.

Directions:
Pepto-Bismol® Original Liquid, Original & Cherry Flavor Chewable Tablets, and Caplets
[Original Liquid]
• shake well before using
• for accurate dosing, use dose cup
[Original Tablet, Cherry Tablets]
• chew or dissolve in mouth
[Caplets]
• swallow with water, do not chew

• adults and children 12 years and over: 1 dose (2 Tbsp or 30 ml; 2 tablets or 2 caplets) every 1/2 to 1 hour as needed
• do not exceed 8 doses (16 Tbsp or 240 ml); 16 tablets or capsules in 24 hours
• use until diarrhea stops but not more than 2 days
• children under 12 years: ask a doctor
• drink plenty of clear fluids to help prevent dehydration caused by diarrhea
Pepto-Bismol® Maximum Strength Liquid
• shake well before use
• for accurate dosing, use dose cup
• adults and children 12 years and over: 1 dose (2 Tbsp 30 ml) every 1 hour as needed
• do not exceed 4 doses (8 Tbsp or 120 ml) in 24 hours
• use until diarrhea stops but not more than 2 days
• children under 12 years: ask a doctor
• drink plenty of clear fluids to help prevent dehydration caused by diarrhea

How Supplied: Pepto-Bismol® Original and Maximum Strength Liquids are pink. Pepto-Bismol® Original Liquid is available in: 4, 8, 12 and 16 fl oz bottles. Pepto-Bismol® Maximum Strength Liquid is available in: 4, 8 and 12 fl oz bottles. Pepto-Bismol® Original and Cherry Flavor Tablets are pink, round, chewable tablets imprinted with a debossed triangle and "Pepto-Bismol" on one side. Tablets are available in: boxes of 30 and 48. Pepto-Bismol® Caplets are pink and imprinted with "Pepto-Bismol" on one side. Caplets are available in bottles of 24 and 40.
• avoid excessive heat (over 104°F or 40°C)
• protect liquids from freezing
Questions: 1-800-717-3786
www.pepto-bismol.com
Shown in Product Identification Guide, page 507

PRILOSEC OTC® TABLETS
(Procter & Gamble)
[prī-lō-sĕk]

Drug Facts

Active Ingredient: **Purpose:**
(in each tablet)
Omeprazole magnesium delayed-release tablet 20.6 mg (equivalent to 20 mg omeprazole) .... Acid reducer

Use:
• treats frequent heartburn (occurs 2 or more days a week)
• not intended for immediate relief of heartburn; this drug may take 1 to 4 days for full effect

Warnings:
Allergy alert: Do not use if you are allergic to omeprazole
Do not use if you have trouble or pain swallowing food, vomiting with blood, or bloody or black stools.

These may be signs of a serious condition. See your doctor.

Ask a doctor before use if you have
- had heartburn over 3 months. This may be a sign of a more serious condition.
- heartburn with **lightheadedness, sweating or dizziness**
- chest pain or shoulder pain with shortness of breath; sweating; pain spreading to arms, neck or shoulders; or lightheadedness
- frequent **chest pain**
- frequent wheezing, particularly with heartburn
- unexplained weight loss
- nausea or vomiting
- stomach pain

Ask a doctor or pharmacist before use if you are taking
- warfarin (blood-thinning medicine)
- prescription antifungal or anti-yeast medicines
- diazepam (anxiety medicine)
- digoxin (heart medicine)
- tacrolimus (immune system medicine)
- atazanavir (medicine for HIV infection)

Stop use and ask a doctor if
- your heartburn continues or worsens
- you need to take this product for more than 14 days
- you need to take more than 1 course of treatment every 4 months

If pregnant or breast-feeding, ask a health professional before use.

Keep out of reach of children. In case of overdose, get medical help or contact a Poison Control Center right away.

Directions:
- adults 18 years of age and older
- this product is to be used once a day (every 24 hours), every day for 14 days
- it may take 1 to 4 days for full effect, although some people get complete relief of symptoms within 24 hours
  14-Day Course of Treatment
  - swallow 1 tablet with a glass of water before eating in the morning
  - take every day for 14 days
  - do not take more than 1 tablet a day
  - do not chew or crush the tablets
  - do not crush tablets in food
  - do not use for more than 14 days unless directed by your doctor
  Repeated 14-Day Courses (if needed)
  - you may repeat a 14-day course every 4 months
  - **do not take for more than 14 days or more often than every 4 months unless directed by a doctor**
- children under 18 years of age: ask a doctor

Other Information:
- read the directions, warnings and package insert before use
- keep the carton and package insert. They contain important information.
- store at 20–25°C (68–77°F)
- keep product out of high heat and humidity
- protect product from moisture

How Prilosec OTC Works For Your Frequent Heartburn

Prilosec OTC works differently from other OTC heartburn products, such as antacids and other acid reducers. Prilosec OTC stops acid production at the source – the **acid pump** that produces stomach acid. Prilosec OTC is to be used once a day (every 24 hours), every day for 14 days.

What to Expect When Using Prilosec OTC

Prilosec OTC is a different type of medicine from antacids and other acid reducers. Prilosec OTC may take 1 to 4 days for full effect, although some people get complete relief of symptoms within 24 hours. Make sure you take the entire 14 days of dosing to treat your frequent heartburn.

Safety Record

For years, doctors have prescribed Prilosec to treat acid-related conditions in millions of people safely.

Who Should Take Prilosec OTC

This product is for adults (18 years and older) with **frequent heartburn**-when you have heartburn 2 or more days a week.
- Prilosec OTC is **not** intended for those who have heartburn infrequently, one episode of heartburn a week or less, or for those who want immediate relief of heartburn.

Tips for Managing Heartburn
- Do not lie flat or bend over soon after eating.
- Do not eat late at night or just before bedtime.
- Certain foods or drinks are more likely to cause heartburn, such as rich, spicy, fatty and fried foods, chocolate, caffeine, alcohol and even some fruits and vegetables.
- Eat slowly and do not eat big meals.
- If you are overweight, lose weight.
- If you smoke, quit smoking.
- Raise the head of your bed.
- Wear loose-fitting clothing around your stomach.

Inactive Ingredients:

glyceryl monostearate, hydroxypropyl cellulose, hypromellose, iron oxide, magnesium stearate, methacrylic acid copolymer, microcrystalline cellulose, paraffin, polyethylene glycol 6000, polysorbate 80, polyvinylpyrrolidone, sodium stearyl fumarate, starch, sucrose, talc, titanium dioxide, triethyl citrate

How Supplied:

Prilosec OTC is available in 14 tablet, 28 tablet and 42 tablet sizes. These sizes contain one, two and three 14-day courses of treatment, respectively. Do not use for more than 14 days in a row unless directed by your doctor. For the 28 count (two 14-day courses) and the 42 count (three 14-day courses), you may repeat a 14-day course every 4 months.

Questions? 1-800-289-9181

Shown in Product Identification Guide, page 507

THERMA-CARE®
(Procter & Gamble)
Therapeutic Heat Wraps

Lower Back/Hip

PLEASE READ ALL INSTRUCTIONS AND WARNINGS BEFORE USE. ADDITIONAL WARNINGS ARE INCLUDED IN THE PACKAGE INSERT. TO REDUCE THE RISK OF BURNS, FIRE, AND PERSONAL INJURY, THIS PRODUCT MUST BE USED IN ACCORDANCE WITH THE USE INSTRUCTIONS AND WARNINGS. THERMACARE® BACK/HIP IS DESIGNED TO FIT THE FOLLOWING PANT/WAIST SIZES

Women's Pant Size	Men's Pant Size
Size 4 up to size 20	28 inches to 47 inches

Uses: Provides temporary relief of minor muscular and joint aches and pains associated with overexertion, strains, sprains, and arthritis.

Directions: Tear open pouch when ready to use. It may take up to 30 minutes for ThermaCare® to reach its therapeutic temperature. Place on pain area on lower back or hip with darker discs toward skin. Over-tightening may cause discomfort. Adjust as needed. For maximum effectiveness, we recommend you wear ThermaCare® for 8 hours. Do not wear for more than 8 hours in any 24-hour period.

WARNING: **THIS PRODUCT CAN CAUSE BURNS. CHECK SKIN FREQUENTLY DURING USE. IF YOU FIND IRRITATION OR A BURN, REMOVE PRODUCT IMMEDIATELY.**

55 OR OLDER: YOUR RISK OF BURNING INCREASES AS YOU AGE. IF YOU ARE 55 YEARS OF AGE OR OLDER, WEAR THERMACARE® OVER A LAYER OF CLOTHING, NOT DIRECTLY AGAINST YOUR SKIN, AND DO NOT WEAR WHILE SLEEPING.

ASK A DOCTOR BEFORE USE if you have
- DIABETES
- poor circulation or heart disease
- rheumatoid arthritis
- or are pregnant

ADDITIONAL WARNINGS: Each heat disc contains iron (~2 grams), which can be harmful if ingested. If ingested, rinse mouth with water and call a Poison Control Center immediately. If heat disc contents come in contact with your skin or eyes, rinse right away with water. Never heat product in a microwave or attempt to reheat as wrap could catch fire. Keep out of reach of children and pets. **DO NOT MICROWAVE**

WHEN USING THIS PRODUCT check skin frequently for signs of burns or blisters – if found stop use

Continued on next page

Therma-Care—Cont.

- if product feels too hot – stop use or wear over clothing
- do not place extra pressure, a tight waistband or belt over the product
- do not use for more than 8 hours in a 24-hour period

DO NOT USE with pain rubs, medicated lotions, creams or ointments

- on unhealthy, damaged or broken skin
- on areas of bruising or swelling that have occurred within 48 hours
- on people unable to follow all use instructions
- on areas of the body where you can't feel heat
- with other forms of heat
- on people unable to remove the product, including children, infants, and some elderly

STOP USE AND ASK A DOCTOR if you experience any discomfort, burning, swelling, rash or other changes in your skin that persist where the wrap is worn

- if after 7 days your pain gets worse or remains unchanged as this may be a sign of a more serious condition

Menstrual

PLEASE READ ALL INSTRUCTIONS AND WARNINGS BEFORE USE. ADDITIONAL WARNINGS ARE INCLUDED IN THE PACKAGE INSERT. TO REDUCE THE RISK OF BURNS, FIRE, AND PERSONAL INJURY, THIS PRODUCT MUST BE USED IN ACCORDANCE WITH THE USE INSTRUCTIONS AND WARNINGS.

Uses: Provides temporary relief of minor menstrual cramp pain and associated back aches.

Directions: Tear open pouch when ready to use. It may take up to 30 minutes for ThermaCare® to reach its therapeutic temperature. Peel away paper to reveal adhesive side. Place on pain area with adhesive side against underwear and not against the skin. Attach firmly. For maximum effectiveness, we recommend you wear ThermaCare® for 8 hours. Do not wear for more than 8 hours in any 24-hour period.

WARNING: **THIS PRODUCT CAN CAUSE BURNS. CHECK SKIN FREQUENTLY DURING USE. IF YOU FIND IRRITATION OR A BURN, REMOVE PRODUCT IMMEDIATELY.**

55 OR OLDER: YOUR RISK OF BURNING INCREASES AS YOU AGE. IF YOU ARE 55 YEARS OF AGE OR OLDER DO NOT USE DURING SLEEP.

ASK A DOCTOR BEFORE USE if you have

- DIABETES
- poor circulation or heart disease
- rheumatoid arthritis
- or are pregnant

ADDITIONAL WARNINGS: Each heat disc contains iron (~2 grams), which can be harmful if ingested. If ingested, rinse mouth with water and call a Poison Control Center immediately. If heat disc contents come in contact with your skin or eyes, rinse right away with water. Never heat product in a microwave or attempt to reheat as wrap could catch fire. Keep out of reach of children and pets.
DO NOT MICROWAVE

WHEN USING THIS PRODUCT check skin frequently for signs of burns or blisters – if found stop use

- if product feels too hot – stop use or wear over clothing
- do not place extra pressure, a tight waistband or belt over the product
- do not use for more than 8 hours in a 24-hour period

DO NOT USE with pain rubs, medicated lotions, creams or ointments

- on unhealthy, damaged or broken skin
- on areas of bruising or swelling that have occurred within 48 hours
- on people unable to follow all use instructions
- on areas of the body where you can't feel heat
- with other forms of heat
- on people unable to remove the product, including children, infants, and some elderly

STOP USE AND ASK A DOCTOR if you experience any discomfort, burning, swelling, rash or other changes in your skin that persist where the wrap is worn

- if after 4 days your pain gets worse or remains unchanged as this may be a sign of a more serious condition

Neck/Shoulder/ Wrist

PLEASE READ ALL INSTRUCTIONS AND WARNINGS BEFORE USE. ADDITIONAL WARNINGS ARE INCLUDED IN THE PACKAGE INSERT. TO REDUCE THE RISK OF BURNS, FIRE, AND PERSONAL INJURY, THIS PRODUCT MUST BE USED IN ACCORDANCE WITH THE USE INSTRUCTIONS AND WARNINGS.

Uses: Provides temporary relief of minor muscular and joint aches and pains associated with overexertion, strains, sprains, and arthritis.

Directions: Tear open pouch when ready to use. It may take up to 30 minutes for ThermaCare® to reach its therapeutic temperature. Peel away paper to reveal adhesive side. Place on pain area with adhesive against the skin. Attach firmly. Be careful when applying to the wrist – do not overlap the heat cells. For maximum effectiveness, we recommend you wear ThermaCare® for 8 hours. Do not wear for more than 8 hours in any 24-hour period.

WARNING: **THIS PRODUCT CAN CAUSE BURNS. CHECK SKIN FREQUENTLY DURING USE. IF YOU FIND IRRITATION OR A BURN, REMOVE PRODUCT IMMEDIATELY.**

55 OR OLDER: YOUR RISK OF BURNING INCREASES AS YOU AGE. IF YOU ARE 55 YEARS OF AGE OR OLDER DO NOT USE DURING SLEEP.

ASK A DOCTOR BEFORE USE if you have

- DIABETES
- poor circulation or heart disease

- rheumatoid arthritis,
- or are pregnant

ADDITIONAL WARNINGS: Each heat disc contains iron (~2 grams), which can be harmful if ingested. If ingested, rinse mouth with water and call a Poison Control Center immediately. If heat disc contents come in contact with your skin or eyes, rinse right away with water. Never heat product in a microwave or attempt to reheat as wrap could catch fire. Keep out of reach of children and pets.
DO NOT MICROWAVE

WHEN USING THIS PRODUCT check skin frequently for signs of burns or blisters – if found stop use

- if product feels too hot – stop use or wear over clothing
- do not place extra pressure over the product
- do not use for more than 8 hours in a 24-hour period

DO NOT USE with pain rubs, medicated lotions, creams or ointments

- on unhealthy, damaged or broken skin
- on areas of bruising or swelling that have occurred within 48 hours
- on people unable to follow all use instructions
- on areas of the body where you can't feel heat
- with other forms of heat
- on people unable to remove the product, including children, infants, and some elderly

STOP USE AND ASK A DOCTOR if you experience any discomfort, burning, swelling, rash or other changes in your skin that persist where the wrap is worn

- if after 7 days your pain gets worse or remains unchanged as this may be a sign of a more serious condition

Knee/Elbow

PLEASE READ ALL INSTRUCTIONS AND WARNINGS BEFORE USE. ADDITIONAL WARNINGS ARE INCLUDED IN THE PACKAGE INSERT. TO REDUCE THE RISK OF BURNS, FIRE, AND PERSONAL INJURY, THIS PRODUCT MUST BE USED IN ACCORDANCE WITH THE USE INSTRUCTIONS AND WARNINGS.

Uses: Provides temporary relief of minor muscular and joint aches and pains associated with overexertion, strains, sprains, and arthritis.

Directions: Tear open pouch when ready to use. It may take up to 30 minutes for ThermaCare® to reach its therapeutic temperature. Peel away paper to reveal adhesive tabs. Using adhesive is optional if you have sensitive skin or have body hair around the knee or elbow area.

Knee: Do not place heat cells on the back of the knee. Bend knee slightly and place opening over kneecap. Secure tabs to skin (optional). Wrap straps around knee and fasten. Over-tightening may cause discomfort. Adjust as needed.

Elbow: Do not place heat cells on the inside of the bend of the arm. Bend elbow slightly and place opening over elbow. Secure tabs to skin (optional). Wrap straps around elbow and fasten. Over-tightening may cause discomfort. Adjust as needed. For maximum effectiveness, we recommend you wear ThermaCare® for 8 hours. Do not wear for more than 8 hours in any 24-hour period.

WARNING: THIS PRODUCT CAN CAUSE BURNS. CHECK SKIN FREQUENTLY DURING USE. IF YOU FIND IRRITATION OR A BURN, REMOVE PRODUCT IMMEDIATELY.

55 OR OLDER: YOUR RISK OF BURNING INCREASES AS YOU AGE. IF YOU ARE 55 YEARS OF AGE OR OLDER, WEAR THERMACARE® OVER A TOWEL OR CLOTH SUCH AS A WASHCLOTH, NOT DIRECTLY AGAINST YOUR SKIN, AND DO NOT WEAR WHILE SLEEPING.

ASK A DOCTOR BEFORE USE if you have
• DIABETES
• poor circulation or heart disease
• rheumatoid arthritis
• or are pregnant

ADDITIONAL WARNINGS: Each heat disc contains iron (~2 grams), which can be harmful if ingested. If ingested, rinse mouth with water and call a Poison Control Center immediately. If heat disc contents come in contact with your skin or eyes, rinse right away with water. Never heat product in a microwave or attempt to reheat as wrap could catch fire. Keep out of reach of children and pets.
DO NOT MICROWAVE

WHEN USING THIS PRODUCT check skin frequently for signs of burns or blisters – if found stop use
• if product feels too hot – stop use or wear over clothing
• do not place extra pressure or tight clothing over the product
• do not use for more than 8 hours in a 24-hour period

DO NOT USE with pain rubs, medicated lotions, creams or ointments
• on unhealthy, damaged or broken skin
• on areas of bruising or swelling that have occurred within 48 hours
• on people unable to follow all use instructions
• on areas of the body where you can't feel heat
• with other forms of heat
• on people unable to remove the product, including children, infants, and some elderly

STOP USE AND ASK A DOCTOR if you experience any discomfort, burning, swelling, rash or other changes in your skin that persist where the wrap is worn
• if after 7 days your pain gets worse or remains unchanged as this may be a sign of a more serious condition.

QUESTIONS
1-800-323-3383 or visit
www.thermacare.com

How Supplied:
Available in boxes of 2 (Knee/Elbow), 2 or 3 (Lower Back/Hip), or 3 (Menstrual & Neck/Shoulder/Wrist) or in single use pouches.
Shown in Product Identification Guide, page 507

THERMACARE®
(Procter & Gamble)
Therapeutic Heat Wraps
Arthritis

Arthritis Hand/Wrist
PLEASE READ ALL INSTRUCTIONS AND WARNINGS BEFORE USE. ADDITIONAL WARNINGS ARE INCLUDED IN THE PACKAGE INSERT. TO REDUCE THE RISK OF BURNS, FIRE, AND PERSONAL INJURY, THIS PRODUCT MUST BE USED IN ACCORDANCE WITH THE USE INSTRUCTIONS AND WARNINGS.

Uses: Provides temporary relief of minor muscular and joint aches and pains associated with overexertion, strains, sprains, and arthritis.

Directions: Tear open pouch when ready to use. It may take up to 30 minutes for ThermaCare to reach its therapeutic temperature. Do not place the heat cells on the palm of the hand. Place on pain area on back of hand with thumb through slit and darker discs toward skin. Wrap straps under palm of hand and fasten. Over-tightening may cause discomfort. Adjust as needed. Be careful when applying to the hand and wrist – do not overlap the heat cells. For maximum effectiveness, we recommend you wear ThermaCare for 12 hours. Do not wear for more than 12 hours in any 24-hour period. Please keep in mind as you use this product, that due to differences in body temperature not everyone senses heat on the hand/wrist the same. Therefore, the product may not feel as warm as you might expect.

WARNING: THIS PRODUCT CAN CAUSE BURNS. CHECK SKIN FREQUENTLY DURING USE. IF YOU FIND IRRITATION OR A BURN, REMOVE PRODUCT IMMEDIATELY.

55 OR OLDER: YOUR RISK OF BURNING INCREASES AS YOU AGE. IF YOU ARE 55 YEARS OF AGE OR OLDER, DO NOT USE DURING SLEEP.

ADDITIONAL WARNINGS: Each heat disc contains iron (~2 grams), which can be harmful if ingested. If ingested, rinse mouth with water and call a Poison Control Center immediately. If heat disc contents come in contact with your skin or eyes, rinse right away with water. Never heat product in a microwave or attempt to reheat, as wrap could catch fire. Keep out of reach of children and pets.
DO NOT MICROWAVE

ASK A DOCTOR BEFORE USE if you have
• DIABETES
• poor circulation or heart disease

• rheumatoid arthritis
• or are pregnant

WHEN USING THIS PRODUCT check skin frequently for signs of burns or blisters – if found, stop use
• if product feels too hot – stop use or wear over clothing
• do not place extra pressure over the product
• do not use for more than 12 hours in a 24-hour period

DO NOT USE with pain rubs, medicated lotions, creams or ointments
• on unhealthy, damaged or broken skin
• on areas of bruising or swelling that have occurred within 48 hours
• on people unable to follow all use instructions
• on areas of the body where you can't feel heat
• with other forms of heat
• on people unable to remove the product, including children, infants, and some elderly

STOP USE AND ASK A DOCTOR if you experience any discomfort, burning, swelling, rash or other changes in your skin that persist where the wrap is worn
• if after 7 days your pain gets worse or remains unchanged, as this may be a sign of a more serious condition

Arthritis Neck/Shoulder/Wrist
PLEASE READ ALL INSTRUCTIONS AND WARNINGS BEFORE USE. ADDITIONAL WARNINGS ARE INCLUDED IN THE PACKAGE INSERT. TO REDUCE THE RISK OF BURNS, FIRE, AND PERSONAL INJURY, THIS PRODUCT MUST BE USED IN ACCORDANCE WITH THE USE INSTRUCTIONS AND WARNINGS.

Uses: Provides temporary relief of minor muscular and joint aches and pains associated with overexertion, strains, sprains, and arthritis.

Directions: Tear open pouch when ready to use. It may take up to 30 minutes for ThermaCare to reach its therapeutic temperature. Peel away paper to reveal adhesive side. Place on pain area with adhesive against the skin. Attach firmly. Be careful when applying to the wrist – do not overlap the heat cells. For maximum effectiveness, we recommend you wear ThermaCare for 12 hours. Do not wear for more than 12 hours in any 24-hour period.

WARNING: THIS PRODUCT CAN CAUSE BURNS. CHECK SKIN FREQUENTLY DURING USE. IF YOU FIND IRRITATION OR A BURN, REMOVE PRODUCT IMMEDIATELY.

55 OR OLDER: YOUR RISK OF BURNING INCREASES AS YOU AGE. IF YOU ARE 55 YEARS OF AGE OR OLDER, DO NOT USE DURING SLEEP

ADDITIONAL WARNINGS: Each heat disc contains iron (~2 grams), which can be harmful if ingested. If ingested, rinse

Continued on next page

Thermacare—Cont.

mouth with water and call a Poison Control Center immediately. If heat disc contents come in contact with your skin or eyes, rinse right away with water. Never heat product in a microwave or attempt to reheat, as wrap could catch fire. Keep out of reach of children and pets.
DO NOT MICROWAVE

ASK A DOCTOR BEFORE USE if you have
• DIABETES
• poor circulation or heart disease
• rheumatoid arthritis
• or are pregnant

WHEN USING THIS PRODUCT check skin frequently for signs of burns or blisters – if found, stop use
• if product feels too hot – stop use or wear over clothing
• do not place extra pressure over the product
• do not use for more than 12 hours in a 24-hour period

DO NOT USE with pain rubs, medicated lotions, creams or ointments
• on unhealthy, damaged or broken skin
• on areas of bruising or swelling that have occurred within 48 hours
• on people unable to follow all use instructions
• on areas of the body where you can't feel heat
• with other forms of heat
• on people unable to remove the product, including children, infants, and some elderly

STOP USE AND ASK A DOCTOR if you experience any discomfort, burning, swelling, rash or other changes in your skin that persist where the wrap is worn
• if after 7 days your pain gets worse or remains unchanged, as this may be a sign of a more serious condition

Arthritis Knee/Elbow
PLEASE READ ALL INSTRUCTIONS AND WARNINGS BEFORE USE. ADDITIONAL WARNINGS ARE INCLUDED IN THE PACKAGE INSERT. TO REDUCE THE RISK OF BURNS, FIRE, AND PERSONAL INJURY, THIS PRODUCT MUST BE USED IN ACCORDANCE WITH THE USE INSTRUCTIONS AND WARNINGS.

Uses: Provides temporary relief of minor muscular and joint aches and pains associated with overexertion, strains, sprains, and arthritis.

Directions: Tear open pouch when ready to use. It may take up to 30 minutes for ThermaCare to reach its therapeutic temperature. Peel away paper to reveal adhesive tabs. Using adhesive is optional if you have sensitive skin or have body hair around the knee or elbow area.

Knee: Do not place heat cells on the back of the knee. Bend knee slightly and place opening over kneecap. Secure tabs to skin (optional). Wrap straps around knee and fasten. Over-tightening may cause discomfort. Adjust as needed.

Elbow: Do not place heat cells on the inside of the bend of the arm. Bend elbow slightly and place opening over elbow. Secure tabs to skin (optional). Wrap straps around elbow and fasten. Over-tightening may cause discomfort. Adjust as needed. For maximum effectiveness, we recommend you wear ThermaCare for 12 hours. Do not wear for more than 12 hours in any 24-hour period.

WARNING: THIS PRODUCT CAN CAUSE BURNS. CHECK SKIN FREQUENTLY DURING USE. IF YOU FIND IRRITATION OR A BURN, REMOVE PRODUCT IMMEDIATELY.

55 OR OLDER: YOUR RISK OF BURNING INCREASES AS YOU AGE. IF YOU ARE 55 YEARS OF AGE OR OLDER, WEAR THERMACARE OVER A TOWEL OR CLOTH SUCH AS A WASHCLOTH, NOT DIRECTLY AGAINST YOUR SKIN, AND DO NOT WEAR WHILE SLEEPING.

ADDITIONAL WARNINGS: Each heat disc contains iron (~2 grams), which can be harmful if ingested. If ingested, rinse mouth with water and call a Poison Control Center immediately. If heat disc contents come in contact with your skin or eyes, rinse right away with water. Never heat product in a microwave or attempt to reheat, as wrap could catch fire. Keep out of reach of children and pets.
DO NOT MICROWAVE

ASK A DOCTOR BEFORE USE if you have
• DIABETES
• poor circulation or heart disease
• rheumatoid arthritis
• or are pregnant

WHEN USING THIS PRODUCT check skin frequently for signs of burns or blisters – if found, stop use
• if product feels too hot – stop use or wear over clothing
• do not place extra pressure or tight clothing over the product
• do not use for more than 12 hours in a 24-hour period

DO NOT USE with pain rubs, medicated lotions, creams or ointments
• on unhealthy, damaged or broken skin
• on areas of bruising or swelling that have occurred within 48 hours
• on people unable to follow all use instructions
• on areas of the body where you can't feel heat
• with other forms of heat
• on people unable to remove the product, including children, infants, and some elderly

STOP USE AND ASK A DOCTOR if you experience any discomfort, burning, swelling, rash or other changes in your skin that persist where the wrap is worn
• if after 7 days your pain gets worse or remains unchanged, as this may be a sign of a more serious Condition

QUESTIONS?
**1-800-323-3383 or visit
www.thermacare.com**

How Supplied:
Available in boxes of 2 (Hand/Wrist & Knee/Elbow) or 3 (Neck/Shoulder/Wrist) or in single use pouches.
Shown in Product Identification Guide, page 507

VICKS® FORMULA 44®
(Procter & Gamble)
Cough Relief
Cough Suppressant
Alcohol 5%

• Maximum Strength
• Non-Drowsy
• For Adults & Children

Drug Facts:

Active Ingredients:
(per 15 ml tablespoon)   **Purpose:**
Dextromethorphan HBr
30 mg .... Cough suppressant

Use: temporarily relieves cough due to minor throat and bronchial irritation associated with a cold

Warnings:
Do not use if you are now taking a prescription monoamine oxidase inhibitor (MAOI) (certain drugs for depression, psychiatric or emotional conditions, or Parkinson's disease), or for 2 weeks after stopping the MAOI drug. If you do not know if your prescription drug contains an MAOI, ask a doctor or pharmacist before taking this product.
Ask a doctor before use if you have:
• cough that occurs with too much phlegm (mucus)
• persistent or chronic cough such as occurs with smoking, asthma, or emphysema
Stop use and ask a doctor if:
• cough lasts more than 7 days, comes back, or occurs with fever, rash, or headache that lasts. These could be signs of a serious condition.
If pregnant or breast feeding, ask a health professional before use.
Keep out of reach of children. In case of overdose, get medical help or contact a Poison Control Center right away.

Directions:
• use dose cup, teaspoon (tsp), or tablespoon (TBSP)
• do not exceed 4 doses per 24 hours

adults and children 12 years and over	1 TBSP (15 ml) every 6-8 hours
children 6 to under 12 years	1½ tsp (7½ ml) every 6-8 hours
children under 6 years	ask a doctor

Other Information:
• **each tablespoon contains** sodium 28 mg
• store at room temperature

Inactive Ingredients: alcohol, carboxymethylcellulose sodium, citric acid, FD&C Blue No. 1, FD&C Red No. 40, flavor, high fructose corn syrup, polyethylene oxide, polyoxyl 40 stearate, propylene glycol, purified water, saccharin sodium, sodium benzoate, sodium citrate.

How Supplied: Available in 4, 6, 8 and 10 OZ.

Questions? 1-800-342-6844

Shown in Product Identification Guide, page 508

VICKS® FORMULA 44D®
(Procter & Gamble)
COUGH & HEAD CONGESTION RELIEF
Cough Suppressant/Nasal Decongestant
Alcohol 5%

Drug Facts
Active Ingredients:
(in each 15 ml tablespoon)   Purpose:

Dextromethorphan HBr
  20 mg .... Cough suppressant
Phenylephrine HCl
  10 mg .... Nasal decongestant

Uses: temporarily relieves these cold symptoms:
• cough
• nasal congestion

Warnings:

Do not use if you are now taking a prescription monoamine oxidase inhibitor (MAOI) (certain drugs for depression, psychiatric or emotional conditions, or Parkinson's disease), or for 2 weeks after stopping the MAOI drug. If you do not know if your prescription drug contains an MAOI, ask a doctor or pharmacist before taking this product.

Ask a doctor before use if you have
• heart disease
• thyroid disease
• diabetes
• high blood pressure
• cough that occurs with too much phlegm (mucus)
• cough that lasts or is chronic such as occurs with smoking, asthma, or emphysema
• trouble urinating due to enlarged prostate gland
• a sodium-restricted diet
When using this product, do not take more than directed.
Stop use and ask a doctor if
• you get nervous, dizzy or sleepless
• symptoms do not get better within 7 days or are accompanied by fever
• cough lasts more than 7 days, comes back, or occurs with fever, rash, or headache that lasts.
  These could be signs of a serious condition.
If pregnant or breast-feeding, ask a health professional before use.
Keep out of reach of children. In case of overdose, get medical help or contact a Poison Control Center right away.

Directions:
• use dose cup, teaspoon (tsp), or tablespoon (TBSP)
• do not exceed 6 doses per 24 hours

adults and children 12 years and over	1 TBSP (15 ml) every 4 hours
children 6 to under 12 years	1½ tsp (7½ ml) every 4 hours
children under 6 years	ask a doctor

Other Information:
• **each tablespoon contains** sodium 35 mg
• store at room temperature

Inactive Ingredients: alcohol, carboxymethylcellulose sodium, citric acid, FD&C Blue No. 1, FD&C Red No. 40, flavor, glycerin, propylene glycol, purified water, saccharin sodium, sodium benzoate, sodium chloride, sorbitol, sucrose

Questions? 1-800-342-6844

How Supplied: Available in 4, 6, 8, and 10 OZ

Shown in Product Identification Guide, page 508

VICKS® FORMULA 44E®
(Procter & Gamble)
Cough & Chest Congestion Relief
Cough Suppressant/Expectorant
Alcohol 5%

• Non-Drowsy
• For Adults & Children

Drug Facts:

Active Ingredients:
(per 15 ml tablespoon)   Purpose:
Dextromethorphan HBr
  20 mg .... Cough suppressant
Guaifenesin
  200 mg .... Expectorant

Uses:
• temporarily relieves cough due to the common cold
• helps loosen phlegm and thin bronchial secretions to rid the bronchial passageways of bothersome mucus

Warnings:
Do not use
• if you are now taking a prescription monoamine oxidase inhibitor (MAOI) (certain drugs for depression, psychiatric or emotional conditions, or Parkinson's disease), or for 2 weeks after stopping the MAOI drug. If you do not know if your prescription drug contains an MAOI, ask a doctor or pharmacist before taking this product.
Ask a doctor before use if you have:
• a sodium restricted diet
• persistent or chronic cough such as occurs with smoking, asthma, chronic bronchitis or emphysema

• cough that occurs with too much phlegm (mucus)
Stop use and ask a doctor if:
• cough lasts more than 7 days, comes back, or occurs with fever, rash, or headache that lasts. These could be signs of a serious condition.
If pregnant or breast-feeding, ask a health professional before use.
Keep out of reach of children. In case of overdose, get medical help or contact a Poison Control Center right away.

Directions:
• use dose cup, teaspoon (tsp), or tablespoon (TBSP)
• do not exceed 6 doses per 24 hours

adults and children 12 years and over	1 TBSP (15 ml) every 4 hours
children 6 to under 12 years	1½ tsp (7½ ml) every 4 hours
children under 6 years	ask a doctor

Other Information:
• **each tablespoon contains** sodium 28 mg
• store at room temperature

Inactive Ingredients: alcohol, carboxymethylcellulose sodium, citric acid, FD&C Blue No. 1, FD&C Red No. 40, flavor, high fructose corn syrup, polyethylene oxide, polyoxyl 40 stearate, propylene glycol, purified water, saccharin sodium, sodium benzoate, sodium citrate.

How Supplied: Available in 4, 6, 8 and 10 OZ.
Questions? 1-800-342-6844

Shown in Product Identification Guide, page 508

VICKS® FORMULA 44M®
(Procter & Gamble)
COUGH, COLD & FLU RELIEF
Cough Suppressant/Antihistamine/
Pain Reliever/Fever Reducer
Alcohol 10%

Drug Facts
Active Ingredients:
(in each 5 ml teaspoon)   Purpose:
Acetaminophen
  162.5 mg .... Pain reliever/
                                          fever reducer
Chlorpheniramine maleate
  1 mg .... Antihistamine
Dextromethorphan HBr
  7.5 mg .... Cough suppressant

Uses temporarily relieves cough/cold/flu symptoms:
• cough due to minor throat and bronchial irritation
• sneezing
• headache
• sore throat
• fever
• runny nose

Continued on next page

Vicks Formula 44M—Cont.

Warnings:

Alcohol warning: If you consume 3 or more alcoholic drinks every day, ask your doctor whether you should take acetaminophen or other pain relievers/fever reducers. Acetaminophen may cause liver damage.

Sore throat warning: If sore throat is severe, persists more than two days, is accompanied or followed by a fever, headache, rash, nausea or vomiting, consult a doctor promptly.

Do not use

- **with other medicines containing acetaminophen**
- if you are now taking a prescription monoamine oxidase inhibitor (MAOI) (certain drugs for depression, psychiatric or emotional conditions, or Parkinson's disease), or for 2 weeks after stopping the MAOI drug. If you do not know if your prescription drug contains an MAOI, ask a doctor or pharmacist before taking this product.

Ask a doctor before use if you have

- glaucoma
- cough that occurs with too much phlegm (mucus)
- a breathing problem or chronic cough that lasts or as occurs with smoking, asthma, chronic bronchitis or emphysema
- trouble urinating due to enlarged prostate gland

Ask a doctor or pharmacist before use if you are taking sedatives or tranquilizers.

When using this product

- **do not use more than directed**
- excitability may occur, especially in children
- drowsiness may occur
- avoid alcoholic drinks
- be careful when driving a motor vehicle or operating machinery
- alcohol, sedatives, and tranquilizers may increase drowsiness

Stop use and ask a doctor if

- pain or cough gets worse or lasts more than 7 days
- fever gets worse or lasts more than 3 days
- redness or swelling is present
- new symptoms occur
- cough comes back or occurs with rash or headache that lasts.

These could be signs of a serious condition.

If pregnant or breast-feeding, ask a health professional before use.

Keep out of reach of children.

Overdose warning: Taking more than the recommended dose can cause serious health problems. In case of overdose, get medical help or contact a Poison Control Center right away. Quick medical attention is critical for adults as well as for children even if you do not notice any signs or symptoms.

Directions:

- take only as recommended — see Overdose warning
- use dose cup or teaspoon (tsp)
- do not exceed 4 doses per 24 hours

adults and children 12 years and over	4 tsp (20 ml) every 6 hours
children under 12 years	ask a doctor

Other Information:

- **each teaspoon contains** sodium 8 mg
- store at room temperature

Inactive Ingredients: alcohol, carboxymethylcellulose sodium, citric acid, FD&C Blue No. 1, FD&C Red No. 40, flavor, high fructose corn syrup, polyethylene glycol, polyethylene oxide, propylene glycol, purified water, saccharin sodium, sodium citrate

Questions? 1-800-342-6844

How Supplied:

Available in 4, 6, 8, and 10 OZ
Shown in Product Identification Guide, page 508

**CHILDREN'S VICKS® NYQUIL®
(Procter & Gamble)
Cold & Cough Relief
Antihistamine/Cough Suppressant**

Children's NyQuil was specially formulated with three effective ingredients to relieve nighttime cough and runny nose so children can rest. Children's NyQuil® is alcohol free and analgesic free and has a pleasant cherry flavor.

Drug Facts

**Active Ingredients:
(in each 15 ml tablespoon)   Purpose:**
Chlorpheniramine maleate
    2 mg .... Antihistamine
Dextromethorphan HBr
    15 mg .... Cough suppressant

Uses: temporarily relieves cold symptoms:

- cough due to minor throat and bronchial irritation
- sneezing
- runny nose

Warnings:

Do not use if you are now taking a prescription monoamine oxidase inhibitor (MAOI) (certain drugs for depression, psychiatric or emotional conditions, or Parkinson's disease), or for 2 weeks after stopping the MAOI drug. If you do not know if your prescription drug contains an MAOI, ask a doctor or pharmacist before taking this product.

Ask a doctor before use if you have

- glaucoma
- cough that occurs with too much phlegm (mucus)

- a breathing problem or chronic cough that lasts or as occurs with smoking, asthma, chronic bronchitis, or emphysema
- trouble urinating due to enlarged prostate gland
- a sodium-restricted diet

Ask a doctor or pharmacist before use if you are taking sedatives or tranquilizers.

When using this product

- **do not use more than directed**
- excitability may occur, especially in children
- marked drowsiness may occur
- avoid alcoholic drinks
- be careful when driving a motor vehicle or operating machinery
- alcohol, sedatives, and tranquilizers may increase drowsiness

Stop use and ask a doctor if

- cough lasts more than 7 days, comes back, or occurs with fever, rash, or headache that lasts. These could be signs of a serious condition.

If pregnant or breast-feeding, ask a health professional before use.

Keep out of reach of children. In case of overdose, get medical help or contact a Poison Control Center right away.

Directions:

- use dose cup or tablespoon (TBSP)
- do not exceed 4 doses per 24 hours

adults and children 12 years and over	2 TBSP (30 ml) every 6 hours
children 6 to 11 years	1 TBSP (15 ml) every 6 hours
children under 6 years	ask a doctor

Other Information:

- **each tablespoon contains** sodium 71 mg
- store at room temperature

Inactive Ingredients: citric acid, FD&C Red No. 40, flavor, potassium sorbate, propylene glycol, purified water, sodium citrate, sucrose

Questions? 1-800-362-1683

How Supplied: Available in 4 and 6 OZ
Shown in Product Identification Guide, page 507

**VICKS® Cough Drops
(Procter & Gamble)
Menthol Cough Suppressant/
Oral Anesthetic
Menthol and Cherry Flavors**

CONSUMER INFORMATION: Vicks Cough Drops provide fast and effective relief. Each drop contains effective medicine to suppress your impulse to cough as it dissolves into a soothing syrup to relieve your sore throat.

Drug Facts:

Menthol:

Active Ingredient:	**Purpose:**
(per drop)	

Menthol 3.3 mg .... Cough suppressant/
oral anesthetic

Cherry:

Active Ingredient:	**Purpose:**
(per drop)	

Menthol 1.7 mg .... Cough suppressant/
oral anesthetic

Uses: Temporarily relieves:
• sore throat
• coughs due to colds or inhaled irritants

Warnings:

Ask a doctor before use if you have:
• cough associated with excessive phlegm (mucus)
• persistent or chronic cough such as those caused by asthma, emphysema, or smoking
• a severe sore throat accompanied by difficulty in breathing or that lasts more than 2 days
• a sore throat accompanied or followed by fever, headache, rash, swelling, nausea or vomiting

Stop use and ask a doctor if:
• you need to use more than 7 days
• cough lasts more than 7 days, comes back, or occurs with fever, rash, or headache that lasts. These could be signs of a serious condition.

If pregnant or breast-feeding, ask a health professional before use.

Keep out of reach of children.

Directions:
• under 5 yrs.: ask a doctor (menthol)
• adults & children 5 yrs. & older: allow 2 drops to dissolve slowly in mouth (cherry)
• adults & children 5 yrs. & older: allow 3 drops to dissolve slowly in mouth
Cough: may be repeated every hour.
Sore Throat: may be repeated every 2 hours.

Other Information:
• store at room temperature

Inactive Ingredients:
Menthol: Ascorbic acid, caramel, corn syrup, eucalyptus oil, sucrose.
Cherry: Ascorbic acid, citric acid, corn syrup, eucalyptus oil, FD&C Blue No. 1, flavor, FD&C Red No. 40, sucrose.

How Supplied: Vicks® Cough Drops are available in boxes of 20 triangular drops. Each red or green drop is debossed with "V."
Questions? 1-800-707-1709

**FACED WITH AN
Rx SIDE EFFECT?**
Turn to the
Companion Drug Index
for products that
provide symptomatic
relief.

**VICKS® DAYQUIL® LIQUID
(Procter & Gamble)**

**VICKS® DAYQUIL® LIQUICAPS®
Multi-Symptom Cold/Flu Relief
Nasal Decongestant/Pain Reliever/
Cough Suppressant/Fever Reducer
Non-drowsy**

Drug Facts

Active Ingredients:

(in each 15 ml tablespoon)	**Purpose:**

Acetaminophen
  325 mg ..... Pain reliever/fever reducer
Dextromethorphan HBr
  10 mg .... Cough suppressant
Phenylephrine HCl
  5 mg .... Nasal decongestant

Uses: temporarily relieves common cold/flu symptoms:
• nasal congestion
• cough due to minor throat and bronchial irritation
• sore throat
• headache
• minor aches and pains
• fever

Warnings:

Alcohol warning: If you consume 3 or more alcoholic drinks every day, ask your doctor whether you should take acetaminophen or other pain relievers/fever reducers. Acetaminophen may cause liver damage.

Sore throat warning: If sore throat is severe, persists for more than two days, is accompanied or followed by a fever, headache, rash, nausea, or vomiting, consult a doctor promptly.

Do not use
• **with other medicines containing acetaminophen**
• if you are now taking a prescription monoamine oxidase inhibitor (MAOI) (certain drugs for depression, psychiatric or emotional conditions, or Parkinson's disease), or for 2 weeks after stopping the MAOI drug. If you do not know if your prescription drug contains an MAOI, ask a doctor or pharmacist before taking this product.

Ask a doctor before use if you have
• heart disease
• thyroid disease
• diabetes
• high blood pressure
• trouble urinating due to enlarged prostate gland
• cough that occurs with too much phlegm (mucus)
• persistent or chronic cough as occurs with smoking, asthma, or emphysema
• a sodium-restricted diet

When using this product, do not use more than directed

Stop use and ask a doctor if
• you get nervous, dizzy or sleepless
• symptoms get worse or last more than 5 days (children) or 7 days (adults)
• fever gets worse or lasts more than 3 days

• redness or swelling is present
• new symptoms occur
• cough comes back, or occurs with rash or headache that lasts.
These could be signs of a serious condition.

If pregnant or breast-feeding, ask a health professional before use.

Keep out of reach of children.

Overdose warning: Taking more than the recommended dose can cause serious health problems. In case of overdose, get medical help or contact a Poison Control Center right away. Quick medical attention is critical for adults as well as for children even if you do not notice any signs or symptoms.

Directions:
• take only as recommended — see Overdose warning
• use dose cup or tablespoon (TBSP)
• do not exceed 5 doses (children) or 6 doses (adults) per 24 hours

adults and children 12 years and over	2 TBSP (30 ml) every 4 hours
children 6 to under 12 years	1 TBSP (15 ml) every 4 hours
children under 6 years	ask a doctor

• **when using other DayQuil or NyQuil products, carefully read each label to insure correct dosing**

Other Information:
• **each tablespoon contains** sodium 50 mg
• store at room temperature

Inactive Ingredients: carboxymethylcellulose sodium, citric acid, disodium EDTA, FD&C Yellow No. 6, flavor, glycerin, propylene glycol, purified water, saccharin sodium, sodium benzoate, sodium chloride, sodium sitrate, sorbitol sucraoofe

Questions? 1-800-251-3374

How Supplied:
Available in 6, 10, and 12 OZ, twin pack and quad pack.

Drug Facts

Active ingredients

(in each LiquiCap)	**Purpose:**

Acetaminophen
  325 mg ..... Pain reliever/fever reducer
Dextromethorphan HBr
  10 mg .... Cough suppressant
Phenylephrine HCl
  5 mg .... Nasal decongestant

Uses:
temporarily relieves common cold/flu symptoms:
• nasal congestion
• cough due to minor throat and bronchial irritation

Continued on next page

Vicks DayQuil—Cont.

- sore throat
- headache
- minor aches and pains
- fever

Warnings:

Alcohol warning: If you consume 3 or more alcoholic drinks every day, ask your doctor whether you should take acetaminophen or other pain relievers/fever reducers. Acetaminophen may cause liver damage.

Sore throat warning: If sore throat is severe, persists for more than two days, is accompanied or followed by a fever, headache, rash, nausea, or vomiting, consult a doctor promptly.

Do not use
- **with other medicines containing acetaminophen**
- if you are now taking a prescription monoamine oxidase inhibitor (MAOI) (certain drugs for depression, psychiatric or emotional conditions, or Parkinson's disease), or for 2 weeks after stopping the MAOI drug. If you do not know if your prescription drug contains an MAOI, ask a doctor or pharmacist before taking this product.

Ask a doctor before use if you have
- heart disease
- thyroid disease
- diabetes
- high blood pressure
- trouble urinating due to enlarged prostate gland
- cough that occurs with too much phlegm (mucus)
- persistent or chronic cough as occurs with smoking, asthma, or emphysema

When using this product, do not use more than directed

Stop use and ask a doctor if
- you get nervous, dizzy or sleepless
- symptoms get worse or last more than 5 days (children) or 7 days (adults)
- fever gets worse or lasts more than 3 days
- redness or swelling is present
- new symptoms occur
- cough comes back, or occurs with rash or headache that lasts.

These could be signs of a serious condition.

If pregnant or breast-feeding, ask a health professional before use.

Keep out of reach of children.

Overdose warning: Taking more than the recommended dose can cause serious health problems. In case of overdose, get medical help or contact a Poison Control Center right away. Quick medical attention is critical for adults as well as for children even if you do not notice any signs or symptoms.

Directions:
- take only as recommended — see Overdose warning
- do not exceed 6 doses per 24 hours

adults and children 12 years and over	2 LiquiCaps with water every 4 hours
children under 12 years	ask a doctor

- **when using other DayQuil or NyQuil products, carefully read each label to insure correct dosing**

Other Information:
- store at room temperature

Inactive Ingredients: FD&C Red No. 40, FD&C Yellow No. 6, gelatin, glycerin, polyethylene glycol, povidone, propylene glycol, purified water, sorbitol special, titanium dioxide

Questions? 1-800-251-3374

How Supplied:
Available in boxes of 2, 12, 20, 24, 40, and 60.

Shown in Product Identification Guide, page 507

VICKS® NYQUIL® COUGH
(Procter & Gamble)
Antihistamine
Cough Suppressant
All Night Cough Relief
Cherry Flavor

alcohol 10%

Drug Facts:

Active Ingredients: **Purpose:**
(per 15 ml tablespoon)
Dextromethorphan HBr
   15 mg .... Cough suppressant
Doxylamine succinate
   6.25 mg .... Antihistamine

Uses: temporarily relieves cold symptoms
- cough
- runny nose and sneezing

Warnings:

Do not use if you are now taking a prescription monoamine oxidase inhibitor (MAOI) (certain drugs for depression, psychiatric or emotional conditions, or Parkinson's disease), or for 2 weeks after stopping the MAOI drug. If you do not know if your prescription drug contains an MAOI, ask a doctor or pharmacist before taking this product.

Ask a doctor before use if you have:
- asthma
- emphysema
- breathing problems
- excessive phlegm (mucus)
- glaucoma
- chronic bronchitis
- persistent or chronic cough
- cough associated with smoking
- trouble urinating due to enlarged prostate gland

Ask a doctor or pharmacist before use if you are taking sedatives or tranquilizers.

When using this product:

- **do not use more than directed**
- marked drowsiness may occur
- avoid alcoholic drinks
- excitability may occur, especially in children
- be careful when driving a motor vehicle or operating machinery
- alcohol, sedatives, and tranquilizers may increase drowsiness

Stop use and ask a doctor if:
- cough lasts more than 7 days, comes back, or occurs with fever, rash, or headache that lasts.
  These could be signs of a serious condition.

If pregnant or breast-feeding, ask a health professional before use.

Keep out of reach of children. In case of overdose, get medical help or contact a Poison Control Center right away.

Directions:
- use dose cup or tablespoon (TBSP)
- do not exceed 4 doses per 24 hours

adults and children 12 years and over	2 TBSP (30 ml) every 6 hours
children under 12 years	ask a doctor

- **when using other DayQuil or NyQuil products, carefully read the label to insure correct dosing.**

Other Information:
- **each tablespoon contains** sodium 18 mg
- store at room temperature

Inactive Ingredients: alcohol, citric acid, FD&C Blue No. 1, FD&C Red No. 40, flavor, high fructose corn syrup, polyethylene glycol, propylene glycol, purified water, saccharin sodium, sodium citrate

How Supplied: Available in 1 FL OZ (30 ml) 6 FL OZ (177 ml), 10 FL OZ (295 ml), and 12 FL OZ (354 ml) plastic bottles with child-resistant, tamper-evident cap and calibrated Medicine cup.
Questions? 1-800-362-1683
Shown in Product Identification Guide, page 508

VICKS® NYQUIL® D
(Procter & Gamble)
Cold & Flu Multi-Symptom Relief
Nasal Decongestant/
Cough Suppressant/Pain Reliever/
Fever Reducer/Antihistamine
Alcohol 10%

Drug Facts:

Active Ingredients: **Purpose:**
(in each 15 ml tablespoon)
Acetaminophen
500 mg .... Pain reliever/fever reducer
Dextromethorphan HBr
15 mg .... Cough suppressant
Doxylamine succinate
6.25 mg .... Antihistamine

Pseudoephedrine HCl
30 mg .... Nasal decongestant

Uses: temporarily relieves common cold/flu symptoms:
* nasal congestion
* cough due to minor throat and bronchial irritation
* sore throat
* headache
* minor aches and pain
* fever
* runny nose and sneezing

Warnings

Alcohol warning: If you consume 3 or more alcoholic drinks every day, ask your doctor whether you should take acetaminophen or other pain relievers/fever reducers. Acetaminophen may cause liver damage.

Sore throat warning: If sore throat is severe, persists for more than two days, is accompanied or followed by fever, headache, rash, nausea, or vomiting, consult a doctor promptly.

Do not use
* **with other medicines containing acetaminophen**
* if you are now taking a prescription monoamine oxidase inhibitor (MAOI) (certain drugs for depression, psychiatric or emotional conditions, or Parkinson's disease), or for 2 weeks after stopping the MAOI drug. If you do not know if your prescription drug contains an MAOI, ask a doctor or pharmacist before taking this product.

Ask a doctor before use if you have
* heart disease
* thyroid disease
* diabetes
* glaucoma
* high blood pressure
* cough that occurs with too much phlegm (mucus)
* a breathing problem or chronic cough that lasts or as occurs with smoking, asthma, chronic bronchitis or emphysema
* trouble urinating due to enlarged prostate gland

Ask a doctor or pharmacist before use if you are taking sedatives or tranquilizers.

When using this product
* **do not use more than directed**
* excitability may occur, especially in children
* marked drowsiness may occur
* avoid alcoholic drinks, be careful when driving a motor vehicle or operating machinery
* alcohol, sedatives, and tranquilizers may increase drowsiness

Stop use and ask a doctor if
* redness or swelling is present
* symptoms do not get better within 7 days or are accompanied by a fever
* you get nervous, dizzy or sleepless
* fever gets worse or lasts more than 3 days

* new symptoms occur
* cough lasts more than 7 days, comes back, or occurs with fever, rash, or headache that lasts. These could be signs of a serious condition.

If pregnant or breast-feeding, ask a health professional before use.

Keep out of reach of children.

Overdose warning: Taking more than the recommended dose can cause serious health problems. In case of overdose, get medical help or contact a Poison Control Center right away. Quick medical attention is critical for adults as well as for children even if you do not notice any signs or symptoms.

Directions:
* take only as recommended - see Overdose warning
* use dose cup or tablespoon (TBSP)
* do not exceed 4 doses per 24 hours

adults and children 12 years and over	2 TBSP (30 ml) every 6 hours
children under 12 years	ask a doctor

* **when using other DayQuil or NyQuil products, carefully read each label to insure correct dosing**

Other information:
* **each tablespoonful contains** sodium 18 mg
* store at room temperature

Inactive ingredients: alcohol, citric acid, D&C Yellow No. 10, FD&C Green No. 3, FD&C Yellow No. 6, flavor, high fructose corn syrup, polyethylene glycol, propylene glycol, purified water, saccharin sodium, sodium citrate

Questions? 1-800-362-1683

How Supplied: Available in 10 OZ

VICKS® NYQUIL® LIQUICAPS®
(Procter & Gamble)

VICKS® NYQUIL® LIQUID
Multi-Symptom Cold/Flu Relief
Cough Suppressant/Antihistamine/
Pain Reliever/Fever Reducer

Drug Facts:

Active ingredients:
(in each LiquiCap)　　　　　　　**Purpose:**
Acetaminophen
325 mg .... Pain reliever/fever reducer
Dextromethorphan HBr
15 mg .... Cough suppressant
Doxylamine succinate
6.25 mg .... Antihistamine

Uses: temporarily relieves common cold/flu symptoms:

* cough due to minor throat and bronchial irritation
* sore throat
* headache
* minor aches and pains
* fever
* runny nose and sneezing

Warnings:

Alcohol warning: If you consume 3 or more alcoholic drinks every day, ask your doctor whether you should take acetaminophen or other pain relievers/fever reducers. Acetaminophen may cause liver damage.

Sore throat warning: If sore throat is severe, persists for more than two days, is accompanied or followed by fever, headache, rash, nausea, or vomiting, consult a doctor promptly.

Do not use
* **with other medicines containing acetaminophen**
* if you are now taking a prescription monoamine oxidase inhibitor (MAOI) (certain drugs for depression, psychiatric or emotional conditions, or Parkinson's disease), or for 2 weeks after stopping the MAOI drug. If you do not know if your prescription drug contains an MAOI, ask a doctor or pharmacist before taking this product.

Ask a doctor before use if you have
* glaucoma
* cough that occurs with too much phlegm (mucus)
* a breathing problem or chronic cough that lasts or as occurs with smoking, asthma, chronic bronchitis or emphysema
* trouble urinating due to enlarged prostate gland

Ask a doctor or pharmacist before use if you are taking sedatives or tranquilizers.

When using this product
* **do not use more than directed**
* excitability may occur, especially in children
* marked drowsiness may occur
* avoid alcoholic drinks
* be careful when driving a motor vehicle or operating machinery
* alcohol, sedatives, and tranquilizers may increase drowsiness

Stop use and ask a doctor if
* pain or cough gets worse or lasts more than 7 days
* fever gets worse or lasts more than 3 days
* redness or swelling is present
* new symptoms occur
* cough comes back or occurs with rash or headache that lasts.

These could be signs of a serious condition.

If pregnant or breast-feeding, ask a health professional before use.

Keep out of reach of children.

Overdose warning: Taking more than the recommended dose can cause serious health problems. In case of overdose, get

Continued on next page

Vicks NyQuil—Cont.

medical help or contact a Poison Control Center right away. Quick medical attention is critical for adults as well as for children even if you do not notice any signs or symptoms.

Directions:
- take only as recommended – see Overdose warning
- do not exceed 4 doses per 24 hours

adults and children 12 years and over	2 LiquiCaps with water every 6 hours
children under 12 years	ask a doctor

- **when using other DayQuil or NyQuil products, carefully read each label to insure correct dosing**

Other information:
- store at room temperature

Inactive ingredients: D&C Yellow No. 10, FD&C Blue No. 1, gelatin, glycerin, polyethylene glycol, povidone, propylene glycol, purified water, sorbitol special, titanium dioxide

Questions? 1–800–362–1683

How Supplied:
Available in boxes of 2, 12, 20, 24, 40 and 60.

Drug Facts

Active Ingredients:
(in each 15 ml tablespoon)   Purpose:

Acetaminophen
500 mg .... Pain reliever/fever reducer
Dextromethorphan HBr
15 mg .... Cough suppressant
Doxylamine succinate
6.25 mg .... Antihistamine

Uses: temporarily relieves common cold/flu symptoms:
- cough due to minor throat and bronchial irritation
- sore throat
- headache
- minor aches and pain
- fever
- runny nose and sneezing

Warnings:

Alcohol warning: If you consume 3 or more alcoholic drinks every day, ask your doctor whether you should take acetaminophen or other pain relievers/fever reducers. Acetaminophen may cause liver damage.

Sore throat warning: If sore throat is severe, persists for more than two days, is accompanied or followed by fever, headache, rash, nausea, or vomiting, consult a doctor promptly.

Do not use
- **with other medicines containing acetaminophen**

- if you are now taking a prescription monoamine oxidase inhibitor (MAOI) (certain drugs for depression, or emotional conditions, or Parkinson's disease), or for 2 weeks after stopping the MAOI drug. If you do not know if your prescription drug contains an MAOI, ask a doctor or pharmacist before taking this product.

Ask a doctor before use if you have
- glaucoma
- cough that occurs with too much phlegm (mucus)
- a breathing problem or chronic cough that lasts or as occurs with smoking, asthma, chronic bronchitis or emphysema
- trouble urinating due to enlarged prostate gland

Ask a doctor or pharmacist before use if you are taking sedatives or tranquilizers.

When using this product
- **do not use more than directed**
- excitability may occur, especially in children
- marked drowsiness may occur
- avoid alcoholic drinks
- be careful when driving a motor vehicle or operating machinery
- alcohol, sedatives, and tranquilizers may increase drowsiness

Stop use and ask a doctor if
- pain or cough gets worse or lasts more than 7 days
- fever gets worse or lasts more than 3 days
- redness or swelling is present
- new symptoms occur
- cough comes back or occurs with rash or headache that lasts.

These could be signs of a serious condition.

If pregnant or breast-feeding, ask a health professional before use.

Keep out of reach of children.

Overdose warning: Taking more than the recommended dose can cause serious health problems. In case of overdose, get medical help or contact a Poison Control Center right away. Quick medical attention is critical for adults as well as for children even if you do not notice any signs or symptoms.

Directions:
- take only as recommended – see Overdose warning
- use dose cup or tablespoon (TBSP)
- do not exceed 4 doses per 24 hours

adults and children 12 years and over	2 TBSP (30 ml) every 6 hours
children under 12 years	ask a doctor

- **when using other DayQuil or NyQuil products, carefully read each label to insure correct dosing**

Other information:
- **each tablespoon contains** sodium 18 mg [original] or 19 mg [cherry]
- store at room temperature

Inactive Ingredients [original] alcohol, citric acid, D&C Yellow No. 10, FD&C Green No. 3, FD&C Yellow No. 6, flavor, high fructose corn syrup, polyethylene glycol, propylene glycol, purified water, saccharin sodium, sodium citrate [cherry] alcohol, citric acid, FD&C Blue No. 1, FD&C Red No. 40, flavor, high fructose corn syrup, polyethylene glycol, propylene glycol, purified water, saccharin sodium, sodium citrate

Questions? 1–800–362–1683

How Supplied:
Available in 6, 10, 12 and 16 OZ, twin, triple and quad pack.

Shown in Product Identification Guide, page 507

PEDIATRIC VICKS® FORMULA 44e®
(Procter & Gamble)
Cough & Chest Congestion Relief
Cough Suppressant/Expectorant

- Non-drowsy
- Alcohol-free
- Aspirin-free

Drug Facts:

Active Ingredient: Purpose:
(per 15 ml tablespoon
Dextromethorphan
HBr 10 mg .... Cough suppressant
Guaifenesin 100 mg .... Expectorant

Uses:
- temporarily relieves cough due to the common cold
- helps loosen phlegm and thin bronchial secretions to rid bronchial passageways of bothersome mucus

Warnings:

Do not use if you are now taking a prescription monoamine oxidase inhibitor (MAOI) (certain drugs for depression, psychiatric or emotional conditions, or Parkinson's disease), or for 2 weeks after stopping the MAOI drug. If you do not know if your prescription drug contains an MAOI, ask a doctor or pharmacist before taking this product.

Ask a doctor before use if you have:
- a sodium restricted diet
- persistent or chronic cough such as occurs with smoking, asthma, chronic bronchitis or emphysema
- cough that occurs with too much phlegm (mucus)

Stop use and ask a doctor if:
- cough lasts more than 7 days, comes back, or occurs with fever, rash, or headache that lasts. These could be signs of a serious condition.

If pregnant or breast-feeding, ask a health professional before use.

Keep out of reach of children. In case of overdose, get medical help or contact a Poison Control Center right away.

Directions:
- use dose cup or tablespoon (TBSP)
- do not exceed 6 doses per 24 hours

adults and children 12 years and over	2 TBSP (30 ml) every 4 hours
children 6 to under 12 years	1 TBSP (15 ml) every 4 hours
children 2 to under 6 years	½ TBSP (7½ ml) every 4 hours
children under 2	ask a doctor

Other Information:
- **each tablespoon contains** sodium 27 mg
- store at room temperature

Inactive Ingredients: carboxymethylcellulose sodium, citric acid, FD&C Red No. 40, flavor, high fructose corn syrup, polyethylene oxide, polyoxyl 40 stearate, propylene glycol, purified water, saccharin sodium, sodium benzoate, sodium citrate.

How Supplied: Available in 4 OZ.
Questions? 1-800-342-6844
Shown in Product Identification Guide, page 507

PEDIATRIC VICKS® FORMULA 44m®
(Procter & Gamble)
Multi-Symptom Cough & Cold Relief
Antihistamine/Cough Suppressant

- **Alcohol-free**
- **Aspirin-free**

Drug Facts

Active Ingredients:
(per 15 ml tablespoon)   Purpose:

Chlorpheniramine maleate
   2 mg .... Antihistamine
Dextromethorphan HBr
   15 mg .... Cough suppressant

Uses: temporarily relieves cough/cold symptoms:
- cough
- sneezing
- runny nose

Warnings:

Do not use if you are now taking a prescription monoamine oxidase inhibitor (MAOI) (certain drugs for depression, psychiatric or emotional conditions, or Parkinson's disease), or for 2 weeks after stopping the MAOI drug. If you do not know if your prescription drug contains an MAOI, ask a doctor or pharmacist before taking this product.

Ask a doctor before use if you have
- glaucoma
- a sodium-restricted diet
- a breathing problem or chronic cough that lasts or as occurs with smoking, asthma, chronic bronchitis, or emphysema

- cough that occurs with too much phlegm (mucus)
- trouble urinating due to enlarged prostate gland

Ask a doctor or pharmacist before use if you are taking sedatives or tranquilizers.

When using this product
- **do not use more than directed**
- excitability may occur, especially in children
- drowsiness may occur
- avoid alcoholic drinks
- be careful when driving a motor vehicle or operating machinery
- alcohol, sedatives, and transquilizers may increase drowsiness

Stop use and ask a doctor if
- symptoms do not get better within 7 days or are accompanied by a fever
- cough lasts more than 7 days, comes back, or occurs with fever, rash, or headache that lasts. These could be signs of a serious condition.

If pregnant or breast-feeding, ask a health professional before use.

Keep out of reach of children. In case of overdose, get medical help or contact a Poison Control Center right away.

Directions:
- use dose cup or tablespoon (TBSP)
- do not exceed 4 doses per 24 hours

adults and children 12 yrs and over	2 TBSP (30 ml) every 6 hours
children 6 to under 12 years	1 TBSP (15 ml) every 6 hours
children under 6 years	ask a doctor

Other Information:
- **each tablespoon contains** sodium 27 mg
- store at room temperature

Inactive Ingredients: carboxymethylcellulose sodium, citric acid, FD&C Red No. 40, flavor, high fructose corn syrup, polyethylene oxide, polyoxyl 40 stearate, propylene glycol, purified water, saccharin sodium, sodium benzoate, sodium citrate

Questions? 1-800-342-6844

How Supplied: 4 FL OZ
Shown in Product Identification Guide, page 507

VICKS® SINEX®
(Procter & Gamble)
Nasal Spray for Sinus Relief
[sī 'nĕx]
Nasal Decongestant

Drug Facts:

Active Ingredient: Purpose:
Phenylephrine
HCl 0.5% .... Nasal decongestant

Uses: Temporarily relieves nasal congestion due to

- colds
- hay fever
- upper respiratory allergies

Warnings:
Ask a doctor before use if you have:
- heart disease
- thyroid disease
- diabetes
- high blood pressure
- trouble urinating due to enlarged prostate gland

When using this product:
- **do not exceed recommended dosage**
- use of this container by more than one person may cause infection
- temporary burning, stinging, sneezing, or increased nasal discharge may occur
- frequent or prolonged use may cause nasal congestion to recur or worsen

Stop use and ask a doctor if:
- symptoms persist for more than 3 days

If pregnant or breast-feeding, ask a health professional before use.

Keep out of reach of children. In case of accidental ingestion, get medical help or contact a poison control center right away.

Directions:

Nasal Spray:
- adults & children 12 yrs. & older: 2 or 3 sprays in each nostril without tilting your head, not more often than every 4 hours.
- under 12 yrs. ask a doctor

Ultra Fine Mist: Remove protective cap. Before using for the first time, prime the pump by firmly depressing its rim several times. Hold container with thumb at base and nozzle between first and second fingers. Without tilting your head, insert nozzle into nostril. Fully depress rim with a firm, even stroke and inhale deeply.
- adults & children 12 yrs. & older: 2 or 3 sprays in each nostril, not more often than every 4 hours.
- under 12 yrs.: ask a doctor

Other Information:
- store at room temperature

Inactive Ingredients: Benzalkonium chloride, camphor, chlorhexidine gluconate, citric acid, disodium EDTA, eucalyptol, menthol, purified water, tyloxapol

How Supplied: Available in ¹/₂ FL OZ (14.7 ml) plastic squeeze bottle and ¹/₂ FL OZ (14.7 ml) measured dose Ultra Fine mist pump. Note: This container is properly filled when approximately half full. Air space equal to one half of volume is necessary to propel the fine spray.
Questions? 1-800-873-8276

FACED WITH AN Rx SIDE EFFECT?
Turn to the Companion Drug Index for products that provide symptomatic relief.

VICKS® SINEX® 12 HOUR
(Procter & Gamble)
[sĭ 'něx]
[Nasal Spray]
[Ultra Fine Mist] for Sinus Relief
Nasal Decongestant

Drug Facts:

Active Ingredient: **Purpose:**
Oxymetazoline HCl
  0.05% .... Nasal decongestant

Uses: Temporarily relieves nasal congestion due to
- colds
- hay fever
- upper respiratory allergies

Warnings:
Ask a doctor before use if you have:
- heart disease
- thyroid disease
- diabetes
- high blood pressure
- trouble urinating due to enlarged prostate gland

When using this product:
- **do not exceed recommended dosage**
- temporary burning, stinging, sneezing, or increased nasal discharge may occur
- frequent or prolonged use may cause nasal congestion to recur or worsen
- use of this container by more than one person may cause infection

Stop use and ask a doctor if:
- symptoms persist for more than 3 days

If pregnant or breast-feeding, ask a health professional before use.
Keep out of reach of children. In case of accidental ingestion, get medical help or contact a poison control center right away.

Directions:
Nasal Spray:
- adults & children 6 yrs. & older (with adult supervision): 2 or 3 sprays in each nostril without tilting your head, not more often than every 10 to 12 hours. Do not exceed 2 doses in 24 hours.
- under 6 yrs.: ask a doctor

Ultra Fine Mist:
  Remove protective cap. Before using for the first time, prime the pump by firmly depressing its rim several times. Hold container with thumb at base and nozzle between first and second fingers. Without tilting your head, insert nozzle into nostril. Fully depress rim with a firm, even stroke and inhale deeply.
- adults & children 6 yrs. & older (with adult supervision): 2 or 3 sprays in each nostril, not more often than every 10 to 12 hours. Do not exceed 2 doses in 24 hours.
- under 6 yrs.: ask a doctor

Other Information:
- store at room temperature

Inactive Ingredients: Benzalkonium chloride, camphor, chlorhexidine gluconate, disodium EDTA, eucalyptol, menthol, potassium phosphate, purified water, sodium chloride, sodium phosphate, tyloxapol.

How Supplied: Available in ½ FL OZ (14.7 ml) plastic squeeze bottle and ½ FL OZ (14.7 ml) measured-dose Ultra Fine mist pump.
Questions? 1-800-873-8276

VICKS® VAPOR INHALER
(Procter & Gamble)
Levmetamfetamine/Nasal Decongestant

Drug Facts

Active Ingredient: **Purpose:**
(per inhaler)
Levmetamfetamine
  50mg .... Nasal decongestant

Uses: Temporarily relieves nasal congestion due to:
- a cold
- hay fever or other upper respiratory allergies

Warnings:
When using this product:
- **do not exceed recommended dosage**
- temporary burning, stinging, sneezing, or increased nasal discharge may occur
- frequent or prolonged use may cause nasal congestion to recur or worsen
- do not use for more than 7 days
- do not use container by more than one person as it may spread infection
- use only as directed

Stop use and ask a doctor if:
- symptoms persist

If pregnant or breast-feeding, ask a health professional before use.
Keep out of reach of children. If swallowed, get medical help or contact a poison control center right away.

Directions:
The product delivers in each 800 ml air 0.04 to 0.15 mg of levmetamfetamine.
- do not use more often than every 2 hours
- under 6 yrs.: ask a doctor
- 6–11 yrs.: with adult supervision, 1 inhalation in each nostril.
- 12 yrs. & older: 2 inhalation in each nostril.

Other Information:
- store at room temperature
- keep inhaler tightly closed.
- This inhaler is effective for a minimum of 3 months after first use.

Inactive Ingredients: Bornyl acetate, camphor, lavender oil, menthol, methyl salicylate.

How Supplied: Available as a cylindrical plastic nasal inhaler.
Net weight: 0.007 OZ (204 mg).
TAMPER EVIDENT: Use only if imprinted wrap is intact.
Questions? 1-800-873-8276
Dist. by Procter & Gamble, Cincinnati OH 45202. ©2001 42438038

VICKS® VAPORUB®
(Procter & Gamble)
VICKS® VAPORUB® CREAM
(greaseless)
(Procter & Gamble)
[vā 'pō-rub]
Cough
Suppressant/Topical Analgesic

Drug Facts

Active Ingredients:
Vicks® VapoRub®:
Active Ingredients: **Purpose:**
Camphor 4.8% .... Cough suppressant, & topical analgesic
Eucalyptus oil
  1.2% .... Cough suppressant
Menthol 2.6% .... Cough suppressant, & topical analgesic

Vicks® VapoRub®:
Active Ingredient: **Purpose:**
Camphor 5.2% .... Cough suppressant, & topical analgesic
Eucalyptus oil
  1.2% .... Cough suppressant
Menthol 2.8% .... Cough suppressant, & topical analgesic

Uses:
- on chest and throat, temporarily relieves cough due to the common cold
- on muscles and joints, temporarily relieves minor aches and pains

Warnings:
Failure to follow these warnings could result in serious consequences.
For external use only; avoid contact with eyes.
Do not use:
- by mouth
- with tight bandages
- in nostrils
- on wounds or damaged skin

Ask a doctor before use if you have:
- cough that occurs with too much phlegm (mucus)
- persistent or chronic cough such as occurs with smoking, asthma or emphysema

When using this product, do not:
- heat
- microwave
- add to hot water or any container where heating water. May cause splattering and result in burns.

Stop use and ask a doctor if:
- muscle aches/pains persist more than 7 days or come back
- cough lasts more than 7 days, comes back, or occurs with fever, rash, or headache that lasts.
  These could be signs of a serious condition.

If pregnant or breast-feeding, ask a health professional before use.
Keep out of reach of children. If swallowed, get medical help or contact a Poison Control Center right away.

Directions:
- **See important warnings under "When using this product"**
- under 2 yrs.: ask a doctor
- adults and children 2 yrs. & older: Rub

a thick layer on chest & throat or rub on sore aching muscles. If desired, cover with a warm, dry cloth. Keep clothing loose about throat/chest to help vapors reach the nose/mouth. Repeat up to three times per 24 hours or as directed by a doctor.

Other Information:
• store at room temperature

Inactive Ingredients:
Vicks® VapoRub®: Cedarleaf oil, nutmeg oil, special petrolatum, thymol, turpentine oil
Vicks® VapoRub® Cream: Carbomer 954, cedarleaf oil, cetyl alcohol, cetyl palmitate, cyclomethicone copolyol, dimethicone copolyol, dimethicone, EDTA, glycerin, imidazolidinyl urea, isopropyl palmitate, methylparaben, nutmeg oil, peg-100 stearate, propylparaben, purified water, sodium hydroxide, stearic acid, stearyl alcohol, thymol, titanium dioxide, turpentine oil

How Supplied:
Vicks VapoRub®: Available in 1.76 oz (50 g) 3.53 oz (100 g) and 6 oz (170 g) plastic jars 0.45 oz (12 g) tin.
Vicks® VapoRub® Cream: Available in 2.99 oz (85 g) tube.
Questions? 1-800-873-8276
www.vicks.com
Vicks® VapoRub® 50142932
Vicks® VapoRub® Cream 50117758
US Pat. 5,322,689
Made in Mexico by Procter & Gamble
Manufactura, S. de R.L. de C.V.
Dist. by Procter & Gamble,
Cincinnati OH 45202

VICKS® VAPOSTEAM®
(Procter & Gamble)
[vă 'pō "stēm]
Liquid Medication for
Hot Steam Vaporizers.
Camphor/Cough Suppressant

Drug Facts:

Active Ingredient: **Purpose:**
Camphor 6.2% .... Cough suppressant

Uses: Temporarily relieves cough associated with a cold.

Warnings:
Failure to follow these warnings could result in serious consequences.
For external use only. Caution: Not for internal use.
Flammable Keep away from fire or flame. For steam inhalation only.
Ask a doctor before use if you have:
• a persistent or chronic cough such as occurs with smoking, emphysema or asthma
• cough that occurs with too much phlegm (mucus)
When using this product do not
• heat
• microwave

• use near an open flame
• take by mouth
• direct steam from the vaporizer too close to the face
• add to hot water or any container where heating water except when adding to cold water only in a hot steam vaporizer. May cause splattering and result in burns.
Stop use and ask a doctor if:
• cough lasts more than 7 days, comes back, or occurs with fever, rash, or headache that lasts.
These could be signs of a serious condition.
Keep out of reach of children. In case of eye exposure (flush eyes with water); or in case of accidental ingestion; seek medical help or contact a Poison Control Center right away.

Directions:
see important warnings under "When using this product"
• under 2 yrs.: ask a doctor
• adults & children 2 yrs. & older: use 1 tablespoon of solution for each quart of water or 1½ teaspoonsful of solution for each pint of water
• add solution directly to cold water only in a hot steam vaporizer
• follow manufacturer's directions for using vaporizer. Breathe in medicated vapors. May be repeated up to 3 times a day.

Other Information:
• close container tightly and store at room temperature away from heat.

Inactive Ingredients: Alcohol 78%, cedarleaf oil, eucalyptus oil, laureth-7, menthol, nutmeg oil, poloxamer 124, silicone.

How Supplied: Available in 4 FL OZ (118 ml) and 8 FL OZ (236 ml) bottles.
Questions? 1-800-873-8276
Made in Mexico by Procter & Gamble
Manufactura S. de R.L. de C.V.
Dist. by Procter & Gamble
Cincinnati OH 45202
50144018

Reese Pharmaceutical Company
10617 FRANK AVENUE
CLEVELAND, OH 44106

Direct Inquiries to:
Voice - (800) 321-7178
Fax - (216) 231-6444
http://www.reesepharmaceutical.com

REESE'S PINWORM TREATMENTS
(Reese)
[rēsĭs]

Directions for Use: For the treatment of pinworms. Read package insert carefully before taking this medication. Take

according to directions. Do not exceed recommended dosage unless directed by a doctor. Medication should be taken only one time as a single dose: do not repeat treatment unless directed by a doctor. When one individual in a household has pinworms, the entire household should be treated unless otherwise advised. These products can be taken any time of day, with or without food. If you are pregnant, nursing a baby, or have liver disease, do not take this product unless directed by a doctor.

DOSAGE GUIDE		
under 25 lbs or 2 yrs of age, consult a doctor		
WEIGHT LBS.	DOSAGE	
	Teaspoons	Caplets
25–37	1/2	2
38–62	1	4
63–87	1-1/2	6
88–112	2	8
113–137	2-1/2	10
138–162	3	12
163–187	3-1/2	14
188 & over	4	16

Warnings: Keep this and all drugs out of the reach of children. In case of accidental overdose, seek professional assistance or contact a poison control center immediately.

How Supplied:
Oral Suspension Liquid
NDC: 10956-618-01
Each 1 mL contains: pyrantel pamoate 144mg
(equivalent of 50 mg pyrantel base)
Pre-Measured Caplet
NDC: 10956-658-24
Packaged in boxes of 24 caplets.
Each caplet contains: pyrantel pamoate 180mg
(equivalent of 62.5 mg pyrantel base)
Shown in Product Identification Guide, page 508

UNKNOWN DRUG?
Consult the
Product Identification Guide
(Gray Pages)
for full-color photos of
leading over-the-counter
medications

Schering-Plough Healthcare Products

556 MORRIS AVENUE
SUMMIT, NJ 07901-1330

Direct Product Requests to:
Schering-Plough HealthCare Products
556 Morris Avenue
Summit, NJ 07901-1330

For Medical Emergencies Contact:
Consumer Relations Department
P.O. Box 377
Memphis, TN 38151
(901) 320-2988 (Business Hours)
(901) 320-2364 (After Hours)

CLARITIN-D 12 HOUR NON-DROWSY
(Schering-Plough Healthcare)
pseudoephedrine sulfate 120 mg/nasal decongestant
Loratadine 5 mg/antihistamine

CLARITIN-D NON-DROWSY 24 HOUR
pseudoephedrine sulfate 240 mg/nasal decongestant
Loratadine 10 mg/antihistamine

FOR CLARITIN-D 12 HOUR NON-DROWSY

Drug Facts
Active Ingredients
(in each tablet):   **Purpose:**
Loratadine 5 mg .... Antihistamine
Pseudoephedrine sulfate
  120 mg .... Nasal decongestant

Uses:
- temporarily relieves these symptoms due to hay fever or other upper respiratory allergies:
  - sneezing
  - itchy, watery eyes
  - runny nose
  - itching of the nose or throat
- temporarily relieves nasal congestion due to the common cold, hay fever or other upper respiratory allergies
- reduces swelling of nasal passages
- temporarily relieves sinus congestion and pressure
- temporarily restores freer breathing through the nose

Warnings:
Do not use
- if you have ever had an allergic reaction to this product or any of its ingredients
- if you are now taking a prescription monoamine oxidase inhibitor (MAOI) (certain drugs for depression, psychiatric, or emotional conditions, or Parkinson's disease), or for 2 weeks after stopping the MAOI drug. If you do not know if your prescription drug contains an MAOI, ask a doctor or pharmacist before taking this product.

Ask a doctor before use if you have
- heart disease
- thyroid disease
- high blood pressure
- diabetes
- trouble urinating due to an enlarged prostate gland
- liver or kidney disease. Your doctor should determine if you need a different dose.

When using this product do not take more than directed.
Taking more than directed may cause drowsiness.

Stop use and ask a doctor if
- an allergic reaction to this product occurs. Seek medical help right away.
- symptoms do not improve within 7 days or are accompanied by a fever
- nervousness, dizziness or sleeplessness occurs

If pregnant or breast-feeding, ask a health professional before use.

Keep out of reach of children. In case of overdose, get medical help or contact a Poison Control Center right away.

Directions: • do not divide, crush, chew or dissolve the tablet

adults and children 12 years and over	1 tablet every 12 hours; not more than 2 tablets in 24 hours
children under 12 years of age	ask a doctor
consumers with liver or kidney disease	ask a doctor

Other Information:
- **each tablet contains:** calcium 30 mg
- **safety sealed:** do not use if the individual blister unit imprinted with Claritin-D® 12 Hr. is open or torn
- **store between 15° and 25° C (59° and 77°F)**
- keep in a dry place

Inactive Ingredients: croscarmellose sodium, dibasic calcium phosphate, hypromellose, lactose monohydrate, magnesium stearate, pharmaceutical ink, povidone, titanium dioxide

Questions or comments?:
1-800-CLARITIN (1-800-252-7484) or **www.claritin.com**

How Supplied: Boxes of 10, 20, and 30 count tablets.

FOR CLARITIN-D NON-DROWSY 24 HOUR

Drug Facts
Active Ingredients
(in each tablet):   **Purpose:**
Loratadine 10 mg .... Antihistamine
Pseudoephedrine sulfate
  240 mg .... Nasal decongestant

Uses:
- temporarily relieves these symptoms due to hay fever or other upper respiratory allergies:
  - sneezing
  - itchy, watery eyes
  - runny nose
  - itching of the nose or throat
- temporarily relieves nasal congestion due to the common cold, hay fever or other upper respiratory allergies
- reduces swelling of nasal passages
- temporarily relieves sinus congestion and pressure
- temporarily restores freer breathing through the nose

Warnings:
Do not use
- if you have ever had an allergic reaction to this product or any of its ingredients
- if you are now taking a prescription monoamine oxidase inhibitor (MAOI) (certain drugs for depression, psychiatric, or emotional conditions, or Parkinson's disease) or for 2 weeks after stopping the MAOI drug. If you do not know if your prescription drug contains an MAOI, ask a doctor or pharmacist before taking this product.

Ask a doctor before use if you have
- heart disease
- thyroid disease
- high blood pressure
- diabetes
- trouble urinating due to an enlarged prostate gland
- liver or kidney disease. Your doctor should determine if you need a different dose.

When using this product do not take more than directed.
Taking more than directed may cause drowsiness.

Stop use and ask a doctor if
- an allergic reaction to this product occurs. Seek medical help right away.
- symptoms do not improve within 7 days or are accompanied by a fever
- nervousness, dizziness or sleeplessness occurs

If pregnant or breast-feeding, ask a health professional before use.

Keep out of reach of children. In case of overdose, get medical help or contact a Poison Control Center right away.

Directions:
- do not divide, crush, chew or dissolve the tablet

adults and children 12 years and over	1 tablet daily with a full glass of water; not more than 1 tablet in 24 hours
children under 12 years of age	ask a doctor
consumers with liver or kidney disease	ask a doctor

Other Information:

- **each tablet contains:** calcium 25 mg
- **safety sealed:** do not use if the individual blister unit imprinted with Claritin-D® 24 hour is open or torn
- store between 20° C to 25° C (68° F to 77° F)
- protect from light and store in a dry place

Inactive Ingredients: carnauba wax, dibasic calcium phosphate, ethylcellulose, hydroxypropyl cellulose, hypromellose, magnesium stearate, pharmaceutical ink, polyethylene glycol, povidone, silicon dioxide, sugar, titanium dioxide, white wax

Questions or comments?:
1-800-CLARITIN (1-800-252-7484) or www.claritin.com

How Supplied: Boxes of 5, 10, and 15 count tablets.
Shown in Product Identification Guide, page 508

CLARITIN® CHILDRENS 24 HOUR NON DROWSY ALLERGY SYRUP GRAPE

Drug Facts
Active Ingredient
(in each 5 mL teaspoonful)　　*Purpose*
Loratadine 5 mg .... Antihistamine

Uses: temporarily relieves these symptoms due to hay fever or other upper respiratory allergies:
- runny nose
- sneezing
- Itchy, watery eyes
- Itching of the nose or throat

Warnings:

Do not use if you have ever had an allergic reaction to this product or any of its ingredients.

Ask a doctor before use if you have liver or kidney disease. Your doctor should determine if you need a different dose.

When using this product do not take more than directed. Taking more than directed may cause drowsiness.

Stop use and ask a doctor if an allergic reaction to this product occurs. Seek medical help right away.

If pregnant or breast-feeding, ask a health professional before use.
Keep out of reach of children. In case of overdose, get medical help or contact a Poison Control Center right away.

Directions:

adults and children 6 years and over	2 teaspoonfuls daily; do not take more than 2 teaspoonfuls in 24 hours
children 2 to under 6 years of age	1 teaspoonful daily; do not take more than 1 teaspoonful in 24 hours
consumers with liver or kidney disease	ask a doctor

Other information:
- **each teaspoonful contains:** sodium 6 mg
- packaged with tamper-evident bottle cap. Do not use if breakable ring is separated or missing.
- store between 20° to 25° C (68° to 77° F)

Inactive ingredients:
edetate disodium, flavor, glycerin, maltitol, phosphoric acid, polyethylene glycol, propylene glycol, sodium benzoate, sodium phosphate monobasic, sorbitol, sucralose, water

Questions or comments?
1-800-CLARITIN (1-800-252-7484) or www.claritin.com

How Supplied: 4 FL OZ (120 mL)
Shown in Product Identification Guide, page 508

CLARITIN® CHILDRENS 24 HOUR NON DROWSY CHEWABLES GRAPE

Drug Facts
Active ingredient
(in each tablet)　　*Purpose*
Loratadine 5 mg .... Antihistamine

Uses: temporarily relieves these symptoms due to hay fever or other upper respiratory allergies:
- runny nose
- sneezing
- itchy, watery eyes
- itching of the nose or throat

Warnings:

Do not use if you have ever had an allergic reaction to this product or any of its ingredients.

Ask a doctor before use if you have liver or kidney disease. Your doctor should determine if you need a different dose.

When using this product do not take more than directed. Taking more than directed may cause drowsiness.

Stop use and ask a doctor if an allergic reaction to this product occurs. Seek medical help right away.

If pregnant or breast-feeding, ask a health professional before use.
Keep out of reach of children. In case of overdose, get medical help or contact a Poison Control Center right away.

Directions:

adults and children 6 years and over	chew 2 tablets daily; not more than 2 tablets in 24 hours
children 2 to under 6 years of age	chew 1 tablet daily; not more than 1 tablet in 24 hours
children under 2 years of age	ask a doctor
consumers with liver or kidney disease	ask a doctor

Other information:
- phenylketonurics: contains phenylalanine 1.4 mg per tablet
- safety sealed. Do not use if the individual blister unit imprinted with Children's Claritin® is open or torn
- store between 20° to 25°C (68° to 77°F)

Inactive ingredients:
aspartame, citric acid anhydrous, colloidal silicon dioxide, D&C red No. 27 aluminum lake, FD&C blue No. 2 aluminum lake, flavor, magnesium stearate, mannitol, microcrystalline cellulose, sodium starch glycolate, stearic acid

Questions or comments?
1-800-CLARITIN (1-800-252-7484) or www.claritin.com

How Supplied: 5 chewable tablets
Shown in Product Identification Guide, page 508

CLARITIN 24 HOUR NON-DROWSY REDITABS
Orally Disintegrating Tablets
(Schering-Plough Healthcare)
loratadine 10 mg/antihistamine

CLARITIN 24 HOUR NON-DROWSY TABLETS
Loratadine 10 mg/antihistamine

FOR CLARITIN REDITABS

Drug Facts

Active Ingredient
(in each tablet):　　**Purpose:**
Loratadine 10 mg .... Antihistamine

Uses: temporarily relieves these symptoms due to hay fever or other upper respiratory allergies:
- runny nose
- itchy, watery eyes
- sneezing
- itching of the nose or throat

Warnings:
Do not use if you have ever had an allergic reaction to this product or any of its ingredients.
Ask a doctor before use if you have liver or kidney disease. Your doctor should determine if you need a different dose.
When using this product do not take more than directed. Taking more than directed may cause drowsiness.

Continued on next page

Claritin—Cont.

Stop use and ask a doctor if an allergic reaction to this product occurs. Seek medical help right away.
If pregnant or breast-feeding, ask a health professional before use.
Keep out of reach of children. In case of overdose, get medical help or contact a Poison Control Center right away.

Directions:
- place 1 tablet on tongue: tablet disintegrates with or without water

adults and children 6 years and over	1 tablet daily: not more than 1 tablet in 24 hours
children under 6 years of age	ask a doctor
consumers with liver or kidney disease	ask a doctor

Other Information:
- safety sealed: do not use if the individual blister unit imprinted with Claritin® Reditabs® is open or torn
- store between 20° to 25° C (68° to 77° F)
- Use tablet immediately after opening individual blister

Inactive Ingredients:
anhydrous citric acid, gelatin, mannitol, mint flavor

Questions or comments?:
1-800-CLARITIN (1-800-252-7484) or www.claritin.com

How Supplied: Boxes of 4, 10, 20, and 30 count tablets.

FOR CLARITIN 24 HOUR NON-DROWSY TABLETS

Drug Facts
Active Ingredient (in each tablet): **Purpose:**

Loratadine 10 mg .... Antihistamine

Uses: temporarily relieves these symptoms due to hay fever or other upper respiratory allergies:
- runny nose
- itchy, watery eyes
- sneezing
- itching of the nose or throat

Warnings:
Do not use if you have ever had an allergic reaction to this product or any of its ingredients.
Ask a doctor before use if you have liver or kidney disease. Your doctor should determine if you need a different dose.
When using this product do not take more than directed. Taking more than directed may cause drowsiness.
Stop use and ask a doctor if an allergic reaction to this product occurs. Seek medical help right away.
If pregnant or breast-feeding, ask a health professional before use.

Keep out of reach of children. In case of overdose, get medical help or contact a Poison Control Center right away.

Directions:

adults and children 6 years and over	1 tablet daily: not more than 1 tablet in 24 hours
children under 6 years of age	ask a doctor
consumers with liver or kidney disease	ask a doctor

Other Information:
- safety sealed: do not use if the individual blister unit imprinted with Claritin® is open or torn
- store between 20° to 25° C (68° to 77° F)
- protect from excessive moisture

Inactive Ingredients:
corn starch, lactose monohydrate, magnesium stearate

Questions or comments?:
1-800-CLARITIN (1-800-252-7484) or www.claritin.com

How Supplied: Boxes of 4, 10, 20, and 30 count tablets.

Shown in Product Identification Guide, page 508

Hyland's, A Division of Standard Homeopathic Company
210 WEST 131ST STREET
BOX 61067
LOS ANGELES, CA 90061

Direct Inquiries to:
Jay Borneman
(800) 624-9659 Ext. 20

HYLAND'S BACKACHE WITH ARNICA
(Standard Homeopathic)

Active Ingredients: BENZOICUM ACIDUM 3X HPUS, COLCHICUM AUTUMNALE 3X HPUS, SULPHUR 3X HPUS, ARNICA MONTANA 6X HPUS, RHUS TOXICODENDRON 6X HPUS.

Inactive Ingredients: Lactose, N.F.

Indications: A homeopathic medicine for the temporary relief of symptoms of low back pain due to strain or overexertion.

Directions: Adults and children over 12 years of age: Take 1–2 caplets with water every 4 hours or as needed.

Warnings: Do not use if imprinted cap band is broken or missing. If symptoms persist for more than seven days or worsen, contact a licensed health care professional. As with any drug, if you are pregnant or nursing a baby, seek the advice of a licensed health care professional before using this product. Keep this and all medications out of the reach of children. In case of accidental overdose, contact a poison control center immediately. In case of emergency, the manufacturer may be reached 24 hours a day, 7 days a week at 800/624-9659.

How Supplied: Bottles of 40 5.5 grain caplets (NDC 54973-2965-2). Store at room temperature.

HYLAND'S CALMS FORTÉ™
(Standard Homeopathic)

Active Ingredients: *Passiflora* (Passion Flower) 1X triple strength HPUS, *Avena Sativa*(Oat) 1X double strength HPUS, *Humulus Lupulus*(Hops) 1X double strength HPUS, *Chamomilla*(Chamomile) 2X HPUS, *Calcarea Phosphorica*(Calcium Phosphate) 3X HPUS, *Ferrum Phosphorica*(Iron Phosphate) 3X HPUS, *Kali Phosphoricum*(Potassium Phosphate) 3X HPUS, *Natrum Phosphoricum*(Sodium Phosphate) 3X HPUS, *Magnesia Phosphoricum*(Magnesium Phosphate) 3X HPUS.

Inactive Ingredients: Lactose, N.F., Calcium Sulfate, Starch (Corn and Tapiocal), Magnesium Stearate.

Indications: Temporary symptomatic relief of simple nervous tension and sleeplessness.

Directions: Adults: As a relaxant: Swallow 1–2 tablets with water as needed, three times daily, preferably before meals. For insomnia: 1 to 3 tablets ½ to 1 hour before retiring. Repeat as needed without danger of side effects. Children: As a relaxant: Swallow 1 tablet with water as needed, three times daily, preferably before meals. For insomnia: 1 to 2 tablets ½ to 1 hour before retiring. Repeat as needed without danger of side effects.

Warning: Do not use if imprinted cap band is broken or missing. If symptoms persist for more than seven days or worsen, consult a licensed health care professional. As with any drug, if you are pregnant or nursing a baby, seek the advice of a licensed health care professional before using this product. Keep this and all medications out of the reach of children. In case of accidental overdose, contact a Poison Control Center immediately. In case of emergency, the manufacturer may be reached 24 hours a day, 7 days a week by calling 800/624-9659.

How Supplied: Bottles of 100 4-grain tablets (NDC 54973-1121-02), 50 4-grain tablets (NDC 54973-1121-01) and 32 5.5-grain caplets (NDC 54973-1121-48). Store at room temperature.

HYLAND'S CALMS FORTE' 4 KIDS
(Standard Homeopathic)

Active Ingredients: ACONITUM NAP. 6X HPUS, CALC. PHOS. 12X HPUS, CHAMOMILLA 6X HPUS, CINA 6X HPUS, LYCOPODIUM 6X HPUS, NAT. MUR. 6X HPUS, PULSATILLA 6X HPUS, SULPHUR 6X HPUS

Inactive Ingredients: Lactose, N.F.

Indications: Temporarily relieves the symptoms restlessness, sleeplessness, night terrors, growing pains, causeless crying, occasional sleeplessness due to travel and lack of focus in children.

Directions: Children ages 2-5: dissolve 2 tablets under tongue every 15 minutes for up to 8 doses until relieved; Then every 4 hours as required.
Children ages 6-11: Dissolve 3 tablets under tongue Every 15 minutes for up to 8 doses until relieved; Then every 4 hours as required.
Children 12 years and over: Dissolve 4 tablets under tongue every 15 minutes for up to 8 does until relieved; then every 4 hours as are required or as recommended by a health care professional

Warnings: Ask a doctor before use if: pregnant or nursing, child is taking any prescription medications. If symptoms don't improve within 7 days, discontinue use and seek the advice of a licensed medical practitioner.
Keep this and all medications out of reach of children. Do not use if imprinted tamper band is broken or missing. In case of accidental overdose, contact a poison control center immediately. In case of emergency, the manufacturer may be contacted 24 hours a day, 7 days a week at 800/624-9659.

How Supplied: Bottles of 125 1 grain tablets (NDC 54973-7518-03). Store at room temperature.

HYLAND'S COLIC TABLETS   OTC
(Standard Homeopathic)

Active Ingredient: *Dioscorea* 3X HPUS, *Chamomilla* 3X HPUS, *Colocynthis* 3X HPUS

Inactive Ingredients: Lactose N.F.

Indications: Temporarily relieves the symptoms of colic and gas pains caused by irritating food, feeding too quickly, swallowing air and similar conditions during teething, colds and other minor upset periods in children.

Directions: For Children up to 2 years: Dissolve 2 tablets on tongue every 15 minutes for up to 8 doses until relieved; then every 2 hours as required. For Children over 2 years: Dissolve 3 tablets as above or as recommended by a licensed health care professional. If you prefer, tablets may be dissolved in a teaspoon of water and then given to the child. Colic Tablets are very soft and dissolve almost instantly

under the tongue. Please note: if your baby has been crying or is very upset, your baby may fall asleep after using this product because the pain has been relieved and your child can rest.

Warnings: Ask a doctor before use if pregnant or nursing. Consult a physician if symptoms persist for more than 7 days or worsen. Keep out of the reach of children. Do not use if imprinted tamper band is broken or missing. In case of accidental overdose, contact a Poison Control Center immediately. In case of emergency, the manufacturer may be contacted 24 hours a day, 7 days a week at 800/624-9659.

How Supplied: Bottle of 125 one-grain, sublingual tablets (NDC 54973-7502-1)

HYLAND'S EARACHE DROPS
(Standard Homeopathic)

Active Ingredients:
Pulsatilla 30C HPUS, Chamomilla 30C HPUS, Sulphur 30C HPUS, Calc Carb 30C HPUS, Belladonna 30C HPUS, Lycopodium 30C HPUS.

Inactive Ingredients:
Citric Acid USP, Purified Water, Sodium Benzoate USP, Vegetable Glycerin USP.

Indications:
Temporarily relieves the symptoms of fever, pain, irritability and sleeplessness associated with earaches after diagnosis by a physician. Relieves common pain and itching of "swimmer's ear." If symptoms persist for more than 48 hours, or if there is a discharge from the ear, discontinue use and contact your physician.

Directions:
Adults and children of all ages: Tilt head sideways and apply 3–4 drops into involved ear 4 times daily or as needed. Tilt ear upward for at least 2 minutes after application or gently place cotton in ear to keep drops in.

Warnings:
Keep away from eyes. Do not take by mouth. Earache drops are only to be used in the ears. Tip of applicator should not enter ear canal. Ask a doctor before use if pregnant or nursing. Consult a physician if symptoms persist for more than 48 hours or if there is discharge from the ear. Keep this and all medications out of reach of children. Do not use if imprinted tamper band is broken or missing. In case of accidental overdose, contact a poison control center immediately. In case of emergency, the manufacturer may be contacted 24 hours a day, 7 days a week at 800/624-9659.

How Supplied: Bottle of .33 ounce (NDC 54973-7516-1)

HYLAND'S EARACHE TABLETS
(Standard Homeopathic)

Active Ingredients: Pulsatilla (Wind Flower) 30C, HPUS; Chamomilla

(Chamomile) 30C, HPUS; Sulphur 30C, HPUS; Calcarea Carbonica (Carbonate of Lime) 30C, HPUS; Belladonna 30C, HPUS; (3 × 10⁻⁶⁰ % Alkaloids) and Lycopodium (Club Moss) 30C, HPUS.

Inactive Ingredients: Lactose NF

Indications: For the relief of symptoms of fever, pain, irritability and sleeplessness associated with earaches in children after diagnosis by a physician. If symptoms persist for more than 48 hours or if there is a discharge from the ear, discontinue use and contact your health care professional.

Directions: Dissolve 4 tablets under the tongue 3 times per day for 48 hours or until symptoms subside. If you prefer, tablets may be dissolved in a teaspoon of water and then given to the child. Earache Tablets are very soft and dissolve almost instantly under the tongue.

Warnings: Do not use if imprinted blisters are broken or damaged. If symptoms persist for more than 48 hours, or if there is a discharge from the ear, discontinue use and consult a licensed health care professional. As with any drug, if you are pregnant or nursing a baby, seek the advice of a licensed health care professional before using this product. Keep this and all medications out of the reach of children. In case of accidental overdose, contact a poison control center immediately. In cases of emergency, the manufacturer may be contacted 24 hours a day, 7 days a week at 800/624-9659.

How Supplied: Blister pack of 40 tablets (NDC 54973-7507-1). Store at room temperature.

HYLAND'S LEG CRAMPS WITH QUININE (Standard Homeopathic)

Active   Ingredients: Cinchona Officinalis 3X, HPUS (Quinine), Viscum Album 3X, HPUS; Gnaphalium Polycephalum 3X, HPUS; Rhus Toxicodendron 6X, HPUS; Aconitum Napellus 6X, HPUS; Ledum Palustre 6X, HPUS; Magnesia Phosphorica 6X, HPUS.

Inactive Ingredients: Lactose, N.F.

Indications: Hyland's Leg Cramps is a traditional homeopathic formula for the relief of symptoms of cramps and pains in lower back and legs often made worse by damp weather. Working without contraindications or side effects, Hyland's Leg Cramps stimulates your body's natural healing response to relieve symptoms. Hyland's Leg Cramps is safe for adults and can be used in conjuction with other medications.

Directions: Adults: Dissolve 2–3 tablets under tongue every 4 hours as needed.

Warnings: Do not use if imprinted cap band is missing or broken. If symptoms persist for more than seven days or

Continued on next page

Hyland's Leg Cramps—Cont.

worsen, contact a licensed health care professional. As with any drug, if you are pregnant or nursing a baby, seek the advice of a licensed health care professional before using this product. Do not use if pregnant, sensitive to quinine or under 12 years of age. Keep this and all medications out of the reach of children. In case of accidental overdose, contact a poison control center immediately. In case of emergency, the manufacturer may be reached 24 hours a day, 7 days a week at 800-624-9659.

How Supplied: Bottles of 100 three grain sublingual tablets (NDC 54973-2956-02), Bottles of 50 three-grain sublingual tablets (NDC 54973-2956-01), Bottles of 40 5.5 grain caplets (NDC 54973-2956-68). Store at room temperature.

HYLAND'S MIGRAINE HEADACHE RELIEF
(Standard Homeopathic)

Active Ingredient: *Glonoinum* 12X HPUS, *Belladonna* 6X HPUS, *Gelsemium* 6X HPUS, *Nux Vomica* 6X HPUS, *Iris Versicolor* 6X HPUS, *Sanguinaria Canadensis* 6X HPUS

Inactive Ingredients: Lactose N.F.

Indications: Temporarily relieves the symptoms of migraine pain.

Directions: Adults and Children over 12 years of age: Dissolve 1 to 2 tablets on tongue every 4 hours or as needed.

Warnings: Ask a doctor before use if pregnant or nursing. Consult a physician if symptoms persist for more than 7 days or worsen. Keep out of the reach of children. Do not use if imprinted tamper band is broken or missing. In case of accidental overdose, contact a Poison Control Center immediately. In case of emergency, the manufacturer may be contacted 24 hours a day, 7 days a week at 800/624-9659.

How Supplied: Bottle of 60 tablets (NDC 54973-3013-01)

HYLAND'S NERVE TONIC
(Standard Homeopathic)

Active Ingredients: Calcarea Phosphorica (Calcium Phosphate) 3X HPUS; Ferrum Phosphorica (Iron Phosphate) 3X HPUS; Kali Phosphoricum (Potassium Phosphate) 3X HPUS; Natrum Phosphoricum (Sodium Phosphate) 3X HPUS; Magnesia Phosphoricum (Magnesium Phosphate) 3X HPUS.

Inactive Ingredients: Lactose, N.F.

Indications: Temporary symptomatic relief of simple nervous tension and stress.

Directions: Adults take 2–6 tablets before each meal and at bedtime. Children: 2 tablets. In severe cases take 3 tablets every 2 hours.

Warnings: Do not use if imprinted cap band is broken or missing. If symptoms persist for more than seven days or worsen, contact a licensed health care professional. As with any drug, if you are pregnant or nursing a baby, seek the advice of a licensed health care professional before using this product. Keep this and all medications out of the reach of children. In case of accidental overdose, contact a poison control center immediately. In cases of emergency, the manufacturer may be contacted 24 hours a day, 7 days a week at 800/624-9659.

How Supplied: Bottles of 32 caplets (NDC 54973-1129-68), Bottles of 500 tablets (NDC 54973-1129-1), Bottles of 1000 tablets (NDC 54973-1129-2), Bottles of 100 tablets (NDC 54973-3014-02)

HYLAND'S RESTFUL LEGS
(Standard Homeopathic)

Active Ingredients: ARSENICUM ALBUM 12X HPUS, LYCOPODIUM 6X HPUS, PULSATILLA 6X HPUS, RHUS TOXICODENDRON 6X HPUS, SULPHUR 6X HPUS, ZINC METALLICUM 12X HPUS.

Inactive Ingredients: Lactose, N.F.

Indications: Temporarily relieves the symptoms of the compelling urge to move legs to relieve sensations of itching, tingling, crawling, and restlessness of legs. Symptoms may occur while sitting or lying down, and improve with activity.

Directions: Adults dissolve 2–3 quick dissolving tablets under tongue every 4 hours or as needed. Children ages 6–12 ½ adult dose.

Warnings: Ask a doctor before use if pregnant or nursing a baby. Consult a physician if symptoms persist for more than 7 days. Keep this and all medications out of reach of children. Do not use if imprinted tamper band is broken or missing. In case of accidental overdose, contact a poison control center immediately. In case of emergency, the manufacturer may be contacted 24 hours a day, 7 days a week at 800/624-9659.

How Supplied: Bottles of 50 3 grain tablets (NDC 54973-2966-1). Store at room temperature.

SMILE'S PRID®
(Standard Homeopathic)

Contains: Acidum Carbolicum 2X HPUS, Ichthammol 2X HPUS, Arnica Montana 3X HPUS, Calendula Off 3X HPUS, Echinacea Ang 3X HPUS, Sulphur 12X HPUS, Hepar Sulph 12X HPUS, Silicea 12X HPUS, Rosin, Beeswax, Petrolatum, Stearyl Alcohol, Methyl & Propyl Paraben.

Indications: Temporary topical relief of pain symptoms associated with boils, minor skin eruptions, redness and irritation. Also aids in relieving the discomfort of superficial cuts, scratches and wounds.

Directions: Wash affected parts with hot water, dry and apply PRID® twice daily on clean bandage or gauze. Do not squeeze or pressure irritated skin area. After irritation subsides, repeat application once a day for several days. Children under two years: consult a physician. CAUTION: If symptoms persist for more than seven days or worsen, or if fever occurs, contact a licensed health care professional. Do not use on broken skin. Keep out of reach of children. In case of accidental ingestion, seek professional assistance or contact a poison control center. For external use only. Avoid contact with eyes.

How Supplied: 18GM tin (NDC 0619-4202-54). Keep in a cool dry place.

HYLAND'S SNIFFLES'N SNEEZES 4 KIDS
(Standard Homeopathic)

Active Ingredients: ACONITUM NAPELLUS 6X HPUS, ALLIUM CEPA 6X HPUS, ZINCUM GLUCONICUM 2X HPUS, GELSENIUM SEMPERVIRENS 6X HPUS.

Inactive Ingredients: Lactose, N.F.

Indications: Temporarily relieves the symptoms of the common cold.

Directions: Children ages 2-5: dissolve 2 tablets under tongue every 15 minutes for up to 8 doses until relieved; then every 4 hours as required. Children ages 6-11: dissolve 3 tablets under tongue every 15 minutes for up to 8 doses until relieved; then every 4 hours as required. Children 12 years and older: dissolve 4 tablets under tongue every 15 minutes for up to 8 doses until relieved; then every 4 hours as required or as recommended by a health care professional.

Warnings: Ask a doctor before use if pregnant or nursing. Consult a physician if: symptoms persist for more than 7 days or worsen. Inflammation, fever or infection develops. Symptoms are accompanied by high fever. (over 101 ° F) Keep this and all medications out of the reach of children. Do not use if imprinted tamper band is broken or missing. In case of accidental overdose, contact a poison control center immediately. In case of emergency, the manufacturer may be contacted 24 hours a day, 7 days a week at 800/624-9659.

How Supplied: Bottles of 125 1 grain tablets (NDC 54973-7519-1). Store at room temperature.

HYLAND'S TEETHING GEL
(Standard Homeopathic)

Active Ingredients: Calcarea Phosphorica (Calcium Phosphate) 12X, HPUS; Chamomilla (Chamomile) 6X, HPUS; Coffea Cruda (Coffee) 6X, HPUS; and Belladonna 6X, HPUS (Alkaloids 0.0000003%)

Inactive Ingredients: Deionized water, Vegetable Glycerin, Hydroxyethyl Cellulose, Methyl Paraben and Propyl Paraben.

Indications: A homeopathic combination for the temporary relief of symptoms of simple restlessness and wakeful irritability due to cutting teeth.

Directions: Apply to gums as necessary. If symptoms persist for more than seven days or worsen, discontinue use and contact your health care professional. Please note, if your baby has been crying or has been very upset, your baby may fall asleep after using this product because the pain has been relieved and your child can rest.

Warnings: Do not use if tube tip is broken or missing. If symptoms persist for more than seven days or if irritation persists, inflammation develops or fever or infection develop, discontinue use and consult a licensed health care professional. As with any drug, if you are pregnant or nursing a baby, seek the advice of a licensed health care professional before using this product. Keep this and all medications out of the reach of children. In case of accidental overdose, contact a poison control center immediately. In case of emergency, the manufacturer may be contacted 24 hours a day, 7 days a week at 800/624-9659.

How Supplied: Tubes of 1/3 OZ. (NDC 54973-7504-3). Store at room temperature.

HYLAND'S TEETHING TABLETS
(Standard Homeopathic)

Active Ingredients: *Calcarea Phosphorica* (Calcium Phosphate) 3X HPUS, *Chamomilla* (Chamomile) 3X HPUS, *Coffea Cruda* (Coffee) 3X HPUS, *Belladonna* 3X HPUS (Alkaloids 0.0003%).

Inactive Ingredients: Lactose N.F.

Indications: A homeopathic combination for the temporary relief of symptoms of simple restlessness and wakeful irritability due to cutting teeth.

Directions: Dissolve 2 to 3 tablets under the tongue 4 times per day. If you prefer, tablets may first be dissolved in a teaspoon of water and then given to the child. If the child is restless or wakeful, 2 tablets every hour for 6 doses or as recommended by a licensed health care professional. Teething Tablets are very soft and dissolve almost instantly under the tongue. Please note, if your baby has been crying or has been very upset, your baby may fall asleep after using this product because the pain has been relieved and your child can rest.

Warning: Do Not use if imprinted cap band is broken or missing. If symptoms persist for more than seven days, or if irritation persist, inflammation develops or fever or infection develop, discontinue use and consult a licensed health care professional. As with any drug, if you are pregnant or nursing a baby, seek the advice of a health care professional before using this product. Keep this and all medications out of the reach of children. In case of accidental overdose, contact a poison control center immediately. In case of emergency, the manufacturer may be contacted 24 hours a day, 7 days a week at 800/624-9659.

How Supplied: Bottles of 125—one grain sublingual tablets (NDC 54973-7504-01). Store at room temperature.

IVYBLOCK®
(Standard Homeopathic)

Active Ingredient: *Bentoquatam* 5% (skin protectant)

Inactive Ingredients: *Bentonite, Benzyl Alcohol, Diisopropyl Adipate, Methylparaben, Purified Water, SDA 40 Denatured Alcohol* (25% By Weight)

Indications: Helps prevent poison ivy, oak and sumac rash when applied before exposure.

Directions: Shake well before use. Apply 15 minutes before risk of exposure. Avoid intentional contact with poison ivy, oak, and sumac. For adults and children 6 and older: apply every 4 hours for continued protection or sooner if needed. For children under 6 years: ask a doctor before use. Remove with soap and water after risk of exposure.

Warnings: For external use only. Keep away from fire or flame. Do not use if you are allergic to any ingredients, or have an open rash. When using this product, do not get into eyes. If contact occurs, rinse eyes thoroughly with water. Keep out of reach of children. If swallowed, get medical help or contact a Poison Control Center right away.

How Supplied: Bottle of 4 ounces (NDC 62333-111-40)

UAS Laboratories
9953 VALLEY VIEW ROAD
EDEN PRAIRIE, MN 55344

Direct Inquiries to:
Dr. S.K Dash
(952) 935-1707
FAX:(952) 935-1650

DDS®-ACIDOPHILUS
(UAS Labs)
Capsule, Tablet & Powder free of dairy products, corn, soy, and preservatives

Description: DDS®-Acidophilus is the source of a special strain of Lactobacillus acidophilus free of dairy products, corn, soy and preservatives. Each capsule or tablet contains 2.5 billion viable DDS®-1 L.acidophilus at the time of manufacturing. One gram of powder contains 5 billion viable DDS®-1 L.acidophilus.

Indications and Usages: An aid in implanting the gut with beneficial Lactobacillus acidophilus under conditions of digestive disorders, acne, yeast infections, and following antibiotic therapy.

Administration: One to two capsules or tablets twice daily before meals. One-fourth teaspoon powder can be substituted for two capsules or tablets.

How Supplied: Bottles of 100 capsules or tablets. 12 bottles per case. Powder is available in 2.5 oz. bottle; 12 bottles per case.

Storage: Keep refrigerated under 40°F.

EDUCATIONAL MATERIAL

DDS®-Acidophilus

Booklet describing superior-strain Acidophilus without dairy products, corn, soy, or preservatives. Five billion viable DDS®-1. L.acidopohilus per gram.

Upsher-Smith Laboratories, Inc
6701 EVENSTAD DRIVE
MAPLE GROVE, MN 55369

Direct Inquiries to:
Professional Services:
(800) 654-2299

AMLACTIN® Moisturizing Lotion and Cream
(Upsher-Smith)
[ăm-lăk-tĭn]
Cosmetic Lotion and Cream

Description: AMLACTIN® Moisturizing Lotion and Cream are special formulations of 12% lactic acid neutralized with ammonium hydroxide to provide a lotion or cream pH of 4.5–5.5. Lactic acid, an alpha-hydroxy acid, is a naturally occur-

Continued on next page

Amlactin—Cont.

ring humectant for the skin. AMLACTIN® moisturizes and softens rough, dry skin.

How Supplied: 225g (8oz) plastic bottle: List No. 0245-0023-22
400g (14oz) plastic bottle: List No. 0245-0023-40
140g (4.9oz) tube: List No. 0245-0024-14

AMLACTIN AP® Anti-Itch
Moisturizing Cream
(Upsher-Smith)
[ăm-lăk'-tĭn]
1% Pramoxine HCl

Description: AMLACTIN AP® Anti-Itch Moisturizing Cream is a special formulation containing 12% lactic acid neutralized with ammonium hydroxide to provide a cream pH of 4.5–5.5 with pramoxine HCl. Lactic acid, an alpha-hydroxy acid, is a naturally occurring humectant which moisturizes and softens rough, dry skin. Pramoxine HCl, USP, 1% is an effective antipruritic ingredient used to relieve itching associated with dry skin.

How Supplied: 140g (4.9oz) tube: NDC No. 0245-0025-14

AMLACTIN XL®
(Upsher-Smith)
Moisturizing Lotion
ULTRAPLEX® Formulation
[ăm-lăk'-tĭn]

Description: AmLactin XL® Moisturizing Lotion is a clinically proven moisturizer which provides powerful mosturizing for rough, dry skin. AmLactin XL® Moisturizing Lotion contains ULTRAPLEX® formulation, a proprietary blend of alpha-hydroxy moisturizing compounds.

How Supplied: 160g (5.6oz) tube: List No. 0245-0022-16

Wellness International
Network, Ltd.
5800 DEMOCRACY DRIVE
PLANO, TX 75024

Direct Inquiries to:
Product Inquiries
(972) 312-1100
E-mail: winproducts@winltd.com

BIOLEAN ACCELERATOR™
Herbal & Amino Acid Formulation

Description: Accelerator™ is a unique blend of herbal extracts and amino acids that, when used in conjunction with BIOLEAN II® or BIOLEAN Free®, prolongs their adaptogenic and thermogenic properties while adding powerful restorative properties. The restorative properties of the amino acids and herbal extracts in Accelerator are a strong complement to the energetic and thermogenic properties of BIOLEAN II and BIOLEAN Free. When used together, these products provide a well-balanced approach to weight loss, increased energy and detoxification.

Directions: For maximum effectiveness, use in conjunction with BIOLEAN II or BIOLEAN Free. As a dietary supplement, take one tablet in the morning with BIOLEAN II or BIOLEAN Free. If desired, Accelerator may also be taken in the afternoon with or without additional BIOLEAN II or BIOLEAN Free. Maximum absorption will be attained if taken with low-calorie food.

Warnings: CAUTION PHENYLKE-TONURICS: Contains 200mg phenylalanine per serving. Not for use by children. Consult your physician before using this product if you are taking appetite suppressing drugs or antidepressants, or if you are pregnant or lactating. If symptoms of allergy develop, discontinue use.

Ingredients: Proprietary herbal extract 250mg (Cuscuta Seed, Black Sesame Seed, Rehmannia Root, Achyranthes Root, Cornus Fruit, Chinese Yam, Eclipta Herb, Rosehips, Ligustrum Fruit, Mulberry Fruit, Polygonati Rhizome, Fo Ti Poria Cocos, Euryale Seed, Alisma Rhizome, Moutan Bark, Phellodendron Bark, Anemarrhena Rhizome, Schisandra Berry, Royal Jelly), L-Phenylalanine 200mg, L-Tyrosine 200mg, Calcium Carbonate, Calcium Phosphate Dibasic, Hydroxypropyl Cellulose, Croscarmelose Sodium, Magnesium Stearate, and Silicon Dioxide.

How Supplied: One bottle contains 56 tablets.

Additional Information: For additional information on ingredients or uses, please visit winltd.com.

These statements have not been evaluated by the Food & Drug Administration. This product is not intended to diagnose, treat, cure or prevent any disease.

BIOLEAN II®
Herbal & Amino Acid
Dietary Supplement

Description: BIOLEAN II® is a dietary supplement for weight loss, appetite suppression and increased energy without the side effects found in many supplements of this nature. BIOLEAN II has a proprietary synergistic blend of natural herbal extracts and pharmaceutical-grade amino acids that promote a multi-faceted approach to fat loss. Key ingredients such as Advantra Z®, guarana seed extract, green tea leaf extract and L-carnitine work together to increase the metabolic rate and encourage fat loss by elevating rates of thermogenesis and lipolysis.

Directions: Recommended Use: AM Serving - As a dietary supplement, take 1 white tablet and 2 green tablets with low calorie food. PM Serving - Take 1 green tablet with low calorie food. If using BIOLEAN II for the first time, limit daily intake to 1 white tablet and 1 green tablet on days 1 and 2, and 1 white tablet and 2 green tablets on day 3. Needs may vary with each individual.

Warnings: CAUTION PHENYLKE-TONURICS: Contains 196mg phenylalanine per AM serving. Not for use by children under the age of 18, pregnant or lactating women. If you have heart disease, thyroid disease, diabetes, high blood pressure, depression or other psychiatric condition, glaucoma, difficulty urinating, prostate enlargement, or seizure disorder, if you are using a monoamine oxidase inhibitor (MAOI), consult a health professional before using this product. Exceeding recommended serving may cause serious adverse effects. Discontinue use and consult your health professional if dizziness, sleeplessness, severe headache, heart palpitations or other similar symptoms occur. The recommended dose of this product contains about as much caffeine as a cup of coffee. Limit the use of caffeine-containing medications, food, or beverages while taking this product because too much caffeine may cause nervousness, irritability, sleeplessness, and occasionally, rapid heart beat. If allergic symptoms develop, discontinue use immediately.

Ingredients: Calcium (as calcium carbonate, calcium phosphate dibasic), Proprietary Blend: [Caffeine (as Guarana Seed 50% Extract, Yerba Mate Leaf 10% Extract, Green Tea Leaf 40% Extract), Citrus Aurantium Fruit 30% Extract (Advantra Z®), Schizandra Berry, Gymnema Sylvestre Leaf 25% Extract, Rehmannia Root, Hawthorne Root, Jujube Seed, Alisma Root, Angelicae dahuricae Radix, Epemidium grandiflorum Radix, Poria Cocos Mushroom, Rhubarb Root, Angelicae sinensis Radix, Codonopsis Root, Eucommia Bark, Panax notoginseng Radi], L-Tyrosine, L-Phenylalanine, L-Carnitine (as L-Carnitine Bitartrate), **Herbal Blend:** Calcium Carbonate, Starch, Stearic Acid, Cellulose, Hydroxypropylcellulose, Croscarmelose Sodium, Magnesium Stearate, Silicon Dioxide, **Amino Acid:** Calcium Phosphate Dibasic, Stearic acid, Silicon Dioxide, Croscarmelose Sodium, Hydroxypropylcellulose, Magnesium Stearate, Ethylcellulose.
Advantra Z® - registered trademark of Nutratech, Inc./Zhishin, LLC licensor of U.S. Patents.

How Supplied: One box contains 28 packets, with 1 white tablet and 3 green tablets per packet.

Additional Information: For additional information on ingredients or uses, please visit winltd.com.

BIOLEAN FREE®
Herbal & Amino Acid Dietary Supplement

Description: BIOLEAN Free® is a dietary supplement designed to reduce body fat, suppress the appetite, provide a healthy feeling of fullness, and improve metabolism of dietary carbohydrates, fats, and proteins. BIOLEAN Free utilizes a strategic blend of vitamins, minerals, amino acids and herbal extracts that enhance fat utilization and energy production through several metabolic pathways. Key ingredients such as quebracho, green tea leaf extract, yerba maté and spices such as ginger and tumeric work together to promote healthy lipolysis, curb cravings, stimulate thermogenesis and increase energy without disrupting the healthy sleep cycle.

Directions: As a dietary supplement, take 4 tablets in mid- to late-morning with low-calorie food. Some persons may require less than 4 tablets, or may prefer taking 3 tablets mid-morning and 1 additional tablet mid-afternoon to achieve optimum results. Do not exceed recommended daily amounts. Needs may vary with each individual.

Warnings: Not for use by children under the age of 18, pregnant or lactating women. Consult your physician before using this product if you are taking appetite suppressing drugs or cardiovascular medication. Consult your physician if you have hypertension, heart disease, arrhythmias, prostatic hypertrophy, glaucoma, liver disease, renal disease or diabetes. Do not use if you have hyperthyroidism, psychosis, Parkinson's Disease, or are taking monoamine oxidase inhibitors (MAOI). Limit the use of caffeine-containing medications, food, or beverages while taking this product because too much caffeine may cause nervousness, irritability, sleeplessness, and occasionally, rapid heart beat. If allergic symptoms develop, discontinue use immediately.

Ingredients: Niacin 40mg (as niacinamide), Vitamin B6 16mg (as pyridoxine HCL), Chromium 400mcg (as chromium Chelavite® chloride), Potassium 100mg (as potassium citrate), Standardized botanical caffeine [Guarana seed (22% methylxanthines), Yerba mate leaf extract (10% methylxanthines), Green tea leaf extract (10% methylxanthines)], Korean ginseng root extract (4% ginsenosides), Uva ursi leaf (20% arbutin), Quebracho bark extract (10% quebrachine), Nonirradiated pure herbs and thermogenic spices 1440mg [Gotu kola leaf (Centella asiatica), Ceylon cinnamon bark, Chinese horseradish root, Jamaican ginger root, Turmeric rhizome, Nigerian cayenne pepper (fruit), English mustard seed, Ho shou wu root, Ginkgo biloba leaf (24% ginkgoflavoneslycosides and 6% bilobalides)], L-Tyrosine 500mg, L-Methionine 100mg, Vanadium 400mcg (as BMOV), Dicalcium phosphate, Cellulose, Cellulose gum, Vegetable stearic acid, Silica, Vegetable magnesium stearate and Vegetable resin glaze.

How Supplied: One box contains 28 packets, 4 tablets per packet.

Additional Information: For additional information on ingredients or uses, please visit winltd.com.

BIOLEAN® LIPOTRIM™
All-Natural Dietary Supplement

Description: LipoTrim™ contains 2 dynamic and powerful ingredients that synergistically reduce the storage of new fat and maintain healthy blood glucose levels to assist in weight loss. Garcinia cambogia extract and chromium polynicotinate help reduce the rate of lipogenesis and assist in maintaining healthy blood sugar levels, especially when used in conjunction with either BIOLEAN II® or BIOLEAN Free®. These potent ingredients combine to help discourage accumulation of body fat, as well as to produce an appetite suppressant effect that can contribute to weight loss. Our weight loss products work in conjunction with a sensible diet and moderate exercise.

Directions: As a dietary supplement, take 1 capsule 3 times daily, 30 minutes before each meal. LipoTrim should be used in conjunction with a healthy diet and exercise program.

Warnings: Not for use by children under the age of 18, pregnant or lactating women. Consult your physician before using this product if your diet consists of less than 1,000 calories per day.

Ingredients: Chromium 100mcg (as Chromium Polynicotinate), Garcinia Cambogia Fruit Extract 500mg, Hydroxypropylmethylcellulose, Calcium Sulfate, Starch, and Silicone Dioxide.

How Supplied: One bottle contains 84 easy-to-swallow capsules.

Additional Information: For additional information on ingredients or uses, please visit winltd.com.

BIOLEAN MASS APPEAL™
Amino Acid & Mineral Workout Supplement

Description: Utilizing natural muscle-boosting, **Mass Appeal™** is specifically formulated to enhance athletic performance without side effects. Creatine, the primary ingredient in Mass Appeal, functions as a storage molecule for high-energy phosphate bonds. These high-energy bonds provide greater energy during exercise requiring short periods of intense activity, such as weight lifting, sprinting, and jumping. Creatine causes a "cell volumizing" effect within the muscle by forcing additional water into the muscle cells. This promotes an increase in protein synthesis within the muscle which facilitates growth while slowing down the destructive breakdown of muscle cells that occurs during normal exercise. Mass Appeal also contains the branched chain amino acids (BCAAs) L-leucine, L-valine and L-isoleucine, which also increase protein synthesis and are oxidized inside muscle cells leading to a protein-sparing effect which indirectly increases anabolism by reducing the muscle's need to burn its own proteins during strenuous exercise. Other key ingredients used to protect against muscle catabolism include alpha-ketoglutaric acid and L-glutamine. Two important compounds within Mass Appeal known for their ability to increase oxygen utilization within red blood cells as well as increase flow of these cells into the muscles are inosine and vanadyl sulfate. Vanadyl sulfate not only augments blood flow into muscle tissue but also increases the transport of glucose into these muscles, thusly increasing glycogen storage and exhibiting an additional muscle-sparing effect. Through supplementation, the normal catabolic breakdown of muscle can be minimized and the muscle tissue preserved.

Directions: Adults may take a loading dose of 3 packets in the morning and 2 packets in the late afternoon for one week. This dose may be repeated every 3 months. Following 1 week of the loading dose, begin the maintenance dose of 1 packet daily 2 hours after exercise. Needs may vary with each individual. For individuals desiring enhanced effects, increase the loading dose to 3-4 packets, 3 times per day (morning, afternoon and evening). Following 1 week of this enhanced loading dose, begin the enhanced maintenance dose of 2 packets in the morning and 2 packets in the late afternoon. It is recommended that one maintain a low-fat, high-protein diet; drink at least 8 glasses of water per day; and engage in 30-60 minutes of aerobic and anaerobic exercise 3-4 times per week. For optimal effects, take in conjunction with Phyto-Vite® and Sure2Endure™.

Warnings: Not for use by children under the age of 18, pregnant or lactating women. Consult your physician before using this product if you have any medical conditions. Do not take if you have kidney disease, muscle disease or are on a protein restricted diet. Discontinue immediately if allergic symptoms develop.

Ingredients: Proprietary Supplement Blend 3255mg: Creatine Monohydrate, Inosine (phosphate-bonded), L-Leucine, L-Valine, L-Isoleucine, Alpha-Ketoglutaric Acid, KIC (Calcium Keto-Isocaproate), L-Glutamine, Vanadyl Sulfate; Dicalcium Phosphate, Microcrystalline Cellulose, Stearic Acid, Croscarmellose Sodium, Silica, Magnesium Stearate and film coating (Hydroxypropyl Methylcellulose, Hydroxypropyl Cellulose, Polyethylene Glycol, Titanium Dioxide and Propylene Glycol).

How Supplied: One box contains 28 packets, 4 tablets per packet.

Additional Information: For additional information on ingredients or uses, please visit winltd.com.

These statements have not been evaluated by the Food & Drug Administration. This product is not intended to diagnose, treat, cure or prevent any disease.

BIOLEAN PROXTREME™
Multi-Protein Dietary Supplement

Description: ProXtreme™ is a multi-protein formula containing a scientific blend of ion-exchange whey protein isolates, cross flow ultra filtration isolates, whey protein concentrates, hydrolyzed whey peptides, glutamine peptides and egg albumen. This combination of various protein sources provides 25g of protein per serving while only having 2g of carbohydrates. ProXtreme provides an ideal ratio of essential and non-essential amino acids in their most easily assimilated forms, while also providing high levels of the branched chain amino acids (BCAAs). To increase absorption and digestibility, the proteins in ProXtreme are enzymatically predigested. These proteins are further processed with whey protein to minimize protein cross-linking.

Directions: As a dietary supplement, add 1 packet ProXtreme to 1 cup water, milk, or juice. Stir, shake, or blend thoroughly.

Warnings: Not for use by young children. If you are pregnant or nursing, consult a health professional before using this product.

Ingredients: Sugar 1g, Potassium 240mg, Carbohydrate 2g, Cholesterol 13mg, Sodium 80mg, Protein 25g, Vitamin A 1,125IU, Vitamin C 27mg, Vitamin D 90IU, Vitamin E 14IU, Riboflavin 450mcg, Niacin 5mg, Vitamin B6 450mcg, Folic Acid 63mcg, Vitamin B12 1.4mcg, Biotin 68mcg, Pantothenic Acid 2mg, Calcium 185mg, Chromium 55mcg, Proprietary Amino Acid Blend 1g (Glutamine Peptides, L-Leucine, L-Isoleucine, L-Valine, Zytrix®* 100mg),

Protein Complex (Whey Protein Isolate, Whey Protein Concentrate, Egg Albumen, Whey Peptides, Glutamine Peptides), Cocoa, Natural and Artificial Flavor, Lecithin, Vitamin/Mineral Blend (Ascorbic Acid, Chromium GTF Polynicotinate, d-alpha Tocopheryl Succinate [Natural Vitamin E], Calcium Phosphate Dibasic, Biotin, Vitamin A Palmitate, Niacinamide, d-Calcium Pantothenate, Cholecalciferol, Folic Acid, Pyridoxine Hydrochloride, Riboflavin, Cyanocobalamin), Xanthan Gum, Acesulfame Potassium, Salt, Sucralose.

*Zytrix® is a registered trademark of Custom Nutriceutical Laboratories.

How Supplied: One box contains 7 vanilla and 7 chocolate single serving packets.

Additional Information: For additional information on ingredients or uses, please visit winltd.com.

These statements have not been evaluated by the Food & Drug Administration. This product is not intended to diagnose, treat, cure or prevent any disease.

DHEA PLUS™
Herbal Supplement

Description: DHEA Plus™ uniquely combines dihydroxyepiandrosterone (DHEA), Bioperine® and ginkgo biloba leaf to safely and effectively provide antioxidants, and support the body in a healthy aging process. DHEA, the primary ingredient, is used by the body to manufacture the sex hormones estrogen and testosterone. As DHEA levels decline with age, women produce less estrogen, which is essential for healthy heart function. Additionally, men lose the metabolic boost that testosterone provides and are at increased risk for fat accumulation. Supplemental DHEA can therefore slow this normal hormonal decline. In fact, scientific research has indicated that adequate levels of DHEA in the body can actually slow the normal aging process. A second key ingredient is Bioperine®, which enhances thermogenic activity and can lead to increases in fat mobilization and utilization. To further ward off the forgetfulness associated with the aging process, DHEA Plus includes gingko biloba to augment blood flow throughout the circulatory system and to the brain. Some improvement in cognitive abilities has been noted as well as inhibition of lipid peroxidation, thereby stabilizing the cell wall against free-radical attack.

Directions: As a dietary supplement, take 1 tablet daily with food.

Warnings: Not for use by children under the age of 18, pregnant or lactating women. Consult your physician before using this product if you are taking prescription medications. Persons with a history of prostate cancer should seek medical advice before using this product.

Ingredients: Dihydroxyepiandrosterone 50mg (DHEA), Ginkgo Biloba Leaf 25mg, Bioperine* 5mg (Piper Nigrum L.), Calcium Phosphate Dibasic, Partially Hydrogenated Vegetable Oil, Starch, Magnesium Stearate, Silicon Dioxide and Croscarmellose Sodium.

*Bioperine is a registered trademark of Sabinsa Corporation.

How Supplied: One bottle contains 60 enteric-coated tablets.

Additional Information: For additional information on ingredients or uses, please visit winltd.com.

These statements have not been evaluated by the Food & Drug Administration. This product is not intended to diagnose, treat, cure or prevent any disease.

FOOD FOR THOUGHT®
Mental Performance Drink
Vitamin and Amino Acid Supplement

Description: Food For Thought®, ideal anytime peak mental performance is needed, contains a proprietary blend of amino acids and choline along with powerful antioxidants and B vitamins that are essential in the production of the acetylcholine, the most abundant neurotransmitter in the body. Adequate acetylcholine is vital because of its role in neuromuscular control and cognitive functioning. This neurotransmitter promotes concentration, good memory, and healthy sleep patterns. Food For Thought further enhances its effectiveness through the utilization of essential vitamins and minerals required for promoting the synthesis of the brain neurotransmitter serotonin, which is crucial for maintaining and regulating normal sleep patterns.

Directions: As a dietary supplement, add 1 packet of mix to 6 oz. of chilled water or fruit juice. Stir briskly. Consume 1–2 times per day. Keep in a cool, dry place. For maximum results, combine this product with 1 serving of Winrgy®.

Warnings: Not for use by children under the age of 18, pregnant or lactating women. Persons taking medications should seek medical advice before taking this product. Persons with ulcers or a history of ulcers should consult their physician before using a choline supplement. Do not consume more than four servings per day. Avoid the use of antacids containing aluminum with this product.

Ingredients: Carbohydrates 6g, Sugars 6g, Vitamin C 72mg (as Ascorbic Acid), Vitamin E 30 IU (as DL-Alpha Tocopheryl Acetate), Thiamin 2.9mg (as Thiamin Mononitrate), Riboflavin 2.8mg, Niacin 73mg (as Niacinamide Niacin), Vitamin B6 4.7mg (as Pyridoxine HCL), Vitamin B12 100mg (as Cyanocobalamin), Pantothenic Acid 380mg (as Calcium

Pantothenate), Calcium 34mg (as calcium pantothenate), Zinc 2.9mg (as Zinc Gluconate), Copper 0.4mg (as Copper Gluconate), Chromium 250mcg (as Chromium Aspartate), Choline 770mg (as Choline Bitartrate), Glycine 130mg, Lysine 35mg (as L-Lysine HCL), Fructose, Natural Flavors, Silicon Dioxide and Magnesium Gluconate.

How Supplied: One box contains 28 single serving packets.

Additional Information: For additional information on ingredients or uses, please visit winltd.com.

These statements have not been evaluated by the Food & Drug Administration. This product is not intended to diagnose, treat, cure or prevent any disease.

PHYTO-VITE®
Advanced Antioxidant, Vitamin and Mineral Supplement

Description: Phyto-Vite® is a state-of-the-art nutritional supplement providing chelated minerals, vitamins and a diverse group of antioxidants. The antioxidant coverage provided by Phyto-Vite is both comprehensive and diverse. First, it includes optimal amounts of vitamins A, C, and E as well as the provitamins alpha and beta carotene. The inclusion of these powerful antioxidants provides protection against the oxidative damage caused by free-radicals. Increased immune system support, increased protein and hormone synthesis, increased soft tissue integrity and improved circulation are just a few of the many effects of these antioxidants. Esterified vitamin C is used in Phyto-Vite to ensure quicker uptake and a decreased rate of excretion. Ginkgo biloba has been added to promote healthy brain function and circulation of blood to the brain, as well as to inhibit lipid peroxidation. A phytonutrient blend obtained from entire plant sources has been incorporated into Phyto-Vite to further enhance its antioxidant effects. Key phytonutrients included are lutein, lycopene, soy isoflavones, and allicin. To ensure optimum absorption and maximum antioxidant effects, Phyto-Vite includes the minerals copper, zinc, manganese and selenium in a chelated form. Phyto-Vite has several unique features such as the inclusion of canola oil to ensure proper absorption of fat-soluble vitamins even on an empty stomach, an extended-release formulation to allow flexibility in serving size and a Betacoat™ casing, a beta carotene coating that is designed to provide antioxidant coverage to the tablet itself. This helps to protect the integrity and activity of the product.

Directions: As a dietary supplement, take 6 tablets per day with 8oz. of liquid. Tablets may be taken all at once or staggered throughout the day.

Warnings: If pregnant or lactating, consult physician before using. Accidental overdose of iron-containing products is a leading cause of fatal poisoning in children under 6. Keep this product out of reach of children. In case of accidental overdose, call a doctor or poison control center immediately.

Ingredients: Vitamin A (25,000IU), Vitamin C 500mg, Vitamin D 200IU, Vitamin E 400IU, Vitamin K 70mcg, Thiamin 15mg, Riboflavin 17mg, Niacin 100mg, Vitamin B6 20mg, Folate 400mcg, Vitamin B12 60mcg, Biotin 300mcg, Pantothenic Acid 75mg, Calcium 500mg, Iron 4mg, Phosphorus 250mg, Iodine 150mcg, Magnesium 400mg, Zinc 15mg, Selenium 200mcg, Copper 2mg, Manganese 5mg, Chromium 200mcg, Potassium 70mg, Phytonutrient Blend 800mg (alfalfa leaf, aged garlic bulb concentrate, Pur-Gar® A-10,000 [garlic bulb], soy protein isolate, broccoli floret, cabbage leaf, cayenne pepper fruit, green onion bulb, parsley leaf, tomato, spirulina), canola oil concentrate 100mg, citrus bioflavonoid complex 50mg, rutin 26mg, quercetin dihydrate 24mg, choline 50mg, Inositol 50mg, PABA 25mg, ginkgo biloba leaf standardized extract 20mg, bilberry fruit standardized extract 10mg, catalase enzymes 10mg, grape seed proanthocyanidins 5mg, red grape skin extract 5mg, boron 1mg, dicalcium phosphate, magnesium oxide, calcium carbonate, calcium ascorbate, microcrystalline cellulose, d-alpha-tocopheryl succinate, croscarmellose sodium, stearic acid, potassium citrate, choline bitartrate, beta-carotene, niacinamide, silica, d-calcium pantothenate, magnesium stearate, copper Chelazome® glycinate, zinc Chelazome® glycinate, calcium citrate, calcium lactate, magnesium amino acid chelate, inositol, L-selenomethionine, kelp, manganese Chelazome® glycinate, biotin, pyridoxine HCl, Ferrochel® iron bisglycinate, boron chelate, riboflavin, magnesium citrate, thiamin mononitrate, retinyl palmitate, chromium Chelavite® glycinate, phylloquinone, cyanocobalamin, vanillin, cholecalciferol, folic acid.

How Supplied: One bottle contains 180 hypoallergenic Betacoat™ tablets. This hypoallergenic formula is free of dairy, yeast, wheat, sugar, starch, animal products, dyes, preservatives, artificial flavors and pesticide residues.

Additional Information: For additional information on ingredients or uses, please visit winltd.com.

These statements have not been evaluated by the Food & Drug Administration. This product is not intended to diagnose, treat, cure or prevent any disease.

SATIÉTÉ®
Herbal and Amino Acid Supplement

Description: Satiété® has a synergistic blend of herbs and amino acids that promotes healthy regulation of the neurotransmitter serotonin, supports a healthy appetite and maintains healthy blood sugar levels. Satiete's key ingredient, 5-HTP, derived from griffonia seed extract, is a precursor to serotonin, which regulates normal mood, sleep, appetite and energy levels. Also included is gymnema sylvestre, an important ingredient which has an effect on the oral cavity that reduces appetite for sweets as well as an ability to reduce metabolism of simple carbohydrates in the gastrointestinal system, thus promoting healthy blood sugar levels. Vanadyl sulfate is also included to promote healthy blood sugar levels as part of a weight loss plan. Additional ingredients included to improve energy levels and combat fatigue are St. John's Wort extract, malic acid, and magnesium. The combination of these ingredients provides a positive impact on serotonin function.

Directions: As a dietary supplement, begin dosage by taking 1 tablet 3 per day 30-60 minutes before meals. If needed after 2 weeks of use, increase the dosage to 2 tablets 3 times per day. Do not exceed 9 tablets daily without medical supervision.

Warnings: If you are taking MAO inhibitors, tricyclic antidepressants, SSRI antidepressants (Prozac®, Paxil™, Zoloft®) or prescription diet drugs, do not take this product without medical supervision. If you suffer from liver or kidney diseases, serious gastrointestinal disorders or carcinoid syndrome, do not take this product without medical supervision. If gastrointestinal upset develops and persists, reduce dosage, take only with large meals or discontinue use.

Ingredients: Griffonia Seed Extract (Supplying 95% min. naturally occurring L-5HTP), Gymnema 33mg, Vanadyl Sulfate 7mg, Vitamin B-2 6.5mg, Niacinamide 6.5mg, Magnesium 55mg (Oxide), Vitamin B-1 6.5mg, Vitamin B-6 6.5mg, Malic Acid 100mg, St. John's Wort Extract 50mg, Ginkgo Biloba Extract 20mg, Vitamin B-12 100mcg, Folic Acid 33mg, Microcrystalline Cellulose, Stearic Acid, Croscarmellose Sodium, Magnesium Stearate, Silicon Dioxide, Ethylcellulose and Hydroxypropylcellulose.

How Supplied: One bottle contains 84 hypoallergenic enteric-coated tablets.

Additional Information: For additional information on ingredients or uses, please visit winltd.com.

These statements have not been evaluated by the Food & Drug Administration. This product is not intended to diagnose, treat, cure or prevent any disease.

WINOMEG3COMPLEX™
Highly Concentrated Molecularly Distilled Omega-3 Ethyl Esters Dietary Supplement

Description: WINOmeg3complex™ is a highly purified pharmaceutical-grade

Continued on next page

WINOmeg3complex—Cont.

88% omega-3 ethyl ester supplement, scientifically formulated to promote mood elevation, cardiac health, joint health, cognitive clarity, improved digestion and emotional well being. WINOmeg3complex provides a high concentration of 60% EPA for maximum benefit to the body's normal inflammatory response. Free of dangerous toxins and clinically tested to surpass all international standards for freshness and purity, WINOmeg3complex has three times the EPA and DHA potency of health food grade fish oil. This high concentration and optimal EPA to DHA blend is enhanced with natural lemon oil in the soft gel capsule for great lemon taste. One WINOmeg3complex soft gel capsule supplies 540mg of EPA and 160mg of DHA. The ratio of EPA to DHA is 3.3 to 1; a balance many experts believe is optimal for good health.

Directions: To support and promote cardiac health, joint health, and emotional well-being, take 2 soft-gel capsules per day with a meal. However, certain individuals may realize additional benefits with a higher dosage. Gradually increase dosage until desired benefits are achieved or as directed by a physician.

Warnings: If you are pregnant or on a blood thinner or other anticoagulant, consult your physician before taking this supplement.

Ingredients: Eicosapentaenoic acid 1080mg (EPA), docosahexaenoic acid 320mg (DHA), other omega-3 fatty acids 180mg, other omega-6 fatty acids 60mg, other fatty acids 150mg, gelatin, glycerine, natural flavor and mixed tocopherols.

How Supplied: One bottle contains 60 easy-to-swallow soft-gel capsules enhanced with natural lemon oil.

Additional Information: For additional information on ingredients or uses, please visit winltd.com.

These statements have not been evaluated by the Food & Drug Administration. This product is not intended to diagnose, treat, cure or prevent any disease.

Wyeth Consumer Healthcare
WYETH
FIVE GIRALDA FARMS
MADISON, NJ 07940-0871

Direct Inquiries to:
Wyeth Consumer Healthcare
(800) 322-3129 (9-5 E.S.T)

ADVIL®
(Wyeth Consumer)
Ibuprofen Tablets, USP
Ibuprofen Caplets (Oval-Shaped Tablets)
Ibuprofen Gel Caplets (Oval-Shaped Gelatin Coated Tablets)
Ibuprofen Liqui-Gel Capsules
Pain reliever/Fever Reducer (NSAID)

Active Ingredient: Each tablet, caplet, or gel caplet, contains Ibuprofen 200 mg (NSAID)*
*nonsteroidal anti-inflammatory drug
Each Liqui-gel capsule contains solubilized Ibuprofen equal to 200 mg ibuprofen (NSAID)* (present as the free acid and potassium salt)
*nonsteroidal anti-inflammatory drug

Uses:
temporarily relieves minor aches and pains due to the common cold, headache, toothache, muscular aches, backache, minor pain of arthritis, menstrual cramps; and temporarily reduces fever.

Warnings:
Allergy alert: Ibuprofen may cause a severe allergic reaction, especially in people allergic to aspirin. Symptoms may include:
• hives
• facial swelling
• asthma (wheezing)
• shock
• skin reddening
• rash
• blisters
If an allergic reaction occurs, stop use and seek medical help right away.
Stomach bleeding warning: This product contains a nonsteroidal anti-inflammatory drug (NSAID), which may cause stomach bleeding. The chance is higher if you:
• are age 60 or older
• have had stomach ulcers or bleeding problems
• take a blood thinning (anticoagutant) or steroid drug
• take other drugs containing an NSAID [aspirin, ibuprofen, naproxen, or others]
• have 3 or more alcoholic drinks every day while using this product
• take more or for a longer time than directed
Do not use
• if you have ever had an allergic reaction to any other pain reliever/fever reducer
• right before or after heart surgery
Ask a doctor before use if you have
• problems or serious side effects from taking pain relievers or fever reducers
• stomach problems that last or come back, such as heartburn, upset stomach, or stomach pain
• ulcers
• bleeding problems
• high blood pressure
• heart or kidney disease
• taken a diuretic
• reached age 60 or older

Ask a doctor or pharmacist before use if you are
• taking any other drug containing an NSAID (prescription or nonprescription)
• taking a blood thinning (anticoagulant) or steroid drug
• under a doctor's care for any serious condition
• taking aspirin for heart attack or stroke, because ibuprofen may decrease this benefit of aspirin
• taking any other drug
When using this product
• take with food or milk if stomach upset occurs
• long term continuous use may increase the risk of heart attack or stroke
Stop use and ask a doctor if
• you feel faint, vomit blood, or have bloody or black stools. These are signs of stomach bleeding.
• pain gets worse or lasts more than 10 days
• fever gets worse or lasts more than 3 days
• stomach pain or upset gets worse or lasts
• redness or swelling is present in the painful area
• any new symptoms appear
If pregnant or breast-feeding, ask a health professional before use. It is especially important not to use ibuprofen during the last 3 months of pregnancy unless definitely directed to do so by a doctor because it may cause problems in the unborn child or complications during delivery.
Keep out of reach of children. In case of overdose, get medical help or contact a Poison Control Center right away.

Directions:
• **do not take more than directed**
• **the smallest effective dose should be used**
• do not take longer than 10 days, unless directed by a doctor (see Warnings)
Adults and children 12 years and over:
• take 1 tablet, caplet, gelcap or liquigel capsule every 4 to 6 hours while symptoms persist
• if pain or fever does not respond to 1 tablet, caplet, gelcap, or liquigel capsule, 2 tablets, caplets, gelcaps or liquigel capsules may be used • do not exceed 6 tablets, caplets, gelcaps or liquigel capsules in 24 hours, unless directed by a doctor
Children under 12 years: ask a doctor

Inactive Ingredients:
Tablets and Caplets: acetylated monoglyceride, colloidal silicon dioxide, corn starch, croscarmellose sodium, methylparaben, microcrystalline cellulose, pharmaceutical glaze, pharmaceutical ink, povidone, pregelatinized starch, propylparaben, sodium benzoate, sodium lauryl sulfate, stearic acid, sucrose, synthetic iron oxide, titanium dioxide, white wax
Gel Caplets: colloidal silicon dioxide, corn starch, croscarmellose sodium, FD&C red no. 40, FD&C yellow no. 6, fractionated coconut oil, gelatin, glycerin,

hypromellose, iron oxides, pharmaceutical ink, pregelatinized starch, propyl gallate, sodium lauryl sulfate, starch, stearic acid, titanium dioxide, triacetin

Liqui-Gels: FD& C green no. 3, gelatin, light mineral oil, pharmaceutical ink, polyethylene glycol, potassium hydroxide, purified water, sorbitan, sorbitol.

Other Information:
- **each Liqui-gel capsule contains:** potassium 20 mg
- read all warnings and directions before use. Keep carton (card).
- store at 20–25°C (68–77°F)
- avoid excessive heat 40°C (above 104°F)

How Supplied:
Coated tablets in a 10 ct. vial in packs of 3 and bottles of 24, 50, 100, 150 (non-child resistant), and 200. Coated caplets in bottles of 24, 50, 100, 165 (non-child resistant), and 200.
Gel caplets in bottles of 24, 50, 100, 165 (non-child resistant) and 200.
Liqui-Gels in bottles of 20, 40, 80, 135 (non-child resistant) and 180.

ADVIL® ALLERGY SINUS CAPLETS
(Wyeth Consumer)
ADVIL® MULTI-SYMPTOM COLD CAPLETS
Pain Reliever/Fever Reducer (NSAID)
Nasal Decongestant
Antihistamine

Active Ingredients (in each caplet):
Chlorpheniramine maleate 2 mg
Ibuprofen 200 mg (NSAID)*
Pseudoephedrine HCl 30 mg
*nonsteroidal anti-inflammatory drug

Uses:
- temporarily relieves these symptoms associated with hay fever or other upper respiratory allergies, and the common cold:
  - runny nose • sneezing • headache
  - itchy, watery eyes
  - nasal congestion • minor aches and pains • itching of the nose or throat
  - sinus pressure • fever

Warnings:
Allergy alert: Ibuprofen may cause a severe allergic reaction, especially in people allergic to aspirin. Symptoms may include:
- hives
- facial swelling
- asthma (wheezing)
- shock
- skin reddening
- rash
- blisters
If an allergic reaction occurs, stop use and seek medical help right away.
Stomach bleeding warning: This product contains a nonsteroidal anti-inflammatory drug (NSAID), which may cause stomach bleeding. The chance is higher if you:
- are age 60 or older

- have had stomach ulcers or bleeding problems
- take a blood thinning (anticoagulant) or steroid drug
- take other drugs containing an NSAID [aspirin, ibuprofen, naproxen, or others]
- have 3 or more alcoholic drinks every day while using this product
- take more or for a longer time than directed

Do not use
- if you have ever had an allergic reaction to any other pain reliever/fever reducer
- right before or after heart surgery
- if you are now taking a prescription monoamine oxidase inhibitor (MAOI) (certain drugs for depression, psychiatric, or emotional conditions, or Parkinson's disease), or for 2 weeks after stopping the MAOI drug. If you do not know if your prescription drug contains an MAOI, ask a doctor or pharmacist before taking this product.

Ask a doctor before use if you have
- a breathing problem such as emphysema or chronic bronchitis
- problems or serious side effects from taking pain relievers or fever reducers
- stomach problems that last or come back, such as heartburn, upset stomach, or stomach pain
- ulcers
- bleeding problems
- high blood pressure
- heart or kidney disease
- thyroid disease
- diabetes
- glaucoma
- trouble urinating due to an enlarged prostate gland
- taken a diuretic
- reached age 60 or older

Ask a doctor or pharmacist before use if you are
- taking any other drug containing an NSAID (prescription or nonprescription)
- taking a blood thinning (anticoagulant) or steroid drug
- under a doctor's care for any serious condition
- taking sedatives or tranquilizers
- taking any other product that contains pseudoephedrine, chlorpheniramine or any other nasal decongestant or antihistamine
- taking aspirin for heart attack or stroke, because ibuprofen may decrease this benefit of aspirin
- taking any other drug

When using this product
- take with food or milk if stomach upset occurs
- long term continuous use may increase the risk of heart attack or stroke
- avoid alcoholic drinks
- be careful when driving a motor vehicle or operating machinery
- drowsiness may occur
- alcohol, sedatives, and tranquilizers may increase drowsiness

Stop use and ask a doctor if
- you feel faint, vomit blood, or have bloody or black stools. These are signs of stomach bleeding.

- pain gets worse or lasts more than 10 days
- fever gets worse or lasts more than 3 days
- nasal congestion lasts for more than 7 days
- stomach pain or upset gets worse or lasts
- redness or swelling is present in the painful area
- you get nervous, dizzy, or sleepless
- symptoms continue or get worse
- any new symptoms appear

If pregnant or breast-feeding, ask a health professional before use. It is especially important not to use ibuprofen during the last 3 months of pregnancy unless definitely directed to do so by a doctor because it may cause problems in the unborn child or complications during delivery.

Keep out of reach of children. In case of overdose, get medical help or contact a Poison Control Center right away.

Directions:
- **do not take more than directed**
- **the smallest effective dose should be used**
- do not take longer than 10 days, unless directed by a doctor (see Warnings)
- adults: take 1 caplet every 4–6 hours while symptoms persist.
- do not take more than 6 caplets in any 24-hour period, unless directed by a doctor
- children under 12 years of age: consult a doctor

Other Information:
- read all warnings and directions before use. Keep carton.
- store in a dry place 20–25°C (68–77°F)
- avoid excessive heat above 40°C (104°F)

Inactive Ingredients: carnauba wax, colloidal silicon dioxide, corn starch, croscarmellose sodium, FD&C red no. 40 aluminum lake, FD&C yellow no. 6 aluminum lake, glyceryl behenate, hypromellose, microcrystalline cellulose, pharmaceutical ink, polydextrose, polyethylene glycol, pregelatinized starch, silicon dioxide, titanium dioxide

How Supplied: Allergy sinus caplets in packages of 20 caplets
Multi-symptom cold caplets in packages of 10 caplets

ADVIL® COLD & SINUS
(Wyeth Consumer)
Caplets, and Liqui-Gels
Pain Reliever/Fever Reducer/(NSAID)
Nasal Decongestant

Active Ingredients (in each caplet):
Ibuprofen 200 mg (NSAID)*
Pseudoephedrine HCl 30 mg

*nonsteroidal anti-inflammatory drug

Continued on next page

Advil Cold & Sinus—Cont.

Active Ingredients (in each LiquiGel):

Solubilized Ibuprofen equal to 200 mg ibuprofen (NSAID)* (present as the free acid and potassium salt)
Pseudoephedrine HCl 30 mg

*nonsteroidal anti-inflammatory drug

Uses:

temporarily relieves these symptoms associated with the common cold or flu:
• headache
• fever
• nasal congestion
• sinus pressure
• minor body aches and pains

Warnings

Allergy alert: Ibuprofen may cause a severe allergic reaction, especially in people allergic to aspirin. Symptoms may include:
• hives
• facial swelling
• asthma (wheezing)
• shock
• skin reddening
• rash
• blisters
If an allergic reaction occurs, stop use and seek medical help right away.

Stomach bleeding warning: This product contains a nonsteroidal anti-inflammatory drug (NSAID), which may cause stomach bleeding. The chance is higher if you:
• are age 60 or older
• have had stomach ulcers or bleeding problems
• take a blood thinning (anticoagulant) or steroid drug
• take other drugs containing an NSAID [aspirin, ibuprofen, naproxen, or others]
• have 3 or more alcoholic drinks every day while using this product
• take more or for a longer time than directed

Do not use
• if you have ever had an allergic reaction to any other pain reliever/fever reducer
• right before or after heart surgery
• if you are now taking a prescription monoamine oxidase inhibitor (MAOI) (certain drugs for depression, psychiatric, or emotional conditions, or Parkinson's disease), or for 2 weeks after stopping the MAOI drug. If you do not know if your prescription drug contains an MAOI, ask a doctor or pharmacist before taking this product

Ask a doctor before use if you have
• problems or serious side effects from taking pain relievers or fever reducers
• stomach problems that last or come back, such as heartburn, upset stomach, or stomach pain
• ulcers
• bleeding problems
• high blood pressure
• heart or kidney disease
• thyroid disease
• diabetes

• trouble urinating due to an enlarged prostate gland
• taken a diuretic
• reached age 60 or older

Ask a doctor or pharmacist before use if you are
• taking any other drug containing an NSAID (prescription or nonprescription)
• taking a blood thinning (anticoagulant) or steroid drug
• under a doctor's care for any serious condition
• taking any other product that contains pseudoephedrine or any other nasal decongestant
• taking aspirin for heart attack or stroke, because ibuprofen may decrease this benefit of aspirin
• taking any other drug

When using this product
• take with food or milk if stomach upset occurs
• long term continuous use may increase the risk of heart attack or stroke

Stop use and ask a doctor if
• you feel faint, vomit blood, or have bloody or black stools. These are signs of stomach bleeding.
• pain gets worse or lasts more than 10 days
• fever gets worse or lasts more than 3 days
• nasal congestion lasts for more than 7 days
• symptoms continue or get worse
• stomach pain or upset gets worse or lasts
• redness or swelling is present in the painful area
• you get nervous, dizzy, or sleepless
• any new symptoms appear

If pregnant or breast-feeding, ask a health professional before use. It is especially important not to use ibuprofen during the last 3 months of pregnancy unless definitely directed to do so by a doctor because it may cause problems in the unborn child or complications during delivery.

Keep out of reach of children. In case of overdose, get medical help or contact a Poison Control Center right away.

Directions:
• **do not take more than directed**
• **the smallest effective dose should be used**
• do not take longer than 10 days, unless directed by a doctor (see Warnings)
• adults and children 12 years of age and over:
  • take 1 caplet or liqui-gel every 4 to 6 hours while symptoms persist. If symptoms do not respond to 1 caplet or liqui-gel, 2 caplets or liqui-gels may be used.
  • do not use more than 6 caplets or liqui-gels in any 24-hour period unless directed by a doctor
• children under 12 years of age: consult a doctor

Other Information:
• store at 20–25°C (68–77°F). Avoid excessive heat above 40°C (104°F).

• read all warnings and directions before use. Keep carton.
• **each Liqui-gel contains:** potassium 20 mg

Inactive Ingredients (caplets): acetylated monoglyceride, carnauba wax, colloidal silicon dioxide, croscarmellose sodium, iron oxides, methylparaben, microcrystalline cellulose, pharmaceutical glaze, pharmaceutical ink, povidone, propylparaben, sodium benzoate, sodium lauryl sulfate, starch, stearic acid, sucrose, titanium dioxide

Inactive Ingredients (liqui-gels): D&C yellow no. 10, FD&C red no. 40, fractionated coconut oil, gelatin, pharmaceutical ink, polyethylene glycol, potassium hydroxide, purified water, sorbitan, sorbitol

How Supplied: Advil Cold and Sinus is an oval-shaped, tan-colored caplet, or a liqui-gel. The caplet is supplied in blister packs of 20 and 40. The liqui-gel is available in blister packs of 16.

CHILDREN'S ADVIL® SUSPENSION
(Wyeth Consumer)
Fever Reducer/Pain Reliever (NSAID)

Active Ingredient:
(in each 5 mL)
Ibuprofen 100 mg (NSAID)*
*nonsteroidal anti-inflammatory drug

Uses: temporarily:
• reduces fever
• relieves minor aches and pains due to the common cold, flu, sore throat, headaches and toothaches

Warnings:

Allergy alert: Ibuprofen may cause a severe allergic reaction, especially in people allergic to aspirin. Symptoms may include:
• hives
• facial swelling
• asthma (wheezing)
• shock
• skin reddening
• rash
• blisters
If an allergic reaction occurs, stop use and seek medical help right away.

Stomach bleeding warning: This product contains a nonsteroidal anti-inflammatory drug (NSAID), which may cause stomach bleeding. The chance is higher if the child:
• has had stomach ulcers or bleeding problems
• takes a blood thinning (anticoagulant) or steroid drug
• takes other drugs containing an NSAID [aspirin, ibuprofen, naproxen, or others]
• takes more or for a longer time than directed

Sore throat warning: Severe or persistent sore throat or sore throat accompanied by high fever, headache, nausea,

Dosing Chart

Weight (lb)	Age (years)	Dose (teaspoon)
under 24 lb	under 2 years	ask a doctor
24–35 lb	2–3 years	1 teaspoon
36–47 lb	4–5 years	1½ teaspoons
48–59 lb	6–8 years	2 teaspoons
60–71 lb	9–10 years	2½ teaspoons
72–95 lb	11 years	3 teaspoons

and vomiting may be serious. Consult doctor promptly. Do not use more than 2 days or administer to children under 3 years of age unless directed by doctor.

Do not use
- if the child has ever had an allergic reaction to any other pain reliever/fever reducer
- right before or after heart surgery

Ask a doctor before use if the child has
- problems or serious side effects from taking pain relievers or fever reducers
- stomach problems that last or come back, such as heartburn, upset stomach, or stomach pain
- ulcers
- bleeding problems
- not been drinking fluids
- lost a lot of fluid due to vomiting or diarrhea
- high blood pressure
- heart or kidney disease
- taken a diuretic

Ask a doctor or pharmacist before use if the child is
- taking any other drug containing an NSAID (prescription or nonprescription)
- taking a blood thinning (anticoagulant) or steroid drug
- under a doctor's care for any serious condition
- taking any other drug

When using this product
- take with food or milk if stomach upset occurs
- long term continuous use may increase the risk of heart attack or stroke

Stop use and ask a doctor if
- the child feels faint, vomits blood, or has bloody or black stools. These are signs of stomach bleeding.
- stomach pain or upset gets worse or lasts
- the child does not get any relief within first day (24 hours) of treatment
- fever or pain gets worse or lasts more than 3 days
- redness or swelling is present in the painful area
- any new symptoms appear

Keep out of reach of children. In case of overdose, get medical help or contact a Poison Control Center right away.

Directions:
- **this product does not contain directions or complete warnings for adult use**
- **do not give more than directed**
- do not give longer than 10 days, unless directed by a doctor (see Warnings)

- **shake well before using**
- find right dose on chart below. If possible, use weight to dose; otherwise use age.
- repeat dose every **6–8 hours,** if needed
- do not use more than **4 times a day**
- measure only with the blue dosing cup provided. Blue dosing cup to be used with Children's Advil Suspension only. Do not use with other products. Dose lines account for product remaining in cup due to thickness of suspension.

[See table above]

Other Information:
- one dose lasts 6–8 hours
- store at 20–25°C (68–77°F)

Inactive Ingredients: (FRUIT FLAVOR) artificial flavors, carboxymethylcellulose sodium, citric acid, edetate disodium, FD&C red no. 40, glycerin, microcrystalline cellulose, polysorbate 80, purified water, sodium benzoate, sorbitol solution, sucrose, xanthan gum
Each teaspoon contains: sodium 3 mg

Inactive Ingredients: (GRAPE FLAVOR) acetic acid, artificial flavor, butylated hydroxytoluene, carboxymethylcellulose sodium, citric acid, edetate disodium, FD&C blue no. 1, FD&C red no. 40, glycerin, microcrystalline cellulose, polysorbate 80, propylene glycol, purified water, sodium benzoate, sorbitol solution, sucrose, xanthan gum
Each teaspoon contains: sodium 3 mg

Inactive Ingredients: (BLUE RASPBERRY FLAVOR) carboxymethylcellulose sodium, citric acid, edetate disodium, FD&C blue no. 1, glycerin, microcrystalline cellulose, natural and artificial flavors, polysorbate 80, propylene glycol, purified water, sodium benzoate, sodium citrate, sorbitol solution, sucrose, xanthan gum
Each teaspoon contains: sodium 10 mg

How Supplied: Bottles of 4 fl. oz. in grape, fruit, and blue raspberry flavors.

ADVIL® PM LIQUI-GELS®
ADVIL® PM CAPLETS
(Wyeth Consumer)
Pain reliever (NSAID)/Nighttime sleep-aid

Active Ingredients (in each Liqui-gel capsule):
Diphenhydramine hydrochloride 25 mg
Solubilized ibuprofen equal to 200 mg ibuprofen (NSAID)*

Active Ingredients (in each caplet):
Diphenhydramine citrate 38 mg
Ibuprofen 200 mg (NSAID)*

*nonsteroidal anti-inflammatory drug

Uses:
- for relief of occasional sleeplessness when associated with minor aches and pains
- helps you fall asleep and stay asleep

Warnings:

Allergy alert: Ibuprofen may cause a severe allergic reaction, especially in people allergic to aspirin. Symptoms may include:
- hives
- facial swelling
- asthma (wheezing)
- shock
- skin reddening
- rash
- blisters
If an allergic reaction occurs, stop use and seek medical help right away.

Stomach bleeding warning: This product contains a nonsteroidal anti-inflammatory drug (NSAID), which may cause stomach bleeding. The chance is higher if you:
- are age 60 or older
- have had stomach ulcers or bleeding problems
- take a blood thinning (anticoagulant) or steroid drug
- take other drugs containing an NSAID [aspirin, ibuprofen, naproxen, or others]
- have 3 or more alcoholic drinks every day while using this product
- take more or for a longer time than directed

Do not use
- if you have ever had an allergic reaction to any other pain reliever/fever reducer
- unless you have time for a full night's sleep
- in children under 12 years of age
- right before or after heart surgery
- with any other product containing diphenhydramine, even one used on skin
- if you have sleeplessness without pain

Ask a doctor before use if you have
- a breathing problem such as emphysema or chronic bronchitis
- problems or serious side effects from taking pain relievers or fever reducers
- stomach problems that last or come back, such as heartburn, upset stomach or stomach pain
- ulcers
- bleeding problems
- high blood pressure
- heart or kidney disease
- taken a diuretic
- reached age 60 or older
- glaucoma
- trouble urinating due to an enlarged prostate gland

Continued on next page

Advil PM—Cont.

Ask a doctor or pharmacist before use if you are
- taking sedatives or tranquilizers, or any other sleep-aid
- taking any other drug containing an NSAID (prescription or nonprescription)
- under a doctor's care for any continuing medical illness
- taking any other antihistamines
- taking a blood thinning (anticoagulant) or steroid drug
- taking aspirin for heart attack or stroke, because ibuprofen may decrease this benefit of aspirin
- taking any other drug

When using this product
- drowsiness will occur
- avoid alcoholic drinks
- do not drive a motor vehicle or operate machinery
- take with food or milk if stomach upset occurs
- long term continuous use may increase the risk of heart attack or stroke

Stop use and ask a doctor if
- you feel faint, vomit blood, or have bloody or black stools. These are signs of stomach bleeding.
- pain gets worse or lasts more than 10 days
- sleeplessness persists continuously for more than 2 weeks. Insomnia may be a symptom of a serious underlying medical illness.
- stomach pain or upset gets worse or lasts
- redness or swelling is present in the painful area
- any new symptoms appear

If pregnant or breast-feeding, ask a health professional before use. It is especially important not to use ibuprofen during the last 3 months of pregnancy unless definitely directed to do so by a doctor because it may cause problems in the unborn child or complications during delivery.

Keep out of the reach of children. In case of overdose, get medical help or contact a Poison Control Center right away.

Directions:
- **do not take more than directed**
- do not take longer than 10 days, unless directed by a doctor (see Warnings)
- adults and children 12 years and over: take 2 caplets or capsules at bedtime
- do not take more than 2 caplets or capsules in 24 hours

Other Information:
- **each Liqui-gel capsule contains:** potassium 20 mg
- read all warnings and directions before use. Keep carton (card).
- store at 20–25°C (68–77°F)
- avoid excessive heat above 40°C (104°F)
- protect Liqui-gel capsules from light

Inactive Ingredients:

Liqui-gel capsules
D&C red no. 33, FD&C blue no. 1, fractionated coconut oil, gelatin, pharmaceutical ink, polyethylene glycol, potassium hydroxide, purified water, sorbitans, sorbitol

Caplets
calcium stearate, carnauba wax, colloidal silicon dioxide, corn starch, croscarmellose sodium, FD&C blue no. 2 aluminum lake, glyceryl behenate, hypromellose, lactose monohydrate, microcrystalline cellulose, pharmaceutical ink, polydextrose, polyethylene glycol, pregelatinized starch, sodium lauryl sulfate, sodium starch glycolate, stearic acid, titanium dioxide

How Supplied:
Caplets — Bottle of 20, 40, 80 and 180 caplets

Liqui-gels — Bottle of 16 and 32 capsules

INFANT'S ADVIL®
CONCENTRATED DROPS
(DYE-FREE)
(Wyeth Consumer)
White Grape Flavor
Fever Reducer/Pain Reliever (NSAID)

Active Ingredient:
(in each 1.25 mL)
Ibuprofen 50 mg (NSAID)*
*nonsteroidal anti-inflammatory drug

Uses: temporarily:
- reduces fever
- relieves minor aches and pains due to the common cold, flu, headaches and toothaches

Warnings:

Allergy alert: Ibuprofen may cause a severe allergic reaction, especially in people allergic to aspirin. Symptoms may include:
- hives • facial swelling • asthma (wheezing)
- shock • skin reddening • rash • blisters
If an allergic reaction occurs, stop use and seek medical help right away.

Stomach bleeding warning: This product contains a nonsteroidal anti-inflammatory drug (NSAID), which may cause stomach bleeding. The chance is higher if the child:
- has had stomach ulcers or bleeding problems
- takes a blood thinning (anticoagulant) or steroid drug
- takes other drugs containing an NSAID [aspirin, ibuprofen, naproxen, or others]
- takes more or for a longer time than directed

Do not use
- if the child has ever had an allergic reaction to any other pain reliever/fever reducer
- right before or after heart surgery

Ask a doctor before use if the child has
- problems or serious side effects from taking pain relievers or fever reducers
- stomach problems that last or come back, such as heartburn, upset stomach, or stomach pain
- ulcers
- bleeding problems
- not been drinking fluids
- lost a lot of fluid due to vomiting or diarrhea
- high blood pressure
- heart or kidney disease
- taken a diuretic

Ask a doctor or pharmacist before use if the child is
- taking any other drug containing an NSAID (prescription or nonprescription)
- taking a blood thinning (anticoagulant) or steroid drug
- under a doctor's care for any serious condition
- taking any other drug

When using this product
- take with food or milk if stomach upset occurs
- long term continuous use may increase the risk of heart attack or stroke

Stop use and ask a doctor if
- the child feels faint, vomits blood, or has bloody or black stools. These are signs of stomach bleeding.
- stomach pain or upset gets worse or lasts
- the child does not get any relief within first day (24 hours) of treatment
- fever or pain gets worse or lasts more than 3 days
- redness or swelling is present in the painful area
- any new symptoms appear

Keep out of reach of children. In case of overdose, get medical help or contact a Poison Control Center right away.

Directions:
- **this product does not contain directions or complete warnings for adult use**
- **do not give more than directed**
- do not give longer than 10 days, unless directed by a doctor (see Warnings)
- **shake well before using**
- find right dose on chart below. If possible, use weight to dose; otherwise use age.
- repeat dose every **6–8 hours,** if needed
- do not use more than **4 times a day**
- measure with the dosing device provided. Do not use with any other device.

[See table below]

Dosing Chart		
Weight (lb)	Age (months)	Dose (mL)
under 6 months		ask a doctor
12–17 lb	6–11 months	1.25 mL
18–23 lb	12–23 months	1.875 mL

Other Information:
- one dose lasts 6–8 hours
- store at 20–25°C (68–77°F)

Inactive Ingredients: (WHITE GRAPE FLAVOR) artificial flavor, carboxymethylcellulose sodium, citric acid, edetate disodium, glycerin, microcrystalline cellulose, polysorbate 80, propylene glycol, purified water, sodium benzoate, sorbitol solution, sucrose, xanthan gum

How Supplied: Bottles of ½ fl. oz. in white grape flavor.

ALAVERT®
(Wyeth Consumer)
Loratadine orally disintegrating tablets
Antihistamine

Active Ingredient (in each tablet):
Loratadine 10 mg

Uses:
temporarily relieves these symptoms due to hay fever or other upper respiratory allergies:
- runny nose • sneezing • itchy, watery eyes
- itching of the nose or throat

Warnings:

Do not use if you have ever had an allergic reaction to this product or any of its ingredients

Ask a doctor before use if you have liver or kidney disease. Your doctor should determine if you need a different dose.

When using this product do not use more than directed. Taking more than recommended may cause drowsiness.

Stop use and ask a doctor if an allergic reaction to this product occurs. Seek medical help right away.

If pregnant or breast-feeding, ask a health professional before use.

Keep out of reach of children. In case of overdose, get medical help or contact a Poison Control Center right away.

Directions:
- tablet melts in mouth. Can be taken with or without water.

Age	Dose
adults and children 6 years and over	1 tablet daily; do not use more than 1 tablet daily
children under 6	ask a doctor
consumers who have liver or kidney disease	ask a doctor

Other Information:
- Phenylketonurics: Contains Phenylalanine 8.4 mg per tablet
- store at 20–25°C (68–77°F)
- keep in a dry place

Inactive Ingredients (Loratadine orally disintegrating tablets) (original): artificial & natural flavor, aspartame, citric acid, colloidal silicon dioxide, corn syrup solids, crospovidone, magnesium stearate, mannitol, microcrystalline cellulose, modified food starch, sodium bicarbonate

(orange mint): anhydrous citric acid, aspartame, butylated hydroxyanisole, colloidal silicon dioxide, corn syrup solids, crospovidone, dextrin, ferric oxides, magnesium stearate, maltodextrin, mannitol, microcrystalline cellulose, modified food starch, natural & artificial flavors, sodium bicarbonate

How Supplied: in packages of 6, 12, 24 & 48

ALAVERT® ALLERGY & SINUS D-12 HOUR TABLETS
(Wyeth Consumer)
Loratadine/Pseudoephedrine Sulfate
Extended Release Tablets
Antihistamine/Nasal Decongestant

Active Ingredients (in each tablet):
Loratadine 5 mg
Pseudoephedrine sulfate 120 mg

Uses:
- temporarily relieves these symptoms due to hay fever or other upper respiratory allergies:
  - runny nose
  - sneezing • itchy, watery eyes
  - itching of the nose or throat
- temporarily relieves nasal congestion due to the common cold, hay fever or other respiratory allergies
- reduces swelling of nasal passages
- temporarily relieves sinus congestion and pressure
- temporarily restores freer breathing through the nose

Warnings:

Do not use
- if you have ever had an allergic reaction to this product or any of its ingredients
- if you are now taking a prescription monoamine oxidase inhibitor (MAOI) (certain drugs for depression, psychiatric, or emotional conditions, or Parkinson's disease), or for 2 weeks after stopping the MAOI drug. If you do not know if your prescription drug contains an MAOI, ask a doctor or pharmacist before taking this product.

Ask a doctor before use if you have
- heart disease • high blood pressure
- thyroid disease • diabetes
- trouble urinating due to an enlarged prostate gland
- liver or kidney disease. Your doctor should determine if you need a different dose.

When using this product do not take more than directed. Taking more than directed may cause drowsiness.

Stop use and ask a doctor if
- an allergic reaction to this product occurs. Seek medical help right away.
- symptoms do not improve within 7 days or are accompanied by a fever
- nervousness, dizziness or sleeplessness occurs

If pregnant or breast-feeding, ask a health professional before use.

Keep out of reach of children. In case of overdose, get medical help or contact a Poison Control Center right away.

Directions:
- do not divide, crush, chew or dissolve the tablet

Age	Dose
adults and children 12 years and over	1 tablet every 12 hours; not more than 2 tablets in 24 hours
children under 12 years of age	ask a doctor
consumers with liver or kidney disease	ask a doctor

Other Information:
- **each tablet contains:** calcium 30 mg
- store between 15° and 25°C (59° and 77°F)
- keep in a dry place

Inactive Ingredients: croscarmellose sodium, dibasic calcium phosphate, hypromellose, lactose monohydrate, magnesium stearate, pharmaceutical ink, povidone, titanium dioxide

How Supplied: Blister packs of 12 and 24 tablets.

ANBESOL® MAXIMUM STRENGTH
Gel and Liquid
(Wyeth Consumer)
Oral Anesthetic

ANBESOL JUNIOR® Gel
Oral Anesthetic

BABY ANBESOL® Gel
Grape Flavor
Oral Anesthetic

Active Ingredients: Anbesol is an oral anesthetic which is available in a Maximum Strength gel and liquid. Anbesol Junior, available in a gel, is an oral anesthetic. Baby Anbesol, available in a grape-flavored gel, is an oral anesthetic and is alcohol-free.
Maximum Strength Anbesol Gel and Liquid contain Benzocaine 20%.
Anbesol Junior Gel contains Benzocaine 10%.
Baby Anbesol Gel contains Benzocaine 7.5%.

Uses: **Maximum Strength Anbesol** temporarily relieves pain associated with the following mouth and gum irritations: toothache, canker sores, minor dental procedures, sore gums, braces, and dentures. **Anbesol Junior** temporarily relieves pain associated with the following mouth and gum irritations: braces, sore gums, canker sores, toothaches, and

Continued on next page

Anbesol—Cont.

minor dental procedures. **Baby Anbesol Gel** temporarily relieves sore gums due to teething in infants and children 4 months of age and older.

Warnings: Allergy alert: Do not use these products if you have a history of allergy to local anesthetics such as procaine, butacaine, benzocaine, or other "caine" anesthetics.

Baby Anbesol: Do not use to treat fever and nasal congestion. These are not symptoms of teething and may indicate the presence of infection. If these symptoms persist, consult your doctor.

Maximum Strength Anbesol, Anbesol Junior and Baby Anbesol:

When using this product
- avoid contact with the eyes
- do not exceed recommended dosage
- do not use for more than 7 days unless directed by a doctor/dentist

Stop use and ask a doctor if
- sore mouth symptoms do not improve in 7 days
- irritation, pain, or redness persists or worsens
- swelling, rash, or fever develops

Keep out of reach of children. If more than used for pain is accidentally swallowed, get medical help or contact a Poison Control Center right away.

Directions: Maximum Strength Anbesol: Gel—
- to open tube, cut tip of the tube on score mark with scissors
- adults and children 2 years of age and older: apply to the affected area up to 4 times daily or as directed by a doctor/ dentist
- children under 12 years of age: adult supervision should be given in the use of this product
- children under 2 years of age: consult a doctor/dentist
- for denture irritation:
  - apply thin layer to the affected area
  - do not reinsert dental work until irritation/pain is relieved
  - rinse mouth well before reinserting

Do not refrigerate.

Liquid—
- adults and children 2 years of age and older:
  - wipe liquid on with cotton, or cotton swab, or fingertip
  - apply to the affected area up to 4 times daily or as directed by a doctor/ dentist
- children under 12 years of age: adult supervision should be given in the use of this product
- children under 2 years of age: consult a doctor/dentist

Anbesol Junior Gel:
- to open tube, cut tip of the tube on score mark with scissors
- adults and children 2 years of age and older: apply to the affected area up to 4 times daily or as directed by a doctor/ dentist
- children under 12 years of age: adult su-

pervision should be given in the use of this product
- children under 2 years of age: consult a doctor/dentist

Baby Anbesol Gel:
- to open tube, cut tip of the tube on score mark with scissors
- children 4 months of age and older: apply to the affected area not more than 4 times daily or as directed by a doctor/ dentist
- infants under 4 months of age: no recommended dosage or treatment except under the advice and supervision of a doctor/dentist

Inactive Ingredients:

Maximum Strength Gel: benzyl alcohol, carbomer 934P, D&C yellow no. 10, FD&C blue no. 1, FD&C red no. 40, flavor, glycerin, methylparaben, polyethylene glycol, propylene glycol, saccharin.

Maximum Strength Liquid: benzyl alcohol, D&C yellow no. 10, FD&C blue no. 1, FD&C red no. 40, flavor, methylparaben, polyethylene glycol, propylene glycol, saccharin.

Junior Gel: artificial flavor, benzyl alcohol, carbomer 934P, D&C red no. 33, glycerin, methylparaben, polyethylene glycol, potassium acesulfame

Baby Gel: benzoic acid, carbomer 934P, D&C red no. 33, edetate disodium, FD&C blue no. 1, flavor, glycerin, methylparaben, polyethylene glycol, propylparaben, saccharin, water

Storage: Store at 20–25°C (68–77°F)

How Supplied: Gels in 0.33 oz (9 g) tubes, Maximum Strength Liquid in 0.41 fl oz (12 mL) bottle.

ANBESOL® COLD SORE THERAPY
(Wyeth Consumer)
Fever blister/Cold sore treatment

Active Ingredients:
Allantoin 1%,
Benzocaine 20%,
Camphor 3%,
White petrolatum 64.9%

Uses:
- temporarily relieves pain associated with fever blisters and cold sores
- relieves dryness and softens fever blisters and cold sores

Warnings: For external use only
Allergy alert: Do not use this product if you have a history of allergy to local anesthetics such as procaine, butacaine, benzocaine, or other "caine" anesthetics.
Do not use over deep or puncture wounds, infections, or lacerations. Consult a doctor.
When using this product
- avoid contact with the eyes
- do not exceed recommended dosage
Stop use and ask a doctor if
- condition worsens
- symptoms persist for more than 7 days
- symptoms clear up and occur again within a few days

Keep out of reach of children. If swallowed, get medical help or contact a Poison Control Center right away.

Directions:
- to open tube, cut tip of the tube on score mark with scissors
- adults and children 2 years of age and older: apply to the affected area not more than 3 to 4 times daily
- children under 12 years of age: adult supervision should be given in the use of this product
- children under 2 years of age: consult a doctor

Other Information:
- store at 20–25°C (68–77°F)

Inactive Ingredients: aloe extract, benzyl alcohol, butylparaben, glyceryl stearate, isocetyl stearate, menthol, methylparaben, propylparaben, sodium lauryl sulfate, vitamin E, white wax

How Supplied: 0.33 oz Tube

CHILDREN'S DIMETAPP® Cold & Allergy Elixir
(Wyeth Consumer)
Antihistamine, Nasal Decongestant

Active Ingredients (in each 5 mL teaspoon):
Brompheniramine maleate, USP 1 mg
Phenylephrine HCl, USP 2.5 mg

Uses:
- temporarily relieves nasal congestion due to the common cold, hay fever or other upper respiratory allergies
- temporarily relieves these symptoms due to hay fever (allergic rhinitis):
  - runny nose
  - sneezing
  - itchy, watery eyes
  - itching of the nose or throat
- temporarily restores freer breathing through the nose

Warnings:
Do not use
- in a child under 2 years of age
- if you are now taking a prescription monoamine oxidase inhibitor (MAOI) (certain drugs for depression, psychiatric, or emotional conditions, or Parkinson's disease), or for 2 weeks after stopping the MAOI drug. If you do not know if your prescription drug contains an MAOI, ask a doctor or pharmacist before taking this product.
Ask a doctor before use if you have
- heart disease
- high blood pressure
- thyroid disease
- diabetes
- trouble urinating due to an enlarged prostate gland
- glaucoma
- a breathing problem such as emphysema or chronic bronchitis
Ask a doctor or pharmacist before use if you are taking sedatives or tranquilizers.

When using this product
- **do not use more than directed**
- drowsiness may occur
- avoid alcoholic beverages
- alcohol, sedatives, and tranquilizers may increase drowsiness
- be careful when driving a motor vehicle or operating machinery
- excitability may occur, especially in children

Stop use and ask a doctor if
- you get nervous, dizzy, or sleepless
- symptoms do not get better within 7 days or are accompanied by fever

If pregnant or breast-feeding, ask a health professional before use.

Keep out of reach of children. In case of overdose, get medical help or contact a Poison Control Center right away.

Directions:
- do not take more than 6 doses in any 24-hour period

age	dose
adults and children 12 years and over	4 teaspoons every 4 hours
children 6 to under 12 years	2 teaspoons every 4 hours
children 2 to under 6 years	ask a doctor
children under 2 years	do not use

Other Information
- **each teaspoon contains:** sodium 3 mg.
- store at 20–25°C (68–77°F)
- dosage cup provided

Inactive Ingredients: artificial flavor, citric acid, FD&C blue no. 1, FD&C red no. 40, glycerin, propylene glycol, purified water, sodium benzoate, sodium citrate, sorbitol, sucralose

How Supplied: Purple, grape-flavored liquid in bottles of 4 fl oz, 8 fl oz, and 12 fl oz.

CHILDREN'S DIMETAPP® DM COLD & COUGH Elixir (Wyeth Consumer)
Antihistamine, Cough Suppressant, Nasal Decongestant

Active Ingredients (in each 5 mL teaspoon)
Brompheniramine maleate, USP 1 mg
Dextromethorphan HBr, USP 5 mg
Phenylephrine HCl, USP 2.5 mg

Uses:
- temporarily relieves cough due to minor throat and bronchial irritation occurring with a cold, and nasal congestion due to the common cold, hay fever or other upper respiratory allergies

- temporarily relieves these symptoms due to hay fever (allergic rhinitis):
  - runny nose
  - sneezing
  - itchy, watery eyes
  - itching of the nose or throat
- temporarily restores freer breathing through the nose

Warnings:
Do not use
- in a child under 2 years of age
- if you are now taking a prescription monoamine oxidase inhibitor (MAOI) (certain drugs for depression, psychiatric, or emotional conditions, or Parkinson's disease), or for 2 weeks after stopping the MAOI drug. If you do not know if your prescription drug contains an MAOI, ask a doctor or pharmacist before taking this product.

Ask a doctor before use if you have
- heart disease
- high blood pressure
- thyroid disease
- diabetes
- trouble urinating due to an enlarged prostate gland
- glaucoma
- cough that occurs with too much phlegm (mucus)
- a breathing problem or persistent or chronic cough that lasts such as occurs with smoking, asthma, chronic bronchitis, or emphysema

Ask a doctor or pharmacist before use if you are taking sedatives or tranquilizers.

When using this product
- **do not use more than directed**
- may cause marked drowsiness
- avoid alcoholic beverages
- alcohol, sedatives, and tranquilizers may increase drowsiness
- be careful when driving a motor vehicle or operating machinery
- excitability may occur, especially in children

Stop use and ask a doctor if
- you get nervous, dizzy, or sleepless
- symptoms do not get better within 7 days or are accompanied by fever
- cough lasts more than 7 days, comes back, or is accompanied by fever, rash, or persistent headache. These could be signs of a serious condition

If pregnant or breast-feeding, ask a health professional before use.

Keep out of reach of children. In case of overdose, get medical help or contact a Poison Control Center right away.

Directions:
- do not take more than 6 doses in any 24-hour period

Age	Dose
adults and children 12 years and over	4 teaspoons every 4 hours
children 6 to under 12 years	2 teaspoons every 4 hours
children 2 to under 6 years	ask a doctor
children under 2 years	do not use

Other Information:
- **each teaspoon contains:** sodium 3 mg
- store at 20–25°C (68–77°F).
- dosage cup provided.

Inactive Ingredients: artificial flavor, citric acid, FD&C blue no. 1, FD&C red no. 40, glycerin, propylene glycol, purified water, sodium benzoate, sodium citrate, sorbitol, sucralose

How Supplied: Purple, grape-flavored liquid in bottles of 4 fl oz and 8 fl oz.

CHILDREN'S DIMETAPP® LONG ACTING COUGH PLUS COLD SYRUP (Wyeth Consumer)
Cough suppressant/Antihistamine

Active Ingredients (in each 5 mL teaspoon):
Chlorpheniramine maleate, USP 1.0 mg
Dextromethorphan HBr, USP 7.5 mg

Uses:
- temporarily relieves cough due to minor throat and bronchial irritation as may occur with a cold
- temporarily relieves these symptoms due to hay fever or other upper respiratory allergies:
  - runny nose • sneezing • itchy, watery eyes • itching of the nose or throat

Warnings:
Do not use if you are now taking a prescription monoamine oxidase inhibitor (MAOI) (certain drugs for depression, psychiatric, or emotional conditions, or Parkinson's disease), or for 2 weeks after stopping the MAOI drug. If you do not know if your prescription drug contains an MAOI, ask a doctor or pharmacist before taking this product.

Ask a doctor before use if you have
- trouble urinating due to an enlarged prostate gland
- glaucoma
- a cough that occurs with too much phlegm (mucus)
- a breathing problem or chronic cough that lasts or as occurs with smoking, asthma, chronic bronchitis or emphysema

Ask a doctor or pharmacist before use if you are taking sedatives or tranquilizers.

When using this product
- **do not use more than directed**
- marked drowsiness may occur • avoid alcoholic drinks
- alcohol, sedatives, and tranquilizers may increase drowsiness
- be careful when driving a motor vehicle or operating machinery
- excitability may occur, especially in children

Stop use and ask a doctor if cough lasts more than 7 days, comes back, or is ac-

Continued on next page

Children's Dimetapp—Cont.

companied by fever, rash, or persistent headache. These could be signs of a serious condition.

If pregnant or breast-feeding, ask a health professional before use.

Keep out of reach of children. In case of overdose, get medical help or contact a Poison Control Center right away.

Directions:
• do not take more than 4 doses in any 24-hour period

age	dose
12 years and older	4 teaspoons every 6 hours
6 to under 12 years	2 teaspoons every 6 hours
under 6 years	ask a doctor

Other Information: • **each teaspoon contains:** sodium 3 mg
• store at 20–25°C (68–77°F)
• dosage cup provided

Inactive Ingredients: artificial flavor, anhydrous citric acid, FD&C blue no. 1, FD&C red no. 40, glycerin, propylene glycol, purified water, sodium benzoate, sodium citrate, sorbitol, sucralose

How Supplied: Bottles of 4 fl. oz.

CHILDREN'S DIMETAPP® COLD & ALLERGY CHEWABLE TABLETS
(Wyeth Consumer)
Antihistamine/Nasal decongestant

Active Ingredients (in each tablet):
Brompheniramine maleate, USP 1 mg
Phenylephrine HCl, USP 2.5 mg

Uses:
• temporarily relieves nasal congestion due to the common cold, hay fever or other upper respiratory allergies
• temporarily relieves these symptoms due to hay fever (allergic rhinitis) or other upper respiratory allergies:
  • runny nose
  • sneezing
  • itchy, watery eyes
  • itching of the nose or throat
• temporarily restores freer breathing through the nose

Warnings:
Do not use
• in a child under 2 years of age
• in a child who is taking a prescription monoamine oxidase inhibitor (MAOI) (certain drugs for depression, psychiatric, or emotional conditions, or Parkinson's disease), or for 2 weeks after stopping the MAOI drug. If you do not know if your child's prescription drug contains an MAOI, ask a doctor or pharmacist before giving this product.

Ask a doctor before use if the child has
• heart disease
• high blood pressure
• thyroid disease
• diabetes
• glaucoma
• a breathing problem such as emphysema or chronic bronchitis

Ask a doctor or pharmacist before use if the child is taking sedatives or tranquilizers.

When using this product
• **do not use more than directed**
• drowsiness may occur
• sedatives and tranquilizers may increase drowsiness
• excitability may occur, especially in children

Stop use and ask a doctor if
• the child gets nervous, dizzy, or sleepless
• symptoms do not get better within 7 days or are accompanied by fever

Keep out of reach of children. In case of overdose, get medical help or contact a Poison Control Center right away.

Directions:
• do not give more than 6 doses in any 24-hour period

age	dose
children 6 to under 12 years	2 tablets every 4 hours
children 2 to under 6 years	ask a doctor
children under 2 years	do not use

Other Information:
• store at 20–25°C (68–77°F)

Inactive Ingredients: artificial and natural flavors, carmine, carrageenan, croscarmellose sodium, fructose, fumaric acid, glycine, magnesium stearate, maltodextrin, mannitol, microcrystalline cellulose, modified starch, polyethylene oxide, silicon dioxide, sorbitol, sucralose, tribasic calcium phosphate

How Supplied:
Packages of 20 chewable tablets

TODDLER'S DIMETAPP® COLD AND COUGH DROPS
(Wyeth Consumer)
Cough suppressant/Nasal decongestant

Active Ingredients (in each 0.8 mL):
Dextromethorphan HBr, USP 2.5 mg;
Phenylephrine HCl, USP 1.25 mg

Uses: Temporarily relieves cough occurring with the common cold and temporarily relieves nasal congestion due to the common cold, hay fever, or other upper respiratory allergies

Warnings:
Do not use
• in a child under 2 years of age

• in a child who is taking a prescription monoamine oxidase inhibitor (MAOI) (certain drugs for depression, psychiatric, or emotional conditions, or Parkinson's disease), or for 2 weeks after stopping the MAOI drug. If you do not know if your child's prescription drug contains an MAOI, ask a doctor or pharmacist before giving this product.

Ask a doctor before use if the child has
• heart disease
• high blood pressure
• thyroid disease
• diabetes
• cough that occurs with too much phlegm (mucus)
• cough that lasts or is chronic such as occurs with asthma

When using this product do not use more than directed

Stop use and ask a doctor if
• the child gets nervous, dizzy, or sleepless
• symptoms do not get better within 7 days or are accompanied by fever
• cough lasts more than 7 days, comes back, or is accompanied by fever, rash, or persistent headache. These could be signs of a serious condition.

Keep out of reach of children. In case of overdose, get medical help or contact a Poison Control Center right away.

Directions:
• do not give more than 6 doses in any 24-hour period
• repeat every 4 hours or as directed by a physician
• measure with the dosing device provided. Do not use with any other device.

age	dose
under 2 years	do not use
2 to under 6 years	1.6 mL

Other Information: • store at 20–25°C (68–77°F) • oral dosing device enclosed

Inactive Ingredients: anhydrous citric acid, artificial flavor, glycerin, propylene glycol, purified water, sodium benzoate, sorbitol solution, sucralose

How Supplied: ½ oz bottle with oral dosing device.

FIBERCON® Caplets
(Wyeth Consumer)
Calcium Polycarbophil
Bulk-Forming Laxative

Active Ingredient
(in each caplet):
Calcium polycarbophil 625 mg equivalent to 500 mg polycarbophil

Uses:
• relieves occasional constipation to help restore and maintain regularity
• this product generally produces bowel movement in 12 to 72 hours

Age	Recommended dose	Daily maximum
adults & children 12 years of age and over	2 caplets once a day	up to 4 times a day
children under 12 years	consult a physician	

Warnings:

Choking: Taking this product without adequate fluid may cause it to swell and block your throat or esophagus and may cause choking. Do not take this product if you have difficulty in swallowing. If you experience chest pain, vomiting, or difficulty in swallowing or breathing after taking this product, seek immediate medical attention.

Ask a doctor before use if you have
- abdominal pain, nausea, or vomiting
- a sudden change in bowel habits that persists over a period of 2 weeks

Ask a doctor or pharmacist before use if you are taking any other drug. Take this product 2 or more hours before or after other drugs. All laxatives may affect how other drugs work.

When using this product
- do not use for more than 7 days unless directed by a doctor
- do not take more than 8 caplets in a 24 hour period unless directed by a doctor

Stop use and ask a doctor if rectal bleeding occurs or if you fail to have a bowel movement after use of this or any other laxative. These could be signs of a serious condition.

Keep out of reach of children. In case of overdose, get medical help or contact a Poison Control Center right away.

Directions:

- take each dose of this product with at least 8 ounces (a full glass) of water or other fluid. Taking this product without enough liquid may cause choking. See choking warning.
- FiberCon works naturally so continued use for one to three days is normally required to provide full benefit. Dosage may vary according to diet, exercise, previous laxative use or severity of constipation.

[See table above]

Inactive Ingredients: caramel, crospovidone, hypromellose, magnesium stearate, microcrystalline cellulose, polyethylene glycol, silicon dioxide, sodium lauryl sulfate

Each caplet contains: 140 mg calcium and 10 mg magnesium.

Storage: Protect contents from moisture. Store at 20–25°C (68–77°F)

How Supplied: Film-coated scored caplets.
Package of 36 caplets, and
Bottles of 60, 90 and 140 caplets.

FACED WITH AN Rx SIDE EFFECT?
Turn to the
Companion Drug Index
for products that
provide symptomatic
relief.

PREPARATION H®
(Wyeth Consumer)
Hemorrhoidal Ointment and
Maximum Strength Cream
PREPARATION H®
Hemorrhoidal Suppositories

Active Ingredients: Preparation H is available in ointment, cream, and suppository product forms. The **Ointment** contains Petrolatum 71.9%, Mineral oil 14%, Shark liver oil 3% and Phenylephrine HCl 0.25%.
The **Maximum Strength Cream** contains White petrolatum USP 15%, Glycerin USP 14.4%, Pramoxine HCl USP 1% and Phenylephrine HCl USP 0.25%.
The **Suppositories** contain Cocoa butter 85.5%, Shark liver oil 3%, and Phenylephrine HCl 0.25%.

Uses: Preparation H Ointment and Suppositories
- helps relieve the local itching and discomfort associated with hemorrhoids
- temporarily shrinks hemorrhoidal tissue and relieves burning
- temporarily provides a coating for relief of anorectal discomforts
- temporarily protects the inflamed, irritated anorectal surface to help make bowel movements less painful

Maximum Strength Cream
- for temporary relief of pain, soreness and burning
- helps relieve the local itching and discomfort associated with hemorrhoids
- temporarily shrinks hemorrhoidal tissue
- temporarily provides a coating for relief of anorectal discomforts
- temporarily protects the inflamed, irritated anorectal surface to help make bowel movements less painful

Warnings:

For all product forms:
Ask a doctor before use if you have
- heart disease
- high blood pressure
- thyroid disease
- diabetes
- difficulty in urination due to enlargement of the prostate gland

Ask a doctor or pharmacist before use if you are presently taking a prescription drug for high blood pressure or depression.

When using this product do not exceed the recommended daily dosage unless directed by a doctor.

Stop use and ask a doctor if
- bleeding occurs
- condition worsens or does not improve within 7 days

If pregnant or breast-feeding, ask a health professional before use.

Keep out of reach of children. If swallowed, get medical help or contact a Poison Control Center right away.

Ointment: For external and/or intrarectal use only. Stop use and ask a doctor if introduction of applicator into the rectum causes additional pain.

Maximum Strength Cream: For external use only. When using this product do not put into the rectum by using fingers or any mechanical device or applicator. **Stop use and ask a doctor if** an allergic reaction develops; or if the symptom being treated does not subside or if redness, irritation, swelling, pain, or other symptoms develop or increase.

Suppositories: For rectal use only.

Directions:

Ointment—
- adults: when practical, cleanse the affected area by patting or blotting with an appropriate cleansing wipe. Gently dry by patting or blotting with a tissue or a soft cloth before applying ointment.
- when first opening the tube, puncture foil seal with top end of cap
- apply to the affected area up to 4 times daily, especially at night, in the morning or after each bowel movement
- intrarectal use:
  - remove cover from applicator, attach applicator to tube, lubricate applicator well and gently insert applicator into the rectum
  - thoroughly cleanse applicator after each use and replace cover
- also apply ointment to external area
- regular use provides continual therapy for relief of symptoms
- children under 12 years of age: ask a doctor

Maximum Strength Cream—
- adults: when practical, cleanse the affected area by patting or blotting with an appropriate cleansing wipe. Gently dry by patting or blotting with a tissue or a soft cloth before applying cream.
- when first opening the tube, puncture foil seal with top end of cap
- apply externally or in the lower portion of the anal canal only
- apply externally to the affected area up to 4 times daily, especially at night, in the morning or after each bowel movement
- for application in the lower anal canal: remove cover from dispensing cap. Attach dispensing cap to tube. Lubricate dispensing cap well, then gently insert dispensing cap partway into the anus.
- thoroughly cleanse dispensing cap after each use and replace cover
- children under 12 years of age: ask a doctor

Suppositories—
- adults: when practical, cleanse the affected area by patting or blotting with an appropriate cleansing wipe. Gently dry by patting or blotting with a tissue or a soft cloth before insertion of this product.

Continued on next page

Preparation H—Cont.

- detach one suppository from the strip; remove the foil wrapper before inserting into the rectum as follows:
  - hold suppository with rounded end up
  - carefully separate foil tabs by inserting tip of fingernail at end marked "peel down"
  - slowly and evenly peel apart (do not tear) foil by pulling tabs down both sides, to expose the suppository
  - remove exposed suppository from wrapper
  - insert one suppository into the rectum up to 4 times daily, especially at night, in the morning or after each bowel movement
- children under 12 years of age: ask a doctor

Other Information

Inactive Ingredients: Ointment—benzoic acid, BHA, BHT, corn oil, glycerin, lanolin, lanolin alcohol, methylparaben, paraffin, propylparaben, thyme oil, tocopherol, water, wax
Maximum Strength Cream—aloe barbadensis leaf extract, BHA, carboxymethylcellulose sodium, cetyl alcohol, citric acid, edetate disodium, glyceryl stearate, laureth-23, methylparaben, mineral oil, panthenol, propyl gallate, propylene glycol, propylparaben, purified water, sodium benzoate, steareth-2, steareth-20, stearyl alcohol, tocopherol, vitamin E, xanthan gum
Suppositories—methylparaben, propylparaben, starch
Storage: Store at 20–25°C (68–77°F).

How Supplied: Ointment: Net Wt. 1 oz and 2 oz **Cream:** Net Wt. 0.9 oz and 1.8 oz **Suppositories:** 12's, 24's and 48's.

PREPARATION H® MEDICATED WIPES
(Wyeth Consumer)

Active Ingredient: Witch Hazel 50%

Uses:
- helps relieve the local itching and discomfort associated with hemorrhoids
- temporary relief of irritation and burning
- aids in protecting irritated anorectal areas

Other Uses:
- **for vaginal care**—cleanse the area by gently wiping, patting or blotting. Repeat as needed.
- **for use as a moist compress**—if necessary, first cleanse the area as described below. Fold wipe to desired size and place in contact with tissue for a soothing and cooling effect. Leave in place for up to 15 minutes and repeat as needed.

Warnings:
For external use only
When using this product
- do not exceed the recommended daily dosage unless directed by a doctor

- do not put this product into the rectum by using fingers or any mechanical device or applicator
Stop use and ask a doctor if
- bleeding occurs
- condition worsens or does not improve within 7 days
If pregnant or breast-feeding, ask a health professional before use. **Keep out of reach of children.** If swallowed, get medical help or contact a Poison Control Center right away.

Directions:
Container and Refill:
- remove tab on right side of wipes pouch label and peel back to open
- grab the top wipe at the edge of the center fold and pull out of pouch
- carefully reseal label on pouch after each use to retain moistness
Travel Pack, Container and Refill:
- adults: unfold wipe and cleanse the area by gently wiping, patting or blotting. If necessary, repeat until all matter is removed from the area.
- use up to 6 times daily or after each bowel movement and before applying topical hemorrhoidal treatments, and then discard
- children under 12 years of age: consult a doctor

Other Information
- store at 20-25°C (68-77°F)
- for best results, flush only one or two wipes at a time

Inactive Ingredients: aloe barbadensis gel, capryl/capramidopropyl betaine, citric acid, diazolidinyl urea, glycerin, methylparaben, propylene glycol, propylparaben, sodium citrate, water.

How Supplied: Containers of 48 wipes. Refills of 48 wipes. 10 count portable pack.

PRIMATENE® Mist
(Wyeth Consumer)
Epinephrine Inhalation Aerosol
Bronchodilator

Active Ingredient: (in each inhalation)
Epinephrine 0.22 mg

Uses:
- for temporary relief of occasional symptoms of mild asthma:
  - wheezing
  - tightness of chest
  - shortness of breath

Warnings:
Asthma alert: Because asthma can be life threatening, see a doctor if you
- are not better in 20 minutes
- get worse
- need 12 inhalations in any day
- use more than 9 inhalations a day for more than 3 days a week
- have more than 2 asthma attacks in a week
For inhalation only
Do not use
- unless a doctor said you have asthma

- if you are now taking a prescription monoamine oxidase inhibitor (MAOI) (certain drugs taken for depression, psychiatric or emotional conditions, or Parkinson's disease), or for 2 weeks after stopping the MAOI drug. If you do not know if your prescription drug contains an MAOI, ask a doctor or pharmacist before taking this product.
Ask a doctor before use if you have
- ever been hospitalized for asthma
- heart disease
- high blood pressure
- diabetes
- thyroid disease
- seizures
- narrow angle glaucoma
- a psychiatric or emotional condition
- trouble urinating due to an enlarged prostate gland
Ask a doctor or pharmacist before use if you are
- taking prescription drugs for asthma, obesity, weight control, depression, or psychiatric or emotional conditions
- taking any drug that contains phenylephrine, pseudoephedrine, ephedrine, or caffeine (such as for allergy, cough-cold, or pain)
When using this product
- **increased blood pressure or heart rate can occur, which could lead to more serious problems such as heart attack and stroke. Your risk may increase if you take more frequently or more than the recommended dose.**
- nervousness, sleeplessness, rapid heart beat, tremor, and seizure may occur. If these symptoms persist or get worse, consult a doctor right away.
- avoid caffeine-containing foods or beverages
- avoid dietary supplements containing ingredients reported or claimed to have a stimulant effect.
- do not puncture or throw into incinerator. Contents under pressure.
- do not use or store near open flame or heat above 120°F (49°C). May cause bursting.
Contains CFC 12, 114, substances which harm public health and environment by destroying ozone in the upper atmosphere.
If pregnant or breast-feeding, ask a health professional before use.
Keep out of reach of children. In case of overdose, get medical help or contact a Poison Control Center right away.

Directions:
- **do not exceed dosage**
- supervise children using this product
- adults and children 4 years and over: start with one inhalation, then wait at least 1 minute. If not relieved, use once more. Do not use again for at least 3 hours.
- children under 4 years of age: ask a doctor

Directions For Use of Mouthpiece:
The Primatene Mist mouthpiece, which is enclosed in the Primatene Mist 15 mL

size (not the refill size), should be used for inhalation only with Primatene Mist.

1. Take plastic cap off mouthpiece. (For refills, use mouthpiece from previous purchase.)
2. Take plastic mouthpiece off bottle.
3. Place short end of mouthpiece on bottle.
4. Turn bottle upside down. Place thumb on bottom of mouthpiece over circular button and forefinger on top of vial. Empty the lungs as completely as possible by exhaling.
5. Place mouthpiece in mouth with lips closed around opening. Inhale deeply while squeezing mouthpiece and bottle together. Release immediately and remove unit from mouth, then complete taking the deep breath, drawing medication into your lungs, holding breath as long as comfortable.
6. Exhale slowly keeping lips nearly closed. This helps distribute the medication in the lungs.
7. For storage, place long end of mouthpiece back on bottle and cover with plastic cap.

Care of the Mouthpiece:

The Primatene Mist mouthpiece should be washed after each use with hot, soapy water, rinsed thoroughly and dried with a clean, lint-free cloth.

Other Information:

• store at room temperature, between 20–25°C (68–77°F) • contains no sulfites

Inactive Ingredients: ascorbic acid, dehydrated alcohol (34%), dichlorodifluoromethane (CFC 12), dichlorotetrafluoroethane (CFC 114), hydrochloric acid, nitric acid, purified water

How Supplied:

$\frac{1}{2}$ Fl oz (15 mL) With Mouthpiece.
$\frac{1}{2}$ Fl oz (15 mL) Refill

ROBITUSSIN® Chest Congestion
(Wyeth Consumer)
Expectorant

Active Ingredient: (in each 5 mL teaspoon)
Guaifenesin, USP 100 mg

Uses: helps loosen phlegm (mucus) and thin bronchial secretions to make coughs more productive

Warnings:
Ask a doctor before use if you have
• cough that occurs with too much phlegm (mucus)
• cough that lasts or is chronic such as occurs with smoking, asthma, chronic bronchitis, or emphysema

Stop use and ask a doctor if cough lasts more than 7 days, comes back, or is accompanied by fever, rash, or persistent headache. These could be signs of a serious condition.

If pregnant or breast-feeding, ask a health professional before use.

Keep out of reach of children. In case of overdose, get medical help or contact a Poison Control Center right away.

Directions:
• do not take more than 6 doses in any 24-hour period
• adults and children 12 years and over: 2–4 teaspoons every 4 hours
• children 6 years to under 12 years: 1–2 teaspoons every 4 hours
• children 2 years to under 6 years: ½–1 teaspoon every 4 hours
• children under 2 years: ask a doctor

Other Information:
• **each teaspoon contains:** sodium 2 mg
• store at 20–25°C (68–77°F)
• alcohol-free
• dosage cup provided

Inactive Ingredients: artificial flavor, caramel, citric acid, FD&C red no. 40, glycerin, high fructose corn syrup, liquid glucose, menthol, propylene glycol, purified water, saccharin sodium, sodium benzoate

How Supplied: Bottles of 4 fl oz, 8 fl oz.

ROBITUSSIN® COUGH DROPS
(Wyeth Consumer)
Menthol Eucalyptus, Cherry and Honey Flavors

ROBITUSSIN® HONEY COUGH® DROPS
Honey-Lemon Tea, Natural Honey Center

ROBITUSSIN® SUGAR FREE
Throat Drops
Natural Citrus
Oral anesthetic/Cough suppressant
Menthol

Active Ingredients:
Robitussin Cough Drops: (in each drop)
Menthol Eucalyptus:
Menthol, USP 10 mg
Cherry and Honey-Lemon:
Menthol, USP 5 mg
Robitussin Honey Cough Drops: (in each drop)
Natural Honey Center and *Honey Lemon Tea*
Menthol, USP 5 mg
Robitussin Sugar Free Throat Drops: (in each drop)
Menthol, USP 2.5 mg

Uses:
• temporarily relieves
  • occasional minor irritation, pain, sore mouth, and sore throat
  • cough associated with a cold or inhaled irritants

Warnings:
Sore throat warning: Severe or persistent sore throat or sore throat accompanied by high fever, headache, nausea, and vomiting may be serious. Consult a doctor

right away. Do not use more than 2 days or give to children under 3 years of age unless directed by a doctor.

Ask a doctor before use if you have
• cough that occurs with too much phlegm (mucus)
• cough that lasts or is chronic such as occurs with smoking, asthma, or emphysema

For ROBITUSSIN SUGAR FREE Throat Drops:

When using this product excessive use may have a laxative effect.

For All ROBITUSSIN Cough and Throat Drops:

Stop use and ask a doctor if cough lasts more than 7 days, comes back, or is accompanied by fever, rash, or persistent headache. These could be signs of a serious condition.

If pregnant or breast-feeding, ask a health professional before use.

Keep out of reach of children.

Directions:

ROBITUSSIN Cough Drops (Menthol Eucalyptus, Cherry, Honey-Lemon Tea, Natural Honey Center and Honey Lemon Drops)
• adults and children 4 years and over: allow 1 drop to dissolve slowly in the mouth
• for sore throat: may be repeated every 2 hours, as needed, or as directed by a doctor
• for cough: may be repeated every 2 hours, as needed, or as directed by a doctor
• children under 4 years of age: ask a doctor

ROBITUSSIN Sugar Free Throat Drops:
• adults and children 4 years and over: allow 2 drops to dissolve slowly in the mouth
• for sore throat: may be repeated every 2 hours, as needed, up to 9 drops per day, or as directed by a doctor
• for cough: may be repeated every 2 hours, as needed, up to 9 drops per day, or as directed by a doctor
• children under 4 years of age: ask a doctor

For ROBITUSSIN Sugar Free Throat Drops:
• **phenylketonurics:** contains phenylalanine 3.37 mg per drop
• does not promote tooth decay
• product may be useful in a diabetic's diet on the advice of a doctor.

Exchange Information*

3 Drops = FREE Exchange
9 Drops = 1 Fruit

* The dietary exchanges are based on Exchange Lists for Meal Planning. Copyright 1995 by the American Diabetes Association Inc. and the American Dietetic Association.

Continued on next page

Robitussin Drops—Cont.

Other Information:
Store at 20–25°C (68–77°F)

Inactive ingredients:

ROBITUSSIN Cough Drops:

Menthol Eucalyptus: corn syrup, eucalyptus oil, flavor, sucrose
Cherry: corn syrup, FD&C red no. 40, flavor, methylparaben, propylparaben, sodium benzoate, sucrose
Honey-Lemon: citric acid, corn syrup, D&C yellow no. 10, FD&C yellow no. 6, honey, lemon oil, methylparaben, povidone, propylparaben, sodium benzoate, sucrose

ROBITUSSIN Honey Cough Drops:

Natural Honey Center: caramel, corn syrup, glycerin, high fructose corn syrup, honey, natural herbal flavor, sorbitol, sucrose
Honey Lemon Tea: caramel, citric acid, corn syrup, honey, natural flavor, sucrose, tea extract

ROBITUSSIN Sugar Free Throat Drops:
aspartame, canola oil, citric acid, D&C yellow no. 10 aluminum lake, FD&C blue no. 1, isomalt, maltitol, natural flavor

How Supplied:

ROBITUSSIN Cough Drops:
All 3 flavors of Robitussin Cough Drops are available in bags of 25 drops.

ROBITUSSIN Honey Cough Drops:
Honey Lemon Tea in bags of 25 drops. Natural Honey Center in bags of 20 drops.

ROBITUSSIN Sugar Free Throat Drops:
Natural Citrus in packages of 18 drops.

ROBITUSSIN® CoughGels®
(Wyeth Consumer)
Long-Acting
Cough Suppressant

Active Ingredient (in each liquid-filled capsule):
Dextromethorphan HBr, USP 15 mg

Use:
temporarily relieves cough due to minor throat and bronchial irritation as may occur with a cold.

Warnings:

Do not use if you are now taking a prescription monoamine oxidase inhibitor (MAOI) (certain drugs for depression, psychiatric, or emotional conditions, or Parkinson's disease), or for 2 weeks after stopping the MAOI drug. If you do not know if your prescription drug contains an MAOI, ask a doctor or pharmacist before taking this product.

Ask a doctor before use if you have
• a cough that occurs with too much phlegm (mucus)
• a cough that lasts or is chronic as occurs with smoking, asthma, or emphysema

Stop use and ask a doctor if cough lasts for more than 7 days, comes back, or is accompanied by fever, rash, or persistent headache. These could be signs of a serious condition.

If pregnant or breast-feeding, ask a health professional before use.

Keep out of reach of children. In case of overdose, get medical help or contact a Poison Control Center right away.

Directions:
• do not take more than 8 capsules in any 24-hour period
• adults and children 12 years and over: take 2 capsules every 6 to 8 hours, as needed
• children under 12 years: ask a doctor

Other Information:
• store at 20–25°C (68–77°F)
• avoid excessive heat above 40°C (104°F)
• protect from light

Inactive Ingredients:
FD&C blue no. 1, FD&C red no. 40, fractionated coconut oil, gelatin, glycerin, mannitol, pharmaceutical ink, polyethylene glycol, povidone, propyl gallate, propylene glycol, purified water, sorbitol, sorbitol anhydrides

How Supplied:
Packages of 20 liquid-filled capsules

ROBITUSSIN® Cough & Allergy
Nasal Decongestant, Cough Suppressant, Antihistamine

Active Ingredients: (in each 5mL teaspoon)
Chlorpheniramine maleate, USP 2 mg
Dextromethorphan HBr, USP 10 mg
Phenylephrine HCl, USP 5 mg

Uses:
• temporarily relieves these symptoms due to hay fever (allergic rhinitis):
  • runny nose
  • sneezing
  • itchy, watery eyes
  • itching of the nose or throat
  • nasal congestion
• temporarily controls cough due to minor throat and bronchial irritation associated with inhaled irritants
• temporarily restores freer breathing through the nose

Warnings:

Do not use • in a child under 2 years of age • if you are now taking a prescription monoamine oxidase inhibitor (MAOI) (certain drugs for depression, psychiatric, or emotional conditions, or Parkinson's disease), or for 2 weeks after stopping the MAOI drug. If you do not know if your prescription drug contains an MAOI, ask a doctor or pharmacist before taking this product.

Ask a doctor before use if you have:
• heart disease
• high blood pressure
• thyroid disease

• diabetes
• trouble urinating due to an enlarged prostate gland
• glaucoma
• a cough that occurs with too much phlegm (mucus)
• a breathing problem or persistent or chronic cough that lasts such as occurs with smoking, asthma, chronic bronchitis, or emphysema

Ask a doctor or pharmacist before use if you are taking sedatives or tranquilizers.

When using this product:
• **do not use more than directed**
• marked drowsiness may occur
• avoid alcoholic beverages
• alcohol, sedatives, and tranquilizers may increase drowsiness
• be careful when driving a motor vehicle or operating machinery
• excitability may occur, especially in children

Stop use and ask a doctor if:
• you get nervous, dizzy, or sleepless
• symptoms do not get better within 7 days or are accompanied by fever
• cough lasts more than 7 days, comes back, or is accompanied by fever, rash, or persistent headache. These could be signs of a serious condition.

If pregnant or breast-feeding, ask a health professional before use.

Keep out of reach of children. In case of overdose, get medical help or contact a Poison Control Center right away.

Directions:
• do not take more than 6 doses in any 24-hour period
• adults and children 12 years and over: 2 teaspoons every 4 hours
• children 6 to under 12 years: 1 teaspoon every 4 hours
• children 2 to under 6 years: ask a doctor
• children under 2 years: do not use

Other Information:
• **each teaspoon contains:** sodium 3 mg
• store at 20–25°C (68–77°F)
• alcohol free
• dosage cup provided

Inactive Ingredients:
anhydrous citric acid, artificial and natural flavor, FD&C red no. 40, glycerin, lactic acid, menthol, propylene glycol, purified water, sodium benzoate, sodium citrate, sorbitol solution, sucralose

How Supplied:
Bottles of 4 fl. oz.

ROBITUSSIN® Head & Chest
Congestion PE (Wyeth Consumer)
Nasal Decongestant, Expectorant

Active Ingredients:
(in each 5 mL teaspoon):
Guaifenesin, USP 100 mg
Phenylephrine HCl, USP 5 mg

Uses: • helps loosen phlegm (mucus) and thin bronchial secretions to make coughs more productive • temporarily relieves nasal congestion due to a cold

Warnings:

Do not use
- in a child under 2 years of age
- if you are now taking a prescription monoamine oxidase inhibitor (MAOI) (certain drugs for depression, psychiatric, or emotional conditions, or Parkinson's disease), or for 2 weeks after stopping the MAOI drug. If you do not know if your prescription drug contains an MAOI, ask a doctor or pharmacist before taking this product.

Ask a doctor before use if you have
- heart disease • high blood pressure
- thyroid disease • diabetes
- trouble urinating due to an enlarged prostate gland
- cough that occurs with too much phlegm (mucus)
- cough that lasts or is chronic such as occurs with smoking, asthma, chronic bronchitis, or emphysema

When using this product do not use more than directed.

Stop use and ask a doctor if
- you get nervous, dizzy, or sleepless
- symptoms do not get better within 7 days or are accompanied by fever
- cough lasts more than 7 days, comes back, or is accompanied by fever, rash, or persistent headache. These could be signs of a serious condition.

If pregnant or breast-feeding, ask a health professional before use.

Keep out of reach of children. In case of overdose, get medical help or contact a Poison Control Center right away.

Directions:
- do not take more than 6 doses in any 24-hr period
- adults and children 12 yrs and over: 2 teaspoons every 4 hours
- children 6 to under 12 yrs: 1 teaspoon every 4 hours
- children 2 to under 6 yrs: ½ teaspoon every 4 hours
- children under 2 yrs: do not use

Other Information:
- store at 20–25°C (68–77°F)
- alcohol-free
- dosage cup provided

Inactive Ingredients:
artificial & natural flavor, citric acid, FD&C red no. 40, glycerin, lactic acid, menthol, propylene glycol, purified water, sodium benzoate, sorbitol, sucralose

How Supplied: Bottles of 4 fl oz

FACED WITH AN Rx SIDE EFFECT?
Turn to the Companion Drug Index for products that provide symptomatic relief.

ROBITUSSIN® COUGH DM (Wyeth Consumer)
ROBITUSSIN® SUGAR FREE COUGH
ROBITUSSIN® COUGH DM INFANT DROPS
ROBITUSSIN® COUGH & CONGESTION
Cough Suppressant, Expectorant

Active Ingredients: (in each 5 mL teaspoon: Robitussin Cough DM, Robitussin Sugar Free Cough)
Dextromethorphan HBr, USP 10 mg
Guaifenesin, USP 100 mg

Active Ingredients: (in each 2.5 mL Robitussin Cough DM Infant Drops)
Dextromethorphan HBr, USP 5 mg
Guaifenesin, USP 100 mg

Active Ingredients: (in each 5 mL teaspoon: Robitussin Cough & Congestion)
Dextromethorphan HBr, USP 10 mg
Guaifenesin, USP 200 mg

Uses:
- temporarily relieves cough due to minor throat and bronchial irritation as may occur with a cold
- helps loosen phlegm (mucus) and thin bronchial secretions to drain bronchial tubes

Warnings:

Do not use if you or your child are now taking a prescription monoamine oxidase inhibitor (MAOI) (certain drugs for depression, psychiatric, or emotional conditions, or Parkinson's disease), or for 2 weeks after stopping the MAOI drug. If you do not know if your child's or your prescription drug contains an MAOI, ask a doctor or pharmacist before taking this product or giving it to your child.

Ask a doctor before use if you or your child has
- cough that occurs with too much phlegm (mucus)
- cough that lasts or is chronic such as occurs with smoking, asthma, chronic bronchitis, or emphysema

Stop use and ask a doctor if cough lasts more than 7 days, comes back, or is accompanied by fever, rash, or persistent headache. These could be signs of a serious condition.

If pregnant or breast-feeding, ask a health professional before use.

Keep out of reach of children. In case of overdose, get medical help or contact a Poison Control Center right away.

Directions: (Robitussin Cough DM, Robitussin Sugar Free Cough, Robitussin Cough & Congestion):
- do not take more than 6 doses in any 24-hour period
- adults and children 12 years and over: 2 teaspoons every 4 hours
- children 6 to under 12 years: 1 teaspoon every 4 hours
- children 2 to under 6 years: ½ teaspoon every 4 hours
- children under 2 years: ask a doctor
- shake well before using (Robitussin Cough & Congestion)

Directions: (Robitussin Cough DM Infant Drops):
- repeat every 4 hrs
- do not use more than 6 doses in any 24-hr period
- choose dosage by weight (if weight not known, choose by age)
- measure with the dosing device provided. Do not use with any other device.
- 24–47 lbs (2 to under 6 years): 2.5 mL
- under 24 lbs (under 2 years): ask a doctor

Inactive Ingredients: (Robitussin Cough DM): citric acid, FD&C red no. 40, flavors, glucose, glycerin, high fructose corn syrup, menthol, saccharin sodium, sodium benzoate, water

Inactive Ingredients: (Robitussin Sugar Free Cough): acesulfame potassium, citric acid, flavors, glycerin, methylparaben, polyethylene glycol, povidone, propylene glycol, saccharin sodium, sodium benzoate, water

Inactive Ingredients: (Robitussin Cough DM Infant Drops): artificial flavors, citric acid, FD&C red no. 40, glycerin, high fructose corn syrup, magnasweet, maltitol solution, maltol, polyethylene glycol, povidone, propylene glycol, purified water, saccharin sodium, sodium benzoate, sodium chloride, sodium citrate

Inactive Ingredients: (Robitussin Cough & Congestion): Carboxymethylcellulose sodium, citric acid, D&C red no. 33, FD&C red no. 40, glycerin, high fructose corn syrup, menthol, microcrystalline cellulose, natural and artificial flavors, polyethylene glycol, povidone, propylene glycol, purified water, saccharin sodium, sodium benzoate, sorbitol solution, xanthan gum

Other Information:
- **each 2.5 mL contains:** sodium 5 mg (Robitussin Cough DM Infant Drops)
- **each teaspoon contains:** sodium 5 mg (Robitussin Cough & Congestion)
- store at 20–25°C (68–77°F)
- alcohol-free
- dosage cup or oral dosing device provided

How Supplied: Robitussin DM (cherry-colored) in bottles of 4, 8 and 12 fl oz
Robitussin Sugar Free Cough in bottles of 4 fl oz
Robitussin DM Infant Drops in 1 fl oz bottles
Robitussin Cough and Congestion in bottles of 4 and 8 fl oz

ROBITUSSIN® COUGH Long Acting (Wyeth Consumer)
ROBITUSSIN® PEDIATRIC COUGH Long Acting
Cough Suppressant

Active ingredients (in each 5 mL teaspoon Robitussin Cough Long Acting):

Continued on next page

Robitussin Cough—Cont.

Dextromethorphan HBr, USP 15 mg
(in each 5 mL tsp Robitussin Pediatric Cough Long Acting):
Dextromethorphan HBr, USP 7.5 mg

Use: temporarily relieves cough due to minor throat and bronchial irritation as may occur with a cold

Warnings:

Do not use if you are now taking a prescription monoamine oxidase inhibitor (MAOI) (certain drugs for depression, psychiatric, or emotional conditions, or Parkinson's disease), or for 2 weeks after stopping the MAOI drug. If you do not know if your prescription drug contains an MAOI, ask a doctor or pharmacist before taking this product.

Ask a doctor before use if you have

- cough that occurs with too much phlegm (mucus)
- cough that lasts or is chronic such as occurs with smoking, asthma, or emphysema

Stop use and ask a doctor if cough lasts more than 7 days, comes back, or is accompanied by fever, rash, or persistent headache. These could be signs of a serious condition.

If pregnant or breast-feeding, ask a health professional before use.

Keep out of reach of children. In case of overdose, get medical help or contact a Poison Control Center right away.

Directions:

- do not take more than 4 doses in any 24-hour period

Robitussin Cough Long Acting

- adults and children 12 years and over: 2 teaspoons every 6 to 8 hours, as needed
- children under 12 years: ask a doctor

Robitussin Pediatric Cough Long Acting

- choose dosage by weight (if weight is not known, choose by age)
- under 24 lbs (under 2 years): ask a doctor
- 24–47 lbs (2 to under 6 years): 1 teaspoon every 6 to 8 hours
- 48–95 lbs (6 to under 12 years): 2 teaspoons every 6 to 8 hours
- 96 lbs and over (12 years and older): 4 teaspoons every 6 to 8 hours

Other Information:

- store at 20–25°C (68–77°F)
- dosage cup provided

Inactive Ingredients: (Robitussin Cough Long Acting): alcohol, citric acid, FD&C red no. 40, flavors, glucose, glycerin, high fructose corn syrup, menthol, saccharin sodium, sodium benzoate, water

(Robitussin Pediatric Cough Long Acting): artificial flavor, citric acid, FD&C red no. 40, glycerin, high fructose corn syrup, propylene glycol, purified water, saccharin sodium, sodium benzoate, sodium chloride, sodium citrate
- **each teaspoon contains:** sodium 5 mg

How Supplied:

Robitussin Cough Long Acting (dark red-colored) in bottles of 4 fl oz.
Robitussin Pediatric (cherry-colored) in bottles of 4 fl oz.

ROBITUSSIN® Cough & Cold (Wyeth Consumer) Long-Acting
ROBITUSSIN® Pediatric Cough & Cold Long-Acting
Cough Suppressant, Antihistamine

Active Ingredients (in each 5 mL teaspoon Robitussin Cough & Cold Long Acting):

Dextromethorphan HBr, USP 15 mg
Chlorpheniramine maleate, USP 2 mg
(in each 5 mL tsp Robitussin Pediatric Cough & Cold Long Acting):
Dextromethorphan HBr, USP 7.5 mg
Chlorpheniramine maleate, USP 1 mg

Uses:

- temporarily relieves cough due to minor throat and bronchial irritation as may occur with a cold
- temporarily relieves these symptoms due to hay fever or other upper respiratory allergies:
  - runny nose
  - sneezing
  - itchy, watery eyes
  - itching of the nose or throat

Warnings:

Do not use if you are now taking a prescription monoamine oxidase inhibitor (MAOI) (certain drugs for depression, psychiatric, or emotional conditions, or Parkinson's disease), or for 2 weeks after stopping the MAOI drug. If you do not know if your prescription drug contains an MAOI, ask a doctor or pharmacist before taking this product.

Ask a doctor before use if you have

- trouble urinating due to an enlarged prostate gland
- glaucoma
- a cough that occurs with too much phlegm (mucus)
- a breathing problem or chronic cough that lasts or as occurs with smoking, asthma, chronic bronchitis or emphysema

Ask a doctor or pharmacist before use if you are taking sedatives or tranquilizers.

When using this product

- **do not use more than directed**
- marked drowsiness may occur
- avoid alcoholic drinks
- alcohol, sedatives, and tranquilizers may increase drowsiness
- be careful when driving a motor vehicle or operating machinery
- excitability may occur, especially in children

Stop use and ask a doctor if cough lasts more than 7 days, comes back, or is accompanied by fever, rash, or persistent headache. These could be signs of a serious condition.

If pregnant or breast-feeding, ask a health professional before use.

Keep out of reach of children. In case of overdose, get medical help or contact a Poison Control Center right away.

Directions:

- repeat dose every 6 hrs, as needed.
- do not take more than 4 doses in any 24-hour period

Robitussin Cough & Cold Long-Acting:

- adults and children 12 years and over: 2 teaspoons
- children under 12 years: ask a doctor

Robitussin Pediatric Cough & Cold Long-Acting:

- choose dosage by weight (if weight is not known, choose by age)
- under 48 lbs (under 6 years): ask a doctor
- 48–95 lbs (6 to under 12 years): 2 teaspoons
- 96 lbs and over (12 years and older): 4 teaspoons

Other Information: • store at 20–25°C (68–77°F) • dosage cup provided

Inactive Ingredients (Robitussin Cough & Cold Long Acting): artificial & natural flavor, citric acid, FD&C red no. 40, glycerin, lactic acid, menthol, propylene glycol, purified water, sodium benzoate, sodium citrate, sorbitol, sucralose

Inactive Ingredients (Robitussin Pediatric Cough & Cold Long Acting): artificial & natural flavor, citric acid, FD&C red no. 40, glycerin, lactic acid, propylene glycol, purified water, sodium benzoate, sodium citrate, sorbitol, sucralose
- **each teaspoon contains:** sodium 3 mg

How Supplied:

Robitussin Cough & Cold Long Acting: Red syrup in bottles of 4 fl oz
Robitussin Pediatric Cough & Cold Long Acting: (bright red) in bottles of 4 fl oz

---

ROBITUSSIN® Cough & Cold CF Liquid (Wyeth Consumer)
ROBITUSSIN® Cough & Cold CF Pediatric Drops
Cough Suppressant/Expectorant/ Nasal decongestant

Active Ingredients: (in each 5 mL teaspoon Robitussin Cough & Cold CF)
Dextromethorphan HBr, USP ...... 10 mg
Guaifenesin, USP .... 100 mg
Phenylephrine HCl, USP .... 5 mg
(in each 2.5mL Robitussin Cough & Cold CF Pediatric Drops)
Dextromethorphan HBr, USP .... 5 mg
Guaifenesin, USP .... 100 mg
Phenylephrine HCl, USP .... 2.5 mg

Uses:

- temporarily relieves these symptoms occurring with a cold:
  - nasal congestion
  - cough due to minor throat and bronchial irritation
- helps loosen phlegm (mucus) and thin bronchial secretions to drain bronchial tubes

Warnings:

Do not use:

- in a child under 2 years of age
- if you or your child are now taking a prescription monoamine oxidase inhibitor (MAOI) (certain drugs for depression, psychiatric, or emotional conditions, or Parkinson's disease), or for 2 weeks after stopping the MAOI drug. If you do not know if your child's or your prescription drug contains an MAOI, ask a doctor or pharmacist before taking this product or giving it to your child.

Ask a doctor before use if you or your child has

- heart disease
- high blood pressure
- thyroid disease
- diabetes
- trouble urinating due to an enlarged prostate gland
- cough that occurs with too much phlegm (mucus)
- cough that lasts or is chronic such as occurs with smoking, asthma, chronic bronchitis or emphysema

When using this product do not use more than directed.

Stop use and ask a doctor if

- you or your child gets nervous, dizzy, or sleepless
- symptoms do not get better within 7 days or are accompanied by fever
- cough lasts more than 7 days, comes back, or is accompanied by fever, rash, or persistent headache. These could be signs of a serious condition.

If pregnant or breast-feeding, ask a health professional before use.

Keep out of reach of children. In case of overdose, get medical help or contact a Poison Control Center right away.

Directions: (Robitussin Cough & Cold CF):

- do not take more than 6 doses in any 24-hour period
- adults and children 12 years and over: 2 teaspoons every 4 hours
- children 6 years to under 12 years: 1 teaspoon every 4 hours
- children 2 years to under 6 years: ½ teaspoon every 4 hours
- children under 2 years: do not use

Directions: (Robitussin Cough & Cold CF Pediatric Drops):

- do not use more than 6 doses in any 24-hour period
- repeat every 4 hours
- choose dosage by weight (if weight is not known, choose by age)
- measure with the dosing device provided. Do not use with any other device.
- 24–47 lbs (2 to under 6 yrs): 2.5 mL
- under 24 lbs (under 2 yrs): do not use

Other Information:

- store at 20–25°C (68–77°F)
- alcohol-free
- dosage cup or oral dosing device provided

Inactive Ingredients: (Robitussin Cough & Cold CF) artificial and natural flavor, citric acid, FD&C red no. 40, glycerin, lactic acid, menthol, propylene glycol, purified water, sodium benzoate, sorbitol, sucralose (Robitussin Cough & Cold CF Pediatric Drops) anhydrous citric acid, artificial & natural flavor, FD&C red no. 40, glycerin, lactic acid, polyethylene glycol, propylene glycol, purified water, sodium benzoate, sodium citrate, sorbitol solution, sucralose

How Supplied: Robitussin Cough & Cold CF (red-colored) in bottles of 4, 8, and 12 fl oz. Robitussin Cough & Cold CF Pediatric Drops in 1 fl oz bottles

---

ROBITUSSIN® NIGHT TIME COUGH AND COLD
(Wyeth Consumer)

ROBITUSSIN NIGHT TIME PEDIATRIC COUGH AND COLD
Antihistamine/Cough Suppressant/Nasal Decongestant

Active ingredient (in each 5 mL teaspoon)

Diphenhydramine HCl, USP 6.25 mg
Phenylephrine HCl, USP 2.5 mg

Uses:

- temporarily relieves these symptoms occurring with a cold, hay fever, or other upper respiratory allergies:
  - nasal congestion • cough
  - runny nose • sneezing
  - itchy, watery eyes • itching of the nose or throat

Warnings:

Do not use

- in a child under 2 years of age
- if you or your child are now taking a prescription monoamine oxidase inhibitor (MAOI) (certain drugs for depression, psychiatric, or emotional conditions, or Parkinson's disease), or for 2 weeks after stopping the MAOI drug. If you do not know if your prescription drug contains an MAOI, ask a doctor or pharmacist before taking this product.
- with any other product containing diphenhydramine, even one used on skin

Ask a doctor before use if you have

- heart disease • high blood pressure
- thyroid disease • diabetes
- trouble urinating due to an enlarged prostate gland • glaucoma
- cough that occurs with too much phlegm (mucus)
- a breathing problem or chronic cough that lasts or as occurs with smoking, asthma, chronic bronchitis, or emphysema

Ask a doctor or pharmacist before use if you are taking sedatives or tranquilizers

When using this product

- do not use more than directed
- marked drowsiness may occur • avoid alcoholic drinks
- alcohol, sedatives, and tranquilizers may increase drowsiness
- be careful when driving a motor vehicle or operating machinery
- excitability may occur, especially in children

Stop use and ask a doctor if

- you get nervous, dizzy, or sleepless
- symptoms do not get better within 7 days or are accompanied by fever
- cough lasts more than 7 days, comes back, or is accompanied by fever, rash or persistent headache. These could be signs of a serious condition.

If pregnant or breast-feeding, ask a health professional before use.

Keep out of reach of children. In case of overdose, get medical help or contact a Poison Control Center right away.

Directions:

- do not take more than 6 doses in any 24-hour period
- do not exceed recommended dosage.

Age	Dose
adults and children 12 years and over	4 teaspoons every 4 hours
children 6 years to under 12 years	2 teaspoons every 4 hours
children 2 years to under 6 years	ask a doctor
children under 2 years	do not use

Other information • each teaspoon contains: sodium 3 mg

- store at 20-25°C (68-77°F)

Inactive ingredients (Robitussin Night Time Cough & Cold) anhydrous citric acid, artificial flavor, FD&C red no. 40, glycerin, menthol, polyethylene glycol, propyl gallate, propylene glycol, purified water, sodium benzoate, sodium citrate, sorbitol solution, sucralose.

(Robitussin Night Time Pediatric Cough & Cold) artificial & natural flavor, citric acid, FD&C red no. 40, glycerin, lactic acid, propylene glycol, purified water, sodium benzoate, sodium citrate, sorbitol, sucralose

How Supplied:

Robitussin Night Time Cough and Cold — bottles of 4 fl. oz.
Robitussin Night Time Pediatric Cough and Cold — bottles of 4 fl. oz.

SECTION 8

DIETARY AND HERBAL SUPPLEMENT INFORMATION

This section presents information on natural remedies and nutritional supplements marketed under
the Dietary Supplement Health and Education Act of
1994. It is made possible through the courtesy of the
manufacturers whose products appear on the following pages. The information concerning each product
has been prepared, edited, and approved by the manufacturer's professional staff.

Products found in this section include vitamins, minerals, herbs and other botanicals, amino acids, other
substances intended to supplement the diet, and concentrates, metabolites, constituents, extracts, and
combinations of these ingredients. The descriptions
of these products are designed to provide all information necessary for informed use, including, when
applicable, active ingredients, inactive ingredients,
actions, warnings, cautions, interactions, symptoms
and treatment of oral overdosage, dosage and
directions for use, and how supplied. Descriptions in

this section must be in full compliance with the
Dietary Supplement Health and Education Act, which
permits claims regarding a product's effect on the
structure or functioning of the body, but forbids
claims regarding a product's ability to treat, diagnose, cure, or prevent any specific disease. Descriptions of products marketed under the act do not
receive formal evaluation or approval from the Food
and Drug Administration.

In compiling this section, the publisher has emphasized the necessity of describing products comprehensively. The descriptions seen here include all information made available by the manufacturer. The
publisher does not warrant or guarantee any product
described here, and does not perform any independent analysis of the information provided. Inclusion of
a product in this book does not represent an endorsement, and the publisher does not necessarily advocate the use of any product listed.

A&Z Pharmaceutical Inc.
180 OSER AVENUE, SUITE 300
HAUPPAUGE, NY 11788

Direct Inquiries to:
(631) 952-3800

D-CAL™
(A & Z Pharmaceutical)
Calcium Supplement with Vitamin D
Chewable Caplets

Ingredients: Calcium Carbonate, Vitamin D, Sorbitol, Flavor, D&C Red #27 Lake, Magnesium Stearate. No sugar, No salt, No lactose, No preservative.

Supplement Facts
Serving Size One Caplet

Each Caplet Contains		% Daily Value
Calcium (as calcium carbonate)	300 mg	30%
Vitamin D	100 IU	25%

Recommended Intake: Take two caplets daily for adult and one caplet for child, or as directed by your physician.

Warnings: KEEP OUT OF REACH OF CHILDREN. Do not accept if safety seal under cap is broken or missing.

Actions: D-Cal™ provides a concentrated form of calcium to help build healthy bones. It contains Vitamin D to help the body absorb calcium. D-Cal™ can also help prevent osteoporosis. It is helpful to pregnant and nursing women, children's growth, and calcium deficiency at all ages.

How Supplied: Bottles of 30 and 60 caplets

Awareness Corporation dba Awareness Life
25 SOUTH ARIZONA PLACE,
SUITE 500
CHANDLER, AZ 85225

Direct Inquiries to:
1-800-69AWARE
Website: http://www.awarenesslife.net

AWARENESS CLEAR™
(Awareness Corporation)

Description: May help with general digestion.*

Ingredients: Proprietary blend of Oregano Leaf, Clove Flowers, Black Walnut Seed Husk, Peppermint Leaf, Nigella, Grapefruit, Winter Melon Seed, Gentian, Hyssop Leaf, Crampbark, Thyme Leaf, Fennel.

Directions: Take 2 capsules a day each morning on an empty stomach, 1–2 hours before eating with 1 glass of water

Warnings: Do not use if Pregnant or Breastfeeding. Keep out of reach of children.

How Supplied: 90 Vegetarian Capsules per Bottle

*These statements have not been evaluated by the Food and Drug Administration. These products are not intended to diagnose, treat, cure, or prevent any disease.
Shown in Product Identification Guide, page 503

DAILY COMPLETE®
(Awareness Corporation)

Description: Liquid Supplement. 100% vegetarian ingredients delivers 211 vitamins, minerals, antioxidants, enzymes, fruits and vegetables, amino acids and herbs, in one ounce liquid a day (great orange taste) Helps to Provide Energy & Reduce Stress Levels*.

Ingredients: Rich in Vitamins & Minerals, Ionic Plant Minerals, Botanical Antioxidants with Phenalgin™, 32 Fruit & Vegetable Whole Juice Complex, Whole Superfood Green complex, 34 Mediterranean Herbs, Essential Fatty Acid Complex, Special Ocean Vegetable Blend

Directions: Take 1 ounce (30 ml) per day, during or immediately after a meal

Warnings: Do not use if pregnant or breast-feeding. Keep out of reach of children.

How Supplied: 30 ounces per Bottle, Clinically Tested Ingredients.
Shown in Product Identification Guide, page 502

EXPERIENCE®
(Awareness Corporation)

Description: Promotes Regularity & Cleanses the Colon*

Ingredients: Proprietary Blend of Senna, Blonde Psyllium Seed Husk, Fennel Seed, Cornsilk, Solomon's seal, Rhubarb Root, Kelp

Directions: Take 1 to 2 Capsules before bedtime with a full glass of water.

Warnings: Do not use if pregnant or breast-feeding or if you have colitis. Keep out of reach of children

How Supplied: 90 Capsules per bottle, Clinically tested

PURE GARDENS CREAM®
(Awareness Corporation)

Description: Natural botanical cream may help to improve appearance of dry skin, fine lines and helps to tone the skin.

Ingredients: Apple oil, vitamin C, vitamin E, Aloe Vera Leaf, Almond Oil, Cold Press Virgin Olive Oil, Sesame Oil, Chamomile Flowers Oil, Calendula Officinalis Oil, Beeswax, Jojoba Oil, Linseed Oil.

Directions: Application for both face and body. External use only

How Supplied: 2 ounce jar, Clinically tested

PURETRIM™ MEDITERRANEAN WELLNESS SHAKE
(Awareness Corporation)

Description: Vegetarian Natural Wholefood High Protein Low Carb Energy Shake. No Dairy, No Soy

Ingredients: Vegetable Pea & Brown Rice Protein, Antioxidants, Prebiotics, Essential Fatty Acids & Enzyme Active Greens

Directions: Mix contents in 10 oz. of cold water.

Warnings: Not for use by pregnant or lactating women. Must be 18 years or older to use.

How Supplied: 10 Packets (Net Wt 500 g)
Shown in Product Identification Guide, page 502

SYNERGYDEFENSE® CAPSULES
(Awareness Corporation)

Description: Improves Digestion, Boosts the Immune System, & strengthens the body's natural defenses*.

Ingredients: Proprietary Blend of Enzymes, Probiotics, Antioxidants, Prebiotics

Directions: Take 1 capsule with a glass of water during or before your largest meal of the day. Take once or twice a daily.

Warnings: Do not use if pregnant or lactating. If under 18, consult a physician before use.

How Supplied: 30 Vegetarian Capsules individually sealed

*These statements have not been evaluated by the Food and Drug Administration. These products are not intended to diagnose, treat, cure, or prevent any disease.

Beach Pharmaceuticals
DIVISION OF BEACH
PRODUCTS, INC.
EXECUTIVE OFFICE:
5220 SOUTH MANHATTAN AVENUE
TAMPA, FL 33611

Direct Inquiries to:
Richard Stephen Jenkins, Executive V.P.
(813) 839-6565
Clete Harmon, Sr. V.P., Regulatory and
Business Affairs
(864) 277-7282

Manufacturing and Distribution:
1700 Perimeter Road
Greenville, SC 29605
(800) 845-8210

BEELITH TABLETS
(Beach)
**magnesium supplement with
pyridoxine HCl**

Description: Each tablet contains magnesium oxide 600 mg and pyridoxine hydrochloride (Vitamin B_6) 25 mg equivalent to Vitamin B_6 20 mg.

Supplement Facts
Serving Size: 1 Tablet

	Amount Per Tablet	% Daily Value
Vitamin B_6 (pyridoxine HCl)	20 mg	1000%
Magnesium (from magnesium oxide)	362 mg	90%

Inactive Ingredients: FD&C Yellow No. 6, hydroxypropyl methylcellulose, magnesium stearate, microcrystalline cellulose, polyethylene glycol, sodium starch glycolate, titanium dioxide.
May also contain D&C Yellow No. 10, FD&C Yellow No. 5 (Tartrazine), hydroxypropyl cellulose, polydextrose, stearic acid and/or triacetin.

Indications: As a dietary supplement for patients with magnesium and/or Vitamin B_6 deficiencies resulting from malnutrition, alcoholism, magnesium depleting drugs, chemotherapy, and inadequate nutritional intake or absorption. Also, increases urinary magnesium levels.

Dosage: One tablet daily or as directed by a physician.

Warnings: Do not take this product if you are presently taking a prescription drug without consulting your physician or other health professional. If you have kidney disease, take only under the supervision of a physician. Excessive dosage may cause laxation. If pregnant or breast-feeding, ask a health professional before use.

KEEP OUT OF THE REACH OF CHILDREN.

How Supplied: Golden yellow, film-coated tablet with the letters **BP** and the number **132** imprinted on each tablet. Packaged in bottles of 100 (Item No. 0486-1132-01) tablets.

Beutlich LP, Pharmaceuticals
1541 SHIELDS DRIVE
WAUKEGAN, IL 60085-8304

Direct Inquiries to:
(847) 473-1100
(800) 238-8542 in the U.S. and Canada
M-Th: 7:30 a.m. - 4:00 p.m. CT
FAX: (847) 473-1122
http://www.beutlich.com
E-mail: beutilich@beutlich.com

PERIDIN-C®
(Beutlich LP)
Vitamin C Supplement
Dietary supplement helps alleviate hot flashes by improving capillary strength and maintaining vascular integrity, reducing the physiologic potential for flushing.[*]
Suggested Use for Hot Flashes[*] - 2 tablets, 3 times per day after meals. Reduce servings gradually after one month until effective daily intake is determined.

Ingredients:
Vitamin C (as ascorbic acid) – 200 mg.
Natural Citrus Bioflavonoids Complex (as Hesperidin Complex standardized to contain 45% total bioflavonoids) – 150 mg.
Natural Citrus Bioflavonoid (as Hesperidin Methyl Chalcone) – 50 mg.

Other ingredients: hypromellose, microcrystalline cellulose, crospovidone, stearic acid, polydextrose, titanium dioxide, yellow 6 lake, polyethylene glycol, magnesium stearate, silicon dioxide, triacetin, carnauba wax and polysorbate 80.

How Supplied:
Bottles of 100 tablets – Product # 0283-0597-01

[*]This statement has not been evaluated by the Food and Drug Administration. This product is not intended to diagnose, treat, cure or prevent any disease.

Dannmarie, LLC
2005 PALMER AVENUE, #200
LARCHMONT, NY 10538

Direct Inquiries to:
Phone: (877) 425-8767
http://www.premcal.com
info@premcal.com

PREMCAL
(Dannmarie)

Description: PremCal is a combination calcium and vitamin D nutritional supplement. PremCal is indicated in those requiring higher than the currently recommended doses of vitamin D such as vitamin D deficiency, premenstrual syndrome, osteoporosis, osteomalacia or malabsorption.

Ingredients: PremCal tablets are supplied in 3 different strengths of vitamin D3 (Light- 500 IU; Regular- 1000 IU; Extra strength -2000 IU) with a constant amount of calcium 500 mg as calcium carbonate and 15 mg of magnesium oxide. Each tablet also contains hypromellose, croscarmellose sodium, malto dextrin, povidone, stearic acid, magnesium stearate, triacetin, polyethylene glycol, silicon dioxide. Free of sugar, soy, wheat, gluten, corn, shellfish, and artificial colors.

Directions: One tablet two times a day with meals or as recommended by your physician.

Warnings: Do not take more than two tablets per day unless directed by your physician. Do not use with prolonged or intense exposure to sunlight unless directed by your physician. Do not use if you have a calcium disorder such as primary hyperparathyroidism, hypercalciuria, elevated calcium levels, kidney stones or kidney disease without consulting your physician.

How Supplied: PremCal Light, Regular and Extra strength are supplied in bottles of 180 tablets. UPC#8-80569-00013-6 (PremCal-Light):UPC#8-80569-00010-5 (PremCal-Regular): UPC#8-80569 00016-7 (PremCal-Extra strength).

Eniva Nutraceutics
9702 ULYSSES STREET NE
MINNEAPOLIS, MN 55434

Direct Inquiries:
Phone: 763-795-8870
Fax: 763-795-8890
www.eniva.com

EFACOR™
(Eniva Nutraceutics)
**Omega-3 Essential Fatty
Acids - Dietary Supplement
(Concentrated EPA and DHA)**

Description: ENIVA EFACOR™ provides pharmaceutical-grade potency and purity in a specialized, natural Omega-3 EFA dietary supplement containing high-dose EPA and DHA. Its formula provides these strongly researched substances with a synergistic blend of other Omega-3 derivatives in a pleasant tasting lemon-lime softgel. Manufactured under strict

Continued on next page

Efacor—Cont.

GMP standards, EFACOR™ is ultra-pure and free of environmental contaminants.

Uses:

Omega-3s, especially EPA and DHA, have been shown to support:
- Cardiovascular Function*
- Neurologic Function and Mood*
- Immune and Joint Function *
- Vision and Ocular Function *
- Weight Management and Skin*†

ENIVA EFACOR™ (2 gelcaps) meets the American Heart Association's (AHA) recommendation of providing 1,000 mg of EPA and DHA daily for cardiovascular health and the FDA's requirement for supporting the statement: Daily intake of Omega-3 in the form of EPA and DHA may reduce the risk of coronary heart disease. FDA evaluated the data and determined that, although there is scientific evidence supporting the claim, the evidence is not conclusive.

---

* This statement has not been evaluated by the Food and Drug Administration. This product is not intended to diagnose, treat, cure, or prevent any disease.
† Along with a proper diet and exercise.

Supplement Facts

Serving Size: 2 Softgels
Servings Per Container: 30

	Amount Per Serving	% Daily Value*
Calories (energy)	20	
Calories From Fat	20	
Total Fat	2 g	3%
Saturated Fat	0 g	0%
Polyunsaturated Fat	1.5 g	†
Monounsaturated Fat	0 g	†
Cholesterol	0 mg	0%
Omega-3 Fatty Acids	1,120 mg	†
EPA (Eicosapentaenoic Acid)	680 mg	†
DHA (Docosahexaenoic Acid)	340 mg	†
Other Omega-3s (includes DPA/ETA)	100 mg	†

* Percent Daily Values are based on a 2,000 calorie diet.
† Daily Values not established.

Ingredients: Ingredients: Highly refined and concentrated omega-3 fish oil, capsule (gelatin, glycerin and purified water), natural lemon and lime flavor, proprietary antioxidant blend (consisting of rosemary extract, ascorbyl palmitate and natural tocopherols).

Dosing: Adult Directions: Two softgels daily, preferably 10 minutes before a meal.
Children (4+) Directions: One softgel daily.

Safety Information: As with all dietary supplements, contact your doctor before use, especially if you are pregnant or lactating, suspect a medical condition or are taking prescription drugs. Do not consume if you are allergic to fish, fish components or any substance in the ingredient listing. Although ENIVA EFACOR™ is manufactured from natural and safe pharmaceutical-grade ingredients, rare sensitivity may develop; should this occur, discontinue use. ENIVA EFACOR™ is not habit forming. Keep this and all dietary supplements out of the reach of children.

How Supplied: Vegetable gel capsule – translucent yellow. Capsule can be bitten to access liquid if person has difficulty swallowing capsule. Lemon-lime flavor. Bottle of 60 softgel capsules. Bottle opens with a tear-off, tamper-resistant plastic cap and contains an inner safety seal. Do not consume if seals are not secure.

Storage: Best if refrigerated upon receipt and after opening. Avoid freezing and excessive heat.

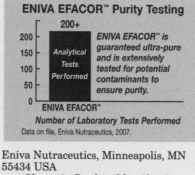

ENIVA EFACOR™ Purity Testing

ENIVA EFACOR™ is guaranteed ultra-pure and is extensively tested for potential contaminants to ensure purity.

Number of Laboratory Tests Performed
Data on file, Eniva Nutraceutics, 2007.

Eniva Nutraceutics, Minneapolis, MN 55434 USA
Shown in Product Identification Guide, page 503

VIBE®
(Eniva Nutraceutics)
Liquid Multi-Nutrient Supplement

Description: Leading medical researchers and clinicians recommend individuals ingest a multi-nutrient dietary supplement on a daily basis. The Eniva VIBE® liquid nutraceutical not only meets medical recommendations in terms of nutrient content, but it has been specifically formulated for rapid absorption and bioavailability due to the predigested nature of its pharmaceutical-grade liquid contents.

Uses/Mechanism: Due to the predigested nature of the vitamins and minerals in the VIBE® nutraceutical, nutrient absorption and cellular bioavailability of nutrients appear to be enhanced. This results in the support of body structure and function.* Through mechanisms not fully elucidated, the antioxidant capacity of VIBE® appears to have an impact on free radicals and their associated metabolism.*

- Scientific evidence suggests consumption of antioxidant vitamins may reduce the risk of certain forms of cancer. However, FDA has determined this evidence is limited and not conclusive.
- As part of a well-balanced diet that is low in saturated fat and cholesterol, Folic Acid, Vitamin B6 and B12 may reduce the risk of vascular disease. However, the FDA has determined this evidence is limited and not conclusive.

Supplement Facts

Serving Size: 1 Fluid Ounce
Servings Per Container: 32

	Amount Per Serving	% Daily Value
Calories	30	
Total Carbohydrate	6 g	2%**
Sugars	4 g	†
Vitamin A	2,000 IU	40%
Vitamin C	120 mg	200%
Vitamin D	500 IU	125%
Vitamin E	30 IU	100%
Thiamin Vitamin B1	1.5 mg	100%
Riboflavin Vitamin B2	1.7 mg	100%
Niacin	18 mg	90%
Vitamin B6	2 mg	100%
Folic Acid	400 mcg	100%
Vitamin B12	12 mcg	200%
Biotin	300 mcg	100%
Pantothenic Acid	10 mg	100%
Calcium	100 mg	10%
Phosphorus	20 mg	2%
Iodine	150 mcg	100%
Magnesium	155 mg	39%
Zinc	5 mg	33%
Selenium	25 mcg	36%
Copper	.5 mg	25%
Manganese	1.8 mg	90%
Chromium	120 mcg	100%
Potassium	175 mg	5%

Trace Minerals Proprietary Blend	3.0 mg	†

Boron, Germanium, Sulfur, Vanadium

AntiOX2®* Phytonutrient Proprietary Blend	6,500 mg	†

Natural Extracts: Cranberry, Raspberry, Blueberry, Blackberry, Strawberry, Cherry, Carrot, Acai Berry, Elderberry, Hibiscus (flower), Lemon, Lime, Apple, Orange, Blackcurrant, Oregano, Chokeberry, Grape, Pumpkin, Tomato, Pomegranate, Wolfberry (gojiberry), Stevia (leaf), Grape Seed Extract; Citrus Bioflavonoids

HeartPRO™* Proprietary Blend	280 mg	†

D-Ribose, CoQ10, L-Carnitine, Malic Acid, Isolated Lecithin, Mixed Tocopherols

CollaMAX®*   3,500 mg †
Proprietary Blend
Green Tea Leaf Extract (water
decaffeinated), L-Lysine, L-Proline, Aloe
Vera Gel, Glucosamine HCl (vegetable),
Glycine, Alanine, Valine, Isoleucine,
Leucine

** Percent Daily Values are based on a
2,000 calorie diet.
† Daily Value not established.

Ingredients: Ingredients: Purified water, natural extracts and flavors (from
blackberry, and/or apple, and/or chokeberry, and/or elderberry, and/or blueberry,
and/or blackcurrant, and/or stevia [leaf],
and/or oregano, and/or tomato, and/or
hibiscus, and/or carrot, and/or pumpkin,
and/or cherry, and/or grape, and/or
cranberry, and/or green tea leaf extract
[water decaffeinated], and/or lemon, and/
or lime, and/or aloe vera gel, and/or grape
seed extract, and/or pomegranate, and/or
wolfberry [gojiberry], and/or acai berry,
and/or strawberry, and/or raspberry, and/
or orange), natural sugars (beet and/or
molasses), magnesium (from magnesium
citrate, and/or magnesium malate, and/or
magnesium sulfate, and/or magnesium
glycerophosphate, and/or magnesium
chloride), citric acid, malic acid, potassium (from potassium citrate, and/or potassium chloride, and/or potassium
iodide, and/or potassium lactate), calcium
(from calcium citrate, and/or calcium
malate, and/or calcium chloride, and/or
calcium glycerophosphate), ascorbic acid,
l-lysine, l-proline, d-alpha-tocopherol
acetate (with mixed tocopherols), sorbic
and/or benzoic acid(s) (protect freshness),
d-ribose, niacin, zinc (from zinc sulfate,
and/or zinc chloride), l-carnitine
fumarate, calcium panthothenate, boron
(sodium borate), glucosamine hcl
(vegetable), vitamin A palmitate, natural
gums (arabic, xanthan, guar), folic acid,
manganese (from manganous chloride,
and/or manganese sulfate), pyridoxine
hcl, riboflavin phosphate, thiamin hcl,
copper (from copper sulfate, and/or
copper gluconate), cholecalciferol, isolated soy lecithin, chromium (from
chromium chloride), biotin, sorbimacro-
gol, CoQ10 (ubidecarenone), vegetable
glycerin, germanium (from germanium
sesquioxide), selenium (from sodium selenate, and/or selenium chloride),
vanadium (from vanadyl sulfate), cyanocobalamin, and/or n-methyl-cobalamin.
May contain rosemarinic acid.

• No Stimulants
• No Artificial Colors
• No Artificial Flavors
• VIBE® is a Decaffeinated Product
• Vegetarian Friendly
• No Fish Ingredients

Dosing: Adult: Ingest 1-2 ounces daily.
Do not exceed 3 ounces per day. For best
results, ingest half dose in the a.m. hours
and the other half in p.m. hours, unless
otherwise directed by a physician.

Safety Information: As with all dietary
supplements, contact your doctor before
use, especially if you are pregnant or lac-

tating, suspect a medical condition or are
taking prescription drugs. Do not consume if you are allergic to any substance
in the ingredient listing. Although Eniva
VIBE® is manufactured from natural and
safe pharmaceutical-grade ingredients,
rare sensitivity may develop; should this
occur, discontinue use. Eniva VIBE® is
not habit forming. Keep this and all
dietary supplements out of the reach of
children.

Storage: Keep refrigerated upon receipt
and after opening. Avoid freezing and excessive heat. Due to natural contents,
product should be consumed within 40
days after opening. It is normal and ex-
pected with natural extracts and ingredients some settling may occur. Shake well
before using.

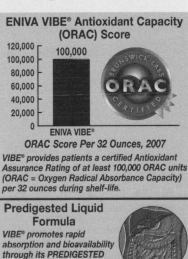

**ENIVA VIBE® Antioxidant Capacity
(ORAC) Score**

ORAC Score Per 32 Ounces, 2007
*VIBE® provides patients a certified Antioxidant
Assurance Rating of at least 100,000 ORAC units
(ORAC = Oxygen Radical Absorbance Capacity)
per 32 ounces during shelf-life.*

**Predigested Liquid
Formula**
*VIBE® promotes rapid
absorption and bioavailability
through its PREDIGESTED
LIQUID formula to support
proper body function.**

**ENIVA VIBE® Certified Safety
Assurance Testing**
• *Heavy Metals*
• *Pesticides / Herbicides*
• *Full Microbiologic, Including Mold & Yeast*
• *Fungal Toxin Screen (mycotoxin)*
• *Allergen & Food Additive Screening*
• *GMO Testing*
Data on file, Eniva Nutraceutics, 2007.

ENIVA VIBE® Quality Testing
• *Ingredient Potency Testing & Verification*
• *Antioxidant ORAC Analysis*
• *Shelf-Life Stability*
• *Biomass Assays*
• *Particle Size Analysis*
Data on file, Eniva Nutraceutics, 2007.

* This statement has not been evaluated
by the Food and Drug Administration.
This product is not intended to diagnose,
treat, cure, or prevent any disease.

Eniva Nutraceutics, Minneapolis, MN
55434 USA
*Shown in Product Identification
Guide, page 503*

4Life Research
9850 S. 300 W
SANDY, UT 84070

Direct Inquiries to:
Ph: (801) 562-3600
Fax: (801) 562-3699
Email: productsupport@4life.com
Website: www.4life.com

4LIFE TRANSFER FACTOR PLUS®
TRI-FACTOR™ FORMULA

Description: Transfer factors are small
peptides of approximately 44 amino acids
that "transfer" cell-mediated immunity
from immune donors to non-immune recipients. 4Life Transfer Factor® products
are derived from egg yolk and cow
colostrum extracts that contain antigen
information. NanoFactor™ concentrate
contains molecules smaller than transfer
factors, stimulating T-Cell activity and
providing additional immune information
to non-immune recipients. Combined,
these compounds comprise the Tri-Factor
Formula, which offers the broadest
spectrum immune support available. The
extraction of 4Life Transfer Factor is
protected by US patents 6,468,534;
6,866,868; with other patents pending.
NanoFactor Technology has several patents pending.
Transfer Factor and NanoFactor educate
the immune system to recognize self
from non-self, thus supporting healthy
immune system balance. Because they in-
struct the immune system to act appro-
priately, these compounds are effective
in supporting normal inflammation response in the body, a key to healthy body
system function.
4Life Transfer Factor Plus Tri-Factor
Formula combines Transfer Factor
E-XF™ and NanoFactor with a proprietary formulation of innate and adaptive
immune system enhancers such as
Inositol Hexaphosphate, Cordyceps, Beta
Glucans, Maitake and Shiitake Mush-
rooms. These ingredients work together
to trigger and enhance the various
immune protective mechanisms of the
body. Clinical studies show that 4Life
Transfer Factor Plus Tri-Factor Formula
can increase Natural Killer cell activity up
to 437 percent above baseline,* and that
NanoFactor stimulates T-Cell activity to
improve the immune system's ability to
stay in balance.

*Blind Independent study conducted by
Dr. Anatoli Vorobiev, Head of Immunology,
at the Russian Academy of Medical
Science.

Summary of Research: In 1949
transfer factors were discovered by Dr.
H. Sherwood Lawrence. Since that time
hundreds of studies have been completed
involving the effect of transfer factors on

Continued on next page

4Life Transfer Factor Plus—Cont.

various diseases. Due to new studies conducted in Russia, the Russian Health Ministry has approved 4Life Transfer Factor and 4Life Transfer Factor Plus to be the first supplements used by doctors and hospitals in Russia. Many of these studies and papers can be accessed through PubMed or other clinical study portals.

NanoFactor research is currently in the forefront of immune science. Scientists have long known that molecules, smaller than transfer factors, existed in colostrum extract but there was no evidence to suggest immune activity. Advanced technology in filtration and testing has enabled 4Life scientists to extract these molecules, test them, and determine their immune activity, specifically an increase in ATP among T-helper cells and cytotoxic T-cells.

Recommended Dose: 600mg Tri-Factor Formula daily. If used in combination with other immune ingredients, such as Transfer Factor Plus Tri-Factor Formula, less may be taken. No toxicity level of Tri-Factor has been found.

4Life Transfer Factor® Products Include:

4Life Transfer Factor® Tri-Factor™ Formula

4Life Transfer Factor Plus® Tri-Factor™ Formula

4Life Transfer Factor® RioVida™ Tri-Factor Formula

4Life provides Targeted Transfer Factor® products to support the following structures and functions of the body: heart, endocrine, male prostate, women's breast and gynecologic, brain and memory health.

Greek Island Labs

**7620 E. MCKELLIPS ROAD
SUITE 4 PMB 86
SCOTTSDALE, AZ 85257**

Direct Inquiries to:
Website: http://www.greekislandlabs.com
(888) 841-7363

**NATURALJOINT™
(Greek Island Labs)**
dietary supplement

Description: Natural Dietary Supplement that Promotes Healthy Joints Supports Flexibility & Mobility*

Ingredients: Proprietary Greek Blend of 37 Natural Ingredients

Directions: 1 Capsules daily with meal

Warnings: Keep out of reach of children. Consult your doctor prior to using this product if you are taking any prescription medication

How Supplied: 30 Capsules (Vegetarian) Per Box

*The statements have not been reviewed or approved by the Food & Drug Administration. This product is not intended to diagnose, treat, cure or prevent any disease

Mannatech, Inc.

**600 S. ROYAL LANE
SUITE 200
COPPELL, TX 75019**

Direct Inquiries to:
Customer Service
(972) 471-8111
https://www.mannatech.com/Country.aspx

**ADVANCED AMBROTOSE™
(Mannatech)
A Glyconutritional Dietary Supplement**

Supplement Facts:

**Advanced Ambrotose™ powder:
Serving Size: 1 scoop (670 mg) mixed with 8 fluid oz. water or juice twice daily
Powder canister: 75g or 150g**

Amount Per Serving	% Daily Value
670 mg	*

*Daily Value not established

**Advanced Ambrotose™ capsules:
Serving Size: two capsules (.67g active components) twice daily
Capsules per container: 120**

Amount Per Serving	% Daily Value
2 capsules	*

*Daily Value not established

Ingredients:

Advanced Ambrotose™ powder
Arabinogalactan (from *Larix* spp. Wood), Aloe Vera (inner leaf gel powder), Rice Starch, Ghatti Gum, Gum Tragacanth, Glucosamine HCl (vegetarian), Wakame (*Undaria pinnatifida*) Algae Extract

Advanced Ambrotose™ capsules
Arabinogalactan (from *Larix* spp. Wood), Aloe Vera (inner leaf gel powder), Rice Starch, Ghatti Gum, Gum Tragacanth, Glucosamine HCl (vegetarian), Wakame (*Undaria pinnatifida*) Algae Extract
Other ingredients: Vegetable capsules, vegetable stearic acid
For additional information on ingredients, visit www.glycoscience.org

Use: Advanced Ambrotose™ is designed to support effective cell-to-cell communication. This stabilized preparation contains a high proportion of very high-molecular-weight polysaccharides, which are responsible for the immune stimulation properties of aloe.**

Directions: The recommended intake of Advanced Ambrotose™ powder is 1 scoop

(670 mg) mixed with 8 fluid oz. water or juice twice daily; the recommended intake of Advanced Ambrotose™ capsules is two capsules twice daily. If desired, consumers may begin by taking less than the recommended intake. If well tolerated, the consumer may gradually increase to the recommended intake. The amount needed by each individual may vary with time, age, genetic makeup, metabolic rate and activities, stress level, current dietary intake, and health challenges of the moment. A health care professional experienced with the use of Advanced Ambrotose™ complex may be helpful.

Warning: Anyone who is taking medication may wish to advise his/her physician about the use of any dietary supplements. **KEEP BOTTLE TIGHTLY CLOSED. STORE IN A COOL, DRY PLACE.**

How Supplied: Bottle of 75g or 150g powder. Bottle of 120 capsules.

**This statement has not been evaluated by the Food and Drug Administration. This product is not intended to diagnose, treat, cure or prevent any disease.
Mannatech Inc.
600 S. Royal Lane, Suite 200
Coppell, Texas 75019
https://www.mannatech.com/Country.aspx
Shown in Product Identification Guide, page 503

**AMBROTOSE®
(Mannatech)
A Glyconutritional Dietary Supplement**

Supplement Facts:

**Ambrotose® powder:
Serving Size 0.44 g (approx. ¼ teaspoon)
Powder canister: 100g**

Amount Per Serving	% Daily Value
0.44g	*

*Daily Value not established.

**Ambrotose® capsules:
Serving Size: one capsule (2 times daily)
Capsules per container: 60**

Amount Per Serving	% Daily Value
1 capsule	*

*Daily Value not established.

Ingredients:

**Ambrotose® Powder
Ambrotose® complex**
(Internationally patented)
Arabinogalactan (Larix *decidua*) (gum), rice starch, Manapol® aloe vera gel extract (inner leaf gel), gum ghatti, Glucosamine HCl, and gum tragacanth.

Ambrotose® capsules
Ambrotose® complex
(Internationally patented)
Arabinogalactan (Larix *decidua*) (gum), aloe vera (inner leaf gel), gum ghatti and gum tragacanth.
Other ingredients: Brown rice flour, silicon dioxide, stearic acid, gelatin.
For additional information on ingredients, visit www.glycoscience.org

Use: Ambrotose® complex is a proprietary formula designed to help provide saccharides used in glycoconjugate synthesis to promote cellular communication and immune support.** Consumers who are healthy may notice improved concentration, more energy, better sleep, improved athletic performance, and a greater sense of well-being.

Directions: The recommended intake of Ambrotose® powder is ¼ teaspoon two times a day; the recommended intake of Ambrotose® capsules is one capsule two times daily. If desired, you may begin by taking less than the recommended intake. If well tolerated, you may gradually increase to the recommended intake. Children between the ages of 12 and 48 months with growth/nutritional problems (failure to thrive) have been given 1 tablespoon a day of Ambrotose powder for 3 months with no adverse effects. The amount needed by each individual may vary with time, age, genetic makeup, metabolic rate, and activities, stress level, current dietary intake, and health challenges of the moment. A health care professional experienced with use of Ambrotose complex may be helpful.

Warning: Anyone who is taking medication may wish to advise his/her physician. One teaspoon of Ambrotose® powder (equivalent to approximately 12 Ambrotose® capsules) contains the amount of glucose equivalent to 1/25 teaspoon of sucrose (table sugar)
KEEP BOTTLE TIGHTLY CLOSED. STORE IN A COOL, DRY PLACE.

How Supplied: Bottle of 3.50 oz (100g) powder. Bottle of 60 (150mg) capsules.
** This statement has not been evaluated by the Food and Drug Administration. This product is not intended to diagnose, treat, cure or prevent any disease.

Mannatech Inc.
600 S. Royal Lane, Suite 200
Coppell, Texas 75019
https://www.mannatech.com/country.asp
Shown in Product Identification Guide, page 503

AMBROTOSE AO™
(Mannatech)
[ăm-brō-tōs]
Glyco-Antioxidant Supplement

[See table above]
For additional information on ingredients, Visit www.glycoscience.org

Use: Ambrotose AO™ capsules help protect both water and fat soluble portions of cells from free radical attacks

Supplement Facts:
Serving Size - 1 Capsule

	Amount Per Serving	% Daily Value
Vitamin E (as mixed d-alpha-, d-beta, d-delta and d-gamma tocopherols)	18 IU	60%
Mtech AO Blend®	113mg	
Quercetin dihydrate		*
Grape pomace extract		*
Green tea extract (leaf)		*
Australian Bush Plum (Terminalia ferdinandiana) (fruit)		*
Ambrotose Phyto Formula®	331mg	
Gum Arabic		*
Xanthan Gum		*
Gum Tragacanth		*
Gum Ghatti		*
Aloe vera (inner leaf gel powder)		*
Phyt•Aloe® Complex		*
Broccoli (flower/stalk), Brussels sprout (aerial part), Cabbage (leaf), Carrot (root), Cauliflower (flower/stalk), Garlic (bulb), Kale (leaf), Onion (bulb), Tomato (fruit), Turnip (root), Papaya (fruit), Pineapple juice powder (fruit)		

Other Ingredients: Vegetable capsule

---

*Daily value not established.

---

while supporting your immune system.** Defend your health by supporting overall immune function through the natural glyconutrients in Ambrotose™ phytoformula.** Protect against the daily onslaught of toxins, poor food, stress and the environment, all of which contribute to the increase in free radicals that can accelerate the aging process.**

** **This statement has not been evaluated by the Food and Drug Administration. This product is not intended to diagnose, treat, cure or prevent any disease.**

Directions: The recommended intake of Ambrotose AO™ capsules is one capsule two times daily.

Oxygen Radical Absorption Capacity (ORAC) can be used to assess the antioxidant status of human blood and serum. One recent study reported that increasing fruit and vegetable consumption from the usual five to an experimental ten servings per day over two weeks can increase serum ORAC values by roughly 13%.[1] In an open-label pilot study of 12 healthy human volunteers, the antioxidant effects of increasing amounts of supplementation with Ambrotose AO™ were evaluated. A battery of tests was selected in order to assess both oxidative damage and protection. Independent companies were contracted to conduct blood and urine chemistry tests and statistical data analyses. An increase in $ORAC_{\beta-PE}$, a measure of oxidative protection, was found at all three doses: 19.1% at 500 mg per day, 37.4% at 1.0 g per day, and 14.3% at 1.5 g per day. A trend of decreased urinary lipid hydroperoxides/creatinine, a marker of oxidative damage, was observed as well. No significant trends were found in regard to urinary alkenal or 8-OHdG levels.[2] Thus, over the same time period, 1.0 g per day of Ambrotose AO™ provided over twice the antioxidant protection (37.4%) provided by 5 servings of fruits and vegetables (13%).

1. Cao G; Booth SL; Sadowski JA; Prior RL;. Increases in human plasma antioxidant capacity after consumption of controlled diets high in fruit and vegetables. *Am J Clin Nutr.* 1998 Nov; 68: 1081-1087.
2. Boyd S, Gary K, Koepke CM, et al. An open-label pilot study of the antioxidant activity in humans of Ambrotose AO™: Results. *GlycoScience & Nutrition (Official Publication of GlycoScience.org: The Nutrition Science Site).* 2003;4(6).
   Shown in Product Identification Guide, page 503

PLUS
(Mannatech)
Herbal-Amino Acid Dietary Supplement

Supplement Facts:
Serving Size - 1 Caplet (3 times daily)

	Amount Per Serving	% Daily Value
Iron	1mg	5
Wild Yam (root) Standardized for 25mg Phytosterols	200mg	*
L-Glutamic acid	200mg	*
L-Glycine	200mg	*
L-Lysine	200mg	*
L-Arginine	100mg	*

Continued on next page

Plus—Cont.

Boron	3mg	*
Beta Sitosterol	25mg	*
Ambrotose®	2.5mg	*

Complex
(patent pending)
Arabinogalactan (Larix decidua) (gum), Aloe vera (inner leaf gel powder), gum ghatti and gum tragacanth.

Other Ingredients: Microcrystalline cellulose, stearic acid, croscarmellose sodium, silicon dioxide, magnesium stearate, coating.

---

*Daily value not established.

For additional information on ingredients, visit www.glycoscience.org

Use: PLUS caplets provide nutrients to help support the endocrine system's natural production and balance of hormones.** A well-functioning endocrine system works in harmony with the body's immune system, helps support the efficient metabolism of fat, and supports natural recovery from physical or emotional stress.** The nutritional components of PLUS caplets are wild yam extract, amino acids, and beta sitosterol. PLUS caplets contain no hormones.

Directions: The recommended intake of PLUS caplets is one caplet three times daily.
**KEEP BOTTLE TIGHTLY CLOSED.
STORE IN A COOL, DRY PLACE.**

How Supplied: Bottle of 90 caplets.

** This statement has not been evaluated by the Food and Drug Administration. This product is not intended to diagnose, treat, cure or prevent any disease.

Shown in Product Identification Guide, page 503

Mayor Pharmaceutical Laboratories

**2401 S. 24TH STREET
PHOENIX, AZ 85034**

Direct Inquiries to:
Medical Director
(602)-244-8899
www.VitaMist.com

VITAMIST®   **OTC**
INTRA-ORAL SPRAY
Nutraceuticals/Dietary Supplements

Product Overview: **Multi-Vitamin Formulations:** VitaMist is available in 5 unique multivitamin formulations, each designed for the needs of a specific population grouping – Multiple, for the general adult propulation; Pre-Natal, for pregnant and lactating mothers and for anyone considering pregnancy; Children's Multiple, for children aged 4 – 12; Women's Health and Men's Formula, for adult women and men.

Anti-Oxidant: a unique blend of antioxidant vitamins A, C, and E together with grape seed extract, lycopene and lutein, to fight the damaging effects of free radicals.

ArthriFlex: a great tasting and powerful combination of glucosamine together with vitamins C and D, and the minerals calcium, manganese, and boron.

C+Zinc / Cold Weather Formula: unique spray formulation delivering zinc, vitamins C and E and the amino acid lysine.

D-Stress: multi-herbal formula with additional B-complex vitamins.

Heart Healthy / Folacin: with folic acid, vitamin B6 and vitamin B12. Medical research has demonstrated that these three vitamins can reduce blood levels of homocysteine, an indicator of coronary artery disease.

Immune / Echinacea+G: ease your sore throat with the great, soothing taste of honey and lemon, while providing Echinacea, goldenseal, vitamin E, and garlic extract.

ReVitalizer: for that energy boost when you need it fast. An enhanced multivitamin formulation with B-complex vitamins, vitamins A, C, and E, and a proprietary herbal extract.

Sleep: poor sleep affects more than 63 million Americans. VitaMist® "Sleep" offers a safe and effective natural alternative to prescription sleep aids, with melatonin, 5-HTP and amino acids blended with herbal extracts.

B12 / B12-500: B12 deficiency can have far-reaching consequences. VitaMist® offers this spray in two different strengths, 60 micrograms (1000%) and 500 micrograms (8333%).

St. John's Wort: This popular herb is available as a spray with added vitamin B12, ginkgo biloba, and folic acid.

E+Selenium: two important anti-oxidant nutrients with a delicious cotton-candy taste.

VitaSight™: eye-friendly nutrients, including vitamins A, C, and E, together with betacarotene, zinc and more.

Colloidal Minerals: more than 70 trace and essential minerals from natural sources – in a fresh, minty spray.

Smoke-Less™: unique herbal combination with additional nutrients.

PMS and LadyMate: special care for the nutritional needs of women throughout the month.

Slender-Mist®: dietary snack replacements containing a combination of vital nutrients. Available in four different flavors.

Blue-Green Sea Spray: with spirulina extract, omega-3 fatty acids from flaxseed oil, and vitamin E.

Re-Leaf: a natural herbal blend of more than 10 herbs designed to provide relief.

Osteo-CalMag: herbal supplement with added vitamin D, calcium, and magnesium.

Pine Bark and Grape Seed: powerful proanthocyanidins from natural sources in a convenient, easy to use, spray.

Performance 3 / Before, During, After: three performance sprays designed for the needs of physical activity. Use Before your work-out, During your routine, and After, as you cool-down.

CardioCare™: heart smart spray with vitamins C and E, and the amino acids lysine and proline, together with coenzyme Q10.

DHEA: the body's key hormone (dehydroepiandrosterone) in both men's and women's formulations.

GinkgoMist: an herb revered for its memory- and circulatory-enhancing properties. Now available in a spray formulation with vitamin B12, acetyl-L-carnitine, choline, inositol, phosphatidylserine and niacin.

Ex. O.: powerful spray containing a blend of cayenne and peppermint as well as additional herbs reported to aid allergy control.

Description: VitaMist® products are patented intra-oral sprays for the delivery of vitamins, minerals, and other nutritional supplements, directly into the oral cavity. A 55 microliter spray delivers high concentrations of nutrients directly onto the mouth's sensitive tissue. The buccal mucosa transfers the nutrients into the bloodstream. (U.S. Patent 4,525,341 – Foreign patents issued and pending.)

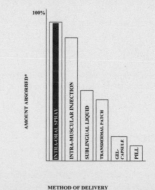

METHOD OF DELIVERY
*Representative of the product class.

Benefits:
• Spray supplementation provides an absorption rate approximately nine times greater than that of pills.

- Once the formula is sprayed into the mouth and swallowed, the nutrients reach the bloodstream within minutes.
- No fillers or binders are added; the body receives only pure ingredients.
- An alternative method of supplementation for those that cannot take pills, or simply do not enjoy swallowing pills.
- Convenient administration; no water needed.

Recommended Dosage: The recommended dosage for all VitaMist® spray dietary supplements is a total of 8 sprays per day (ideally 2 sprays, 4 times per day).

How Supplied: VitaMist® spray dietary supplements are supplied in convenient, easy to use, safety-sealed containers fitted with a natural pump. Each container provides approximately 240 sprays, a 30-day supply. VitaMist® sprays are not pressurized.

Memory Secret
**1221 BRICKELL AVENUE
SUITE 1540
MIAMI, FL 33131**

Direct Inquiries to:
(866) 673-2738
Fax: (305) 675-2279

INTELECTOL® MEMORY ENHANCER (Memory Secret) VINPOCETINE TABLETS MEMORY SECRET

Description: INTELECTOL® is the purest form of Vinpocetine available. Vinpocetine is a derivative of Vincamine, which is extracted from the Periwinkle plant (*Vinca Minor, Vinca Pervinca*). Research suggests that Vinpocetine helps to maintain healthy blood circulation in the brain and supports certain neurotransmitters in the memory process.* Vinpocetine supports and protects brain blood vessel health and aids mental function.*

Directions: As a dietary supplement, take 2 tablets twice daily with meals. Vinpocetine should be taken as part of an on-going regimen with exercise, a healthy diet and keeping active the mind. Do not use if tamper-evident seal is broken.

Cautions: Take product with food to avoid stomach upset. Not recommended for use by pregnant women, nursing mothers or anyone under 18 years old. Consult a doctor or health care professional before use if you have any medical condition or if taking any medication. Not recommended for use by anyone with hemophilia, heart problems or low blood pressure. **Keep out of reach of children.** Store in a cool, dry place.

Supplement Facts
Serving Size 2 tablets
Servings Per Container: 25

	Amount Per Serving	% DV
Vinpocetine (from Periwinkle seed extract)	10 mg	*

*Daily Value not established.
Other Ingredients: Lactose, hydroxypropylcellulose, magnesium stearate and talc.

---

*These statements have not been evaluated by the Food & Drug Administration. This product is not intended to diagnose, treat, cure, or prevent any disease.

Distributed by: The Memory Secret, Inc.
1221 Brickell Ave., Suite 1540, Miami, FL 33131/USA
memorysecret™
www.memorysecret.net
Shown in Product Identification Guide, page 504

Mission Pharmacal Company
**10999 IH 10 WEST, SUITE 1000
SAN ANTONIO, TX 78230-1355**

Direct Inquiries to:
P.O. Box 786099
San Antonio, TX 78278-6099
(800) 292-7364

CALCET® TRIPLE CALCIUM + VITAMIN D (Mission Pharmacal) Dietary Supplement

Description: For low-calcium Leg cramps* and to help reduce the risk of osteoporosis.
*The unique triple calcium formula found in Calcet is recommended by doctors and pharmacists for the relief of leg cramps in pregnancy, leg cramps in athletes and occasional leg cramps people get at night. Calcet is ideal if you need additional calcium to help fight osteoporosis or because of a milk allergy. Regular exercise and a healthy diet with enough calcium helps teens and young adult white and Asian women maintain good bone health and may reduce their high risk of osteoporosis later in life. Adequate calcium intake is important, but daily intakes above about 2,000 mg are not likely to provide any additional benefit.

---

*These statements have not been evaluated by the Food and Drug Administration. This product is not intended to diagnose, treat, cure or prevent any disease.

Supplement Facts
Serving Size: 2 tablets

	Amount Per Serving	% Daily Value
Vitamin D_3 (as cholecalciferol)	200 IU	50%
Calcium (as calcium carbonate, calcium gluconate, calcium lactate)	300 mg	30%

Ingredients: Calcium carbonate, calcium gluconate, calcium lactate, polyethylene glycol, hydroxypropyl methylcellulose, croscarmellose sodium, color added, magnesium stearate, FD & C Yellow 5 lake, magnesium silicate, vitamin D_3.

Directions for Use: Take two tablets at bedtime and two tablets upon waking. Do not exceed 4 tablets a day except on the advice or recommendation of your physician, pharmacist or health professional.

Warnings: KEEP THIS PRODUCT OUT OF THE REACH OF CHILDREN.

How Supplied: 100 coated tablets, UPC 0178-0251-01.
STORE AT ROOM TEMPERATURE.

CITRACAL® CAPLETS
**Calcium Citrate with Vitamin D
Dietary Supplement
(Mission Pharmacal)**

Description: Citracal® helps ensure women will have the strong bones necessary to take on a life filled with activity and ambitions. Regular exercise and a healthy diet with enough calcium helps teen and young adult white and Asian women maintain good bone health and may reduce their high risk of osteoporosis later in life. Adequate calcium intake is important, but daily intakes above about 2,000 mg are not likely to provide any additional benefit.

Serving Size: 2 caplets

	Amount Per Serving	%Daily Value
Vitamin D_3 (as cholecalciferol)	400 IU	100%
Calcium (as calcium citrate)	630 mg	63%

Ingredients: Calcium citrate, polyethylene glycol, croscarmellose sodium, polyvinyl alcohol-part hydrolyzed, color added, magnesium silicate, magnesium stearate, vitamin D_3.

Continued on next page

Citracal Caplets—Cont.

Directions for Use: Take 1 to 2 caplets two times daily or as recommended by your physician, pharmacist, or health professional.

Other Information: STORE AT ROOM TEMPERATURE. KEEP OUT OF THE REACH OF CHILDREN.

How Supplied: 60 coated caplets, UPC 0178-0815-60; 120 coated caplets, UPC 0178-0815-12.

Novartis Consumer Health, Inc.
**200 KIMBALL DRIVE
PARSIPPANY, NJ 07054-0622**

Direct Inquiries to:
Consumer & Professional Affairs
(800) 452-0051
Fax: (800) 635-2801
Or write to the above address

BENEFIBER® FIBER SUPPLEMENT
(Novartis Consumer Health, Inc.)

Description:
Doctors agree that fiber is an important part of a healthy diet. However most people only get half the daily recommended amount of fiber.* Now it's easier than ever to add fiber to your diet with Benefiber®, a 100% natural fiber that you can mix with almost anything. It's
• Taste-free • Grit-free • Non-thickening so it won't alter the taste or texture of your foods or beverages.
Be creative with Benefiber®. Try it in your coffee, juice, yogurt, your baked goods, favorite recipes or whatever you desire. You won't even know it's there!

*The American Dietetic Association recommends a healthy diet include 25-35 grams of fiber a day.

Supplement Facts
Serving Size: 2 tsp (3.5g)

Amount Per Serving	%DV*
Calories 15	
Sodium 0mg	0%
Total Carbohydrate 4g	1%
Dietary Fiber 3g	12%
Soluble Fiber 3g	†
Sugars 0g	†

* Percent Daily Values (DV) are based on a 2,000 calorie diet.
† Daily Value not established.

Ingredients: Wheat dextrin
Gluten Free (less than 10 ppm gluten)

Directions
Stir 2 teaspoons of Benefiber into 4-8 oz. of any beverage or soft food (hot or cold). Stir well until dissolved.
Not recommended for carbonated beverages.

AGE	SERVINGS	
12 yrs. to adult	2 tsp	3 times daily[1]
6 to 11 yrs.	1 tsp	3 times daily[2]
Under 6 yrs.	Ask a doctor before use	

[1] Not to exceed 6 tsp per day
[2] Not to exceed 3 tsp per day
tsp = teaspoon
Keep out of reach of children.
If you are pregnant or nursing a baby, ask a health professional before use.

Tamper Evident Feature: Do Not Use if printed inner seal is broken or missing.

Other Information:
Store at controlled room temperature 20-25°C (68-77°F). Protect from moisture. Use within 6 months of opening.

Questions? Call **1-800-452-0051**
24 hours a day, 7 days a week or visit us at www.Benefiber.com for recipe ideas and additional information.

How Supplied: Available in 2.8 oz (20 Servings), 5.4 oz (38 Servings), 8.6 oz (62 Servings), 12.3 oz (90 Servings), 16.7 oz (125 Servings) and 25.6 oz (190 Servings) bottles.
Shown in Product Identification Guide, page 504

BENEFIBER® CAPLETS
(Novartis Consumer Health, Inc.)
Fiber supplement

Supplement Facts
Serving Size: 3 Caplets

Amount Per Serving	%DV*
Calories 15	
Sodium 0mg	0%
Total Carbohydrate 4g	1%
Dietary Fiber 3g	12%
Soluble Fiber 3g	†
Sugars 0g	†

* Percent Daily Values (DV) are based on a 2,000 calorie diet.
† Daily Value not established.

Ingredients: Wheat dextrin, microcrystalline cellulose, magnesium stearate, colloidal silicon dioxide
Gluten Free (less than 10 ppm gluten)

Directions:
Adults: Take 3 caplets up to 3 times daily to supplement the fiber content of your diet. Swallow with liquid. Do not exceed 9 caplets per day.
Keep out of reach of children.
If you are pregnant or nursing a baby, ask a health professional before use.

Tamper Evident Feature:
Do Not Use if inner seal imprinted with **"SEALED for YOUR PROTECTION"** is broken or missing.

Benefiber® guarantees your satisfaction or your money back.

Questions? Call **1-800-452-0051**
24 hours a day, 7 days a week or visit us at www.benefiber.com for additional information.

Other Information:
Store at controlled room temperature 20-25°C (68–77°F). Protect from excessive heat and moisture.

How Supplied:
Available in 72 ct. and 114 ct. bottles.
Shown in Product Identification Guide, page 504

BENEFIBER® FIBER SUPPLEMENT
**Sugar Free Orange Creme Chewables
Sugar Free Assorted Fruit Chewables
(Novartis Consumer Health, Inc.)**

Benefiber® Chewable Tablets are an easy way to add fiber to your diet. Because there's no need for water or mixing, you can take them virtually anywhere, anytime.

Supplement Facts
Serving Size: 3 Tablets

Amount Per Serving	%DV*
Calories 30	
Sodium 0mg	0%
Total Carbohydrate 8g	1%
Dietary Fiber 3g	12%
Soluble Fiber 3g	†
Sugars 0g	†

*Percent Daily Values (DV) are based on a 2,000 calorie diet.
†Daily Value not established.

Sugar Free Orange Creme Chewables

Ingredients: Wheat dextrin, sorbitol, corn starch, microcrystalline cellulose, dextrates, citric acid, natural and artificial flavor (soy), magnesium stearate, silicon dioxide, sucralose, yellow 6 aluminum lake, aspartame, acesulfame potassium
Gluten Free (less than 20 ppm gluten)

Sugar Free Assorted Fruit Chewables

Ingredients: Wheat dextrin, sorbitol, corn starch, microcrystalline cellulose, dextrates, citric acid, natural and artificial flavor (soy), magnesium stearate, silicon dioxide, sucralose, aspartame, acesulfame potassium, red 40 lake, yellow 6 lake, blue 1 lake
Gluten Free (less than 20 ppm gluten)

Directions: Adults: Chew 3 tablets up to 3 times daily to supplement the fiber content of your diet.

Age	Servings
12 yrs to adult	3 tablets up to 3 times daily[1]
6 to 11 yrs.	1 ½ tablets up to 3 times daily[2]
Under 6 yrs.	Ask your doctor before use

[1]Not to exceed 9 tablets per day
[2]Not to exceed 4 ½ tablets daily

Phenylketonurics:
Contains Phenylalanine

Keep out of reach of children. If you are pregnant or nursing a baby, ask a health professional before use.

Tamper Evident Feature: Do Not Use if inner seal imprinted with **"SEALED for YOUR PROTECTION"** is broken or missing. Store at controlled room temperature 20-25°C (68-77°F). Protect from excessive heat and moisture. Benefiber® guarantees your satisfaction or your money back.

Questions? Call **1-800-452-0051** 24 hours a day, 7 days a week or visit us at **www.benefiber.com** for additional information.

How Supplied: Orange Creme available in bottles of 36 and 100 ct tablets. Assorted Fruit available in 100 ct tablets.
Shown in Product Identification Guide, page 504

BENEFIBER® FIBER SUPPLEMENT PLUS B VITAMINS & FOLIC ACID
(Novartis Consumer Health, Inc.)
Caplets

Benefiber® Plus B Vitamins & Folic Acid provides the same amount of fiber as the leading fiber supplement[1] plus an excellent source of Vitamins B6, B12 and Folic Acid. Getting the recommended level of these important nutrients, as part of a diet low in saturated fat and cholesterol, can help promote a healthy heart and energy & vitality.*
Benefiber Plus B Vitamins & Folic Acid Caplets contain 100% natural fiber ingredient and are convenient and easy-to-use.

Supplement Facts
Serving Size: 3 Caplets

Amount Per Serving	%DV*
Calories 15	
Sodium 0mg	0%
Total Carbohydrate 4g	1%
Dietary Fiber 3g	12%
Soluble Fiber 3g	†
Sugars 0g	†
Vitamin B$_6$ 0.7mg	35%
Folic Acid 134mcg	34%
Vitamin B$_{12}$ 2mcg	33%

* Percent Daily Values (DV) are based on a 2,000 calorie diet.
† Daily Value not established.

Ingredients: Wheat dextrin, microcrystalline cellulose, magnesium stearate, colloidal silicon dioxide, modified food starch, pyroxidine hydrochloride (Vit. B$_6$), sodium citrate, citric acid, folic acid, sodium benzoate, sorbic acid, cyanocobalamin (Vit. B$_{12}$)
Gluten Free (less than 10ppm gluten)
Store at controlled room temperature 20-25°C (68-77°F). Protect from excessive heat and moisture.

Directions: Adults: Take 3 caplets up to 3 times daily to supplement the fiber content of your diet. Swallow with liquid. Do not exceed 9 caplets per day.
Keep out of reach of children.
If you are pregnant or nursing a baby, ask a health professional before use.

Tamper Evident Feature: Do Not Use if inner seal imprinted with **"SEALED for YOUR PROTECTION"** is broken or missing.
Benefiber® guarantees your satisfaction or your money back.
Questions? Call **1-800-452-0051** 24 hours a day, 7 days a week or visit us at **www.benefiber.com** for additional information.

---

[1]Metamucil Caplets offer 3 grams of dietary fiber. Metamucil® is a registered trademark of The Procter & Gamble Company.
* This statement has not been evaluated by the Food and Drug Administration. This product is not intended to diagnose, treat, cure or prevent any disease.

How Supplied:
Available in 60 ct. bottles.
Shown in Product Identification Guide, page 504

BENEFIBER® FIBER SUPPLEMENT PLUS B VITAMINS & FOLIC ACID
(Novartis Consumer Health, Inc.)
Non-Thickening Powder

Benefiber® Plus B Vitamins & Folic Acid provides the same amount of fiber as the leading fiber supplement[1] plus an excellent source of Vitamins B6, B12, and Folic Acid. Getting the recommended level of these important nutrients, as part of a diet low in saturated fat and cholesterol, can help promote a healthy heart and energy & vitality.*
Benefiber Plus B Vitamins & Folic Acid contains 100% natural fiber ingredient that will not alter the taste or texture of your favorite foods or beverages since it is
• Taste-Free • Sugar-Free • Grit-Free
Be creative with Benefiber. Try it in your juice, yogurt, whatever you desire.
You won't even know it's there!

Supplement Facts
Serving Size: 2 tsp (3.8g)

Amount Per Serving	%DV*
Calories 15	
Sodium 0mg	0%
Total Carbohydrate 4g	1%
Dietary Fiber 3g	12%
Soluble Fiber 3g	†
Sugars 0g	†
Vitamin B$_6$ 0.7mg	35%
Folic Acid 134mcg	34%
Vitamin B$_{12}$ 2mcg	33%

* Percent Daily Values (DV) are based on a 2,000 calorie diet.
† Daily Value not established.

Ingredients: Wheat dextrin, modified food starch, pyridoxine hydrochloride (Vit. B$_6$), folic acid, sodium citrate, citric acid, silicon dioxide, sodium benzoate, sorbic acid, cyanocobalamin (Vit. B$_{12}$)
Gluten Free (less than 10ppm gluten)
Store at controlled room temperature 20-25°C (6B-77°F). Protect from moisture. Use within 6 months of opening.

Tamper Evident Feature: Do Not Use if inner seal imprinted with **"SEALED for YOUR PROTECTION"** is broken or missing.

Packaged by weight, not volume. Contents may settle during shipping and handling.
Benefiber® guarantees your satisfaction or your money back.
Questions? Call **1-800-452-0051** 24 hours a day, 7 days a week or visit us at **www.benefiber.com** for recipe ideas and additional information.

Directions: Stir 2 teaspoons of Benefiber into 4 - 8 oz. of your favorite beverage or soft food. Stir well until dissolved.
Not recommended for carbonated beverages.

Age	Servings		
12 yrs. to adult	2 tsp	3 times daily[2]	
6 to 11 yrs.	1 tsp	3 times daily[3]	
Under 6 yrs.	Ask your doctor before use		

[2]Not to exceed 6 tsp per day.
[3]Not to exceed 3 tsp per day.
tsp = teaspoon

Keep out of reach of children.
If you are pregnant or nursing a baby, ask a health professional before use.

---

[1]Metamucil Powders offer 3 grams of dietary fiber. Metamucil® is a registered trademark of The Procter & Gamble Company.

* This statement has not been evaluated by the Food and Drug Administration.

Continued on next page

Benefiber Plus Powder—Cont.

This product is not intended to diagnose, treat, cure or prevent any disease.

How Supplied: Available in 6.4 oz powder bottles.

Shown in Product Identification Guide, page 504

BENEFIBER® FIBER SUPPLEMENT PLUS CALCIUM
(Novartis Consumer Health, Inc.)
Wild Berry Chewables
Artificially Flavored

Benefiber® Plus Calcium Chewable Tablets are an easy way to add fiber and calcium to your diet. These great tasting tablets provide as much fiber per 3 tablet serving as the leading bulk fiber powder† and as much calcium as an 8 oz glass of milk to promote bone health. Because there is no need for water or mixing, you can take them virtually anywhere, anytime.*

Supplement Facts
Serving Size: 3 Tablets

Amount Per Serving	%DV*
Calories 30	
Total Carbohydrate 8g	3%
Dietary Fiber 3g	12%
Soluble Fiber 3g	†
Sugars 0g	†
Calcium 300mg	30%

* Percent Daily Values (DV) are based on a 2,000 calorie diet.
† Daily Value not established.

Ingredients: Wheat dextrin, sorbitol, corn starch, calcium carbonate, microcrystalline cellulose, dextrates, citric acid, artificial flavors (soy), maltodextrin, magnesium stearate, powdered cellulose, silicon dioxide, mineral oil, sucralose, red 40 aluminum lake, aspartame, acesulfame potassium, blue 1 aluminum lake. Gluten Free (less than 20ppm gluten)

Directions: Adults: Chew 3 tablets up to 3 times daily to supplement the fiber content of your diet.

Age	Servings
12 yrs. to adult	3 tablets up to 3 times daily[1]
6 to 11 yrs.	1 1/2 tablets up to 3 times daily[2]
Under 6 yrs.	Ask your doctor before use

[1]Not to exceed 9 tablets per day
[2]Not to exceed 4 1/2 tablets per day

Phenylketonurics: **Contains Phenylalanine.**

Keep out of reach of children.
If you are pregnant or nursing a baby, ask a health professional before use.

Tamper Evident Feature: Do Not Use if inner seal imprinted with **"SEALED for YOUR PROTECTION"** is broken or missing. Store at controlled room temperature 20-25°C (68-77°F). Protect from excessive heat and moisture.
Benefiber® guarantees your satisfaction or your money back.
Questions? Call **1-800-452-0051** 24 hours a day, 7 days a week or visit us at **www.benefiber.com** for additional information.

† Metamucil Powders offer 3 grams of dietary fiber. Metamucil® is a registered trademark of The Procter & Gamble Company.
*This statement has not been evaluated by the Food and Drug Administration. This product is not intended to diagnose, treat, cure or prevent any disease.

How Supplied: Available in 90 ct. bottles.
Shown in Product Identification Guide, page 504

Procter & Gamble
P.O. BOX 559
CINCINNATI, OH 45201

Direct Inquiries to:
Consumer Relations
(800) 832-3064

ALIGN DAILY PROBIOTIC SUPPLEMENT
(Procter & Gamble)

Description: Align contains Bifantis (*Bifidobacterium infantis* 35624), a purified strain of healthy (probiotic) bacteria. Align is a daily dietary supplement that works naturally to help build and maintain a healthy, balanced digestive system. Align comes as an easy-to-swallow capsule that, when taken just once a day, every day, provides a natural defense against episodic constipation, diarrhea, urgency, gas, and bloating. Each capsule of Align contains 1×10^9 (one billion) live bacteria when manufactured, and continues to provide an effective level until at least the "best by" date. Align capsules are calorie-free, and contain no artificial sweeteners, gluten or lactose. Align with Bifantis is clinically proven and is recommended by some of the world's leading gastroenterologists.

Uses: Align Daily Probiotic Supplement helps build and maintain a strong and healthy digestive system. Align may be especially helpful for people who desire a natural defense against episodes of digestive upsets such as constipation, diarrhea, urgency, gas and bloating. Taking

Align daily can help restore the natural balance of healthy bacteria in the digestive system.

Warnings: Keep out of reach of children. In case of accidental ingestion, contact your doctor or contact a Poison Control Center.

Directions: Take one capsule daily. Keep capsules in original packaging for best results. Store at room temperature.

How Supplied: 28 capsules.

Other ingredients: microcystalline cellulose, hydroxypropylmethylcellulose capsule USP grade, magnesium stearate, sugar, sodium caseinate, sodium citrate dihydrate, propyl gallate, FD&C blue #2. Align contains milk and soy ingredients. Align is lactose free.

Questions? 1-800-208-0112 or AlignGI.com
Shown in Product Identification Guide, page 507

METAMUCIL® DIETARY FIBER SUPPLEMENT
(Procter & Gamble)
[*met uh-mū sil*]
(psyllium husk)
Also see Metamucil Fiber Laxative in Nonprescription Drugs section

Description: Metamucil contains psyllium husk (from the plant *Plantago ovata*), a concentrated source of soluble fiber which can be used to increase one's dietary fiber intake. When used as part of a diet low in saturated fat and cholesterol, 7g per day of soluble fiber from psyllium husk (the amount in 3 doses of Metamucil) may reduce the risk of heart disease by lowering cholesterol. Each dose of Metamucil powder and Metamucil Fiber Wafers contains approximately 3.4 grams of psyllium husk (or 2.4 grams of soluble fiber). A listing of ingredients and nutrition information is available in the listing of Metamucil Fiber Laxative in the Nonprescription Drug section. Metamucil Smooth Texture Sugar-Free Unflavored, Metamucil capsules and Metamucil plus Calcium capsules contains no sugar and no artificial sweeteners. Metamucil Plus Calcium Capsules also helps build strong bones. Metamucil Smooth Texture Sugar-Free Orange Flavor and Berry Burst Flavor contains aspartame (phenylalanine content of 25 mg and 16 mg per dose respectively). Metamucil powdered products are gluten-free.
Fibersure from the makers of Metamucil, is an all natural, clear-mixing powder that is flavor-free, non-thickening and quickly dissolves in water or most other liquids and won't change the flavor or texture. Fibersure is made of 100% Inulin (a natural vegetable fiber), and can easily be included into cooking and baking.
[See table on next page]

Uses: Metamucil Dietary Fiber Supplement can be used as a concentrated source

Metamucil Dietary Fiber Supplements

Versions/Flavors	Ingredients (alphabetical order)	Sodium mg/dose	Calcium mg/dose	Potassium mg/dose	Calories kcal/dose	Total Carbohydrate g/dose	Dietary Fiber/ (Soluble) g/dose	Serving (Weight in gms)	How Supplied
Capsules plus Calcium	Psyllium husk, Calcium carbonate, Geltain, Crosprovidone, Titanium dioxide, Polysorbate 80, Caramel color, Red 40 Lake, Blue 1 Lake, Yellow 6 Lake	0	300	30	10	12	3 (2.4)	5 capsules (2.6)	Bottles: 75 ct, 120 ct, 150 ct.
Fibersure	Inulin	0	0	0	25	6	5 (5)	1 heaping teaspoon (5.8)	Bottles: 34 servings, 57 servings, 100 servings.
Smooth Texture Orange Flavor Metamucil Powder	Citric Acid, FD&C Yellow #6, Natural and Artificial Flavor, Psyllium Husk, Sucrose	5	7	30	45	12	3 (2.4)	1 rounded tablespoon ~12g	Canisters: Doses: 48, 72, 114, 188; Cartons: 30 single-dose packets.
Smooth Texture Sugar-Free Orange Flavor Metamucil Powder	Aspartame, Citric Acid, FD&C Yellow #6, Maltodextrin, Natural and Artificial Flavor, Psyllium Husk	5	7	30	20	5	3 (2.4)	1 rounded teaspoon ~5.8g	Canisters: Doses: 30, 48, 72, 114, 180, 220; Cartons: 30 single-dose packets.
Smooth Texture Sugar-Free Unflavored Metamucil Powder	Citric Acid, Maltodextrin, Psyllium Husk	4	7	30	20	5	3 (2.4)	1 rounded teaspoon ~5.4g	Canisters: Doses: 48, 72 114.
Smooth Texture Sugar-Free Berry Bust	Psyllium Husk, Maltodextrin, Natural And Artificial Flavor, Citric Acid, Malic Acid, Acesulfame Potassium, Aspartame, FD&C Red No. 40, FD&C Blue No. 1	5	7	30	20	5	3 (2)	1 rounded teaspoon (5.8g)	Canisters: 48, 72, 114.
Coarse Milled Unflavored Metamucil Powder	Psyllium Husk, Sucrose	3	6	30	25	7	3 (2.4)	1 rounded teaspoon ~7g	Canisters: Doses: 48, 72 114.
Coarse Milled Orange Flavor Metamucil Powder	Citric Acid, FD&C Yellow #6, Natural and Artificial Flavor, Psyllium Husk, Sucrose	5	6	30	40	11	3 (2.4)	1 rounded tablespoon ~11g	Canisters: Doses: 48,72 114.
Metamucil Capsules	Caramel color, FD&C Blue No. 1 Aluminum Lake, FD&C Red No. 40 Aluminum Lake, FD&C Yellow No. 6 Aluminum Lake, gelatin, polysorbate 80, psyllium husk	0	5	30	10	3	3 (2.4)	6 capsules 3.2g	Bottles: 100 ct, 160 ct, 300 ct
Wafers **Apple** Metamucil Wafers	(1)	20	14	60	120	17	6	2 wafers 24 g	Cartons: 12 doses
Cinnamon Metamucil Wafers	(2)	20	14	60	120	17	6	2 wafers 24 g	Cartons: 12 doses

(1) ascorbic acid, brown sugar, cinnamon, corn oil, corn starch, fructose, lecithin, molasses, natural and artificial flavors, oat hull fiber, psyllium husk, sodium bicarbonate, sucrose, water, wheat flour

(2) ascorbic acid, cinnamon, corn oil, corn starch, fructose, lecithin, molasses, natural and artificial flavors, nutmeg, oat hull fiber, oats, psyllium husk, sodium bicarbonate, sucrose, water, wheat flour

Continued on next page

Metamucil—Cont.

of soluble fiber to increase the dietary intake of fiber. Diets low in saturated fat and cholesterol that include 7 grams of soluble fiber per day from psyllium husk, as in Metamucil, may reduce the risk of heart disease by lowering cholesterol. One adult dose of Metamucil has 2.4 grams of this soluble fiber. Consult a doctor if you are considering use of this product as part of a cholesterol-lowering program.

Warnings: Read entire Drug Facts section in listing for Metamucil Fiber Laxative in the Nonprescription Drug section.

Directions: Adults 12 yrs. & older: 1 dose in 8 oz of liquid *3 times daily.*
Capsules: 2–6 capsules for increasing daily fiber intake; 6 capsules for cholesterol lowering use. Up to three times daily. Under 12 yrs.: Consult a doctor. See mixing directions in Drug Facts in listing for Metamucil Fiber Laxative in the Nonprescription Drug section.
NOTICE: Mix this product with at least 8 oz (a full glass) of liquid. Taking without enough liquid may cause choking. Do not take if you have difficulty swallowing.
Capsules plus Calcium: 2-5 capsules as an easy way to increase daily fiber and calcium intake. May be taken up to 4 times daily. Under 12 yrs: Consult a doctor.
Fibersure: Stir 1 heaping teaspoon briskly in 8 oz or more water or other beverages. Product dissolves best in room temperature or warmer liquid. Not recommended for carbonated beverages. Add desired amount directly to foods as you prepare them. For best results use in moist foods or recipes.
For listing of ingredients and nutritional information for Metamucil Dietary Fiber Supplement, and for laxative indications and directions for use, see Metamucil Fiber Laxative in the Nonprescription Drug section.
Notice to Health Care Professionals: To minimize the potential for allergic reaction, health care professionals who frequently dispense powdered psyllium products should avoid inhaling airborne dust while dispensing these products. Handling and Dispensing: To minimize generating airborne dust, spoon product from the canister into a glass according to label directions.

How Supplied: Powder: canisters and cartons of single-dose packets. Capsules: 100 and 160 count bottles. For complete ingredients and sizes for each version, see Metamucil Table 1, page 718, Nonprescription Drug section.

Questions? 1-800-983-4237

Shown in Product Identification Guide, page 507

Tahitian Noni International
**333 WEST RIVER PARK DRIVE
PROVO, UT 84604 USA**

Direct Inquiries to:
Phone: (801) 234-1000
Website: http://www.tahitiannoni.com

**TAHITIAN NONI® Leaf Serum
(Tahitian Noni Int'l)
TAHITIAN NONI® Leaf Serum Soothing Gel**

Description: In an exclusive process known only to Tahitian Noni International, we've extracted the juice of the long-treasured noni leaf and made it into a soothing balm. Especially for skin that's been exposed to the elements, this serum will condition and revitalize irritated, wind-chaffed, or sunburned skin with lasting relief.

Ingredients: TAHITIAN NONI® Exclusive Noni Leaf Formula [Purified Water, *Morinda citrifolia* (Noni) Leaf Juice, *Morinda citrifolia* (Noni) Leaf Extract, *Vanilla tahitensis* (Tahitian Vanilla) Fruit Extract], Pentylene Glycol, Propylene Glycol, SD Alcohol 40-B, PEG-400 Laurate and Laureth-4, Sodium Dehydroacetate, Disodium EDTA, Phenoxyethanol, Fragrance, Acrylates/C10-30 Alkyl Acrylate Crosspolymer, Potassium Hydroxide.

Suggested Use: Smooth over irritated skin as needed.

Storage: Keep tightly closed in a dry place; do not expose to excessive heat.

How Supplied:
1, 3 and 6 packs of cream, 1 oz/30 ml Packaged for Tahitian Noni International, a subsidiary of Morinda, Inc. Provo, UT 84604. USA.

References
Su C, Palu 'AK et al., TNI Patent Pending. A Noni leaf extract demonstrated significant wound healing effects in the mouse cutaneous assay by doubling the wound closure rate.
Su C, Palu 'AK et al., TNI Patent Pending Noni leaf extracts and Noni leaf juice inhibited the proliferation of a human epidermoid carcinoma cell line, A431, with an IC_{50} 76 ug/ml and 0.2% respectively.
Mannetje L. Morinda citrifolia L. in: Plant-Resources of South-East Asia (Edit.: E. Westphal, P. and C. M. Jansen). Pudoc Wageningen 1989, p. 185-187. A Noni leaf preparation is used as a tonic and antiseptic. Leaves are placed directly on wounds and the leaf juice produces pain-killing effects.
Saludes JP et al., Antitubercular constituents from the hexane fraction of Morinda citrifolia Linn. (Rubiaceae). Phytother. Res. 2002. (16): 683-685

Ethanol and hexane fractions from Morinda citrifolia leaf showed antitubercular activity by killing 89% of the bacteria *in vitro*, comparable to 97% kill by the anti-TB drug rifampicin at the same concentration.
Zin ZM et al., Antioxidant activities of chromatographic fractions obtained from roots, fruit and leave of Mengkudu (Morinda citrifolia L.). Food Chemistry 2006. 94: 169-178.
Methanol fractions from defatted Noni leaf juice showed strong antioxidant activities comparable to that of alpha-tocopherol.

* This statement has not been evaluated by the Food and Drug Administration. This product is not intended to diagnose, treat, cure or prevent any disease

Shown in Product Identification Guide, page 508

**TAHITIAN NONI® LIQUID DIETARY SUPPLEMENT
(Tahitian Noni Int'l)**

Description: TAHITIAN NONI® Juice has a heritage, a pedigree that distinguishes it from every other product on the market. This pedigree extends back 2,000 years to the people who used the noni fruit for its benefits. The countless benefits of this unique fruit can only be enjoyed if the fruit is revealed in its most pure form. Our proprietary formulation captures this precisely. It's no wonder that TAHITIAN NONI Juice touches the lives of millions worldwide. You'll find 2,000 years of goodness in every bottle of TAHITIAN NONI Juice! Always look for the TAHITIAN NONI Juice Footprint: Your only assurance of quality, purity, and authenticity.

Supplement Facts

Serving Size: 1 fluid ounce (30 ml)
Servings Per Container 33

Amount Per Serving	%Daily Value*
Calories 13	
Total Carbohydrate 3g	1%
Surgars 2g	†

*Percent Daily Values are based on a 2,000 calorie diet.
†Daily Value not established.

Ingredients: Reconstituted *Morinda citrifolia* fruit juice from pure juice puree from French Polynesia, natural grape juice concentrate, natural blueberry juice concentrate, and natural flavors. Not made from dried or powdered *Morinda citrifolia*.

How Supplied: 1 FL. OZ./30 mL daily. Preferably before meals
Shake well before using and refrigerate after opening
Do not use if seal around cap is broken

Packaged by Tahitian Noni International, a subsidiary of Morinda, Inc. Provo, UT 84604. USA.

References

Morinda citrifolia (Noni): a literature review and recent advances in Noni research. Acta Pharmacol Sin. 2002 Dec; 23(12):1127-41.

In a human clinical study, TAHITIAN NONI® Juice has been shown to have significant antioxidant activity by lowering free radical levels in the blood. Research has also revealed that TAHITIAN NONI® Juice and noni fruit have positive effects on immune system performance. Significant anti-inflammatory activity has also been demonstrated in several studies.

Effects of Morinda citrifolia on quality of life and auditory function in postmenopausal women. J Altern Complement Med. 2004 Oct; 10(5): 737-9.

A pilot clinical study in postmenopausal women revealed several potential health benefits including improved physical function (physical energy/strength) and mental health quality of life parameters, as well as auditory functions.

The inhibitory effects of Morinda citrifolia L. noni on phosphodiesterase enzymes: The possible mechanisms for increasing energy and improving diabetic conditions. Afa K. Palu, et al. CIPAM 2006 Abstracts. IVth International Conference on Aromatic and Medicinal Plants from French Overseas Regions. Tahiti. July 10-13, 2006. p. 12.

Experimental research reveals one biological mechanism by which TAHITIAN NONI® Juice helps increase overall physical energy of consumers.

Palu 'AK et al., Morinda citrifolia L., Noni has Cholesterol Lowering Potential. The 47th Annual Meeting of Society for Economic Botany. Chiang Mai, Thailand June 5-9, 2006.

Bioassay investigations showed TAHITIAN NONI® Juice (TNJ) inhibited HMG-CoA Reductase, an enzyme involved in human cholesterol biosynthesis by 50, 81 and 83%, respectively. This might explain how TNJ lowers cholesterol in smokers.

Noni Juice May Lower Cholesterol and Triglycerides in Adult Smokers. Wang MY et al., American Heart Association 46th Annual Conference on Cardiovascular Disease Epidemiology and Prevention Meeting Report. Phoenix, Ariz., March 2 2006.

Smokers drinking 4 ounces of TAHITIAN NONI® Juice daily for 4 weeks in a double blind placebo control clinical trial showed a decrease in averages of cholesterol from 235.2 mg/dL to 190.2 mg/dL and triglycerides from 242.5 mg/dL to 193.5 mg/dL.

Palu 'AK et al., Morinda citrifolia L. Noni: An angiotensin converting enzyme inhibitor. The 232nd ACS National Meeting, San Francisco, CA, Sept. 10-14, 2006.

TAHITIAN NONI® Juice inhibited ACE enzymes and blocked AT_1 and AT_2 receptors concentration-dependently. A pilot clinical study of 10 hypertensive subjects showed consuming 4 ounces of TNJ a day for 1 month lowered blood pressure from averages of 144/83 (pre-test) to 132/76 (post-test).

A Safety Review of Noni Fruit Juice. Journal of Food Science 2006 October; 71(8):R100-R106.

Several preclinical safety tests and a human clinical safety study have revealed no adverse health effects, even at high doses (more than 3/4 liter per day in humans and up to 80 mL/kg in animals). The available data, along with more than 200 years of documented food use in the tropics, substantiate its continued use as a safe food.

TAHITIAN NONI® Juice Is Safe for Human Consumption. The EFSA Journal 2006, 376:1-12.

The European Food Safety Authority (EFSA) reports, "From a toxicological point of view, noni juice has been adequately tested. . . . It is unlikely that consumption of noni juice, at the observed levels of intake, induces adverse human liver effects."

TAHITIAN NONI® Juice Does Not Contain Athletic Banned Substances. www.consumerlab.com/results/tahitian_noni.asp

Analysis of TNJ revealed the absence of all performance-enhancing substances banned by the World Anti Doping Association.

TAHITIAN NONI® Juice Not a Significant Source of Potassium.

A case report stated that the potassium content of noni juice was 56.3 mEq/L, or 65 mg/ounce, and may be a "surreptitious" source of potassium for patients with renal kidney disease. **(Mueller et al. Am J Kidney Dis 2000 35:330–2)**. Mueller **(USA Today, March 28, 2000)** clarified his research, stating he did not analyze TAHITIAN NONI® Juice, but rather a different brand of noni juice and that the amount of potassium was only "as much as you'd get in 2 inches of banana." The Potassium content of TAHITIAN NONI® Juice is 40 mg per 1 ounce serving. Compared to Grape juice* 42 mg per 1 ounce serving, Banana* 102 mg per 1 ounce serving and Yogurt* 66 mg per 1 ounce.

---

* Source: USDA Nutrient Database for Standard Reference.

This statement has not been evaluated by the Food and Drug Administration. This product is not intended to diagnose, treat, cure or prevent any disease

Shown in Product Identification Guide, page 508

TAHITIAN NONI® Seed Oil (Tahitian Noni Int'l)

Product Information

This exclusive oil delivers intense moisture and relief to dry or distressed skin. It is designed to help improve skin health issues that come from within.

The first and only essential oil derived from noni seeds. High in linoleic acid, a powerful ally in skin hydration and cellular health.

This world exclusive light oil delivers intense healing moisture and relief to rough, distressed skin. It takes over 50,000 seeds to make just one ounce of this rare and precious oil. Absorbs easily into skin.

Product Benefits

- Hydrates and softens skin to hasten the healing process of distressed skin
- Protects with valuable antioxidants
- An essential building block for healthy looking skin
- High in linoleic acid which helps relieve dry, flaky, or rough skin and helps maintain smooth, moist skin
- Won't clog pores

Featured Ingredients

Pure Noni Seed Oil

Hydrates and softens while protecting skin with valuable antioxidants

Recommended Use

Gently apply a small amount of Noni Seed Oil to distressed skin anywhere healing moisture can be beneficial.

How Supplied:

33 FL oz (10 ml) bottle
Packaged for Tahitian Noni International, a subsidiary of Morinda, Inc. Provo, UT 84604. USA.

References

West BJ, Palu 'AK, Jensen CJ. Noni Seed Oil Analysis. TNI Patent Pending. Noni seed oil analysis reveal that it has natural phytosterols, vitamin E and a significant source of omega-6 fatty acid, an essential fatty acid.

Palu 'AK, Zhou BN, West BJ et al. TNI Patent Pending. Noni seed oil can reduce pain and inflammation due to its significant and selective inhibition of COX-2 enzymes.

Douglas M. Rope, M.D. Midwest Clinical Trials. A study to Asses the Comedogenicity of a Test Product When Applied Topically to the Skin of Healthy Human Subjects. May 19, 2004. Noni seed oil significantly reduced the number of closed comedones (white heads) on the skin of 26 teenage volunteers during a clinical trial.

* Source: USDA Nutrient Database for Standard Reference.

Shown in Product Identification Guide, page 508

FACED WITH AN Rx SIDE EFFECT?

Turn to the Companion Drug Index for products that provide symptomatic relief.

Topical BioMedics, Inc.
PO BOX 494
RHINEBECK, NY 12572-0494

Direct Inquiries to:
Aurora Paradise
Phone: (845) 871-4900
Fax: (845) 876-0818
E-mail: Aparadise@topicalbiomedics.com

TOPRICIN®
(Topical BioMedics, Inc.)

Key Facts:

Topricin® is an odorless non-irritating anti-inflammatory pain relief cream that provides excellent adjunctive support in medical treatments such as post surgical, physical and occupational therapy, chiropractic. Greaseless and contains no lanolin, menthol, capsaicin, or fragrances.

Active Ingredients (HPUS) Arnica Montana 6X, Echinacea 6X, Aesculus 6X, Ruta Graveolens 6X, Lachesis 8X, Rhus Tox 6X Belladonna 6X, Crotalus 8X, Heloderma 8X, Naja 8X, Graphites 6X. Fomitopsis officinalis IX.

Major Uses: Topical relief of inflammation & pain, and a healing treatment for soft tissue & trauma/sports injuries.

Benefits: relieves swelling, stiffness, numbness, tingling and burning pain associated with these soft tissue ailments: carpal tunnel syndrome, other neuropathic pain, arthritis, lower back pain, muscle spasm of the back, neck, legs, and feet, muscle soreness, crushing injury, and sprains. First aid: bruises, minor burns. Use before and after exercise

Directions Apply generously 3-4 times a day or more often if needed making sure to cover the entire joint or area of pain. Massage in until absorbed. Reapply before bed and at the start of the day for best results.

For further information go to www.topicalbiomedics.com

Safety Information: For external use only, use only as directed, if pain persists for more that 7 days or worsens, Consult a doctor. This homeopathic medicine has no known side effects or contraindications. Complies with FDA standards as an OTC medicine. Safe to use for children, adults, pregnant women and the elderly. Paraben free.

Inactive Ingredients purified water, highly refined vegetable oils, glycerin, medium-chain-triglyceride.

How Supplied:
Consumer size 4 oz jar or 2 oz tube
For professional use only: 16 oz or 32 oz pump bottle

Shown in Product Identification Guide, page 508

Wellness International Network, Ltd.
5800 DEMOCRACY DRIVE
PLANO, TX 75024

Direct Inquiries to:
Product Inquiries
(972) 312-1100
E-mail: winproducts@winltd.com

SLEEP-TITE™
(Wellness Int'l)
Herbal Sleep Aid

Description: Sleep-Tite™ is a natural herbal sleep aid formulated to promote a deeper, more restorative sleep. This powerful tool's primary function is to rejuvenate and restore by assisting the body in initiating and maintaining sleep. Sleep-Tite is a blend of 10 all-natural herbs, including California poppy, passion flower, valerian, and skullcap. These herbs help maintain healthy sleep cycles because of their calming effects and ability to relieve muscle tension. Additional ingredients, including hops, celery seed and chamomile all provide a generalized calming effect and are especially helpful for indigestion, gastrointestinal and smooth muscle relaxation. In addition to these calming herbs, Sleep-Tite also contains feverfew, an herb that reduces the body's production of prostaglandin and serotonin, hormones that can lead to the onset of everyday stress headaches. By utilizing this unique blend of herbs to aid in the effective initiation and maintenance of sleep patterns, Sleep-Tite can be consumed by adults, thereby promoting physical and emotional well-being in a safe, active manner.

Directions: As a dietary supplement, take 2 Sleep-Tite caplets approximately 30-60 minutes prior to bedtime. Some persons may require less than 2 caplets to achieve optimum results. Do not exceed recommended nightly amounts. Needs may vary with each individual.

Warnings: Not for use by children under the age of 18, pregnant or lactating women. Consult your physician before using this product if you have any medical condition or are taking antidepressants, sedatives or hypnotic medications. Do not take this product if using Monoamine Oxidase Inhibitors (MAOI). This product may cause drowsiness and should not be taken with alcohol or while operating a vehicle or other machinery. If allergic symptoms develop, discontinue use. Keep out of reach of children.

Ingredients: European Valerian Root 4:1 extract, Celery Seed 4:1 extract, Hops Strobile 4:1 extract, Passion Flower 4:1 extract (whole plant), California Poppy 5:1 extract (aerial parts), Chamomile Flower 5:1 extract, Chinese Fu Ling 5:1 extract (Poria Cocos), Jujube Seed 5:1 extract, Feverfew 5:1 extract (aerial parts), Skullcap (aerial parts), Dicalcium Phosphate, Microcrystalline Cellulose, Croscarmellose Sodium, Stearic Acid, Silica, Magnesium Stearate and Sugar Coat (calcium sulfate, sucrose, kaolin, talc, gelatin, shellac, titanium dioxide, anise oil, beeswax and carnauba wax).

How Supplied: One box contains 28 packets, 2 caplets per packet.

Additional Information: For additional information on ingredients or uses, please visit winltd.com.

These statements have not been evaluated by the Food & Drug Administration. This product is not intended to diagnose, treat, cure or prevent any disease.

STEPHAN™ CLARITY®
(Wellness Int'l)
Vitamin, Mineral and Amino Acid Supplement

Description: Clarity® contains specific vitamins, minerals, amino acids and nutrients important for memory and concentration. Key ingredients such as lecithin, glutamic acid and ginkgo biloba promote increased brain functioning. These nutrients provide fuel for the brain as well as increased blood flow to the entire central nervous system. These ingredients and their effects ensure that Clarity is a natural and effective way to better one's health.

Directions: As a dietary supplement, take 1 capsule 3 times daily with meals.

Warnings: CAUTION PHENYLKETONURICS: Contains 9.2mg phenylalanine per serving.

Ingredients: Proprietary blend (Lecithin, Bee Pollen, L-Glutamic Acid, Ribonucleic Acid Yeast, L-Aspartic Acid, L-Arginine HCl, L-Leucine, L-Lysine HCL, L-Phenylalanine, L-Serine, L-Proline, L-Valine, L-Isoleucine, L-Alanine, L-Glycine, L-Threonine, L-Tyrosine, L-Histidine, L-Cysteine HCl, L-Methionine, Adenosine Triphosphate, Ginkgo Biloba 50:1 Extract), Hydroxypropylmethylcellulose, DL-Alpha Tocopheryl Acetate, Ascorbic Acid, Niacinamide, Stearic Acid, Ethylcellulose, Vitamin A Acetate, D-Calcium Pantothenate, Thiamine HCL, Silicon Dioxide, Dicalcium Phosphate, Pyridoxine HCl, Riboflavin, Folic Acid, Cholecalciferol, Biotin, Cyancobalamin.

How Supplied: One bottle contains 60 easy-to-swallow capsules.

Additional Information: For additional information on ingredients or uses, please visit winltd.com.

These statements have not been evaluated by the Food & Drug Administration. This product is not intended to diagnose, treat, cure or prevent any disease.

STEPHAN™ ELASTICITY®
(Wellness Int'l)
Vitamin, Mineral and Amino Acid Supplement

Description: Elasticity® contains a scientifically balanced mixture of specific amino acids and nutrients established as important for skin tone and texture. Vitamin A and selenium, 2 key ingredients known for their antioxidant properties, help maintain the skin's youthful appearance and provide internal protection against the effects of sun exposure on the skin.

Directions: As a dietary supplement, take 1 capsule 3 times daily with meals.

Warnings: Accidental overdose of iron-containing products is a leading cause of fatal poisoning in children under 6. Keep this product out of reach of children. In case of accidental overdose, call a doctor or poison control center immediately.

Ingredients: Proprietary Blend (Shavegrass Herb, L-Glutamic Acid, Bladderwrack Extract, Ribonucleic Acid Yeast, L-Aspartic Acid, L-Arginine HCl, L-Leucine, L-Lysine HCl, L-Phenylalanine, L-Serine, L-Proline, L-Valine, L-Isoleucine, L-Alanine, L-Glycine, L-Threonine, L-Tyrosine, L-Histidine, L-Cysteine HCl, L-Methionine, Adenosine Triphosphate), Hydroxypropylmethylcellulose, DL-Alpha Tocopheryl Acetate, Ascorbic Acid, Ethylcellulose, Stearic Acid, Silicon Dioxide, Calcium Amino Acid Chelate, Manganese Amino Acid Chelate, Iron Amino Acid Chelate, Magnesium Amino Acid Chelate, Zinc Amino Acid Chelate, Vitamin A Acetate, Selenium Amino Acid Chelate, Chromium Amino Acid Chelate.

How Supplied: One bottle contains 60 easy-to-swallow capsules.

Additional Information: For additional information on ingredients or uses, please visit winltd.com.

These statements have not been evaluated by the Food & Drug Administration. This product is not intended to diagnose, treat, cure or prevent any disease.

STEPHAN™ ELIXIR®
(Wellness Int'l)
Vitamin, Mineral and Amino Acid Supplement

Description: Elixir® is formulated with an exclusive blend of vitamins, minerals and amino acids that provide an overall feeling of well-being and are an important component for healthy living. Key ingredients such as vitamin E and the amino acid cysteine have shown to protect the body from the effects of aging with their powerful antioxidant properties. These antioxidants help protect cells by preventing the damaging effects of free-radicals. Additionally, cysteine is an important component inassisting the body's normal detoxification process.

Directions: As a dietary supplement, take 1 capsule 3 times daily with meals.

Warnings: CAUTION PHENYLKE-TONURICS: Contains 6.9mg phenylalanine per serving. Accidental overdose of iron containing products is a leading cause of fatal poisoning in children under 6. Keep this product out of reach of children. In case of accidental overdose, call a doctor or poison control center immediately.

Ingredients: Proprietary Blend (Isolated Soy Protein, Bee Pollen, Citric Acid, Malic Acid, Ribonucleic Acid Yeast, Ginkgo Biloba Leaf Extract, Adenosine Triphosphate), Hydroxypropylmethylcellulose, Zinc Amino Acid Chelate, Iron Amino Acid Chelate, DL–alpha tocopheryl Acetate, Starch, Ascorbic Acid, Calcium Carbonate, Niacinamide, D-Calcium Pantothenate, Vitamin A Acetate, Silicon Dioxide, Thiamine HCl, Dicalcium Phosphate, Pyridoxine HCl, Riboflavin, Folic Acid, Selenium Amino Acid Chelate, Cholecalciferol, Biotin, Cyanocobalamin.

How Supplied: One bottle contains 60 easy-to-swallow capsules.

Additional Information: For additional information on ingredients or uses, please visit winltd.com.

These statements have not been evaluated by the Food & Drug Administration. This product is not intended to diagnose, treat, cure or prevent any disease.

STEPHAN™ ESSENTIAL®
(Wellness Int'l)
Herbal and Amino Acid Supplement

Description: Essential® contains specific vitamins, minerals, herbs and amino acids that are proactive to cardiovascular and circulatory management. Two primary ingredients, L-carnitine and vitamin E, provide increased energy utilization in the heart and skeletal muscles as well as protective antioxidant effects, thereby supporting the health of the entire circulatory system. Another key ingredient, linoleic acid, also supports heart health by improving blood flow and healthy cardiovascular levels.

Directions: As a dietary supplement, take 1 capsule 3 times daily with meals.

Warnings: CAUTION PHENYLKE-TONURICS: Contains 6.9mg phenylalanine per serving.

Ingredients: Proprietary Blend (Isolated Soy Protein, L-Carnitine Bitartrate, Bee Pollen, Marine Lipid Concentrate, Ribonucleic Acid Yeast, Adenosine Triphosphate), Hydroxypropylmethylcellulose, Magnesium Amino Acid Chelate, Starch, D-Alpha Tocopheryl Succinate, Selenium Amino Acid Chelate, Silicon Dioxide.

How Supplied: One bottle contains 60 easy-to-swallow capsules.

Additional Information: For additional information on ingredients or uses, please visit winltd.com.

These statements have not been evaluated by the Food & Drug Administration. This product is not intended to diagnose, treat, cure or prevent any disease.

STEPHAN™ FEMININE®
(Wellness Int'l)
Vitamin, Mineral and Amino Acid Supplement

Description: Feminine® contains selected vitamins, minerals and amino acids regarded as important to the ever-changing female body. This is achieved through such scientifically researched ingredients as magnesium and boron. Magnesium is important for regulating the flow of calcium between cells and is essential for adequate calcium uptake, which can lead to fewer PMS symptoms such as irritability, depression, headaches, backaches and menstrual cramps. Boron is vital at reducing excretion of both calcium and magnesium. This in turn assists in maintaining healthy bones.

Directions: As a dietary supplement, take 1 capsule 3 times daily with meals.

Warnings: CAUTION PHENYLKE-TONURICS: Contains 9.2mg phenylalanine per serving.

Ingredients: Proprietary blend (Isolated Soy Protein, Magnesium Oxide, Boron Aspartate, Ribonucleic Acid Yeast, Adenosine Triphosphate), Hydroxypropylmethylcellulose, DL-Alpha Tocopheryl Acetate, Starch, Silicon Dioxide, Selenium Amino Acid Chelate.

How Supplied: One bottle contains 60 easy-to-swallow capsules.

Additional Information: For additional information on ingredients or uses, please visit winltd.com.

These statements have not been evaluated by the Food & Drug Administration. This product is not intended to diagnose, treat, cure or prevent any disease.

STEPHAN™ FLEXIBILITY®
(Wellness Int'l)
Vitamin, Mineral and Amino Acid Supplement

Description: Flexibility® is rich in vitamins, minerals and amino acids recognized as beneficial to the health of joints and soft tissues. Two important amino acids utilized in Flexibility include glycine and histidine. These amino acids are known to promote neuromuscular control as well as maintain healthy, flexible joints. Boron, another key ingredient, is vital in protecting joints and vitamin E is added to soothe muscle cramps

Continued on next page

StePHan Flexibility—Cont.

associated with heavy exercise or everyday exertions.

Directions: As a dietary supplement, take 1 capsule 3 times daily with meals.

Warnings: CAUTION PHENYLKETONURICS: Contains 9.2mg phenylalanine per serving.

Ingredients: Proprietary Blend (Boron Gluconate, L-Glutamic Acid, Ribonucleic Acid Yeast, L-Aspartic Acid, L-Arginine HCL, L-Leucine, L-Lysine HCl, Bee Pollen, L-Phenylalanine, L-Serine, L-Proline, L-Valine, L-Isoleucine, L-Alanine, L-Glycine, L-Threonine, L-Tyrosine, L-Histidine, L-Cysteine HCl, L-Methionine, Adenosine Triphosphate), Hydroxypropylmethylcellulose, Zinc Amino Acid Chelate, Calcium Amino Acid Chelate, Stearic Acid, Ascorbic Acid, Whey, D-Alpha Tocopheryl Succinate, Magnesium Stearate, Niacinamide, Silicon Dioxide, Cellulose, Vitamin A Palmitate, D-Calcium Pantothenate, Thiamine HCl, Dicalcium Phosphate, Pyridoxine HCl, Riboflavin, Folic Acid, Selenomethionine, Cholecalciferol, Biotin, Cyanocobalamin.

How Supplied: One bottle contains 60 easy-to-swallow capsules.

Additional Information: For additional information on ingredients or uses, please visit winltd.com.

These statements have not been evaluated by the Food & Drug Administration. This product is not intended to diagnose, treat, cure or prevent any disease.

STEPHAN™ LOVPIL™
(Wellness Int'l)
Vitamin, Herbal and Amino Acid Supplement

Description: Lovpil™ is a nutritional supplement formulated with vitamins, minerals, herbs and amino acids recognized as important for general health and sexual vitality. Damiana, typically thought of as an aphrodisiac by those familiar with its effects, is an important ingredient utilized in Lovpil and is known for its stimulating properties on male virility and libido. Two other key ingredients, arginine and vitamin C, are essential in maintaining healthy sperm counts and protecting sperm from oxidative DNA damage.

Directions: As a dietary supplement, take 1 capsule 3 times daily with meals.

Ingredients: Proprietary Blend (Damiana Leaf, Isolated Soy Protein, Ribonucleic Acid Yeast, Adenosine Triphosphate), Calcium Carbonate, Hydroxypropylmethylcellulose, Ascorbic Acid, Stearic Acid, Zinc Amino Acid Chelate, Magnesium Stearate, Manganese Amino Acid Chelate, Silicon Dioxide, Vitamin A Acetate, Dicalcium Phosphate, Cholecalciferol, Folic acid, Selenomethionine, Cyanocobalamin.

How Supplied: One bottle contains 60 easy-to-swallow capsules.

Additional Information: For additional information on ingredients or uses, please visit winltd.com.

These statements have not been evaluated by the Food & Drug Administration. This product is not intended to diagnose, treat, cure or prevent any disease.

STEPHAN™ MASCULINE®
(Wellness Int'l)
Mineral, Herbal and Amino Acid Supplement

Description: Masculine® contains a special blend of nutrients with vitamins, minerals, herbs and amino acids shown to be essential for healthy male reproductive systems. Zinc, a key ingredient in Masculine, is important in maintaining healthy testosterone levels. Adequate zinc levels are essential to support the health of the male sex glands, increased sexual interest, mental alertness, emotional stability and a healthy, balanced appetite. In many normal males, zinc supplementation was accompanied by increases in sperm count and plasma testosterone.

Directions: As a dietary supplement, take 1 capsule 3 times daily with food.

Ingredients: Proprietary Blend (L-Histidine, Bee Pollen, Parsley Leaf, Ribonucleic Acid, Adenosine Triphosphate), Calcium Carbonate, Zinc Amino Acid Chelate, Hydroxypropylmethylcellulose, Magnesium Amino Acid Chelate, Stearic Acid, Magnesium Stearate.

How Supplied: One bottle contains 60 easy-to-swallow capsules.

Additional Information: For additional information on ingredients or uses, please visit winltd.com.

These statements have not been evaluated by the Food & Drug Administration. This product is not intended to diagnose, treat, cure or prevent any disease.

STEPHAN™ PROTECTOR®
(Wellness Int'l)
Vitamin, Mineral and Amino Acid Supplement

Description: Protector® is a nutritional supplement that combines specific vitamins, minerals and amino acids recognized as important for the health of areas associated with the human immune system. Astragalus is a key ingredient known for improving immune system integrity by relieving stress-induced immune system suppression. Additionally, research indicates that kelp supplies dozens of important nutrients for improved cardiovascular health and function.

Directions: As a dietary supplement, take 1 capsule 3 times daily with meals.

Warnings: CAUTION PHENYLKETONURICS: Contains 9.2mg phenylalanine per serving.

Ingredients: Proprietary Blend (Isolated Soy Protein, Astragalus Root, Bee Pollen, Kelp, Ribonucleic Acid Yeast, Adenosine Triphosphate), Hydroxypropylmethylcellulose, Cellulose, Stearic acid, Magnesium Stearate, Silicon Dioxide.

How Supplied: One bottle contains 60 easy-to-swallow capsules.

Additional Information: For additional information on ingredients or uses, please visit winltd.com.

These statements have not been evaluated by the Food & Drug Administration. This product is not intended to diagnose, treat, cure or prevent any disease.

STEPHAN™ RELIEF®
(Wellness Int'l)
Mineral, Herbal and Amino Acid Supplement

Description: Relief® is formulated with a special combination of nutrients, vitamins, minerals, amino acids and herbs recognized as important to the digestive and excretory systems. Parsley, a key ingredient in Relief, aids digestion with its carminative effects. Also included is psyllium, a gel-forming fiber that promotes both bowel regularity and helps maintain healthy, normal cholesterol levels.

Directions: As a dietary supplement, take 1 capsule 3 times daily with meals.

Ingredients: Proprietary Blend (Psyllium Seed Powder, L-Isoleucine, L-Leucine, L-Valine, Bee Pollen, Bladderwrack Herb 5:1 Extract, Parsley Leaf 4:1 Extract, Ribonucleic Acid Yeast, Adenosine Triphosphate), Hydroxypropylmethylcellulose, Starch, D-Calcium Pantothenate, Silicon Dioxide.

How Supplied: One bottle contains 60 easy-to-swallow capsules.

Additional Information: For additional information on ingredients or uses, please visit winltd.com.

These statements have not been evaluated by the Food & Drug Administration. This product is not intended to diagnose, treat, cure or prevent any disease.

STEPHAN™ TRANQUILITY™
(Wellness Int'l)
Vitamin, Mineral and Amino Acid Supplement

Description: Tranquility™ is a nutritional supplement which contains a blend of vitamins, minerals and amino acids recognized as important to areas involved in stress management. Two primary ingredients are myo-inositol and valerian root, both of which are beneficial in regulating the healthy sleep cycle and stress levels. Additionally, myo-inositol has been shown to support healthy triglyceride and cholesterol levels.

Directions: As a dietary supplement, take 1 capsule 3 times daily with meals.

Warnings: CAUTION PHENYLKE-TONURICS: Contains 9.2mg phenylalanine per serving.

Ingredients: Proprietary Blend (Isolated Soy Protein, Choline Bitartrate, Inositol, Lecithin, Ribonucelic Acid Yeast, Valerian Root Extract, Adenosine Triphosphate), Hydroxypropylmethylcellulose, DL-Alpha Tocopheryl Acetate, Calcium Aspartate, Silicon Dioxide, Ascorbic Acid, Stearic Acid, Niacinamide, Magnesium Amino Acid Chelate, Vitamin A Palmitate, Hydroxypropylcellulose, D-Calcium Pantothenate, Thiamine HCl, Dicalcium Phosphate, Pyridoxine HCl, Riboflavin, Folic Acid, Cholecalciferol, Biotin, Cyanocobalumin.

How Supplied: One bottle contains 60 easy-to-swallow capsules.

Additional Information: For additional information on ingredients or uses, please visit winltd.com.

These statements have not been evaluated by the Food & Drug Administration. This product is not intended to diagnose, treat, cure or prevent any disease.

BIOLEAN SURE2ENDURE™
(Wellness Int'l)
Herbal, Vitamin and Mineral Workout Supplement

Description: Sure2Endure™ is formulated to enhance the body's endurance, stamina, and ability to recover after a workout through an innovative blend of herbs, vitamins and minerals. Among these specially selected ingredients is ciwujia, known to alleviate fatigue and support the immune system. This herb has been shown to improve overall performance in aerobic exercise, endurance activities and weight lifting without any stimulant side effects. Ciwujia increases fat metabolism during exercise by shifting toward the use of fat as an energy source instead of carbohydrates. Additionally, this herb improves endurance by reducing lactic acid production thereby delaying fatigue that can often lead to muscle pain and cramps after a normal workout. Sure2Endure also provides antioxidant coverage and enzyme cofactors to meet the high demands that exercise places on the body. These antioxidants and cofactors scavenge free radicals formed during exercise as well promote carbohydrate metabolism, further leading to increased physical performance. To protect joints during exercise and ensure healthy connective tissue, glucosamine is a key ingredient in Sure2Endure. Since tissue stress and damage are often the re-

sult of strenuous exercise, it is important to maintain proper integrity and recovery of connective tissue. In addition to promoting healthy connective tissue, natural anti-inflammatory compounds bromelain and boswellia are included to further support the health of joints and soft tissues.

Directions: As a dietary supplement, take 3 tablets 1 hour prior to exercise. For optimum performance, use in conjunction with BIOLEAN II® or BIOLEAN Free® 1 hour before exercise. Phyto-Vite® may be taken with this product to maximize the antioxidant effect necessary with exercise. Mass Appeal™ may also be consumed for maximum effectiveness. Needs may vary with each individual.

Warnings: Not for use by children under the age of 18, pregnant or lactating women. Consult your physician before using this product if you have any medical conditions. Discontinue immediately if allergic symptoms develop. Keep out of reach of children. Contains shellfish.

Ingredients: Vitamin C 500mg (as Ascorbic Acid), Vitamin E 100IU (as D-Alpha Tocopheryl Succinate), Thiamin 10mg (as Thiamin Mononitrate), Riboflavin 12mg, Vitamin B6 15mg (as Pyridoxine HCl), Vitamin B12 20mcg (as Cyanocobalamin), Chromium 200mcg (as patented Chelavite® Chromium Dinicotinate Glycinate), Eleuthero, Magnesium L-aspartate, Potassium L-aspartate, Indian Frankincense, Bromelain (600GDU/g), Glucosamine HCl, Dicalcium Phosphate, Microcrystalline Cellulose, Croscarmellose Sodium, Stearic Acid, Silica, Magnesium Stearate and Sugar Coat (calcium sulfate, sucrose, kaolin, talc, gelatin, shellac, titanium dioxide, wintergreen oil, FD&C yellow #5, FD&C blue #1, beeswax and carnauba wax).

How Supplied: One box contains 28 packets, 3 tablets per packet.

Additional Information: For additional information on ingredients or uses, please visit winltd.com.

These statements have not been evaluated by the Food & Drug Administration. This product is not intended to diagnose, treat, cure or prevent any disease.

WINRGY®
(Wellness Int'l)
Energy Drink
Vitamin and Mineral Supplement

Description: Utilizing key ingredients such as riboflavin, vitamin B12, niacin and a proprietary blend of amino acids and caffeine, **Winrgy**® helps promote the alertness and energy required for an active lifestyle. Winrgy incorporates a unique blend of vitamins and minerals that are important in the creation of noradrenaline, a powerful neurotransmitter responsible for regulating alertness and the sleep-wakefulness cycle as well as be-

ing essential for memory and the learning process. Additionally, essential ingredients in Winrgy help the body convert energy from carbohydrates, protein, and fat, as well as combat daily physical and mental fatigue. Unlike caffeine alone, Winrgy offers the raw materials necessary to promote the body's normal production of noradrenaline and is ideal for anytime performance is required.

Directions: As a dietary supplement, add 1 packet of mix to 6 oz. of chilled water or fruit juice. Stir briskly. Consume 1–2 times per day. Keep in a cool, dry place. For maximum results, combine this product with one serving size of Food For Thought®.

Warnings: CAUTION PHENYLKE-TONURICS: Contains phenylalanine. Not for use by children under the age of 18, pregnant or lactating women. Persons taking medications should seek medical advice before taking this product. Do not consume more than 4 servings per day. Avoid the use of antacids containing aluminum with this product.

Ingredients: Carbohydrates 11g, Sugars 10g, Vitamin C 150mg (as Ascorbic Acid), Vitamin E 30IU (as DL-Alpha Tocopheryl Acetate), Thiamin 1.5mg (as Thiamin Mononitrate), Riboflavin 3mg, Niacin 73mg (as Niacinamide), Vitamin B6 13mg (as Pyridoxine HCL), Folate 180mcg (as Folic Acid), Vitamin B12 19mcg (as Cyanocobalamin), Pantothenic Acid 48mg (as Calcium Pantothenate), Zinc 4.5mg (as Zinc Gluconate), Copper 0.62mg (as Copper Gluconate), Manganese 2.6mg (as Manganese Aspartate), Chromium 260mcg (as Chromium Aspartate), Potassium 25mg (as Potassium Aspartate), Phenylalanine 570mg (as L-phenylalanine), Taurine 180mg, Glycine 135mg, Caffeine 80mg, Fructose, Natural Flavor, Citric Acid and Silicon Dioxide.

How Supplied: One box contains 28 single serving packets.

Additional Information: For additional information on ingredients or uses, please visit winltd.com.

These statements have not been evaluated by the Food & Drug Administration. This product is not intended to diagnose, treat, cure or prevent any disease.

FACED WITH AN Rx SIDE EFFECT?
Turn to the
Companion Drug Index
for products that
provide symptomatic
relief.

Wyeth Consumer Healthcare

FIVE GIRALDA FARMS
MADISON, NJ 07940-0871

Direct Inquiries to:
Wyeth Consumer Healthcare
(800) 322-3129 (9-5 E.S.T)

CALTRATE® 600 + D
(Wyeth Consumer)
Calcium Supplement

Supplement Facts
Serving Size 1 Tablet

Amount Per Serving	% DV
Vitamin D 400 IU	100%
Calcium 600 mg	60%

Ingredients: Calcium Carbonate, pregelatinized corn starch. Contains < 2% of: Acacia, Cholecalciferol (Vit.D₃), Croscarmellose Sodium, dl-Alpha Tocopherol, FD&C Yellow 6 Aluminum Lake, Magnesium Stearate, Medium-Chain Triglycerides, Polyethylene Glycol, Polyvinyl Alcohol, Sucrose, Talc, Titanium Dioxide, Tricalcium Phosphate. **Keep out of reach of children.**

Suggested Use: Take one tablet twice daily with food or as directed by your physician. Not formulated for use in children.

As with any supplement, if you are pregnant, nursing, or taking medication, consult your doctor before use.

Storage:
Store at room temperature. Keep bottle tightly closed. Bottle sealed with printed foil under cap. Do Not Use if foil is torn.

How Supplied:
Bottles of 60, 120 tablets

CALTRATE® 600 + D PLUS
Minerals Tablets
(Wyeth Consumer)
CALTRATE® 600 + D PLUS
Minerals Chewables
Calcium Carbonate
Calcium Supplement With Vitamin D & Minerals

Supplement Facts
Serving Size 1 Tablet

Amount Per Serving	%DV
Vitamin D 400 IU	100%
Calcium 600 mg	60%
Magnesium 50 mg	13%
Zinc 7.5 mg	50%
Copper 1 mg	50%
Manganese 1.8 mg	90%
Boron 250 mcg	*

* Daily Value (%DV) not established.

Ingredients: Calcium Carbonate, Starch, Magnesium Oxide. Contains <2% of: Acacia, Cholecalciferol (Vit. D₃), Croscarmellose Sodium, Cupric Sulfate, dl-Alpha Tocopherol, FD&C Blue 1 Aluminum Lake, FD&C Red 40 Aluminum Lake, FD&C Yellow 6 Aluminum Lake, Hypromellose, Magnesium Stearate, Manganese Sulfate, Medium-Chain Triglycerides, Microcrystalline Cellulose, Polysorbate 80, Sodium Borate, Sucrose, Titanium Dioxide, Triacetin, Tricalcium Phosphate, Zinc Oxide.

Chewables
Supplement Facts
Serving Size 1 Tablet

Amount Per Serving	% DV
Calories 10	
Total Carbohydrate 2 g	<1%+
Sugars 2 g	*
Vitamin D 400 IU	100%
Calcium 600 mg	60%
Magnesium 40 mg	10%
Zinc 7.5 mg	50%
Copper 1 mg	50%
Manganese 1.8 mg	90%
Boron 250 mcg	*

* Daily Value (%DV) not established.
+ Percent Daily Value based on a 2,000 calorie diet

Ingredients: Dextrose, Calcium Carbonate, Maltodextrin. Contains <2% of: Adipic Acid, BHT, Cholecalciferol (Vit. D₃), Corn Starch, Crospovidone, Cupric Oxide, dl-Alpha Tocopherol, FD&C Blue 2 Aluminum Lake, FD&C Red 40 Aluminum Lake, FD&C Yellow 6 Aluminum Lake, Gelatin, Hypromellose, Magnesium Oxide, Magnesium Stearate, Manganese Sulfate, Mineral Oil, Modified Starch, Natural and Artificial Flavor, Partially Hydrogenated Soybean Oil, Powdered Cellulose, Sodium Borate, Stearic Acid, Sucrose, Zinc Oxide.

Suggested Use: Take one tablet twice daily with food or as directed by your physician. Not formulated for use in children.

As with any supplement, if you are pregnant, nursing, or taking medication, consult your doctor before use.
Keep out of reach of children.
Store at room temperature. Keep bottle tightly closed.
Bottle sealed with printed foil under cap. Do Not Use if foil is torn.

How Supplied: Tablets; Bottles of 60 & 120
Chewables, Bottles of 60 & 90.
(Orange, cherry and fruit punch flavors)

CENTRUM®
(Wyeth Consumer)
High Potency
Multivitamin/Multimineral Supplement
From A to Zinc®

Supplement Facts
Serving Size 1 Tablet

Each Tablet Contains	% DV
Vitamin A 3500 IU	70%
(29% as Beta Carotene)	
Vitamin C 90 mg	150%
Vitamin D 400 IU	100%
Vitamin E 30 IU	100%
Vitamin K 25 mcg	31%
Thiamin 1.5 mg	100%
Riboflavin 1.7 mg	100%
Niacin 20 mg	100%
Vitamin B₆ 2 mg	100%
Folic Acid 500 mcg	125%
Vitamin B₁₂ 6 mcg	100%
Biotin 30 mcg	10%
Pantothenic Acid 10 mg	100%
Calcium 200 mg	20%
Iron 18 mg	100%
Phosphorus 109 mg	11%
Iodine 150 mcg	100%
Magnesium 100 mg	25%
Zinc 11 mg	73%
Selenium 55 mcg	79%
Copper 0.9 mg	45%
Manganese 2.3 mg	115%
Chromium 35 mcg	29%
Molybdenum 45 mcg	60%
Chloride 72 mg	2%
Potassium 80 mg	2%
Boron 150 mcg	*
Nickel 5 mcg	*
Silicon 2 mg	*
Tin 10 mcg	*
Vanadium 10 mcg	*
Lutein 250 mcg	*
Lycopene 300 mcg	*

*Daily Value (%DV) not established.

Ingredients: Dibasic Calcium Phosphate, Magnesium Oxide, Potassium Chloride, Calcium Carbonate, Microcrystalline Cellulose, Ascorbic Acid (Vit. C), Ferrous Fumarate, dl-Alpha Tocopheryl Acetate (Vit. E). Contains < 2% of: Acacia, Anhydrous Citric Acid, Ascorbyl Palmitate, Beta Carotene, Biotin, Boric Acid, BHT, Calcium Pantothenate, Calcium Stearate, Cholecalciferol (Vit. D), Chromium Picolinate, Corn Starch, Crospovidone, Cupric Sulfate, Cyanocobalamin (Vit. B₁₂), dl-Alpha Tocopherol, FD&C Yellow 6 Aluminum Lake, Folic Acid, Gelatin, Hydrogenated Palm Oil, Hypromellose, Lutein, Lycopene, Maltodextrin, Manganese Sulfate, Medium-Chain Triglycerides, Modified Food Starch, Niacinamide, Nickelous Sulfate, Phytonadione (Vit. K), Polyethylene Glycol, Polyvinyl Alcohol, Potassium Iodide, Pregelatinized Corn Starch, Pyridoxine Hydrochloride (Vit. B₆), Riboflavin (Vit. B₂), Silicon Dioxide, Sodium Ascorbate, Sodium Benzoate, Sodium Citrate, Sodium Metavanadate, Sodium Molybdate, Sodium Selenate, Sorbic Acid, Sucrose, Talc, Thiamine Mononitrate (Vit. B₁), Titanium Dioxide, Tri Calcium Phosphate, Vitamin A Acetate (Vit. A), Zinc Oxide. May also contain <2%: Sodium Aluminum Silicate.

Suggested Use:
Adults – One tablet daily with food. Not formulated for use in children.

As with any supplement, if you are pregnant, nursing, or taking medication, consult your doctor before use.

Warning: Accidental overdose of iron-containing products is a leading cause of fatal poisoning in children under 6. Keep this product out of reach of children. In case of accidental overdose, call a doctor or poison control center immediately.

IMPORTANT INFORMATION: Long-term intake of high levels of vitamin A (excluding that sourced from beta-carotene) may increase the risk of osteoporosis in adults. Do not take this product if taking other vitamin A supplements.

How Supplied: Bottles of 15, 50, 130, 180, 250 tablets
Storage: Store at room temperature. Keep bottle tightly closed.
Bottle sealed with printed foil under cap. Do not use if foil is torn.

CENTRUM® KIDS COMPLETE
(Wyeth Consumer)
DORA the EXPLORER, RUGRATS, SPONGEBOB SQUARE PANTS, & NICKTOONS
Multivitamin/Multimineral Supplement
(Orange, Cherry, Fruit Punch)++

Supplement Facts:
[See table above]

++Combined Ingredients List for 3 flavors

Ingredients: Sucrose, Dibasic Calcium Phosphate, Mannitol (wheat), Calcium Carbonate, Stearic Acid (soybean), Magnesium Oxide, Ascorbic Acid (Vit. C), Pregelatinized Starch, Microcrystalline Cellulose, dl-Alpha Tocopheryl Acetate (Vit. E). Contains < 2% of: Acacia, Aspartame,** Beta Carotene, Biotin, BHT, Calcium Pantothenate, Carbonyl Iron, Carrageenan, Chromic Chloride, Citric Acid, Cupric Oxide, Cyanocobalamin (Vit. B$_{12}$), Dextrose, Ergocalciferol (Vit. D), FD&C Blue 2 Aluminum Lake, FD&C Red 40 Aluminum Lake (sulfite), FD&C Yellow 6 Aluminum Lake, Folic Acid, Gelatin, Glucose, Guar Gum, Lactose (milk), Magnesium Stearate, Malic Acid, Maltodextrin, Manganese Sulfate, Mono- and Di-glycerides, Natural and Artificial Flavors, Niacinamide, Phytonadione (Vit. K), Potassium Iodide, Potassium Sorbate, Purified Water, Pyridoxine Hydrochloride (Vit. B$_6$), Riboflavin (Vit. B$_2$), Silicon Dioxide, Sodium Ascorbate, Sodium Benzoate, Sodium Citrate, Sodium Molybdate, Sodium Silicoaluminate, Sorbic Acid, Starch, Thiamine Mononitrate (Vit. B$_1$), Tocopherol, Tribasic Calcium Phosphate, Vanillin, Vitamin A Acetate (Vit. A), Zinc Oxide.

Suggested Use: Children 2 and 3 years of age, chew approximately ½ tablet daily with food. Children 4 years of age and older, chew 1 tablet daily with food. Not formulated for use in children less than 2 years of age.

Warning: Accidental overdose of iron-containing products is a leading cause of fatal poisoning in children under 6. Keep this product out of reach of children. In case of accidental overdose, call a doctor or poison control center immediately.
CONTAINS ASPARTAME.
** PHENYLKETONURICS: CONTAINS PHENYLALANINE.

Storage: Store at room temperature. Keep bottle tightly closed.
Bottle sealed with printed foil under cap. Do not use if foil is torn.

How Supplied: Assorted Flavors—Uncoated Tablet—Bottles of 60, 100 tablets
Marketed by: Wyeth Consumer Healthcare, Madison, NJ 07940

CENTRUM® PERFORMANCE
Multivitamin/Multimineral Supplement (Wyeth Consumer)

Supplement Facts
Serving Size 1 Tablet

Each Tablet Contains	% DV
Vitamin A 3500 IU	70%
(29% as Beta Carotene)	
Vitamin C 120 mg	200%
Vitamin D 400 IU	100%
Vitamin E 60 IU	200%
Vitamin K 25 mcg	31%
Thiamin 4.5 mg	300%
Riboflavin 5.1 mg	300%
Niacin 40 mg	200%
Vitamin B$_6$ 6 mg	300%
Folic Acid 400 mcg	100%
Vitamin B$_{12}$ 18 mcg	300%
Biotin 50 mcg	17%
Pantothenic Acid 12 mg	120%
Calcium 100 mg	10%
Iron 18 mg	100%
Phosphorus 48 mg	5%
Iodine 150 mcg	100%
Magnesium 40 mg	10%
Zinc 11 mg	73%
Selenium 70 mcg	100%
Copper 0.9 mg	45%
Manganese 4 mg	200%
Chromium 120 mcg	100%
Molybdenum 75 mcg	100%
Chloride 72 mg	2%
Potassium 80 mg	2%
Ginseng Root (*Panax ginseng*) 50 mg Standardized Extract	*
Ginkgo Biloba Leaf (*Ginkgo biloba*) 60 mg Standardized Extract	*
Boron 60 mcg	*
Nickel 5 mcg	*
Silicon 4 mg	*
Tin 10 mcg	*
Vanadium 10 mcg	*

*Daily Value (%DV) not established.

Serving Size: ½ Tablet / 1 Tablet

Amount Per Tablet:	% DV for Children 2 and 3 Years (1/2 Tablet)	% DV for Children 4 Years and Older (1 Tablet)
Calories 5		
Total Carbohydrate <1g	*	<1%+
Vitamin A 3500 IU	70%	70%
(29% as Beta Carotene)		
Vitamin C 60 mg	75%	100%
Vitamin D 400 IU	50%	100%
Vitamin E 30 IU	150%	100%
Vitamin K 10 mcg	*	13%
Thiamin 1.5 mg	107%	100%
Riboflavin 1.7 mg	106%	100%
Niacin 20 mg	111%	100%
Vitamin B$_6$ 2 mg	143%	100%
Folic Acid 400 mcg	100%	100%
Vitamin B$_{12}$ 6 mcg	100%	100%
Biotin 45 mcg	15%	15%
Pantothenic Acid 10 mg	100%	100%
Calcium 108 mg	7%	11%
Iron 18 mg	90%	100%
Phosphorus 50 mg	3%	5%
Iodine 150 mcg	107%	100%
Magnesium 40 mg	10%	10%
Zinc 15 mg	94%	100%
Copper 2 mg	100%	100%
Manganese 1 mg	*	50%
Chromium 20 mcg	*	17%
Molybdenum 20 mcg	*	27%

*Daily Value (%DV) not established.
+Percent Daily Values based on a 2,000 calorie diet.

Continued on next page

Centrum Performance—Cont.

Ingredients: Dibasic Calcium Phosphate, Potassium Chloride, Ascorbic Acid (Vit. C), Microcrystalline Cellulose, Calcium Carbonate, dl-Alpha Tocopheryl Acetate (Vit. E), Magnesium Oxide, Ginseng Root (*Panax ginseng*) Standardized Extract, Ginkgo Biloba Leaf (*Ginkgo biloba*) Standardized Extract, Ferrous Fumarate, Maltodextrin, Niacinamide, Crospovidone, Contains <2% of: Acacia, Anydrous Citric Acid, Ascorbyl Palmitate, Beta Carotene, Biotin, Boric Acid, BHT, Calcium Pantothenate, Cholecalciferol (Vit. D), Chromium Picolinate, Colloidal Silicon Dioxide, Corn Starch, Cupric Sulfate, Cyanocobalamin (Vit. B_{12}), dl-Alpha Tocopherol, Dried Glucose Syrup, FD&C Yellow 6 Aluminum Lake, Folic Acid, Gelatin, Hydrogenated Palm Oil, Hypromellose, Magnesium Stearate, Manganese Sulfate, Medium-Chain Triglycerides, Modified Food Starch, Nickelous Sulfate, Phytonadione (Vit. K), Polyethylene Glycol, Polyvinyl Alcohol, Potassium Iodide, Pregelatinized Corn Starch, Pyridoxine Hydrochloride (Vit. B_6), Riboflavin (Vit. B_2), Silicon Dioxide, Sodium Aluminosilicate, Sodium Ascorbate, Sodium Benzoate, Sodium Citrate, Sodium Metavanadate, Sodium Molybdate, Sodium Selenate, Sorbic Acid, Stannous Chloride, Sucrose, Talc, Thiamin Mononitrate (Vit. B_1), Titanium Dioxide, Tri Calcium Phosphate, Vitamin A Acetate (Vit. A), Zinc Oxide.

Suggested Use: Adults—One tablet daily with food. Not formulated for use in children.

Warning: Accidental overdose of iron-containing products is a leading cause of fatal poisoning in children under 6. Keep this product out of reach of children. In case of accidental overdose, call a doctor or poison control center immediately.

As with any supplement, if you are pregnant, nursing, or taking medication, contact your doctor before use.

IMPORTANT INFORMATION: Long-term intake of high levels of vitamin A (excluding that sourced from beta-carotene) may increase the risk of osteoporosis in adults. Do not take this product if taking other vitamin A supplements.

Store at Room Temperature. Keep bottle tightly closed. Bottle is sealed with printed foil under cap. Do not use if foil is torn.

How Supplied: Bottles of 45, 75, 120 and 150 Tablets.

CENTRUM® SILVER®
(Wyeth Consumer)
Multivitamin/Multimineral Supplement
Specially Formulated for Adults 50+

Supplement Facts
Serving Size 1 Tablet

Each Tablet Contains	% DV
Vitamin A 2500 IU	50%
(40% as Beta Carotene)	
Vitamin C 90 mg	150%
Vitamin D 500 IU	125%
Vitamin E 50 IU	167%
Vitamin K 30 mcg	38%
Thiamin 1.5 mg	100%
Riboflavin 1.7 mg	100%
Niacin 20 mg	100%
Vitamin B_6 3 mg	150%
Folic Acid 500 mcg	125%
Vitamin B_{12} 25 mcg	417%
Biotin 30 mcg	10%
Pantothenic Acid 10 mg	100%
Calcium 220 mg	22%
Phosphorus 110 mg	11%
Iodine 150 mcg	100%
Magnesium 50 mg	13%
Zinc 11 mg	73%
Selenium 55 mcg	79%
Copper 0.9 mg	45%
Manganese 2.3 mg	115%
Chromium 45 mcg	38%
Molybdenum 45 mcg	60%
Chloride 72 mg	2%
Potassium 80 mg	2%
Boron 150 mcg	*
Nickel 5 mcg	*
Silicon 2 mg	*
Vanadium 10 mcg	*
Lutein 250 mcg	*
Lycopene 300 mcg	*

*Daily Value (%DV) not established.

Ingredients: Dibasic Calcium Phosphate, Calcium Carbonate, Potassium Chloride, Microcrystalline Cellulose, Ascorbic Acid (Vit. C), Magnesium Oxide, dl-Alpha Tocopheryl Acetate (Vit. E), Modified Food Starch. Contains < 2% of: Acacia, Anhydrous Citric Acid, Ascorbyl Palmitate, Beta Carotene, Biotin, Boric Acid, BHT, Calcium Pantothenate, Calcium Stearate, Cholecalciferol (Vit. D), Chromium Picolinate, Corn Starch, Crospovidone, Cupric Sulfate, Cyanocobalamin (Vit. B_{12}), dl-Alpha Tocopherol, FD&C Blue 2 Aluminum Lake, FD&C Red 40 Aluminum Lake, FD&C Yellow 6 Aluminum Lake, Folic Acid, Gelatin, Hydrogenated Palm Oil, Hypromellose, Lutein, Lycopene, Manganese Sulfate, Medium-Chain Triglycerides, Niacinamide, Nickelous Sulfate, Phytonadione (Vit. K), Polyethylene Glycol, Polyvinyl Alcohol, Potassium Iodide, Pregelatinized Corn Starch, Pyridoxine Hydrochloride (Vit. B_6), Riboflavin (Vit. B_2), Silicon Dioxide, Sodium Ascorbate, Sodium Benzoate, Sodium Borate, Sodium Citrate, Sodium Metavanadate, Sodium Molybdate, Sodium Selenate, Sorbic Acid, Sucrose, Talc, Thiamine Mononitrate (Vit. B_1), Titanium Dioxide, Tri Calcium Phosphate, Vitamin A Acetate (Vit. A), Zinc Oxide. May also contain < 2%: Maltodextrin, Sodium Aluminum Silicate.

Suggested Use:

Adults – One tablet daily with food. Not formulated for use in children.

As with any supplement, if you are pregnant, nursing, or taking medication, contact your doctor before use.

IMPORTANT INFORMATION: Long-term intake of high levels of vitamin A (excluding that sourced from beta-carotene) may increase the risk of osteoporosis in adults. Do not take this product if taking other vitamin A supplements.

How Supplied: Bottles of 60, 100, 150 tablets

Storage:

Store at Room Temperature. Keep bottle tightly closed. Bottle is sealed with printed foil under cap. Do not use if foil is torn.

GENERIC DRUG INFORMATION

This section presents information on generic nonprescription drugs marketed for home use by consumers.

Pharmaceutical product descriptions in this section must be in compliance with the Code of Federal Regulations' labeling requirements for over-the-counter drugs. The descriptions are designed to provide all information necessary for informed use, including, when applicable, active ingredients, inactive ingredients, indications, actions, warnings, cautions, drug interactions, symptoms and treatment of oral over-

dosage, dosage and directions for use, professional labeling, and how supplied.

In compiling this section, the publisher has emphasized the necessity of describing products comprehensively. The publisher does not warrant or guarantee any product described here, and does not perform any independent analysis of the information. Inclusion of a product in this book does not represent an endorsement, and the publisher does not necessarily advocate the use of any product listed.

ALLERGY ANTIHISTAMINE
Diphenhydramine Hydrochloride

Active ingredient
(in each capsule) **Purpose**
Diphenhydramine
hydrochloride 25 mg .... Antihistamine

Uses
- temporarily relieves these symptoms of hay fever or other upper respiratory allergies:
  - runny nose
  - sneezing
  - itchy nose or throat
  - itchy, watery eyes
- temporarily relieves these symptoms of the common cold:
  - runny nose
  - sneezing

Warnings
Do not use with any other product containing diphenhydramine, even one used on skin

Ask a doctor before use if you have
- trouble urinating due to an enlarged prostate gland
- glaucoma
- a breathing problem such as emphysema or chronic bronchitis

Ask a doctor or pharmacist before use if you are taking tranquilizers or sedatives

When using this product
- excitability may occur, especially in children
- marked drowsiness may occur
- avoid alcoholic drinks
- alcohol, sedatives and tranquilizers may increase drowsiness
- be careful when driving a motor vehicle or operating machinery

If pregnant or breast-feeding, ask a health professional before use.

Keep out of reach of children. In case of overdose, get medical help or contact a Poison Control Center right away.

Directions
- take every 4 to 6 hours, not more than 6 doses in 24 hours

adults and children 12 years and over	1 or 2 capsules
children 6 to under 12 years	1 capsule
children under 6 years	ask a doctor

Other information
- store at room temperature (59°-86°F)
- protect from moisture

Inactive ingredients
benzyl alcohol, butylparaben, D&C red no. 28, D&C yellow no. 10, edetate calcium disodium, edible ink, FD&C blue no. 1, FD&C blue no. 2, FD&C red no. 40, gelatin, lactose, magnesium stearate, methylparaben, polysorbate 80, propylparaben, silicon dioxide, sodium lauryl sulfate, sodium propionate

ANTI-DIARRHEAL CAPLETS
Loperamide Hydrochloride Tablets, 2 mg

Use controls symptoms of diarrhea, including Travelers' Diarrhea

Warnings
Allergy alert: Do not use if you have ever had a rash or other allergic reaction to loperamide HCl

Do not use if you have bloody or black stool

Ask a doctor before use if you have
- fever
- mucus in the stool
- a history of liver disease

Ask a doctor or pharmacist before use if you are taking antibiotics

When using this product
- tiredness, drowsiness or dizziness may occur. Be careful when driving or operating machinery.

Stop use and ask a doctor if
- symptoms get worse
- diarrhea lasts for more than 2 days
- you get abdominal swelling or bulging. These may be signs of a serious condition.

If pregnant or breast-feeding, ask a health professional before use.

Keep out of reach of children. In case of overdose, get medical help or contact a Poison Control Center right away.

Directions
- **drink plenty of clear fluids to help prevent dehydration caused by diarrhea**
- find right dose on chart. If possible, use weight to dose; otherwise, use age.

adults and children 12 years and over	2 caplets after the first loose stool; 1 caplet after each subsequent loose stool; but no more than 4 caplets in 24 hours
children 9-11 years (60-95 lbs)	1 caplet after the first loose stool; 1/2 caplet after each subsequent loose stool; but no more than 3 caplets in 24 hours
children 6-8 years (48-59 lbs)	1 caplet after the first loose stool; 1/2 caplet after each subsequent loose stool; but no more than 2 caplets in 24 hours
children under 6 years (up to 47 lbs)	ask a doctor

Other information
- store between 20-25°C (68-77°F)
- **do not use if carton or blister unit is broken or torn**

- see end panel for lot number and expiration date

Inactive ingredients
anhydrous lactose, carnauba wax, D&C yellow no. 10, FD&C blue no. 1, hypromellose, magnesium stearate, microcrystalline cellulose, polyethylene glycol, pregelatinized starch

Questions? If you have questions of a medical nature, please contact your pharmacist, doctor or health care professional.

CALCIUM ANTACID TABLETS
REGULAR STRENGTH
Antacid, Calcium Supplement

Active ingredient
(in each tablet) **Purpose**
Calcium carbonate 500 mg .... Antacid

Uses
relieves:
- acid indigestion
- heartburn

Warnings
Ask a doctor or pharmacist before use if you are taking a prescription drug. Antacids may interact with certain prescription drugs.

When using this product do not take more than 16 tablets in a 24-hour period, or use the maximum dosage of this product for more than 2 weeks, except under the advice and supervision of a doctor.
Keep out of reach of children.

Directions
- chew 2-4 tablets as symptoms occur, or as directed by a doctor.

CALCIUM SUPPLEMENT

USES: As a daily source of extra calcium.

DIRECTIONS: Chew 2 tablets twice daily.

Supplement Facts
Serving Size: 2 Tablets
Servings Per Container: 75

Amount Per Serving	% Daily Value*
Calories 5	
Sugars 1g	†
Calcium 400 mg	**40%**

*Percent Daily Values are based on a 2,000 calorie diet.
† Daily Value not established.

Other information
- do not use if printed seal under cap is torn or missing.
- store at room temperature.

Inactive ingredients
adipic acid, blue 1, corn starch, crospovidone, dextrose, flavors, magnesium stearate, maltodextrin, red 27, red 30, sucrose, talc, yellow 6, yellow 10.

REV 0705-A

HEARTBURN RELIEF
Cimetidine Tablets USP, 200 mg
Acid Reducer

Active ingredient
(in each tablet)   **Purpose**
Cimetidine 200 mg .... Acid reducer

Uses
- **relieves** heartburn associated with acid indigestion and sour stomach
- **prevents** heartburn associated with acid indigestion and sour stomach brought on by eating or drinking certain food and beverages

Warnings
Allergy alert: Do not use if you are allergic to cimetidine or other acid reducers

Do not use
- if you have trouble or pain swallowing food, vomiting with blood, or bloody or black stools. These may be signs of a serious condition. See your doctor.
- with other acid reducers

Ask a doctor before use if you have
- frequent **chest pain**
- frequent wheezing, particularly with heartburn
- unexplained weight loss
- nausea or vomiting
- stomach pain
- had heartburn over 3 months. This may be a sign of a more serious condition.
- heartburn with **lightheadedness, sweating or dizziness**
- chest pain or shoulder pain with shortness of breath; sweating; pain spreading to arms, neck or shoulders; or lightheadedness

Ask a doctor or pharmacist before use if you are taking
- theophylline (oral asthma medicine)
- warfarin (blood thinning medicine)
- phenytoin (seizure medicine)

If you are not sure you are taking one of these medicines, talk to your doctor or pharmacist.

Stop use and ask a doctor if
- your heartburn continues or worsens
- stomach pain continues
- you need to take this product for more than 14 days

If pregnant or breast-feeding, ask a health professional before use.

Keep out of reach of children. In case of overdose, get medical help or contact a Poison Control Center right away.

Directions
- adults and children 12 years and over:
  - to **relieve** symptoms, swallow 1 tablet with a glass of water
  - to **prevent** symptoms, swallow 1 tablet with a glass of water **right before or any time up to 30 minutes before** eating food or drinking beverages that cause heartburn
  - do not take more than 2 tablets in 24 hours
- children under 12 years: ask a doctor

Other information
- do not use if printed foil under cap is broken or missing
- store at 20°-25°C (68°-77°F)

Inactive ingredients
hypromellose, magnesium stearate, microcrystalline cellulose, polyethylene glycol, polysorbate 80, povidone, pregelatinized starch, sodium lauryl sulfate, sodium starch glycolate, titanium dioxide

Questions? If you have questions of a medical nature, please contact your pharmacist, doctor or health care professional.

NICOTINE POLACRILEX GUM 2 mg (NICOTINE) STOP SMOKING AID

Active ingredient
(in each chewing piece)   **Purpose**
Nicotine polacrilex
2 mg (nicotine) .... Stop smoking aid

Use
- reduces withdrawal symptoms, including nicotine craving, associated with quitting smoking

Warnings
If you are pregnant or breast-feeding, only use this medicine on the advice of your health care provider. Smoking can seriously harm your child. Try to stop smoking without using any nicotine replacement medicine. This medicine is believed to be safer than smoking. However, the risks to your child from this medicine are not fully known.

Do not use
- if you continue to smoke, chew tobacco, use snuff, or use a nicotine patch or other nicotine containing products

Ask a doctor before use if you have
- a sodium-restricted diet
- heart disease, recent heart attack, or irregular heartbeat. Nicotine can increase your heart rate.
- high blood pressure not controlled with medication. Nicotine can increase blood pressure.
- stomach ulcer or diabetes

Ask a doctor or pharmacist before use if you are
- using a non-nicotine stop smoking drug
- taking prescription medicine for depression or asthma. Your prescription dose may need to be adjusted.

Stop use and ask a doctor if
- mouth, teeth, or jaw problems occur
- irregular heartbeat or palpitations occur
- you get symptoms of nicotine overdose such as nausea, vomiting, dizziness, diarrhea, weakness, and rapid heartbeat

Keep out of reach of children and pets. Pieces of nicotine gum may have enough nicotine to make children and pets sick. Wrap used pieces of gum in paper and throw away in the trash. In case of overdose, get medical help or contact a Poison Control Center right away.

Directions
- if you are under 18 years of age, ask a doctor before use
- before using this product, read the enclosed User's Guide for complete directions and other important information
- stop smoking completely when you begin using the gum
- **if you smoke 25 or more cigarettes a day;** use 4 mg nicotine gum
- **if you smoke less than 25 cigarettes a day;** use according to the following 12 week schedule:

Weeks 1 to 6	Weeks 7 to 9	Weeks 10 to 12
1 piece every 1 to 2 hours	1 piece every 2 to 4 hours	1 piece every 4 to 8 hours

- nicotine gum is a medicine and must be used a certain way to get the best results
- chew the gum slowly until it tingles. Then park it between your cheek and gum. When the tingle is gone, begin chewing again, until the tingle returns.
- repeat this process until most of the tingle is gone (about 30 minutes)
- do not eat or drink for 15 minutes before chewing the nicotine gum, or while chewing a piece
- to improve your chances of quitting, use at least 9 pieces per day for the first 6 weeks
- if you experience strong or frequent cravings, you may use a second piece within the hour. However, do not continuously use one piece after another since this may cause you hiccups, heartburn, nausea or other side effects.
- do not use more than 24 pieces a day
- it is important to complete treatment. Stop using the nicotine gum at the end of 12 weeks. If you still feel the need to use nicotine gum, talk to your doctor.

Other information
- **each piece contains:** calcium 115 mg, sodium 8 mg
- store at 20 - 25°C (68 - 77°F)
- protect from light

Inactive ingredients carnauba wax, flavors, gum base, magnesium oxide, sodium bicarbonate, sodium carbonate, talc and xylitol

To remove the gum, tear off single unit.

Peel off backing starting at corner with loose edge.

Continued on next page

Nicotine Polacrilex Gum—Cont.

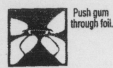

Push gum through foil.

- **Not for sale to those under 18 years of age.**
- **Proof of age required.**
- **Not for sale in vending machines or from any source where proof of age cannot be verified.**

NICOTINE TRANSDERMAL SYSTEM STOP SMOKING AID
Patch

Active ingredient
(in each patch)   **Purpose**
Nicotine, 21 mg delivered
over 24 hours .... Stop smoking aid

Use reduces withdrawal symptoms, including nicotine craving, associated with quitting smoking

Warnings
If you are pregnant or breast-feeding, only use this medicine on the advice of your health care provider. Smoking can seriously harm your child. Try to stop smoking without using any nicotine replacement medicine. This medicine is believed to be safer than smoking. However, the risks to your child from this medicine are not fully known.

Do not use
- if you continue to smoke, chew tobacco, use snuff, use nicotine gum, or use nicotine patch or other nicotine containing products

Ask a doctor before use if you have
- heart disease, recent heart attack, or irregular heartbeat. Nicotine can increase your heart rate.
- high blood pressure not controlled with medication. Nicotine can increase your blood pressure.
- an allergy to adhesive tape or have skin problems, because you are more likely to get rashes

Ask a doctor or pharmacist before use if you are
- using a non-nicotine stop smoking drug
- taking a prescription medicine for depression or asthma. Your prescription dose may need to be adjusted.

When using this product
- do not smoke even when not wearing the patch. The nicotine in your skin will still be entering your bloodstream for several hours after you take off the patch.

- if you have vivid dreams or other sleep disturbances remove this patch at bedtime

Stop use and ask a doctor if
- skin redness caused by the patch does not go away after four days, or if your skin swells, or you get a rash
- irregular heartbeat or palpitations occur
- you get symptoms of nicotine overdose, such as nausea, vomiting, dizziness, weakness and rapid heartbeat

Keep out of reach of children and pets. Used patches have enough nicotine to poison children and pets. If swallowed, get medical help or contact a Poison Control Center right away. Discard used patches in disposal tray. If disposal tray is not enclosed, save pouch to use for patch disposal. Dispose of the used patch by folding sticky ends together and putting in pouch.

Directions
- **If you are under 18 years of age, ask a doctor before use**
- before using this product, read the enclosed self-help guide for complete directions and other information
- stop smoking completely when you begin using the patch
- if you smoke **more than 10 cigarettes per day,** use the following schedule below:

Weeks 1 thru 4	Weeks 5 and 6	Weeks 7 and 8
STEP 1 use one 21 mg patch/day	STEP 2 use one 14 mg patch/day	STEP 3 use one 7 mg patch/day

- if you smoke **10 or less cigarettes per day,** start with **Step 2** for 6 weeks, then **Step 3** for 2 weeks and then stop
- apply one new patch every 24 hours on skin that is dry, clean and hairless
- remove backing from patch and immediately press onto skin. Hold for 10 seconds.
- wash hands after applying or removing patch. Discard used patches in disposal tray. If disposal tray is not enclosed, save pouch to use for patch disposal. Dispose of the used patch by folding sticky ends together and putting in pouch.
- the used patch should be removed and a new one applied to a different skin site at the same time each day
- if you have vivid dreams, you may remove the patch at bedtime and apply a new one in the morning
- do not wear more than one patch at a time
- do not cut patch in half or into smaller pieces
- do not leave patch on for more than 24 hours because it may irritate your skin and loses strength after 24 hours
- **remove patch prior to undergoing any MRI (magnetic resonance imaging) procedures**
- stop using the patch at the end of 8

weeks. If you still feel the need to use the patch talk to your doctor.

Other information
- store at 20-25°C (68-77°F)

Inactive ingredients acrylate adhesive, aluminized polyester, cellulose paper, methacrylic acid copolymer

Comments or Questions?
Call **1-800-585-8682** Weekdays (9am-8pm ET)
- **Not for sale to persons under 18 years of age.**
- **Proof of age required.**
- **Not for sale in vending machines or from any source where proof of age cannot be verified.**
For your family's protection, patches are supplied in child-resistant pouches.

Do not use if individual pouch is open or torn.

Carton shrink wrapped for your protection.

Do not use if shrink wrap is open or torn.

TO INCREASE YOUR SUCCESS IN QUITTING:
1. You must be motivated to quit.
2. Use one patch daily according to directions.
3. Complete the full treatment program.
4. Do not use patch for more than 8 weeks.
5. Use patch with a behavioral support program, such as the one described in the enclosed booklet and on the compact disc.

NON-DROWSY NASAL DECONGESTANT MAXIMUM STRENGTH
Pseudoephedrine Hydrochloride
Nasal Decongestant

Active ingredient
(in each tablet)   **Purpose**
Pseudoephedrine hydrochloride
30 mg .... Nasal decongestant

Uses
- temporarily relieves sinus congestion and pressure
- temporarily relieves nasal congestion due to the common cold, hay fever or other upper respiratory allergies

Warnings
Do not use if you are now taking a prescription monoamine oxidase inhibitor (MAOI) (certain drugs for depression, psychiatric or emotional conditions, or Parkinson's disease), or for 2 weeks after stopping the MAOI drug. If you do not know if your prescription drug contains an MAOI, ask a doctor or pharmacist before taking this product.

Ask a doctor before use if you have
- heart disease
- high blood pressure

- diabetes
- trouble urinating due to an enlarged prostate gland
- thyroid disease

When using this product

- do not use more than directed

Stop use and ask a doctor if

- you get nervous, dizzy or sleepless
- symptoms do not get better within 7 days or occur with fever

If pregnant or breast-feeding, ask a health professional before use.

Keep out of reach of children. In case of overdose, get medical help or contact a Poison Control Center right away.

Directions

- take every 4 to 6 hours, not more than 4 doses in 24 hours

adults and children 12 years and over	2 tablets
children 6 to under 12 years	1 tablet
children under 6 years	ask a doctor

Other information

- **each tablet contains:** calcium 20 mg
- store at 20°-25°C (68°-77°F)

Inactive ingredients carnauba wax, dibasic calcium phosphate, FD&C red no. 40 aluminum lake, hypromellose, magnesium stearate, microcrystalline cellulose, polyethylene glycol, polysorbate 80, silicon dioxide, titanium dioxide

---

NON-DROWSY NASAL DECONGESTANT PE

Phenylephrine HCl Tablets
Nasal Decongestant
Does not Contain Pseudoephedrine

Active ingredient
(in each tablet) **Purpose**
Phenylephrine hydrochloride
10 mg .... Nasal decongestant

Uses

- temporarily relieves sinus congestion and pressure
- temporarily relieves nasal congestion due to the common cold, hay fever or other upper respiratory allergies

Warnings

Do not use if you are now taking a prescription monoamine oxidase inhibitor (MAOI) (certain drugs for depression, psychiatric or emotional conditions, or Parkinson's disease), or for 2 weeks after

stopping the MAOI drug. If you do not know if your prescription drug contains an MAOI, ask a doctor or pharmacist before taking this product.

Ask a doctor before use if you have

- heart disease
- high blood pressure
- diabetes
- trouble urinating due to an enlarged prostate gland
- thyroid disease

When using this product

- do not use more than directed

Stop use and ask a doctor if

- you get nervous, dizzy or sleepless
- symptoms do not improve within 7 days or are accompanied by fever

If pregnant or breast-feeding, ask a health professional before use.

Keep out of reach of children. In case of overdose, get medical help or contact a Poison Control Center right away.

Directions

- take every 4 hours
- do not take more than 6 doses in 24 hours
- adults and children 12 years of age and over: 1 tablet
- children under 12 years of age: ask a doctor

Other information

- store at room temperature (59°-86°F)

Inactive ingredients carnauba wax, dibasic calcium phosphate, FD&C red no. 40 aluminum lake, lecithin, magnesium stearate, microcrystalline cellulose, polyethylene glycol, polyvinyl alcohol, silicon dioxide, talc, titanium dioxide

---

REGULAR STRENGTH PAIN RELIEF TABLETS

Acetaminophen
Pain Reliever - Fever Reducer

SEALED WITH PRINTED FOIL UNDER CAP FOR YOUR PROTECTION

Active ingredient
(in each tablet) **Purpose**
Acetaminophen 325 mg .... Pain reliever/
fever reducer

Uses
temporarily relieves minor aches and pains due to:

- headache
- backache
- the common cold
- menstrual cramps

- muscular aches
- arthritis
- toothache
- reduces fever

Warnings

Overdose warning: Taking more than the recommended dose can cause serious health problems, including liver damage. In case of overdose, get medical help or contact a Poison Control Center right away. Quick medical attention is critical for adults as well as for children even if you do not notice any signs or symptoms.

Alcohol warning: If you consume 3 or more alcoholic drinks every day, ask your doctor whether you should take acetaminophen or other pain relievers/fever reducers. Acetaminophen may cause liver damage.

Do not use with any other product containing acetaminophen

Stop use and ask a doctor if

- pain gets worse or lasts for more than 10 days
- new symptoms occur
- fever gets worse or lasts for more than 3 days
- redness or swelling is present

If pregnant or breast-feeding, ask a health professional before use.

Keep out of reach of children.

Directions

- do not use more than directed (see overdose warning)

adults and children 12 years and over	• take 2 tablets every 4 to 6 hours as needed • do not take more than 12 tablets in 24 hours
children 6-11 years	• take 1 tablet every 4 to 6 hours as needed • do not take more than 5 tablets in 24 hours
children under 6 years	do not use this adult Regular Strength product in children under 6 years of age; this will provide more than the recommended dose (overdose) and could cause serious health problems

Other information

- store at room temperature (59°-86°F)

Inactive ingredients croscarmellose sodium*, povidone, pregelatinized starch, stearic acid

---

*may contain this ingredient

PRODUCT COMPARISON TABLES

This section provides a quick comparison of the ingredients and dosages of common brand-name drugs in 12 therapeutic classes: Acne Products; Allergic Rhinitis Products; Analgesic Products; Antacid and Heartburn Products; Antidiarrheal Products; Antiflatulant Products; Contact Dermatitis Products; Cough, Cold, and Flu Products; Headache/Migraine Products; Laxative Products; Psoriasis Products; and Wound Care Products.

Table 1. ACNE PRODUCTS

Brand Name	Ingredient/Strength	Dose
BENZOYL PEROXIDE		
Clean & Clear Continuous Control Acne Cleanser *(Johnson & Johnson Consumer)*	Benzoyl Peroxide 10%	**Adults & Peds:** Use bid.
Clean & Clear Persa-Gel 10, Maximum Strength *(Johnson & Johnson Consumer)*	Benzoyl Peroxide 10%	**Adults & Peds:** Use qd-tid.
Clearasil Daily Acne Control cream *(Reckitt Benckiser)*	Benzoyl Peroxide 10%	**Adults & Peds:** Use qd-tid.
Clearasil Maximum Strength Acne Treatment vanishing cream *(Reckitt Benckiser)*	Benzoyl Peroxide 10%	**Adults & Peds:** Use qd-tid.
Clearasil Total Control Acne Crisis Clear Up *(Reckitt Benckiser)*	Benzoyl Peroxide 10%	**Adults & Peds:** Use qd-tid.
Clearasil Ultra Acne Treatment tinted cream *(Reckitt Benckiser)*	Benzoyl Peroxide 10%	**Adults & Peds:** Use tid.
Clearasil Ultra Acne Treatment vanishing cream *(Reckitt Benckiser)*	Benzoyl Peroxide 10%	**Adults & Peds:** Use tid.
Neutrogena Clear Pore Cleanser Mask *(Neutrogena)*	Benzoyl Peroxide 3.5%	**Adults & Peds:** Use biw-tiw.
Neutrogena On-the-Spot Acne Treatment vanishing cream *(Neutrogena)*	Benzoyl Peroxide 2.5%	**Adults & Peds:** Use qd initially, then bid-tid.
Oxy 10 Balance Oil-Free Maximum Strength Acne Wash *(GlaxoSmithKline Consumer Healthcare)*	Benzoyl Peroxide 10%	**Adults & Peds:** Use bid-tid.
Oxy Balance Acne Treatment for Sensitive Skin vanishing cream *(GlaxoSmithKline Consumer Healthcare)*	Benzoyl Peroxide 5%	**Adults & Peds:** Use qd-tid.
Oxy Balance Maximum Acne Treatment tinted lotion *(GlaxoSmithKline Consumer Healthcare)*	Benzoyl Peroxide 10%	**Adults & Peds:** Use qd-tid.
Oxy Spot Treatment *(GlaxoSmithKline Consumer Healthcare)*	Benzoyl Peroxide 10%	**Adults & Peds:** Use qd-tid.
PanOxyl Aqua Gel Maximum Strength gel *(Stiefel)*	Benzoyl Peroxide 10%	**Adults & Peds:** Use qd initially, then bid-tid.
PanOxyl Bar 10% Maximum Strength *(Stiefel)*	Benzoyl Peroxide 10%	**Adults & Peds:** Use qd initially, then bid-tid.
PanOxyl Bar 5% *(Stiefel)*	Benzoyl Peroxide 5%	**Adults & Peds:** Use qd initially, then bid-tid.
ZAPZYT Maximum Strength Acne Treatment gel *(Waltman Pharmaceuticals)*	Benzoyl Peroxide 10%	**Adults & Peds:** Use qd-tid.
ZAPZYT Treatment Bar *(Waltman Pharmaceuticals)*	Benzoyl Peroxide 10%	**Adults & Peds:** Use qd-tid.
SALICYLIC ACID		
Aveeno Clear Complexion Cleansing Bar *(Johnson & Johnson Consumer)*	Salicylic Acid 0.5%	**Adults & Peds:** Use daily.
Aveeno Clear Complexion Foaming Cleanser *(Johnson & Johnson Consumer)*	Salicylic Acid 0.5%	**Adults & Peds:** Use daily.
Aveeno Correcting Treatment, Clear Complexion *(Johnson & Johnson Consumer)*	Salicylic Acid 1%	**Adults & Peds:** Use qd-tid.
Bioré Blemish Fighting Cleansing Cloths *(Kao Brands Company)*	Salicylic Acid 0.5%	**Adults & Peds:** Use qd-tid.
Bioré Blemish Fighting Ice Cleanser *(Kao Brands Company)*	Salicylic Acid 2%	**Adults & Peds:** Use qd.

Table 1. ACNE PRODUCTS (cont.)

BRAND NAME	INGREDIENT/STRENGTH	DOSE
Bye Bye Blemish Acne Lemon Scrub *(Beauty Beat)*	Salicylic Acid 1%	**Adults & Peds:** Use qd-tid.
Bye Bye Blemish Anti-Acne Moisturizer *(Beauty Beat)*	Salicylic Acid 0.5%	**Adults & Peds:** Use qd-tid.
Bye Bye Blemish Anti-Acne Serum *(Beauty Beat)*	Salicylic Acid 1%	**Adults & Peds:** Use qd-tid.
Bye Bye Blemish Drying Lotion *(Beauty Beat)*	Salicylic Acid 2%	**Adults & Peds:** Use pm.
Bye Bye Blemish Purifying Acne Mask *(Beauty Beat)*	Salicylic Acid 0.5%	**Adults & Peds:** Use qd.
Clean & Clear Advantage Acne Cleanser *(Johnson & Johnson Consumer)*	Salicylic Acid 2%	**Adults & Peds:** Use qd.
Clean & Clear Advantage Acne Spot Treatment *(Johnson & Johnson Consumer)*	Salicylic Acid 2%	**Adults & Peds:** Use qd.
Clean & Clear Advantage Daily Cleansing Pads *(Johnson & Johnson Consumer)*	Salicylic Acid 2%	**Adults & Peds:** Use qd.
Clean & Clear Blackhead Clearing Astringent *(Johnson & Johnson Consumer)*	Salicylic Acid 1%	**Adults & Peds:** Use qd.
Clean & Clear Blackhead Clearing Daily Cleansing Pads *(Johnson & Johnson Consumer)*	Salicylic Acid 1%	**Adults & Peds:** Use qd.
Clean & Clear Blackhead Clearing Scrub *(Johnson & Johnson Consumer)*	Salicylic Acid 2%	**Adults & Peds:** Use qd.
Clean & Clear Clear Advantage Daily Acne Clearing lotion *(Johnson & Johnson Consumer)*	Salicylic Acid 1%	**Adults & Peds:** Use qd.
Clean & Clear Continuous Control Acne Wash, Oil Free *(Johnson & Johnson Consumer)*	Salicylic Acid 2%	**Adults & Peds:** Use qd.
Clean & Clear Facial Cleansing Bar, Blackhead Clearing *(Johnson & Johnson Consumer)*	Salicylic Acid 0.5%	**Adults & Peds:** Use qd.
Clean & Clear Oil-Free Dual Action Moisturizer lotion *(Johnson & Johnson Consumer)*	Salicylic Acid 0.5%	**Adults & Peds:** Use qd-tid.
Clearasil 3 in 1 Acne Defense Cleanser *(Reckitt Benckiser)*	Salicylic Acid 2%	**Adults & Peds:** Use qd-tid.
Clearasil Acne Fighting Cleansing Wipes *(Reckitt Benckiser)*	Salicylic Acid 2%	**Adults & Peds:** Use qd.
Clearasil Acne Fighting Facial Moisturizer *(Reckitt Benckiser)*	Salicylic Acid 2%	**Adults & Peds:** Use qd-tid.
Clearasil Acne Fighting Foaming Cleanser *(Reckitt Benckiser)*	Salicylic Acid 2%	**Adults & Peds:** Use qd-tid.
Clearasil Blackhead Clearing Pads with Targeted Action *(Reckitt Benckiser)*	Salicylic Acid 2%	**Adults & Peds:** Use qd-tid.
Clearasil Blackhead Clearing Scrub *(Reckitt Benckiser)*	Salicylic Acid 2%	**Adults & Peds:** Use qd.
Clearasil Daily Acne Control Pore Cleansing Pads *(Reckitt Benckiser)*	Salicylic Acid 2%	**Adults & Peds:** Use qd.
Clearasil Daily Blackhead Control Astringent *(Reckitt Benckiser)*	Salicylic Acid 1%	**Adults & Peds:** Use qd.

Table 1. ACNE PRODUCTS (cont.)

BRAND NAME	INGREDIENT/STRENGTH	DOSE
Clearasil Daily Oil Control Cream Cleanser *(Reckitt Benckiser)*	Salicylic Acid 1%	**Adults & Peds:** Use qd.
Clearasil Icewash, Acne Gel Cleanser *(Reckitt Benckiser)*	Salicylic Acid 2%	**Adults & Peds:** Use qd.
Clearasil Maximum Strength Pore Cleansing Pads *(Reckitt Benckiser)*	Salicylic Acid 2%	**Adults & Peds:** Use qd-tid.
Clearasil Oil Control Acne Wash *(Reckitt Benckiser)*	Salicylic Acid 2%	**Adults & Peds:** Use qd.
Clearasil Overnight Acne Defense Gel *(Reckitt Benckiser)*	Salicylic Acid 2%	**Adults & Peds:** Use qd-tid.
Clearasil Total Control Daily Skin Perfecting Treatment *(Reckitt Benckiser)*	Salicylic Acid 0.5%	**Adults & Peds:** Use qd.
Clearasil Total Control Deep Pore Cream Cleanser *(Reckitt Benckiser)*	Salicylic Acid 2%	**Adults & Peds:** Use qd.
Clearasil Ultra Acne Clearing Scrub *(Reckitt Benckiser)*	Salicylic Acid 2%	**Adults & Peds:** Use qd.
Clearasil Ultra Deep Pore Cleansing Pads *(Reckitt Benckiser)*	Salicylic Acid 2%	**Adults & Peds:** Use qd-tid.
L'Oréal Pure Zone Pore Unclogging Scrub Cleanser *(L'Oreal)*	Salicylic Acid 1%	**Adults & Peds:** Use bid.
L'Oréal Pure Zone Skin Clearing Foaming Cleanser *(L'Oreal)*	Salicylic Acid 2%	**Adults & Peds:** Use bid.
Neutrogena Clear Pore Treatment - Night Time *(Neutrogena)*	Salicylic Acid 2%	**Adults & Peds:** Use qd.
Neutrogena Advanced Solutions Acne Mark Fading Peel with CelluZyme *(Neutrogena)*	Salicylic Acid 2%	**Adults & Peds:** Use qw-tiw.
Neutrogena Blackhead Eliminating Astringent *(Neutrogena)*	Salicylic Acid 0.5%	**Adults & Peds:** Use qd.
Neutrogena Blackhead Eliminating Daily Scrub *(Neutrogena)*	Salicylic Acid 2%	**Adults & Peds:** Use prn.
Neutrogena Blackhead Eliminating Treatment Mask *(Neutrogena)*	Salicylic Acid 0.5%	**Adults & Peds:** Use biw-tiw.
Neutrogena Body Clear Body Scrub *(Neutrogena)*	Salicylic Acid 2%	**Adults & Peds:** Use qd.
Neutrogena Body Clear Body Wash *(Neutrogena)*	Salicylic Acid 2%	**Adults & Peds:** Use qd.
Neutrogena Clear Pore Oil-Controlling Astringent *(Neutrogena)*	Salicylic Acid 2%	**Adults & Peds:** Use qd-tid.
Neutrogena Maximum Strength Oil Controlling Pads *(Neutrogena)*	Salicylic Acid 2%	**Adults & Peds:** Use qd-tid.
Neutrogena Multi-Vitamin Acne Treatment *(Neutrogena)*	Salicylic Acid 1.5%	**Adults & Peds:** Use prn.
Neutrogena Oil Free Acne Stress Control Power Clear scrub *(Neutrogena)*	Salicylic Acid 2%	**Adults & Peds:** Use qd.
Neutrogena Oil Free Acne Stress Control Power Foam wash *(Neutrogena)*	Salicylic Acid 2%	**Adults & Peds:** Use qd.
Neutrogena Acne Stress Control 3-in-1 Hydrating Acne Treatment *(Neutrogena)*	Salicylic Acid 2%	**Adults & Peds:** Use qd.
Neutrogena Oil Free Acne Wash Cleansing Cloths *(Neutrogena)*	Salicylic Acid 2%	**Adults & Peds:** Use qd.
Neutrogena Oil Free Acne Wash Cream Cleanser *(Neutrogena)*	Salicylic Acid 2%	**Adults & Peds:** Use qd.

Table 1. ACNE PRODUCTS (cont.)

BRAND NAME	INGREDIENT/STRENGTH	DOSE
Neutrogena Rapid Clear Acne Defense Lotion *(Neutrogena)*	Salicylic Acid 2%	**Adults & Peds:** Use qd-tid.
Neutrogena Rapid Clear Acne Eliminating Gel *(Neutrogena)*	Salicylic Acid 2%	**Adults & Peds:** Use qd-tid.
Neutrogena Skin Clearing Face Wash *(Neutrogena)*	Salicylic Acid 1.5%	**Adults & Peds:** Use bid.
Neutrogena Skin Clearing Moisturizer *(Neutrogena)*	Salicylic Acid 2%	**Adults & Peds:** Use prn.
Noxzema Continuous Clean Clarifying Toner *(Procter & Gamble)*	Salicylic Acid 2%	**Adults & Peds:** Use qd-tid.
Noxzema Continuous Clean Deep Foaming Cleanser *(Procter & Gamble)*	Salicylic Acid 2%	**Adults & Peds:** Use qd.
Noxzema Continuous Clean Microbead Cleanser *(Procter & Gamble)*	Salicylic Acid 2%	**Adults & Peds:** Use qd.
Noxzema Triple Clean Pads *(Procter & Gamble)*	Salicylic Acid 2%	**Adults & Peds:** Use qd-tid.
Olay Daily Facials Clarity Daily Scrub *(Procter & Gamble)*	Salicylic Acid 2%	**Adults & Peds:** Use qd.
Olay Daily Facials Clarity Purifying Toner *(Procter & Gamble)*	Salicylic Acid 2%	**Adults & Peds:** Use qd-tid.
Olay Daily Facials Night Cleansing Cloths *(Procter & Gamble)*	Salicylic Acid 2%	**Adults & Peds:** Use qd-tid.
Olay Daily Facials Self-Foaming Discs *(Procter & Gamble)*	Salicylic Acid 2%	**Adults & Peds:** Use qd-tid.
Oxy Balance Daily Cleansing Pads, Sensitive Skin *(GlaxoSmithKline Consumer Healthcare)*	Salicylic Acid 0.5%	**Adults & Peds:** Use qd-tid.
Oxy Balance Deep Pore Cleansing Pads, Gentle *(GlaxoSmithKline Consumer Healthcare)*	Salicylic Acid 0.5%	**Adults & Peds:** Use qd-tid.
Oxy Deep Pore Acne Medicated Cleansing Pads, Maximum Strength *(GlaxoSmithKline Consumer Healthcare)*	Salicylic Acid 2%	**Adults & Peds:** Use qd-tid.
Oxy Body Wash *(GlaxoSmithKline Consumer Healthcare)*	Salicylic Acid 2%	**Adults & Peds:** Use qd.
Phisoderm Anti-Blemish Gel Facial Wash *(Chattem)*	Salicylic Acid 2%	**Adults & Peds:** Use qd.
St. Ives Medicated Apricot Scrub *(St. Ives Laboratories)*	Salicylic Acid 2%	**Adults & Peds:** Use qd.
Stridex Facewipes to Go with Acne Medication *(Blistex)*	Salicylic Acid 0.5%	**Adults & Peds:** Use qd-tid.
Stridex Triple Action Acne Pads Maximum Strength, Alcohol Free *(Blistex)*	Salicylic Acid 2%	**Adults & Peds:** Use qd-tid.
Stridex Triple Action Acne Pads with Salicylic Acid, Super Scrub *(Blistex)*	Salicylic Acid 2%	**Adults & Peds:** Use qd-tid.
Stridex Triple Action Medicated Acne Pads, Sensitive Skin *(Blistex)*	Salicylic Acid 0.5%	**Adults & Peds:** Use qd-tid.
ZAPZYT Acne Wash Treatment For Face & Body *(Waltman Pharmaceuticals)*	Salicylic Acid 2%	**Adults & Peds:** Use bid.
ZAPZYT Acne Wash with Soothing Aloe & Chamomile *(Waltman Pharmaceuticals)*	Salicylic Acid 2%	**Adults & Peds:** Use qd-tid.
ZAPZYT Pore Treatment Gel *(Waltman Pharmaceuticals)*	Salicylic Acid 2%	**Adults & Peds:** Use qd-tid.

Table 2. ALLERGIC RHINITIS PRODUCTS

BRAND NAME	INGREDIENT/STRENGTH	DOSE
ANTIHISTAMINE		
Alavert 24-Hour Allergy tablets *(Wyeth Consumer Healthcare)*	Loratadine 10mg	**Adults & Peds: ≥6 yrs:** 1 tab qd. **Max:** 1 tab q24h.
Benadryl Allergy capsules *(McNeil Consumer)*	Diphenhydramine HCl 25mg	**Adults: ≥12 yrs:** 1-2 caps q4-6h. **Peds: 6-12 yrs:** 1 cap q4-6h **Max:** 6 doses q24h.
Benadryl Allergy chewable tablets *(McNeil Consumer)*	Diphenhydramine HCl 12.5mg	**Adults: ≥12 yrs:** 2-4 tabs q4-6h. **Peds: 6-12 yrs:** 1-2 tabs q4-6h. **Max:** 6 doses q24h.
Benadryl Allergy liquid *(McNeil Consumer)*	Diphenhydramine HCl 12.5mg/5mL	**Adults: ≥12 yrs:** 2-4 tsps (10-20mL) q4-6h. **Peds: 6-12 yrs:** 1-2 tsp (5-10mL) q4-6h. **Max:** 6 doses q24h.
Benadryl Allergy Ultratabs *(McNeil Consumer)*	Diphenhydramine HCl 25mg	**Adults: ≥12 yrs:** 1-2 tabs q4-6h. **Peds: 6-12 yrs:** 1 tab q4-6h. **Max:** 6 doses q24h.
Benadryl Children's Allergy fastmelt tablets *(McNeil Consumer)*	Diphenhydramine Citrate HCl 19mg	**Adults: ≥12 yrs:** 2-4 tabs q4-6h. **Peds: 6-12 yrs:** 1-2 tabs q4-6h. **Max:** 6 doses q24h.
Chlor-Trimeton 4-Hour Allergy tablets *(Schering-Plough)*	Chlorpheniramine Maleate 4mg	**Adults: ≥12 yrs:** 1 tab q4-6h. **Max:** 6 tabs q24h. **Peds: 6-12 yrs:** ½ tab q4-6h. **Max:** 3 tabs q24h.
Claritin 24 Hour Allergy tablets *(Schering-Plough)*	Loratadine 10mg	**Adults & Peds: ≥6 yrs:** 1 tab qd. **Max:** 1 tab q24h.
Claritin Children's syrup *(Schering-Plough)*	Loratadine 5mg/5mL	**Adults: ≥6 yrs:** 2 tsp qd. **Max:** 2 tsp q24h. **Peds: 2-6 yrs:** 1 tsp qd. **Max:** 1 tsp q24h.
Claritin RediTabs *(Schering-Plough)*	Loratadine 10mg	**Adults & Peds: ≥6 yrs:** 1 tab qd. **Max:** 1 tab q24h.
Dimetapp ND Children's Allergy liquid *(Wyeth Consumer Healthcare)*	Loratadine 5mg/5mL	**Adults: ≥6 yrs:** 2 tsp qd. **Max:** 2 tsp q24h. **Peds: 2-6 yrs:** 1 tsp qd. **Max:** 1 tsp q24h.
Dimetapp ND Children's Allergy tablets *(Wyeth Consumer Healthcare)*	Loratadine 10mg	**Adults & Peds: ≥6 yrs:** **Max:** 1 tab q24h.
Tavist Allergy tablets *(Novartis Consumer Health)*	Clemastine Fumarate 1.34mg	**Adults & Peds: ≥12 yrs:** 1 tab q12h. **Max:** 2 tabs q24h.
Tavist ND 24-Hour Allergy tablets *(Novartis Consumer Health)*	Loratadine 10mg	**Adults & Peds: ≥6 yrs:** 1 tab qd. **Max:** 1 tab q24h.
Triaminic Allerchews *(Novartis Consumer Health)*	Loratadine 10mg	**Adults & Peds: ≥6 yrs:** 1 tab qd. **Max:** 1 tab q24h.
ANTIHISTAMINE COMBINATIONS		
Advil Allergy Sinus caplets *(Wyeth Consumer Healthcare)*	Chlorpheniramine Maleate/Ibuprofen/ Pseudoephedrine HCl 2mg-200mg-30mg	**Adults & Peds: ≥12 yrs:** 1 tab q4-6h. **Max:** 6 tabs q24h.
Alavert D-12 Hour Allergy tablets *(Wyeth Consumer Healthcare)*	Loratadine/Pseudoephedrine Sulfate 5mg-120mg	**Adults & Peds: ≥12 yrs:** 1 tab q12h. **Max:** 2 tabs q24h.
Benadryl Allergy & Sinus Headache caplets *(McNeil Consumer)*	Diphenhydramine HCl/Acetaminophen/ Phenylephrine HCl 12.5mg-325mg-5mg	**Adults & Peds: ≥12 yrs:** 2 caps q4h. **Max:** 12 caps q24h.
Benadryl Severe Allergy & Sinus Headache caplets *(McNeil Consumer)*	Diphenhydramine HCl/Acetaminophen/ Phenylephrine HCl 25mg-325mg-5mg	**Adults & Peds: ≥12 yrs:** 2 tabs q4h. **Max:** 12 tabs q24h.
Benadryl-D Allergy & Sinus Liquid *(McNeil Consumer)*	Diphenhydramine HCl/Pseudoephedrine HCl 12.5mg-30mg/5mL	**Adults & Peds: ≥12 yrs:** 2 tsp q4-6h. **Peds: 6-12 yrs:** 1 tsp q4-6h. **Max:** 4 doses q24h.
Benadryl-D Allergy & Sinus tablets *(McNeil Consumer)*	Diphenhydramine HCl/Phenylephrine HCl 25mg-10mg	**Adults & Peds: ≥12 yrs:** 1 tab q4h. **Max:** 6 tabs q24h.
Claritin-D 12 Hour Allergy & Congestion tablets *(Schering-Plough)*	Loratadine/Pseudoephedrine Sulfate 5mg-120mg	**Adults & Peds: ≥12 yrs:** 1 tab q12h. **Max:** 2 tabs q24h.
Claritin-D 24 Hour Allergy & Congestion tablets *(Schering-Plough)*	Loratadine/Pseudoephedrine Sulfate 10mg-240mg	**Adults & Peds: ≥12 yrs:** 1 tab q12h. **Max:** 1 tabs q24h.

Table 2. ALLERGIC RHINITIS PRODUCTS (cont.)

BRAND NAME	INGREDIENT/STRENGTH	DOSE
Drixoral Allergy Sinus sustained-action tablets (Schering-Plough)	Dexbrompheniramine Maleate/Acetaminophen/ Pseudoephedrine HCl 3mg-500mg-60mg	**Adults & Peds: ≥12 yrs:** 2 tabs q12h. **Max:** 4 tabs q24h.
Sinutab Sinus caplets (McNeil Consumer)	Acetaminophen/Phenylephrine HCl 325mg-5mg	**Adults & Peds: ≥12 yrs:** 2 tabs q4h. **Max:** 12 tabs q24h.
Sudafed PE Sinus & Allergy tablets (McNeil Consumer)	Chlorpheniramine Maleate/Phenylephrine HCl 4mg-10mg	**Adults: ≥12 yrs:** 1 tab q4h. **Peds: 6-12 yrs:** 1/2 tab q4h. **Max:** 6 doses q24h.
Tylenol Allergy Complete Multi-Symptom Cool Burst caplets (McNeil Consumer)	Chlorpheniramine Maleate/Acetaminophen/ Phenylephrine HCl 2mg-325mg-5mg	**Adults & Peds: ≥12 yrs:** 2 tabs q4h. **Max:** 12 tabs q24h.
Tylenol Allergy Complete Nighttime Cool Burst caplets (McNeil Consumer)	DiphenhydramineHCl/Acetaminophen/ Phenylephrine HCl 25mg-325mg-5mg	**Adults & Peds: ≥12 yrs:** 2 tabs q4h. **Max:** 12 tabs q24h.
Tylenol Allergy Complete caplets (McNeil Consumer)	Chlorpheniramine Maleate/Acetaminophen/ Pseudoephedrine HCl 2mg-500mg-30mg	**Adults & Peds: ≥12 yrs:** 2 tabs q4-6h. **Max:** 8 tabs q24h.
Tylenol Allergy Complete Night Time caplets (McNeil Consumer)	Diphenhydramine HCl/Acetaminophen/ Pseudoephedrine HCl 25mg-500mg-30mg	**Adults & Peds: ≥12 yrs:** 2 tabs q4-6h. **Max:** 8 tabs q24h.
Tylenol Severe Allergy caplets (McNeil Consumer)	Diphenhydramine HCl/Acetaminophen 12.5mg-500mg	**Adults & Peds: ≥12 yrs:** 2 tabs q4-6h. **Max:** 8 tabs q24h.
TOPICAL NASAL DECONGESTANTS		
4-Way Fast Acting Nasal Decongestant Spray (Novartis Consumer Health)	Phenylephrine HCl 1%	**Adults & Peds: ≥12 yrs:** Instill 2-3 sprays per nostril q4h.
4-Way Nasal Decongestant Spray, 12 Hour (Novartis Consumer Health)	Phenylephrine HCl 1%	**Adults & Peds: ≥12 yrs:** Instill 2-3 sprays per nostril q4h.
4-Way No Drip Nasal Decongestant Spray (Novartis Consumer Health)	Phenylephrine HCl 1%	**Adults & Peds: ≥12 yrs:** Instill 2-3 sprays per nostril q4h.
Afrin Extra Moisturizing Nasal Spray (Schering-Plough)	Oxymetazoline HCl 0.05%	**Adults & Peds: ≥6 yrs:** Instill 2-3 sprays per nostril q10-12h.
Afrin No Drip Nasal Spray (Schering-Plough)	Oxymetazoline HCl 0.05%	**Adults & Peds: ≥6 yrs:** Instill 2-3 sprays per nostril q10-12h.
Afrin No Drip Sinus Nasal Spray (Schering-Plough)	Oxymetazoline HCl 0.05%	**Adults & Peds: ≥6 yrs:** Instill 2-3 sprays per nostril q10-12h.
Afrin Original Nasal Spray (Schering-Plough)	Oxymetazoline HCl 0.05%	**Adults & Peds: ≥6 yrs:** Instill 2-3 sprays per nostril q10-12h.
Afrin Original Pumpmist Nasal Spray (Schering-Plough)	Oxymetazoline HCl 0.05%	**Adults & Peds: ≥6 yrs:** Instill 2-3 sprays per nostril q10-12h.
Afrin Severe Congestion Nasal Spray (Schering-Plough)	Oxymetazoline HCl 0.05%	**Adults & Peds: ≥6 yrs:** Instill 2-3 sprays per nostril q10-12h.
Afrin Sinus Nasal Spray (Schering-Plough)	Oxymetazoline HCl 0.05%	**Adults & Peds: ≥6 yrs:** Instill 2-3 sprays per nostril q10-12h.
Benzedrex Inhaler (B.F. Ascher)	Propylhexedrine 250 mg	**Adults & Peds: ≥6 yrs:** Inhale 2 sprays per nostril q2h.
Neo-Synephrine 12 Hour Extra Moisturizing Nasal Spray (Bayer Healthcare)	Oxymetazoline HCl 0.05%	**Adults & Peds: ≥6 yrs:** Instill 2-3 sprays per nostril q10-12h.
Neo-Synephrine 12 Hour Nasal Decongestant Spray (Bayer Healthcare)	Oxymetazoline HCl 0.05%	**Adults & Peds: ≥6 yrs:** Instill 2-3 sprays per nostril q10-12h.

Table 2. ALLERGIC RHINITIS PRODUCTS (cont.)

BRAND NAME	INGREDIENT/STRENGTH	DOSE
Neo-Synephrine Extra Strength Nasal Decongestant Drops *(Bayer Healthcare)*	Phenylephrine HCl 1%	**Adults & Peds: ≥12 yrs:** Instill 2-3 drops per nostril q4h.
Neo-Synephrine Extra Strength Nasal Spray *(Bayer Healthcare)*	Phenylephrine HCl 1%	**Adults & Peds: ≥6 yrs:** Instill 2-3 sprays per nostril q4h.
Neo-Synephrine Mild Formula Nasal Spray *(Bayer Healthcare)*	Phenylephrine HCl 0.25%	**Adults & Peds: ≥6 yrs:** Instill 2-3 sprays per nostril q4h.
Neo-Synephrine Regular Strength Nasal Decongestant Spray *(Bayer Healthcare)*	Phenylephrine HCl 0.5%	**Adults & Peds: ≥12 yrs:** Instill 2-3 sprays per nostril q4h.
Nostrilla 12 Hour Nasal Decongestant *(Bayer Healthcare)*	Oxymetazoline HCl 0.05%	**Adults & Peds: ≥6 yrs:** Instill 2-3 sprays per nostril q10-12h.
Vicks Sinex 12 Hour Ultra Fine Mist For Sinus Relief *(Procter & Gamble)*	Oxymetazoline HCl 0.05%	**Adults & Peds: ≥12 yrs:** Instill 2-3 sprays per nostril q10-12h.
Vicks Sinex Long Acting Nasal Spray For Sinus Relief *(Procter & Gamble)*	Oxymetazoline HCl 0.05%	**Adults & Peds: ≥12 yrs:** Instill 2-3 sprays per nostril q10-12h.
Vicks Sinex Nasal Spray For Sinus Relief *(Procter & Gamble)*	Phenylephrine HCl 0.5%	**Adults & Peds: ≥12 yrs:** Instill 2-3 sprays per nostril q4h.
TOPICAL NASAL MOISTURIZERS		
4-Way Saline Moisturizing Mist *(Novartis Consumer Health)*	Water, Boric Acid, Glycerin, Sodium Chloride, Sodium Borate, Eucalyptol, Menthol, Polysorbate 80, Benzalkonium Chloride	**Adults & Peds: ≥2 yrs:** Instill 2-3 sprays per nostril prn.
Ayr Baby's Saline Nose Spray, Drops *(B.F. Ascher)*	Sodium Chloride 0.65%	**Peds:** Instill 2 to 6 drops in each nostril.
Ayr Saline Nasal Gel *(B.F. Ascher)*	Aloe Vera Gel, Carbomer, Diazolidinyl Urea, Dimethicone Copolyrsl, FD&C Blue 1, Geranium Oil, Glycerin, Glyceryl Polymethacrylate, Methyl Gluceth 10, Methylparaben, Poloxamer 184, Propylene Glycol, Propylparaben, Sodium Chloride, Tocopherol Acetate, Triethanolamine, Xanthan Gum, Water	**Adults & Peds: ≥12 yrs:** Apply to nostril prn.
Ayr Saline Nasal Gel, No-Drip Sinus Spray *(B.F. Ascher)*	Water, Sodium Carbomethyl Starch, Propylene Glycol, Glycerin, Aloe Barbadensis Leaf Juice (Aloe Vera Gel), Sodium Chloride, Cetyl Pyridinium Chloride, Citric Acid, Disodium EDTA, Glycine Soja (Soybean Oil), Tocopheryl Acetate, Benzyl Alcohol, Benzalkonium Chloride, Geranium Maculatum Oil	**Adults & Peds: ≥12 yrs:** Use prn as directed.
Ayr Saline Nasal Mist *(B.F. Ascher)*	Sodium Chloride 0.65%	**Adults & Peds: ≥12 yrs:** Instill 2 sprays per nostril prn.
ENTSOL Mist, Buffered Hypertonic Nasal Irrigation Mist *(Bradley Pharmaceuticals)*	Purified Water, Sodium Chloride, Sodium Phosphate Dibasic Edetate Disodium, Potassium Phosphate Monobasic, Benzalkonium Chloride	**Adults & Peds: ≥12 yrs:** Instill 1-2 sprays per nostril prn.
ENTSOL Single Use, Pre-Filled Nasal Wash Squeeze Bottle *(Bradley Pharmaceuticals)*	Purified Water Sodium Chloride, Sodium Phosphate Dibasic, Potassium Phosphate Monobasic	**Adults & Peds: ≥12 yrs:** Use as directed.
ENTSOL Spray, Buffered Hypertonic Saline Nasal Spray *(Bradley Pharmaceuticals)*	Purified Water, Sodium Chloride Phosphate Dibasic, Potassium Phosphate Monobasic	**Adults & Peds: ≥12 yrs:** Instill 1 spray per nostril bid, 6 times daily.
Little Noses Saline Spray/Drops, Non-Medicated *(Vetco)*	Sodium Chloride 0.65%	**Peds:** 2-6 drops per nostril as directed.

Table 2. ALLERGIC RHINITIS PRODUCTS (cont.)

BRAND NAME	INGREDIENT/STRENGTH	DOSE
Ocean Premium Saline Nasal Spray *(Fleming)*	Sodium Chloride 0.65%, Phenylcarbinol, Benzalkonium Chloride	**Adults & Peds: ≥6 yrs:** Instill 2 sprays per nostril prn.
Simply Saline Sterile Saline Nasal Mist *(Blairex)*	Sodium Chloride 0.9%	**Adults & Peds: ≥12 yrs:** Use prn as directed.
SinoFresh Moisturizing Nasal & Sinus Spray *(SinoFresh HealthCare)*	Cetylpyridinium Chloride 0.05%	**Adults & Peds: ≥12 yrs:** Instill 1-3 sprays per nostril qd.
Zicam Nasal Moisturizer *(Zicam)*	Purified Water; High Purity Sodium Chloride; Aloe Vera	**Adults & Peds: ≥12 yrs:** Use as directed.
MISCELLANEOUS		
NasalCrom Allergy Prevention Nasal Spray *(McNeil Consumer)*	Cromolyn Sodium 5.2 mg	**Adults & Peds: ≥6 yrs:** Instill 1 spray per nostril q4-6h.
NasalCrom Nasal Allergy Symptom Controller, Nasal Spray *McNeil Consumer)*	Cromolyn Sodium 5.2 mg	**Adults & Peds: ≥2 yrs:** Instill 1 spray per nostril q4-6h.
Similasan Hay Fever Relief, Non-Drowsy Formula, Nasal Spray *(Similasan)*	Cardiospermum HPUS 6X, Galphimia Glauca HPUS 6X, Luffa Operculata HPUS 6X, Sabadilla HPUS 6x	**Adults & Peds: ≥12 yrs:** Use as directed.
Zicam Allergy Relief, Homeopathic Nasal Solution, Pump *(Zicam)*	Luffa Operculata 4x, 12x, 30x, Galphimia Glauca 12x, 30x, Histaminum Hydrochloricum 12x, 30x, 200x, Sulphur 12x, 30x, 200x	**Adults & Peds: ≥6 yrs:** Instill 2-3 sprays per nostril q4h.

Table 3. ANALGESIC PRODUCTS

Brand Name	Ingredient/Strength	Dose
ACETAMINOPHEN		
Anacin Aspirin Free tablets *(Insight Pharmaceuticals)*	Acetaminophen 500mg	**Adults & Peds:** ≥12 yrs: 2 tab sq6h. **Max:** 8 tabs q24h.
Feverall Childrens' suppositories *(Alpharma)*	Acetaminophen 120mg	**Peds: 3-6 yrs:** 1-2 supp. q4-6h. max 6 supp. q24h.
Feverall Infants' suppositories *(Alpharma)*	Acetaminophen 80mg	**Peds: 3-11 months:** 1 supp. q6h. **12-36 months:** 1 supp. q4h. **Max:** 6 supp. q24h.
Feverall Jr. Strength suppositories *(Alpharma)*	Acetaminophen 325mg	**Peds: 6-12 yrs:** 1 supp. q4-6h. **Max:** 6 supp. q24h.
Tylenol 8 Hour caplets *(McNeil Consumer)*	Acetaminophen 650mg	**Adults & Peds:** ≥12 yrs: 2 tabs q8h prn. **Max:** 6 tabs q24h.
Tylenol 8 Hour geltabs *(McNeil Consumer)*	Acetaminophen 650mg	**Adults & Peds:** ≥12 yrs: 2 tabs q8h prn. **Max:** 6 tabs q24h.
Tylenol Arthritis caplets *(McNeil Consumer)*	Acetaminophen 650mg	**Adults:** 2 tabs q8h prn. **Max:** 6 tabs q24h.
Tylenol Arthritis geltabs *(McNeil Consumer)*	Acetaminophen 650mg	**Adults:** 2 tabs q8h prn. **Max:** 6 tabs q24h.
Tylenol Children's Meltaways tablets *(McNeil Consumer)*	Acetaminophen 80mg	**Peds: 2-3 yrs (24-35 lbs):** 2 tabs. **4-5 yrs (36-47 lbs):** 3 tabs. **6-8 yrs (48-59 lbs):** 4 tabs. **9-10 yrs (60-71 lbs):** 5 tabs. **11 yrs (72-95 lbs):** 6 tabs. May repeat q4h. **Max:** 5 doses q24h.
Tylenol Children's suspension *(McNeil Consumer)*	Acetaminophen 160mg/5mL	**Peds: 2-3 yrs (24-35 lbs):** 1 tsp (5mL). **4-5 yrs (36-47 lbs):** 1.5 tsp (7.5mL). **6-8 yrs (48-59 lbs):** 2 tsp (10mL). **9-10 yrs (60-71 lbs):** 2.5 tsp (12.5mL). **11 yrs (72-95 lbs):** 3 tsp (15mL). May repeat q4h. **Max:** 5 doses q24h.
Tylenol Extra Strength caplets *(McNeil Consumer)*	Acetaminophen 500mg	**Adults & Peds:** ≥12 yrs: 2 tabs q4-6h prn. **Max:** 8 tabs q24h.
Tylenol Extra Strength Cool caplets *(McNeil Consumer)*	Acetaminophen 500mg	**Adults & Peds:** ≥12 yrs: 2 tabs q4-6h prn. **Max:** 8 tabs q24h.
Tylenol Extra Strength gelcaps *(McNeil Consumer)*	Acetaminophen 500mg	**Adults & Peds:** ≥ 12 yrs: 2 caps q4-6h prn. **Max:** 8 caps q24h.
Tylenol Rapid Blast liquid *(McNeil Consumer)*	Acetaminophen 500mg/15mL	**Adults & Peds:** ≥12 yrs: 2 tbl (30mL) q4-6h prn. **Max:** 8 tbl (120mL) q24h.
Tylenol Extra Strength EZ tablets *(McNeil Consumer)*	Acetaminophen 500mg	**Adults & Peds:** ≥12 yrs: 2 tabs q4-6h prn. **Max:** 8 tabs q24h.
Tylenol Extra Strength Go tablets *(McNeil Consumer)*	Acetaminophen 500mg	**Adults & Peds:** ≥12 yrs: 2 tabs q4-6h prn. **Max:** 8 tabs q24h.
Tylenol Infants' suspension *(McNeil Consumer)*	Acetaminophen 80mg/0.8mL	**Peds: 2-3 yrs (24-35 lbs):** 1.6mL q4h prn. **Max:** 5 doses (8mL) q24h.
Tylenol Junior Meltaways tablets *(McNeil Consumer)*	Acetaminophen 160mg	**Peds: 6-8 yrs (48-59 lbs):** 2 tabs. **9-10 yrs (60-71 lbs):** 2.5 tabs. **11 yrs (72-95 lbs):** 3 tabs. **12 yrs (≥96 lbs):** 4 tabs. May repeat q4h. **Max:** 5 doses q24h.
Tylenol Regular Strength tablets *(McNeil Consumer)*	Acetaminophen 325mg	**Adults & Peds:** ≥12 yrs: **2 tabs** q4-6h prn. **Max:** 12 tabs q24h. **Peds: 6-11 yrs:** 1 tab q4-6h. **Max:** 5 tabs q24h.
ACETAMINOPHEN COMBINATIONS		
Anacin Advanced Headache tablets *(Insight Pharmaceuticals)*	Acetaminophen/Aspirin/Caffeine 250mg-250mg-65mg	**Adults & Peds:** ≥12 yrs: 2 tabs q6h. **Max:** 8 tabs q24h.
Excedrin Back & Body caplets *(Novartis Consumer Health)*	Acetaminophen/Aspirin Buffered 250mg-250mg	**Adults & Peds:** ≥12 yrs: 2 tabs **Max:** 8 tabs q24h.

Table 3. ANALGESIC PRODUCTS (cont.)

BRAND NAME	INGREDIENT/STRENGTH	DOSE
Excedrin Extra Strength caplets *(Novartis Consumer Health)*	Acetaminophen/Aspirin/Caffeine 250mg-250mg-65mg	**Adults & Peds: ≥12 yrs:** 2 tabs q6h. **Max:** 8 tabs q24h.
Excedrin Extra Strength geltabs *(Novartis Consumer Health)*	Acetaminophen/Aspirin/Caffeine 250mg-250mg-65mg	**Adults & Peds: ≥12 yrs:** 2 tabs q6h. **Max:** 8 tabs q24h.
Excedrin Extra Strength tablets *(Novartis Consumer Health)*	Acetaminophen/Aspirin/Caffeine 250mg-250mg-65mg	**Adults & Peds: ≥12 yrs:** 2 tabs q6h. **Max:** 8 tabs q24h.
Excedrin Migraine caplets *(Novartis Consumer Health)*	Acetaminophen/Aspirin/Caffeine 250mg-250mg-65mg	**Adults:** 2 tabs prn. **Max:** 2 tabs q24h.
Excedrin Migraine geltabs *(Novartis Consumer Health)*	Acetaminophen/Aspirin/Caffeine 250mg-250mg-65mg	**Adults:** 2 tabs prn. **Max:** 2 tabs q24h.
Excedrin Migraine tablets *(Novartis Consumer Health)*	Acetaminophen/Aspirin/Caffeine 250mg-250mg-65mg	**Adults:** 2 tabs prn. **Max:** 2 tabs q24h.
Excedrin Quicktabs tablets *(Novartis Consumer Health)*	Acetaminophen/Caffeine 500mg-65mg	**Adults & Peds: ≥12 yrs:** 2 tabs q6h. **Max:** 8 tabs q24h.
Excedrin Sinus Headache caplets *(Novartis Consumer Health)*	Acetaminophen/Phenylephrine HCl 325mg-5mg	**Adults & Peds: ≥12 yrs:** 2 tabs q4h. **Max:** 12 tabs q24h.
Excedrin Sinus Headache tablets *(Novartis Consumer Health)*	Acetaminophen/Phenylephrine HCl 325mg-5mg	**Adults & Peds: ≥12 yrs:** 2 tabs q4h. **Max:** 12 tabs q24h.
Excedrin Tension Headache caplets *(Novartis Consumer Health)*	Acetaminophen/Caffeine 500mg-65mg	**Adults & Peds: ≥12 yrs:** 2 tabs q6h. **Max:** 8 tabs q24h.
Excedrin Tension Headache geltabs *(Novartis Consumer Health)*	Acetaminophen/Caffeine 500mg-65mg	**Adults & Peds: ≥12 yrs:** 2 tabs q6h. **Max:** 8 tabs q24h.
Excedrin Tension Headache tablets *(Novartis Consumer Health)*	Acetaminophen/Caffeine 500mg-65mg	**Adults & Peds: ≥12 yrs:** 2 tabs q6h. **Max:** 8 tabs q24h.
Goody's Extra Strength Headache Powders *(GlaxoSmtihKline Consumer Healthcare)*	Acetaminophen/Aspirin/Caffeine 260mg-520mg-32.5mg	**Adults & Peds: ≥12 yrs:** 1 powder q4-6h. **Max:** 4 powders q24h.
Midol Menstrual Headache caplets *(Bayer Healthcare)*	Acetaminophen/Caffeine 500mg-65g	**Adults & Peds: ≥12 yrs:** 2 tabs q6h. **Max:** 8 tabs q24h.
Midol Menstrual Complete caplets *(Bayer Healthcare)*	Acetaminophen/Caffeine/Pyrilamine Maleate 500mg-60mg-15mg	**Adults & Peds: ≥12 yrs:** 2 tabs q6h. **Max:** 8 tabs q24h.
Midol Menstrual Complete caplets *(Bayer Healthcare)*	Acetaminophen/Caffeine/Pyrilamine Maleate 500mg-60mg-15mg	**Adults & Peds: ≥12 yrs:** 2 tabs q6h. **Max:** 8 tabs q24h.
Midol PMS caplets *(Bayer Healthcare)*	Acetaminophen/Pamabrom/Pyrilamine 500mg-25mg-15mg	**Adults & Peds: ≥12 yrs:** 2 tabs q6h. **Max:** 8 tabs q24h.
Midol Teen caplets *(Bayer Healtcare)*	Acetaminophen/Pamabrom 500mg-25mg	**Adults & Peds: ≥12 yrs:** 2 tabs q6h. **Max:** 8 tabs q24h.
Pamprin Multi-Symptom caplets *(Chattem Consumer Products)*	Acetaminophen/Pamabrom/Pyrilamine 500mg-25mg-15mg	**Adults & Peds: ≥12 yrs:** 2 tabs q4-6h. **Max:** 8 tabs q24h.
Premsyn PMS caplets *(Chattem Consumer Products)*	Acetaminophen/Pamabrom/Pyrilamine 500mg-25mg-15mg	**Adults & Peds: ≥12 yrs:** 2 tabs q4-6h. **Max:** 8 tabs q24h.
Tylenol Women's caplets *(McNeil Consumer)*	Acetaminophen/Pamabrom 500mg-25mg	**Adults & Peds: ≥12 yrs:** 2 tabs q4-6h. **Max:** 8 tabs q24h.
Vanquish caplets *(Bayer Healthcare)*	Acetaminophen/Aspirin/Caffeine 194mg-227mg-33mg	**Adults & Peds: ≥12 yrs:** 2 tabs q6h. **Max:** 8 tabs q24h.
ACETAMINOPHEN/SLEEP AID		
Excedrin PM caplets *(Novartis Consumer Health)*	Acetaminophen/Diphenhydramine 500mg-38mg	**Adults & Peds: ≥12 yrs:** 2 tabs qhs.
Excedrin PM geltabs *(Novartis Consumer Health)*	Acetaminophen/Diphenhydramine citrate 500mg-38 mg	**Adults & Peds: ≥12 yrs:** 2 tabs qhs.
Excedrin PM tablets *(Novartis Consumer Health)*	Acetaminophen/Diphenhydramine citrate 500mg-38 mg	**Adults & Peds: ≥12 yrs:** 2 tabs qhs.
Goody's PM Powder *(GlaxoSmithKline Consumer Healthcare)*	Acetaminophen/Diphenhydramine 1000mg-76mg/dose	**Adults & Peds: ≥12 yrs:** 1 packet (2 powders) qhs.

Table 3. ANALGESIC PRODUCTS (cont.)

BRAND NAME	INGREDIENT/STRENGTH	DOSE
Tylenol PM caplets (McNeil Consumer)	Acetaminophen/Diphenhydramine 500mg-25mg	**Adults & Peds: ≥12 yrs:** 2 tabs qhs.
Tylenol PM gelcaps (*McNeil Consumer*)	Acetaminophen/Diphenhydramine 500mg-25mg	**Adults & Peds: ≥12 yrs:** 2 caps qhs.
Tylenol PM geltabs (*McNeil Consumer*)	Acetaminophen/Diphenhydramine 500mg-25mg	**Adults & Peds: ≥12 yrs:** 2 tabs qhs.
Tylenol PM liquid (*McNeil Consumer*)	Acetaminophen/Diphenhydramine 1000g-50mg/30 mL	**Adults & Peds: ≥12 yrs:** 2 tbl (30mL) qhs. **Max:** 8 tbl (120mL) q24h.

NONSTEROIDAL ANTI-INFLAMMATORY DRUGS (NSAIDs)

BRAND NAME	INGREDIENT/STRENGTH	DOSE
Advil caplets (*Wyeth Consumer Healthcare*)	Ibuprofen 200mg	**Adults & Peds: ≥12 yrs:** 1-2 tabs q4-6h. **Max:** 6 tabs q24h.
Advil Children's Chewables tablets (*Wyeth Consumer Healthcare*)	Ibuprofen 50mg	**Peds: 2-3 yr (24-35 lb):** 2 tabs q6-8h. **4-5 yr (36-47 lb):** 3 tabs q6-8h. **6-8 (45-89 lb):** 4 tabs q6-8h. **9-10 yr (60-71 lb):** 5 tabs q6-8h. **11 yr (72-95 lb):** 6 tabs q6-8h. **Max:** 4 doses q24h
Advil Children's suspension (*Wyeth Consumer Healthcare*)	Ibuprofen 100mg/5mL	**Peds: 2-3 yrs (24-35 lbs):** 1 tsp (5mL). **4-5 yrs (36-47 lbs):** 1.5 tsp (7.5mL). **6-8 yrs (48-59 lbs):** 2 tsp (10mL). **9-10 yrs (60-71 lbs):** 2.5 tsp (12.5mL). **11 yrs (72-95 lbs):** 3 tsp (15mL). May repeat q6-8h. **Max:** 4 doses q24h.
Advil gelcaps (*Wyeth Consumer Healthcare*)	Ibuprofen 200mg	**Adults & Peds: ≥12 yrs:** 1-2 caps q4-6h. Max: 6 caps q24h.
Advil Infants' Drops (*Wyeth Consumer Healthcare*)	Ibuprofen 50mg/1.25mL	**Peds: 6-11 months (12-17 lbs):** 1.25mL. **12-23 months (18-23 lbs):** 1.875mL. May repeat q6-8h. **Max:** 4 doses q24h.
Advil Junior Strength tablets (*Wyeth Consumer Healthcare*)	Ibuprofen 100mg	**Peds: 6-10 yrs (48-71 lbs):** 2 tabs. **11 yrs (72-95 lbs):** 3 tabs. May repeat q6-8h. **Max:** 4 doses q24h.
Advil Junior Strength Chewable tablets (*Wyeth Consumer Healthcare*)	Ibuprofen 100mg	**Peds: 6-10 yrs (48-71 lbs):** 2 tabs. **11 yrs (72-95 lbs):** 3 tabs. May repeat q6-8h. **Max:** 4 doses q24h.
Advil Liqui-Gels (*Wyeth Consumer Healthcare*)	Ibuprofen 200mg	**Adults & Peds: ≥12 yrs:** 1-2 caps q4-6h. **Max:** 6 caps q24h.
Advil Migraine capsules (*Wyeth Consumer Healthcare*)	Ibuprofen 200mg	**Adults:** 2 caps prn. **Max:** 2 caps q24h.
Advil tablets (*Wyeth ConsumerHealthcare*)	Ibuprofen 200mg	**Adults & Peds: ≥12 yrs:** 1-2 tabs q4-6h. **Max:** 6 tabs q24h.
Aleve caplets (*Bayer Healthcare*)	Naproxen Sodium 220mg	**Adults: ≥65 yrs:** 1 tab q12h. **Max:** 2 tabs q24h. **Adults & Peds: ≥12 yrs:** 1 tab q8-12h. **Max:** 3 tabs q24h.
Aleve gelcaps (*Bayer Healthcare*)	Naproxen Sodium 220mg	**Adults: ≥65 yrs:** 1 cap q12h. **Max:** 2 caps q24h. **Adults & Peds: ≥12 yrs:** 1 cap q8-12h. **Max:** 3 caps q24h.
Aleve tablets (*Bayer Healthcare*)	Naproxen Sodium 220mg	**Adults: ≥65 yrs:** 1 tab q12h. **Max:** 2 tabs q24h. **Adults & Peds: ≥12 yrs:** 1 tab q8-12h. **Max:** 3 tabs q24h.
Midol Cramps and Body Aches tablets (*Bayer Healthcare*)	Ibuprofen 200mg	**Adults & Peds: ≥12 yrs:** 1-2 tabs q4-6h. **Max:** 6 tabs q24h.
Midol Extended Relief caplets (*Bayer Healthcare*)	Naproxen Sodium 220mg	**Adults & Peds: ≥12 yrs:** 1 tabs q8-12h. **Max:** 3 tabs q24h.

Table 3. ANALGESIC PRODUCTS (cont.)

BRAND NAME	INGREDIENT/STRENGTH	DOSE
Motrin Children's suspension *(McNeil Consumer)*	Ibuprofen 100mg/5mL	**Peds: 2-3 yrs (24-35 lbs):** 1 tsp (5mL). **4-5 yrs (36-47 lbs):** 1.5 tsp (7.5mL). **6-8 yrs (48-59 lbs):** 2 tsp (10mL). **9-10 yrs (60-71 lbs):** 2.5 tsp (12.5mL). **11 yrs (72-95 lbs):** 3 tsp (15mL). May repeat q6-8h. **Max:** 4 doses q24h.
Motrin IB caplets *(McNeil Consumer)*	Ibuprofen 200mg	**Adults & Peds: ≥12 yrs:** 1-2 tabs q4-6h. **Max:** 6 tabs q24h.
Motrin IB gelcaps *(McNeil Consumer)*	Ibuprofen 200mg	**Adults & Peds: ≥12 yrs:** 1-2 tabs q4-6h. **Max:** 6 tabs q24h.
Motrin IB tablets *(McNeil Consumer)*	Ibuprofen 200mg	**Adults & Peds: ≥12 yrs:** 1-2 tabs q4-6h. **Max:** 6 tabs q24h.
Motrin Infants' Drops *(McNeil Consumer)*	Ibuprofen 50mg/1.25mL	**Peds: 6-11 months (12-17 lbs):** 1.25mL. **12-23 months (18-23 lbs):** 1.875mL. May repeat q6-8h. **Max:** 4 doses q24h.
Motrin Junior Strength chewable tablets *(McNeil Consumer)*	Ibuprofen 100mg	**Peds: 6-8 yrs (48-59 lbs):** 2 tabs. **9-10 yrs (60-71 lbs):** 2.5 tabs. **11 yrs (72-95 lbs):** 3 tabs. May repeat q6-8h. **Max:** 4 doses q24h.
Nuprin caplets *(CVS)*	Ibuprofen 200mg	**Adults & Peds: ≥12 yrs:** 1-2 tabs q4-6h. **Max:** 6 tabs q24h.
Nuprin tablets *(CVS)*	Ibuprofen 200mg	**Adults & Peds: ≥12 yrs:** 1-2 tabs q4-6h. **Max:** 6 tabs q24h.
SALICYLATES		
Anacin 81 tablets *(Insight Pharmaceuticals)*	Aspirin 81mg	**Adults & Peds: ≥12 yrs:** 4-8 tabs q4h. **Max:** 48 tabs q24h.
Aspergum chewable tablets *(Schering-Plough)*	Aspirin 227mg	**Adults & Peds: ≥12 yrs:** 2 tabs q4h. **Max:** 16 tabs q24h.
Bayer Aspirin Extra Strength caplets *(Bayer Healthcare)*	Aspirin 500mg	**Adults & Peds: ≥12 yrs:** 1-2 tabs q4-6h. **Max:** 8 tabs q24h.
Bayer Aspirin safety coated caplets *(Bayer Healthcare)*	Aspirin 325mg	**Adults & Peds: ≥12 yrs:** 1-2 tabs q4h or 3 tabs q6h. **Max:** 12 tabs q24h.
Bayer Children's Aspirin chewable tablets *(Bayer Healthcare)*	Aspirin 81mg	**Adults & Peds: ≥12 yrs:** 4-8 tabs q4h. **Max:** 48 tabs q24h.
Bayer Low Dose Aspirin tablets *(Bayer Healthcare)*	Aspirin 81mg	**Adults & Peds: ≥12 yrs:** 4-8 tabs q4h. **Max:** 48 tabs q24h.
Bayer Sugar Free Low Dose Aspirin tablets *(Bayer Healthcare)*	Aspirin 81mg	**Adults & Peds: ≥12 yrs:** 4-8 tabs q4h. **Max:** 48 tabs q24h.
Genuine Bayer Aspirin tablets *(Bayer Healthcare)*	Aspirin 325 mg	**Adults & Peds: ≥12 yrs:** 1-2 tabs q4h or 3 tabs q6h. **Max:** 12 tabs q24h.
Bayer Extra-Strength Plus caplets *(Bayer Healthcare)*	Aspirin 500mg	**Adults & Peds: ≥12 yrs:** 2 tabs q6h. **Max:** 8 tabs q24h.
Doan's Regular Strength caplets *(Novartis Consumer Health)*	Magnesium Salicylate Tetrahydrate 377mg	**Adults & Peds: ≥12 yrs:** 2 tabs q4h. **Max:** 12 tabs q24h.
Ecotrin Adult Low Strength tablets *(GlaxoSmithKline Consumer Healthcare)*	Aspirin 81mg	**Adults:** 4-8 tabs q4h. **Max:** 48 tabs q24h.
Ecotrin Enteric Low Strength tablets *(GlaxoSmithKline Consumer Healthcare)*	Aspirin 81mg	**Adults:** 4-8 tabs q4h. **Max:** 48 tabs q24h.
Ecotrin Enteric Regular Strength tablets *(GlaxoSmtihKline Consumer Healthcare)*	Aspirin 325mg	**Adults & Peds: ≥12 yrs:** 1-2 tabs q4h. **Max:** 12 tabs q24h.
Ecotrin Maximum Strength tablets *(GlaxoSmithKline Consumer Healthcare)*	Aspirin 500mg	**Adults & Peds: ≥12 yrs:** 2 tabs q6h. **Max:** 8 tabs q24h.

Table 3. ANALGESIC PRODUCTS (cont.)

Brand Name	Ingredient/Strength	Dose
Ecotrin Regular Strength tablets *(GlaxoSmithKline Consumer Healthcare)*	Aspirin 325mg	**Adults & Peds: ≥12 yrs:** 1-2 tabs q4h. **Max:** 12 tabs q24h.
Halfprin 162mg tablets *(Kramer Laboratories)*	Aspirin 162mg	**Adults & Peds: ≥12 yrs:** 2-4 tabs q4h. **Max:** 24 tabs q24h.
Halfprin 81mg tablets *(Kramer Laboratories)*	Aspirin 81mg	**Adults & Peds: ≥12 yrs:** 4-8 tabs q4h. **Max:** 48 tabs q24h.
St. Joseph Adult Low Strength chewable tablets *(McNeil Consumer)*	Aspirin 81mg	**Adults & Peds: ≥12 yrs:** 4-8 tabs q4h. **Max:** 48 tabs q24h.
St. Joseph Adult Low Strength tablets *(McNeil Consumer)*	Aspirin 81mg	**Adults & Peds: ≥12 yrs:** 4-8 tabs q4h. **Max:** 48 tabs q24h.
SALICYLATES, BUFFERED		
Ascriptin Maximum Strength tablets *(Novartis Consumer Health)*	Aspirin Buffered with Maalox/Calcium Carbonate 500mg	**Adults & Peds: ≥12 yrs:** 2 tabs q4h. **Max:** 8 tabs q24h.
Ascriptin Regular Strength tablets *(Novartis Consumer Health)*	Aspirin Buffered with Maalox/Calcium Carbonate 325mg	**Adults & Peds: ≥12 yrs:** 2 tabs q4h. **Max:** 12 tabs q24h.
Bayer Extra Strength Plus caplets *(Bayer Healthcare)*	Aspirin Buffered with Calcium Carbonate 500mg	**Adults & Peds: ≥12 yrs:** 1-2 tabs q4-6h. **Max:** 8 tabs q24h.
Bufferin Extra Strength tablets *(Novartis Consumer Health)*	Aspirin Buffered with Calcium Carbonate/ Magnesium Oxide/ Magnesium Carbonate 500mg	**Adults & Peds: ≥12 yrs:** 2 tabs q6h. **Max:** 8 tabs q24h.
Bufferin tablets *(Novartis Consumer Health)*	Aspirin Buffered with Calcium Carbonate/ Magnesium Oxide/ Magnesium Carbonate 325mg	**Adults & Peds: ≥12 yrs:** 2 tabs q4h. **Max:** 12 tabs q24h.
SALICYLATE COMBINATIONS		
Alka-Seltzer effervescent tablets *(Bayer Healthcare)*	Aspirin/Citric Acid/Sodium Bicarbonate 325mg-1000mg-1916mg	**Adults & Peds: ≥12 yrs:** 2 tabs q4h. **Max:** 8 tabs q24h.
Alka-Seltzer Extra Strength effervescent tablets *(Bayer Healthcare)*	Aspirin/Citric Acid/Sodium Bicarbonate 500mg-1000mg-1985mg	**Adults & Peds: ≥12 yrs:** 2 tabs q6h. **Max:** 7 tabs q24h.
Alka-Seltzer Morning Relief effervescent tablets *(Bayer Healthcare)*	Aspirin/Caffeine 500mg-65mg	**Adults & Peds: ≥12 yrs:** 2 tabs q6h. **Max:** 8 tabs q24h.
Anacin Pain Reliever caplets *(Insight Pharmaceuticals)*	Aspirin/Caffeine 400mg-32mg	**Adults & Peds: ≥12 yrs:** 2 tabs q6h. **Max:** 8 tabs q24h.
Anacin Extra Strength tablets *(Insight Pharmaceuticals)*	Aspirin/Caffeine 500mg-32mg	**Adults & Peds: ≥12 yrs:** 2 tabs q6h. **Max:** 8 tabs q24h.
Anacin tablets *(Insight Pharmaceuticals)*	Aspirin/Caffeine 400mg-32mg	**Adults & Peds: ≥12 yrs:** 2 tabs q6h. **Max:** 8 tabs q24h.
Bayer Back & Body Pain caplets *(Bayer Healthcare)*	Aspirin/Caffeine 500mg-32.5mg	**Adults & Peds: ≥12 yrs:** 2 tabs q6h. **Max:** 8 tabs q24h.
BC Arthritis Strength powders *(GlaxoSmtihKline Consumer Healthcare)*	Aspirin/Caffeine/Salicylamide 742mg-38mg-222mg	**Adults & Peds: ≥12 yrs:** 1 powder q3-4h. **Max:** 4 powders q24h.
BC Original powders *(GlaxoSmithKline Consumer Healthcare)*	Aspirin/Caffeine/Salicylamide 650mg-33.3mg-195mg	**Adults & Peds: ≥12 yrs:** 1 powder q 3-4 h.
SALICYLATE/SLEEP AID		
Alka-Seltzer PM Pain Reliever & Sleep Aid, effervescent tablets *(Bayer Healthcare)*	Aspirin/Diphenhydramine Citrate 325mg-38 mg	**Adults & Peds: ≥12 yrs:** 2 tabs qpm.
Bayer PM Relief caplets *(Bayer Healthcare)*	Aspirin/Diphenhydramine 500mg-38.3mg	**Adults & Peds: ≥12 yrs:** 2 tabs qhs.
Doan's Extra Strength PM caplets *(Novartis Consumer Health)*	Magnesium Salicylate Tetrahydrate/ Diphenhydramine 580mg-25mg	**Adults & Peds: ≥12 yrs:** 2 tabs qhs.

Table 4. ANTACID AND HEARTBURN PRODUCTS

Brand Name	Ingredient/Strength	Dose
ANTACID		
Alka-Mints chewable tablets *(Bayer Healthcare)*	Calcium Carbonate 850mg	**Adults & Peds: ≥12 yrs:** 1-2 tabs q2h. **Max:** 9 tabs q24h.
Alka-Seltzer Gold tablets *(Bayer Healthcare)*	Citric Acid/Potassium Bicarbonate/ Sodium Bicarbonate 1000mg-344mg-1050mg	**Adults: ≥60 yrs:** 2 tabs q4h prn. **Max:** 6 tabs q24h. **Adults & Peds: ≥12 yrs:** 2 tabs q4h prn. **Max:** 8 tabs q24h. **Peds: ≤12 yrs:** 1 tab q4h prn. Max: 4 tabs q24h.
Alka-Seltzer Heartburn Relief tablets *(Bayer Healthcare)*	Citric Acid/Sodium Bicarbonate 1000mg-1940mg	**Adults: ≥60 yrs:** 2 tabs q4h prn. **Max:** 4 tabs q24h. **Adults & Peds: ≥12 yrs:** 2 tabs q4h prn. **Max:** 8 tabs q24h.
Alka-Seltzer tablets, Extra-Strength *(Bayer Healthcare)*	Aspirin/Sodium Bicarbonate/Citric Acid 500mg-1985mg-1000mg	**Adults: ≥60 yrs:** 2 tabs q6h prn. **Max:** 3 tabs q24h. **Adults & Peds: ≥12 yrs:** 2 tabs q6h prn. **Max:** 7 tabs q24h.
Brioschi powder *(Brioschi)*	Sodium Bicarbonate/Tartaric Acid 2.69g-2.43g/dose	**Adults & Peds: ≥12 yrs:** 1 capful (6g) dissolved in 4-6 oz water q1h. **Max:** 6 doses q24h.
Dulcolax Milk of Magnesia liquid *(Boehringer Ingelheim Consumer Healthcare)*	Magnesium Hydroxide 400mg/5mL	**Adults & Peds: ≥12 yrs:** 1-3 tsp (5-15mL) qd-qid.
Gaviscon Extra Strength liquid *(GlaxoSmithKline Consumer Healthcare)*	Aluminum Hydroxide/Magnesium Carbonate 254mg-237.5mg/5mL	**Adults:** 2-4 tsp (10-20mL) qid.
Gaviscon Extra Strength tablets *(GlaxoSmithKline Consumer Healthcare)*	Aluminum Hydroxide/Magnesium Carbonate 160mg-105mg	**Adults:** 2-4 tabs qid.
Gaviscon Original chewable tablets *(GlaxoSmithKline Consumer Healthcare)*	Aluminum Hydroxide/Magnesium Trisilicate 80mg-20mg	**Adults:** 2-4 tabs qid.
Gaviscon Regular Strength liquid *(GlaxoSmithKline Consumer Healthcare)*	Aluminum Hydroxide/Magnesium Carbonate 95mg-358mg/5ml	**Adults:** 2-4 tsp (10-20mL) qid.
Gaviscon Acid Breakthrough, chewable tablets *(GlaxoSmithKline Consumer Healthcare)*	Calcium Carbonate 500mg	**Adults:** 2 tabs prn.
Maalox Quick Dissolve Regular Strength chewable tablets *(Novartis Consumer Health)*	Calcium Carbonate 600mg	**Adults:** 1-2 tabs prn. **Max:** 12 tabs q24h.
Mylanta, Children's *(Johnson & Johnson/Merck Consumer)*	Calcium Carbonate 400 mg	**Peds: 6-11 yrs (48-95 lbs):** Take 2 tab prn. **Peds: 2-5 yrs (24-47 lbs):** Take 1 tab prn
Mylanta gelcaps *(Johnson & Johnson/Merck Consumer)*	Calcium Carbonate/Magnesium Hydroxide 550mg-125mg	**Adults:** 2-4 caps prn. **Max:** 12 caps q24h.
Mylanta Supreme Antacid liquid *(Johnson & Johnson/Merck Consumer)*	Calcium Carbonate/Magnesium Hydroxide 400mg-135mg/5mL	**Adults:** 2-4 tsp (10-20mL) qid. **Max:** 18 tsp (90mL) q24h.
Mylanta Ultra chewable tablets *(Johnson & Johnson/Merck Consumer)*	Calcium Carbonate/Magnesium Hydroxide 700mg-300mg	**Adults:** 2-4 tabs qid. **Max:** 10 tabs q24h.
Pepto-Bismol Children's Chewable tablets *(Proctor & Gamble)*	Calcium Carbonate 400 mg	**Peds: 2-5 yrs (24-47 lbs):** Take 1 tab q24h. **Peds: 6-11 yrs (48-95 lbs):** Take 2 tab q24h.
Phillips Milk of Magnesia liquid *(Bayer Healthcare)*	Magnesium Hydroxide 400mg/5mL	**Adults & Peds: ≥12 yrs:** 30-60mL qd. **Peds: 6-11 yrs:** 15-30mL qd. 2-5 yrs: 5-15mL qd.
Rolaids Extra Strength Softchews *(McNeil Consumer)*	Calcium Carbonate 1177mg	**Adults:** 2-3 chews q1h prn. **Max:** 6 chews q24h.
Rolaids Extra Strength tablets *(McNeil Consumer)*	Calcium Carbonate/Magnesium Hydroxide 675mg-135mg	**Adults:** 2-4 tabs q1h prn. **Max:** 10 tabs q24h.
Rolaids tablets *(McNeil Consumer)*	Calcium Carbonate/Magnesium Hydroxide 550mg-110mg	**Adults:** 2-4 tabs q1h prn. **Max:** 12 tabs q24h.
Titralac chewable tablets *(3M Consumer Healthcare)*	Calcium Carbonate 420mg	**Adults:** 2 tabs q2-3h prn. **Max:** 19 tabs q24h.
Tums chewable tablets *(GlaxoSmithKline Consumer Healthcare)*	Calcium Carbonate 500mg	**Adults:** 2-4 tabs q1h prn. **Max:** 15 tabs q24h.

Table 4. ANTACID AND HEARTBURN PRODUCTS (cont.)

BRAND NAME	INGREDIENT/STRENGTH	DOSE
Tums E-X chewable tablets *(GlaxoSmithKline Consumer Healthcare)*	Calcium Carbonate 750mg	**Adults:** 2-4 tabs prn. **Max:** 10 tabs q24h.
Tums Lasting Effects chewable tablets *(GlaxoSmithKline Consumer Healthcare)*	Calcium Carbonate 500mg	**Adults:** 2 tabs prn. **Max:** 15 tabs q24h.
Tums Smooth Dissolve tablets *(GlaxoSmithKline Consumer Healthcare)*	Calcium Carbonate 750mg	**Adults:** 2-4 tabs prn. **Max:** 10 tabs q24h.
Tums Ultra Maximum Strength chewable tablets *(GlaxoSmithKline Consumer Healthcare)*	Calcium Carbonate 1000mg	**Adults:** 2-3 tabs prn. **Max:** 7 tabs q24h.
ANTACID/ANTIFLATULENT		
Gas-X with Maalox capsules *(Novartis Consumer Health)*	Calcium Carbonate/Simethicone 250mg-62.5mg	**Adults:** 2-4 caps prn. **Max:** 8 caps q24h.
Gas-X Extra Strength with Maalox capsules *(Novartis Consumer Health)*	Calcium Carbonate/Simethicone 500mg-125mg	**Adults:** 1-2 caps prn. **Max:** 4 caps q24h.
Gelusil chewable tablets *(McNeil Consumer)*	Aluminum Hydroxide/Magnesium Hydroxide/Simethicone 200mg-200mg-20mg	**Adults:** 2-4 tabs qid.
Maalox Max liquid *(Novartis Consumer Health)*	Aluminum Hydroxide/Magnesium Hydroxide/Simethicone 400mg-400mg-40mg/5mL	**Adults & Peds: ≥12 yrs:** 2-4 tsp (10-20mL) qid. **Max:** 12 tsp (60mL) q24h.
Maalox Max Quick Dissolve Maximum Strength tablets *(Novartis Consumer Health)*	Calcium Carbonate/Simethicone 1000mg-60mg	**Adults:** 1-2 tabs prn. **Max:** 8 tabs q24h.
Maalox Regular Strength liquid *(Novartis Consumer Health)*	Aluminum Hydroxide/Magnesium Hydroxide/Simethicone 200mg-200mg-20mg/5mL	**Adults & Peds: ≥12 yrs:** 2-4 tsp (10-20mL) qid. **Max:** 16 tsp (80mL) q24h.
Mylanta Maximum Strength liquid *(Johnson & Johnson/Merck Consumer)*	Aluminum Hydroxide/Magnesium Hydroxide/Simethicone 400mg-400mg-40mg/5mL	**Adults & Peds: ≥12 yrs:** 2-4 tsp (10-20mL) qid. **Max:** 12 tsp (60mL) q24h.
Mylanta Regular Strength liquid *(Johnson & Johnson/Merck Consumer)*	Aluminum Hydroxide/Magnesium Hydroxide/Simethicone 200mg-200mg-20mg/5mL	**Adults & Peds: ≥12 yrs:** 2-4 tsp (10-20mL) qid. **Max:** 12 tsp (60mL) q24h.
Rolaids Multi-Sympton chewable tablets *(McNeil Consumer)*	Calcium Carbonate/Magnesium Hydroxide/Simethicone 675mg-135mg-60mg	**Adults:** 2 tabs qid prn. **Max:** 8 tabs q24h.
Titralac Plus chewable tablets *(3M Consumer Healthcare)*	Calcium Carbonate/Simethicone 420mg-21mg	**Adults:** 2 tabs q2-3h prn. **Max:** 19 tabs q24h.
BISMUTH SUBSALICYLATE		
Maalox Total Stomach Relief Maximum Strength liquid *(Novartis Consumer Health)*	Bismuth Subsalicylate 525mg/15mL	**Adults & Peds: ≥12 yrs:** 2 tbl (30mL) q1/2-1h. **Max:** 8 tbl (120mL) q24h.
Pepto Bismol chewable tablets *(Procter & Gamble)*	Bismuth Subsalicylate 262mg	**Adults & Peds: ≥12 yrs:** 2 tabs q1/2-1h. **Max:** 8 doses q24h.
Pepto Bismol caplets *(Procter & Gamble)*	Bismuth Subsalicylate 262mg	**Adults & Peds: ≥12 yrs:** 2 tabs q1/2-1h. **Max:** 8 doses q24h.
Pepto Bismol liquid *(Procter & Gamble)*	Bismuth Subsalicylate 262mg/15mL	**Adults & Peds: ≥12 yrs:** 2 tbl (30mL) q1/2-1h. **Max:** 8 doses (240mL) q24h.
Pepto Bismol Maximum Strength liquid *(Procter & Gamble)*	Bismuth Subsalicylate 525mg/15mL	**Adults & Peds: ≥12 yrs:** 2 tbl (30mL) q1h. **Peds:** 9-12 yrs: 1 tbl (15mL) q1h. **6-9 yrs:** 2 tsp (10mL) q1h. **3-6 yrs:** 1 tsp (5mL). **Max:** of 8 doses (240mL) q24h.
H₂-RECEPTOR ANTAGONIST		
Pepcid AC chewable tablets *(Johnson & Johnson/Merck Consumer)*	Famotidine 10mg	**Adults & Peds: ≥12 yrs:** 1 tab qd. **Max:** 2 tabs q24h.
Pepcid AC gelcaps *(Johnson & Johnson/Merck Consumer)*	Famotidine 10mg	**Adults & Peds: ≥12 yrs:** 1 tab qd. **Max:** 2 tabs q24h.

Table 4. ANTACID AND HEARTBURN PRODUCTS (cont.)

BRAND NAME	INGREDIENT/STRENGTH	DOSE
Pepcid AC Maximum Strength tablets *(Johnson & Johnson/Merck Consumer)*	Famotidine 20mg	**Adults & Peds: ≥12 yrs:** 1 tab qd. **Max:** 2 tabs q24h.
Pepcid AC tablets *(Johnson & Johnson/Merck Consumer)*	Famotidine 10mg	**Adults & Peds: ≥12 yrs:** 1 tab qd. **Max:** 2 tabs q24h.
Tagamet HB tablets *(GlaxoSmithKline Consumer Healthcare)*	Cimetidine 200mg	**Adults & Peds: ≥12 yrs:** 1 tab qd. **Max:** 2 tabs q24h.
Zantac 150 tablets *(Boehringer Ingelheim Consumer) Healthcare)*	Ranitidine 150mg	**Adults & Peds: ≥12 yrs:** 1 tab qd. **Max:** 2 tabs q24h.
Zantac 75 tablets *(Boehringer Ingelheim Consumer Healthcare)*	Ranitidine 75mg	**Adults & Peds: ≥12 yrs:** 1 tab qd. **Max:** 2 tabs q24h.
H$_2$-RECEPTOR ANTAGONIST/ANTACID		
Pepcid Complete chewable tablets *(Johnson & Johnson/Merck Consumer)*	Famotidine/Calcium Carbonate/ Magnesium Hydroxide 10mg-800mg-165mg	**Adults & Peds: ≥12 yrs:** 1 tab qd. **Max:** 2 tabs q24h.
PROTON PUMP INHIBITOR		
Prilosec OTC tablets *(Procter & Gamble)*	Omeprazole 20mg	**Adults:** 1 tab qd x 14 days. May repeat 14 day course q 4 months.

Table 5. ANTIDIARRHEAL PRODUCTS

BRAND NAME	INGREDIENT/STRENGTH	DOSE
ABSORBENT AGENTS		
Equalactin chewable tablets *(Numark Laboratories)*	Calcium Polycarbophil 625mg	**Adults: ≥12 yrs:** 2 tabs q30min prn. **Max:** 6 doses q24h. **Peds: 6-12 yrs:** 1 tab q30min. **Max:** 6 doses q24h. **3-6 yrs:** 1 tab q30min. **Max:** 3 doses q24h.
Fibercon caplets *(Lederle Consumer Health)*	Calcium Polycarbophil 625mg	**Adults: ≥12 yrs:** 2 tabs q30min prn. **Max:** 6 doses q24h. **Peds: 6-12 yrs:** 1 tab q30min. **Max:** 6 doses q24h. **3-6 yrs:** 1 tab q30min. **Max:** 3 doses q24h.
Fiber-Lax tablets *(Rugby Laboratories)*	Calcium Polycarbophil 625mg	**Adults: ≥12 yrs:** 2 tabs q30min prn. **Max:** 6 doses q24h. **Peds: 6-12 yrs:** 1 tab q30min. **Max:** 6 doses q24h. **3-6 yrs:** 1 tab q30min. **Max:** 3 doses q24h.
Kapectolin *(Consolidated Midland Corp)*	Kaolin/Pectin 90g-2g/30mL	**Adults:** 60-120mL after each loose bowel movement. **Peds: ≥12 yrs:** 45-60mL after each loose bowel movement. **6-12 yrs:** 30-60mL after each loose bowel movement. **3-6 yrs:** 15-30mL after each loose bowel movement.
Konsyl Fiber tablets *(Konsyl Pharmaceuticals)*	Calcium Polycarbophil 625mg	**Adults: ≥12 yrs:** 2 tabs q30min prn. **Max:** 6 doses q24h. **Peds: 6-12 yrs:** 1 tab q30min. **Max:** 6 doses q24h. **3-6 yrs:** 1 tab q30min. **Max:** 3 doses q24h.
Phillip's Fibercaps *(Bayer Healthcare)*	Calcium Polycarbophil 625mg	**Adults: ≥12 yrs:** 2 tabs q30min prn. **Max:** 6 doses q24h. **Peds: 6-12 yrs:** 1 tab q30min. **Max:** 6 doses q24h. **3-6 yrs:** 1 tab q30min. **Max:** 3 doses q24h.
ANTIPERISTALTIC AGENTS		
Imodium A-D caplet *(McNeil Consumer)*	Loperamide HCl 2mg	**Adults: ≥12 yrs:** 2 caplets after first loose stool; 1 caplet after each subsequent loose stool. **Max:** 4 caplets q24h. **Peds: 9-11 yrs: (60-95 lbs):** 1 caplet after first loose stool; ½ caplet after each subsequent loose stool. **Max:** 3 caplets q24h. **6-8 yrs: (48-59 lbs):** 1 caplet after first loose stool; ½ caplet after each subsequent loose stool. **Max:** 2 caplets q24h.
Imodium A-D E-Z Chews *(McNeil Consumer)*	Loperamide HCl 2mg	**Adults: ≥12 yrs:** 2 tabs after first loose stool; 1 tab after each subsequent loose stool. **Max:** 4 tabs q24h. **Peds: 9-11 yrs: (60-95 lbs):** 1 tab after first loose stool; ½ tab after each subsequent loose stool. **Max:** 3 tabs q24h. **6-8 yrs: (48-59 lbs):** 1 tab after first loose stool; ½ tab after each subsequent loose stool. **Max:** 2 tabs q24h.
Imodium A-D liquid *(McNeil Consumer)*	Loperamide HCl 1mg/7.5mL	**Adults: ≥12 yrs:** 30mL (6 tsp) after first loose stool; 15mL (3 tsp) after each subsequent loose stool. **Max:** 60mL (12 tsp) q24h. **Peds: 9-11 yrs: (60-95 lbs):** 15mL (3 tsp) after first loose stool; 7.5mL (1½ tsp) after each subsequent loose stool. **Max:** 45mL (9 tsp) q24h. **6-8 yrs: (48-59 lbs):** 15 mL (3 tsp) after first loose stool; 7.5mL (1½ tsp) after each subsequent loose stool. **Max:** 30mL (6 tsp) q24h.

Table 5. ANTIDIARRHEAL PRODUCTS (cont.)

BRAND NAME	INGREDIENT/STRENGTH	DOSE
ANTIPERISTALTIC/ANTIFLATULENT AGENTS		
Imodium Advanced caplet *(McNeil Consumer)*	Loperamide HCl/Simethicone 2mg-125mg	**Adults: ≥12 yrs:** 2 tabs after first loose stool; 1 tab after each subsequent loose stool. **Max:** 4 tabs q24h. **Peds: 9-11 yrs: (60-95 lbs):** 1 tab after first loose stool; ½ tab after each subsequent loose stool. **Max:** 3 tabs q24h. **6-8 yrs: (48-59 lbs):** 1 tab after first loose stool; ½ tab after each subsequent loose stool. **Max:** 2 tabs q24h.
Imodium Advanced chewable tablet *(McNeil Consumer)*	Loperamide HCl/Simethicone 2mg-125mg	**Adults: ≥12 yrs:** 2 tabs after first loose stool; 1 tab after each subsequent loose stool. **Max:** 4 tabs q24h. **Peds: 9-11 yrs: (60-95 lbs):** 1 tab after first loose stool; ½ tab after each subsequent loose stool. **Max:** 3 tabs q24h. **6-8 yrs: (48-59 lbs):** 1 tab after first loose stool; ½ tab after each subsequent loose stool. **Max:** 2 tabs q24h.
BISMUTH SUBSALICYLATE		
Kaopectate caplet *(Chattem)*	Bismuth Subsalicylate 262mg	**Adults & Peds: ≥12 yrs:** 2 tabs q½-1h. **Max:** 8 doses q24h.
Kaopectate Extra Strength liquid *(Chattem)*	Bismuth Subsalicylate 525mg/15mL	**Adults: ≥12 yrs:** 2 tbl (30mL). **Peds: 9-12 yrs:** 1 tbl (15mL) q1h prn. **6-9 yrs:** 2 tsp (10mL) q1h prn. **3-6 yrs:** 1 tsp (5mL) q1h prn. **Max:** 8 doses q24h.
Kaopectate liquid *(Chattem)*	Bismuth Subsalicylate 262mg/15mL	**Adults: ≥12 yrs:** 2 tbl (30mL). **Peds: 9-12 yrs:** 1 tbl (15mL) q1h prn. **6-9 yrs:** 2 tsp (10mL) q1h prn. **3-6 yrs:** 1 tsp (5mL) q1h prn. **Max:** 8 doses q24h.
Pepto Bismol chewable tablets *(Procter & Gamble)*	Bismuth Subsalicylate 262mg	**Adults & Peds: ≥12 yrs:** 2 tabs q½-1h. **Max:** 8 doses q24h.
Pepto Bismol caplets *(Procter & Gamble)*	Bismuth Subsalicylate 262mg	**Adults & Peds: ≥12 yrs:** 2 tabs q½-1h. **Max:** 8 doses q24h.
Pepto Bismol liquid *(Procter & Gamble)*	Bismuth Subsalicylate 262mg/15mL	**Adults & Peds: ≥12 yrs:** 2 tbl (30mL) q½-1h. **Max:** 8 doses q24h.
Pepto Bismol Maximum Strength *(Procter & Gamble)*	Bismuth Subsalicylate 525mg/15mL	**Adults: ≥12 yrs:** 2 tbl (30mL). **Peds: 9-12 yrs:** 1 tbl (15mL) q1h prn. **6-9 yrs:** 2 tsp (10mL) q1h prn. **3-6 yrs:** 1 tsp (5mL) q1h prn. **Max:** 8 doses q24h.

Table 6. ANTIFLATULANT PRODUCTS

BRAND NAME	INGREDIENT/STRENGTH	DOSE
ALPHA-GALACTOSIDASE		
Beano Food Enzyme Dietary Supplement drops (AkPharma)	Alpha-Galactosidase Enzyme 150 GalU	**Adults:** Add 5 drops before meals.
Beano Food Enzyme Dietary Supplement tablets (AkPharma)	Alpha-Galactosidase Enzyme 150 GalU	**Adults:** Take 3 tab before meals.
ANTACID/ANTIFLATULENCE		
Gas-X with Maalox capsules (Novartis Consumer Health)	Calcium Carbonate/Simethicone 250mg-62.5mg	**Adults:** 2-4 caps prn. **Max:** 8 caps q24h.
Gas-X Extra Strength with Maalox capsules (Novartis Consumer Health)	Calcium Carbonate/Simethicone Adults: 500mg-125mg	**Adults:** 1-2 caps prn. **Max:** 4 caps q24h.
Gelusil chewable tablets (Pfizer Consumer Healthcare)	Aluminum Hydroxide/Magnesium Hydroxide/Simethicone 200mg-200mg-20mg	**Adults:** 2-4 tabs qid.
Maalox Max liquid (Novartis Consumer Health)	Aluminum Hydroxide/Magnesium Hydroxide/Simethicone 400mg-400mg-40mg/5mL	**Adults & Peds:** ≥12 yo: 2-4 tsp (10-20mL) qid. **Max:** 12 tsp (60mL) q24h.
Maalox Max Quick Dissolve Maximum Strength tablets (Novartis Consumer Health)	Calcium Carbonate/Simethicone 1000mg-60mg	**Adults:** 1-2 tabs prn. **Max:** 8 tabs q24h.
Maalox Regular Strength liquid (Novartis Consumer Health)	Aluminum Hydroxide/Magnesium Hydroxide/Simethicone 200mg-200mg-20mg/5mL	**Adults & Peds:** ≥12 yrs: 2-4 tsp (10-20mL) qid. **Max:** 16 tsp (80mL) q24h.
Mylanta Maximum Strength liquid (Johnson & Johnson/Merck Consumer)	Aluminum Hydroxide/Magnesium Hydroxide/Simethicone 400mg-400mg-40mg/5mL	**Adults & Peds:** ≥12 yrs: 2-4 tsp (10-20mL) qid. **Max:** 12 tsp (60mL) q24h.
Mylanta Regular Strength liquid (Johnson & Johnson/Merck Consumer)	Aluminum Hydroxide/Magnesium Hydroxide/Simethicone 200mg-200mg-20mg/5mL	**Adults & Peds:** ≥12 yrs: 2-4 tsp (10-20mL) qid. **Max:** 24 tsp (120mL) q24h.
Rolaids Antacid & Antigas Soft Chews (McNeil Consumer)	Calcium Carbonate/Simethicone 1177mg-80mg	**Adults:** 2-3 chews hourly prn.
Titralac Plus chewable tablets (3M Consumer Healthcare)	Calcium Carbonate/Simethicone 420mg-21mg	**Adults:** 2 tabs q2-3h prn. **Max:** 19 tabs q24h.
SIMETHICONE		
GasAid Maximum Strength Anti-Gas softgels (McNeil Consumer)	Simethicone 125mg	**Adults:** Take 1-2 cap prn and qhs. **Max:** 4 cap q24h.
Gas-X Infant Drops (Novartis Consumer Health)	Simethicone 20 mg/0.3mL	**Peds:** ≥2 yrs. (≥24 lbs): 0.6mL prn. **Peds:** <2 yrs. (<24 lbs): 0.3mL prn. **Max:** 6 doses q24h.
Gas-X Thin Strips (Novartis Consumer Health)	Simethicone 62.5mg	**Adults:** Allow 2-4 strips to dissolve prn **Max:** 8 strips q24h.
Gas-X Antigas Chewable tablets (Novartis Consumer Health)	Simethicone 80mg	**Adults:** Take 1-2 cap prn and qhs. **Max:** 6 cap q24h.
Gas-X Extra Strength Antigas softgels (Novartis Consumer Health)	Simethicone 125mg	**Adults:** Take 1-2 cap prn and qhs. **Max:** 4 cap q24h.
Gas-X Maximum Strength Antigas softgels (Novartis Consumer Health)	Simethicone 166mg	**Adults:** Take 1-2 cap prn and qhs. **Max:** 3 cap q24h.
Little Tummys Gas Relief drops (Vetco)	Simethicone 20 mg/0.3mL	**Peds:** >2 yrs (>24 lbs): 0.6mL prn. **Peds:** <2 yrs (<24 lbs): 0.3mL prn. **Max:** 12 doses q24h.
Mylanta Gas Maximum Strength Chewable tablets (Johnson & Johnson/Merck Consumer)	Simethicone 125 mg	**Adults:** Chew 1-2 tab prn and qhs.
Mylanta Gas Regular Strength Chewable tablets (Johnson & Johnson/Merck Consumer)	Simethicone 80 mg	**Adults:** Chew 1-2 tab prn and qhs.
Mylicon Infant's Gas Relief drops (Johnson & Johnson/Merck Consumer)	Simethicone 20 mg/0.3mL	**Peds:** ≥2 yrs. (≥24lbs): 0.6mL prn. **Peds:** <2 yrs. (<24lbs): 0.3mL prn. **Max:** 12 doses q24h.

Table 7. CONTACT DERMATITIS PRODUCTS

Brand Name	Ingredient/Strength	Dose
ANTIHISTAMINE		
Benadryl Extra Strength Gel Pump (McNeil Consumer)	Diphenhydramine HCl 2%	**Adults & Peds ≥12 yrs:** Apply to affected area tid-qid.
ANTIHISTAMINE COMBINATION		
Benadryl Extra Strength Cream (McNeil Consumer)	Diphenhydramine HCl/Zinc Acetate 2%-0.1%	**Adults & Peds ≥12 yrs:** Apply to affected area tid-qid.
Benadryl Extra Strength Spray (McNeil Consumer)	Diphenhydramine HCl/Zinc Acetate 2%-0.1%	**Adults & Peds ≥12 yrs:** Apply to affected area tid-qid.
Benadryl Itch Relief Spray (McNeil Consumer)	Diphenhydramine HCl/Zinc Acetate 2%-0.1%	**Adults & Peds ≥2 yrs:** Apply to affected area tid-qid.
Benadryl Itch Relief Stick (McNeil Consumer)	Diphenhydramine HCl/Zinc Acetate 2%-0.1%	**Adults & Peds ≥2 yrs:** Apply to affected area tid-qid.
Benadryl Original Cream (McNeil Consumer)	Diphenhydramine HCl/Zinc Acetate 1%-0.1%	**Adults & Peds ≥2 yrs:** Apply to affected area tid-qid.
CalaGel Anti-Itch Gel (Tec Laboratories)	Diphenhydramine HCl/Zinc Acetate/ Benzenthonium Chloride 2%-0.215%-15%	**Adults & Peds ≥2 yrs:** Apply to affected area tid-qid.
Ivarest Anti-Itch Cream (Blistex)	Diphenhydramine HCl/Calamine 2%-14%	**Adults & Peds ≥2 yrs:** Apply to affected area tid-qid.
ASTRINGENT		
Domeboro Powder Packets (Bayer Healthcare)	Aluminum Acetate/Aluminum Sulfate 938mg-1191mg	**Adults & Peds:** Dissolve 1-2 packets and apply to affected area for 15-30 min tid.
Ivy-Dry Super Lotion Extra Strength (Ivy Corporation)	Zinc Acetate/Benzyl Alcohol 2%-10%	**Adults & Peds: ≥6 yrs:** Apply to affected area qd-tid.
ASTRINGENT COMBINATION		
Aveeno Anti-Itch Cream (Johnson & Johnson Consumer)	Calamine/Pramoxine HCl 3%-1%	**Adults & Peds ≥2 yrs:** Apply to affected area tid-qid.
Aveeno Anti-Itch Lotion (Johnson & Johnson Consumer)	Calamine/Pramoxine HCl/Camphor 3%-1%-0.47%	**Adults & Peds ≥2 yrs:** Apply to affected area tid-qid.
Caladryl Clear Lotion (Johnson & Johnson Consumer)	Zinc Acetate/Pramoxine HCl 0.1%-1%	**Adults & Peds ≥2 yrs:** Apply to affected area tid-qid.
Caladryl Lotion (Johnson & Johnson Consumer)	Calamine/Pramoxine HCl 8%-1%	**Adults & Peds ≥2 yrs:** Apply to affected area tid-qid.
Calamine lotion (generic) (Various)	Calamine/Zinc Oxide 6.971%-6.971%	**Adults & Peds:** Apply to affected area prn.
CLEANSER		
Ivy-Dry Scrub (Ivy Corporation)	Polyethylene, sodium lauryl sulfoacetate, cetearyl alcohol, nonoxynol-9, camellia sinensis oil, phenoxyethanol, methylparaben, propylparaben, triethanolamine, carbomer, erythorbic acid, aloe barbadensis extract, tocopheryl acetate extract, tetrasodium EDTA	**Adults & Peds:** Wash affected area prn.
IvyStat! Gel/Exfoliant (Tec Laboratories)	Hydrocortisone 1% (gel); Cocamidopropylsultaine, PEG-4 laurate, cocamide DEA, polyethylene beads, sodium chloride, benzethonium chloride (cleanser)	**Adults & Peds:** Apply to affected area tid-qid.
CORTICOSTEROID		
Aveeno Anti-Itch Cream 1% (Johnson & Johnson Consumer)	Hydrocortisone 1%	**Adults & Peds ≥2 yrs:** Apply to affected area tid-qid.
Cortaid Advanced 12-Hour Anti-Itch Cream (Johnson & Johnson Consumer)	Hydrocortisone 1%	**Adults & Peds ≥2 yrs:** Apply to affected area tid-qid.
Cortaid Intensive Therapy Cooling Spray (Johnson & Johnson Consumer)	Hydrocortisone 1%	**Adults & Peds ≥2 yrs:** Apply to affected area tid-qid.
Cortaid Intensive Therapy Moisturizing Cream (Johnson & Johnson Consumer)	Hydrocortisone 1%	**Adults & Peds ≥2 yrs:** Apply to affected area tid-qid

Table 7. CONTACT DERMATITIS PRODUCTS (cont.)

BRAND NAME	INGREDIENT/STRENGTH	DOSE
Cortaid Maximum Strength Cream *(Johnson & Johnson Consumer)*	Hydrocortisone 1%	**Adults & Peds ≥2 yrs:** Apply to affected area tid-qid.
Cortaid Maximum Strength Ointment *(Johnson & Johnson Consumer)*	Hydrocortisone 1%	**Adults & Peds ≥2 yrs:** Apply to affected area tid-qid.
Cortizone-10 Cream *(Chattem)*	Hydrocortisone 1%	**Adults & Peds ≥2 yrs:** Apply to affected area tid-qid.
Cortizone-10 Maximum Strength Anti-Itch Ointment *(Chattem)*	Hydrocortisone 1%	**Adults & Peds ≥2 yrs:** Apply to affected area tid-qid.
Cortizone-10 Ointment *(Chattem)*	Hydrocortisone 1%	**Adults & Peds ≥2 yrs:** Apply to affected area tid-qid.
Cortizone-10 Plus Maximum Strength Cream *(Chattem)*	Hydrocortisone 1%	**Adults & Peds ≥2 yrs:** Apply to affected area tid-qid.
Cortizone-10 Quick Shot Spray *(Chattem)*	Hydrocortisone 1%	**Adults & Peds ≥2 yrs:** Apply to affected area tid-qid.
Dermarest Eczema Lotion *(Del Laboratories)*	Hydrocortisone 1%	**Adults & Peds ≥2 yrs:** Apply to affected area tid-qid.
COUNTERIRRITANT		
Gold Bond First Aid Quick Spray *(Chattem)*	Menthol/Benzethonium Chloride 1%-0.13%	**Adults & Peds ≥2 yrs:** Apply to affected area tid-qid.
Gold Bond Medicated Maximum Strength Anti-Itch Cream *(Chattem)*	Menthol/Pramoxine HCl 1%-1%	**Adults & Peds ≥2 yrs:** Apply to affected area tid-qid.
Ivy Block Lotion *(Enviroderm Pharmaceuticals)*	Bentoquatam 5%	**Adults & Peds ≥2 yrs:** Apply q4h for continued protection.
LOCAL ANESTHETIC		
Solarcaine Aloe Extra Burn Relief Gel *(Schering-Plough)*	Lidocaine HCl 0.5%	**Adults & Peds ≥2 yrs:** Apply to affected area tid-qid.
Solarcaine Aloe Extra Spray *(Schering-Plough)*	Lidocaine HCl 0.5%	**Adults & Peds ≥2 yrs:** Apply to affected area tid-qid.
Solarcaine First Aid Medicated Spray *(Schering-Plough)*	Benzocaine/Triclosan 20%-0.13%	**Adults & Peds ≥2 yrs:** Apply to affected area qd-tid.
LOCAL ANESTHETIC COMBINATION		
Bactine First Aid Liquid *(Bayer Healthcare)*	Lidocaine HCl/Benzalkonium Chloride 2.5%-0.13%	**Adults & Peds ≥2 yrs:** Apply to affected area qd-tid.
Bactine Pain Relieving Cleansing Spray *(Bayer Healthcare)*	Lidocaine HCl/Benzalkonium Chloride 2.5%-0.13%	**Adults & Peds ≥2 yrs:** Apply to affected area qd-tid.
Lanacane Maximum Strength Cream *(Combe)*	Benzocaine/Benzethonium Chloride 20%-0.2%	**Adults & Peds ≥2 yrs:** Apply to affected area qd-tid.
Lanacane Maximum Strength Spray *(Combe)*	Benzocaine/Benzethonium Chloride/Ethanol 20%-0.2%-36%	**Adults & Peds ≥2 yrs:** Apply to affected area qd-tid.
Lanacane Original Formula Cream *(Combe)*	Benzocaine/Benzethonium Chloride 6%-0.2%	**Adults & Peds ≥2 yrs:** Apply to affected area qd-tid.
SKIN PROTECTANT		
Aveeno Skin Relief Moisturizing Cream *(Johnson & Johnson Consumer)*	Dimethicone 2.5%	**Adults & Peds:** Apply to affected area prn.
SKIN PROTECTANT COMBINATION		
Aveeno Itch Relief Lotion *(Johnson & Johnson Consumer)*	Dimethicone/Menthol 2.5%-0.1%	**Adults & Peds ≥2 yrs:** Apply to affected area tid-qid.
Gold Bond Extra Strength Medicated Body Lotion *(Chattem)*	Dimethicone/Menthol 5%-0.5%	**Adults & Peds:** Apply to affected area prn.
Gold Bond Medicated Body Lotion *(Chattem)*	Dimethicone/Menthol 5%-0.15%	**Adults & Peds:** Apply to affected area prn.
Gold Bond Medicated Extra Strength Powder *(Chattem)*	Zinc Oxide/Menthol 5%-0.8%	**Adults & Peds ≥2 yrs:** Apply to affected area tid-qid.
Vaseline Intensive Care Lotion Advanced Healing *(Kendall)*	Dimethicone 1%-White Petrolatum	**Adults & Peds:** Apply to affected area prn.

Table 8. COUGH-COLD-FLU PRODUCTS

Brand Name	Analgesic	Antihistamine	Decongestant	Cough Suppressant	Expectorant	Dose
ANTIHISTAMINE + DECONGESTANT						
Actifed Cold & Allergy tablets *(McNeil Consumer)*		Chlorpheniramine Maleate 4mg	Phenylephrine HCl 10mg			**Adults: ≥12 yrs:** 1 tabs q4-6h. **Max:** 4 tabs q4-6h. **Peds: 6-12 yrs:** 1/2 tab q4-6h. **Max:** 2 tabs q24h.
Benadryl Children's Allergy & Cold Fastmelt tablets *(McNeil Consumer)*		Diphenhydramine 19mg	Pseudoephedrine HCl 30mg			**Adults: ≥12 yrs:** 2 tabs q4h. **Max:** 8 tabs q24h. **Peds: 6-12 yrs:** 1 tab q4h. **Max:** 4 tabs q4h.
Benadryl-D Allergy/Sinus tablets *(McNeil Consumer)*		Diphenhydramine HCl 25mg	Phenylephrine HCl 10mg			**Adults & Peds: ≥12 yrs:** 1 tab q4h. **Max:** 6 tab q24h.
Children's Benadryl-D Allergy & Sinus liquid *(McNeil Consumer)*		Diphenhydramine HCl 12.5mg/5mL	Pseudoephedrine HCl 30mg/5mL			**Adults: ≥12 yrs:** 2 tsp (10mL) q4-6h. **Peds: 6-12 yrs:** 1 tsp (5mL) q4-6h. **Max:** 4 doses q24h.
Children's Benadryl Allergy & Cold Fastmelt tablets *(McNeil Consumer)*		Diphenhydramine HCl 19mg	Pseudoephedrine HCl 30mg			**Adult & Peds ≥12 yrs:** 2 tabs q4h. **Max:** 8 tabs q24h. **Peds: 6-12 yrs:** 1 tab q4hr. **Max:** 6 doses q24h.
Dimetapp Children's Cold & Allergy elixir *(Wyeth Consumer Healthcare)*		Brompheniramine Maleate 1mg/5mL	Phenylephrine 2.5mg/5mL			**Adults: ≥12 yrs:** 4 tsp (20mL) q4h. **Peds: 6-12 yrs:** 2 tsp (10mL) q4h. **Max:** 6 doses q24h.
Triaminic Cold & Allergy liquid *(Novartis Consumer Health)*		Chlorpheniramine Maleate 1mg/5mL	Phenylephrine HCl 2.5mg/5mL			**Adults: ≥12 yrs:** 1 tsp (5mL) q4h. **Max:** 6 doses q24h. **Peds: 6-12 yrs:** 2 tsp (10mL).
Triaminic Nighttime Cough & Cold liquid *(Novartis Consumer Health)*		Diphenhydramine HCl 6.25mg/5mL	Phenylephrine HCl 2.5mg/5mL			**Adults: ≥12 yrs:** 1 tsp (5mL) q4h. **Max:** 6 doses q24h. **Peds: 6-12 yrs:** 2 tsp (10mL).
ANTIHISTAMINE + DECONGESTANT + ANALGESIC						
Actifed Cold & Sinus caplets *(McNeil Consumer)*	Acetaminophen 500mg	Chlorpheniramine Maleate 2mg	Pseudoephedrine HCl 30mg			**Adults & Peds: ≥12 yrs:** 2 tabs q6h. **Max:** 8 tabs q24h.
Advil Multi-Symptom Cold caplets *(Wyeth Consumer Healthcare)*	Ibuprofen 200mg	Chlorpheniramine Maleate 2mg	Pseudoephedrine HCl 30mg			**Adults & Peds: ≥12 yrs:** 1 tab q4-6h. **Max:** 6 tabs q24h.
Alka-Seltzer Plus Cold effervescent tablets *(Bayer Healthcare)*	Acetaminophen 250mg	Chlorpheniramine Maleate 2mg	Phenylephrine 5mg			**Adults & Peds: ≥12 yrs:** 2 tabs q4h. **Max:** 8 tabs q24h.
Benadryl Allergy & Cold caplets *(McNeil Consumer)*	Acetaminophen 500mg	Diphenhydramine HCl 12.5mg	Phenylephrine 5mg			**Adults & Peds: ≥12 yrs:** 2 cap q4h. **Max:** 12 q24h. **Peds: 6-12 yrs:** 1 cap q4h. **Max:** 5 tabs q24h.
Benadryl Allergy & Sinus Headache caplets *(McNeil Consumer)*	Acetaminophen 325mg	Diphenhydramine HCl 12.5mg	Phenylephrine 5mg			**Adults & Peds: ≥12 yrs:** 2 tab q4h. **Max:** 12 tab q24h. **Peds: 6-12 yrs:** 1 cap q4h. **Max:** 5 tabs q24h.

Table 8. COUGH-COLD-FLU PRODUCTS (cont.)

Brand Name	Analgesic	Antihistamine	Decongestant	Cough Suppressant	Expectorant	Dose
Benadryl Severe Allergy & Sinus Headache caplets (McNeil Consumer)	Acetaminophen 325mg	Diphenhydramine HCl 25mg	Phenylephrine HCl 5mg			**Adults & Peds: ≥12 yrs:** 2 caps q4h. **Max:** 12 caps q24h.
Comtrex Acute Head Cold caplets (Novartis Consumer Healthcare)	Acetaminophen 500mg	Brompheniramine Maleate 2mg	Pseudoephedrine HCl 30mg			**Adults & Peds: ≥12 yrs:** 2 tabs q6h. **Max:** 8 tabs q24h.
Comtrex Flu Therapy Nighttime liquid (Novartis Consumer Healthcare)	Acetaminophen 1000mg/30mL	Chlorpheniramine Maleate 4mg/30mL	Pseudoephedrine HCl 60mg/30mL			**Adults & Peds: ≥12 yrs:** 2 tbl (30mL) q6h. **Max:** 8 tbl (240mL) q24h.
Comtrex Flu Therapy Day & Night tablets (Novartis Consumer Healthcare)	Acetaminophen 500mg	Chlorpheniramine Maleate 2mg	Pseudoephedrine HCl 30mg			**Adults & Peds: ≥12 yrs:** 2 tabs q6h. **Max:** 4 daytime tabs q24h.
Comtrex Nighttime Acute Head Cold liquid (Bristol-Myers Squibb)	Acetaminophen 1000mg/30mL	Brompheniramine Maleate 4mg/30mL	Pseudoephedrine HCl 60mg/30mL			**Adults & Peds: ≥12 yrs:** 2 tbl (30mL) q6h. **Max:** 8 tbl (240mL) q24h.
Contac Cold & Flu Maximum Strength caplets (GlaxoSmithKline Consumer Healthcare)	Acetaminophen 500mg	Chlorpheniramine Maleate 2mg	Phenylephrine HCl 5mg			**Adults & Peds: ≥12 yrs:** 2 caps q4-6h. **Max:** 8 caps q24h.
Dristan Cold Multi-Symptom tablets (Wyeth Consumer Healthcare)	Acetaminophen 325mg	Chlorpheniramine Maleate 2mg	Phenylephrine HCl 5mg			**Adults & Peds: ≥12 yrs:** 2 tabs q4h. **Max:** 12 caps q24h.
Robitussin Cold & Congestion tablets (Wyeth Consumer Healthcare)	Acetaminophen 325mg	Chlorpheniramine Maleate 2mg	Phenylephrine HCl 5mg			**Adults & Peds: ≥12 yrs:** 2 tabs q4h. **Max:** 12 caps q24h.
Sudafed Sinus PE Nighttime Cold caplets (McNeil Consumer)	Acetaminophen 325mg	Diphenhydramine HCl 25mg	Phenylephrine HCl 5mg			**Adults & Peds: ≥12 yrs:** 2 tabs q4h. **Max:** 12 tabs q24h.
Sudafed PE Severe Cold caplets (McNeil Consumer)	Acetaminophen 325mg	Diphenhydramine HCl 12.5mg	Phenylephrine HCl 5mg			**Adults & Peds: ≥12 yrs:** 2 tabs q4h. **Max:** 12 tabs q24h. **Peds: 6-12 yrs:** 1 tab q4h. **Max:** 5 tabs q24h.
Theraflu Cold & Sore Throat Hot Liquid (Novartis Consumer Health)	Acetaminophen 325mg/packet	Pheniramine Maleate 20mg/packet	Phenylephrine HCl 10mg/packet			**Adults & Peds: ≥12 yrs:** 1 packet q4h. **Max:** 6 packets q24h.
Theraflu Nighttime Severe Cold Hot liquid (Novartis Consumer Health)	Acetaminophen 650mg/packet	Pheniramine Maleate 20mg/packet	Phenylephrine HCl 10mg/packet			**Adults & Peds: ≥12 yrs:** 1 packet q4h. **Max:** 6 packets q24h.
Theraflu Flu & Sore Throat liquid (Novartis Consumer Health)	Acetaminophen 650mg/packet	Pheniramine Maleate 20mg/packet	Phenylephrine HCl 10mg/packet			**Adults & Peds: ≥12 yrs:** 1 packet q4h. **Max:** 6 packets q24h.
Tylenol Children's Plus Cold liquid (McNeil Consumer)	Acetaminophen 160mg/5mL	Chlorpheniramine Maleate 1mg/5mL	Phenylephrine HCl 2.5mg/5mL			**Peds: 6-11 yrs (48-95 lbs):** 2 tsp (10mL) q4h. **Max:** 5 doses q24h.

Table 8. COUGH-COLD-FLU PRODUCTS (cont.)

Brand Name	Analgesic	Antihistamine	Decongestant	Cough Suppressant	Expectorant	Dose
Tylenol Children's Plus Cold & Allergy liquid *(McNeil Consumer)*	Acetaminophen 160mg/5mL	Diphenhydramine HCl 12.5mg/5mL	Phenylephrine HCl 2.5mg/5mL			**Peds: 6-11 yrs (48-95 lbs):** 2 tsp (10mL) q4-6h. **Max:** 4 doses q24h.
Tylenol Children's Plus Cold Nighttime suspension *(McNeil Consumer)*	Acetaminophen 160mg/5mL	Chlorpheniramine Maleate 1mg/5mL	Pseudoephedrine HCl 15mg/5mL			**Peds: 6-12 yrs (48-95 lbs):** 2 tsp (10mL) q4-6h. **Max:** 8 tsp (40mL) q24h.
Tylenol Flu Nighttime gelcaps *(McNeil Consumer)*	Acetaminophen 500mg	Diphenhydramine HCl 25mg	Pseudoephedrine HCl 30mg			**Adults & Peds: ≥12 yrs:** 2 caps q6h. **Max:** 8 caps q24h.
Tylenol Sinus Congestion & Pain Nighttime caplets *(McNeil Consumer)*	Acetaminophen 325mg	Chlorpheniramine Maleate 2mg	Phenylephrine HCl 5mg			**Adults & Peds: ≥12 yrs:** 2 caps q4h. **Max:** 12 caps q24h.
Tylenol Sinus Nighttime caplets *(McNeil Consumer)*	Acetaminophen 500mg	Doxylamine Succinate 6.25mg	Pseudoephedrine HCl 30mg			**Adults & Peds: ≥12 yrs:** 2 tabs q4-6h **Max:** 8 tabs q24h.
COUGH SUPPRESSANT						
Delsym 12 Hour Cough Relief liquid *(Celltech Pharmaceuticals)*				Dextromethorphan Polistrex 30mg/5mL		**Adults: ≥12 yrs:** 2 tsp (10mL) q12h. **Peds: 6-12 yrs:** 1 tsp (5mL) q12h. **2-6 yrs:** 1/2 tsp (2.5mL) q12h. **Max:** 4 doses q24h.
PediaCare Long-Acting Cough liquid *(McNeil Consumer)*				Dextromethorphan HBr 7.5mg/5mL		**Peds: 6-12 yrs:** 2 tsp q6-8h. **2-6 yrs:** 1 tsp q6-8h. **Max:** 4 doses q24h.
Robitussin Cough Long-Acting liquid *(Wyeth Consumer Healthcare)*				Dextromethorphan HBr 15mg/5mL		**Adults & Peds: ≥12 yrs:** 2 tsp (10mL) q6-8h. **Max:** 8 tsp (40mL) q24h.
Robitussin CoughGels liqui-gels *(Wyeth Consumer Healthcare)*				Dextromethorphan HBr 15mg		**Adults & Peds: ≥12 yrs:** 2 caps q6-8h. **Max:** 8 caps q24h.
Robitussin Pediatric Cough liquid *(Wyeth Consumer Healthcare)*				Dextromethorphan HBr 7.5mg/5mL		**Adults: ≥12 yrs (≥96 lbs):** 4 tsp (20mL) q6-8h. **Peds: 6-12 yrs (48-95 lbs):** 2 tsp (10mL) q6-8h. **2-6 yrs:** 1 tsp (5mL) q6-8h. **Max:** 4 doses q24h.
Simply Cough liquid *(McNeil Consumer)*				Dextromethorphan HBr 5mg/5mL		**Peds: 6-12 yrs (48-95 lbs):** 2 tsp (10mL) q4h. **2-6 yrs (24-47 lbs):** 1 tsp (5mL) q4h. **Max:** 4 doses q24h.
Theraflu Long Acting Cough thin strips *(Novartis Consumer Health)*				Dextromethorphan 11mg/strip		**Adults & Peds: ≥12 yrs:** 2 strips q6-8h. **Max:** 8 strips q24h.
Triaminic Long Acting Cough thin strips *(Novartis Consumer Health)*				Dextromethorphan 5.5mg/strip		**Peds: 6-12 yrs:** 2 strips q6-8h. **Max:** 8 strips q24h.
Vicks Day Quil Cough *(Procter & Gamble)*				Dextromethorphan HBr 15mg/15mL		**Adults & Peds: ≥12 yrs:** 2 tbl (30mL) q6-8h. **Peds: 6-12 yrs:** 1 tbl (15mL) q6-8h. **Max:** 4 doses q24h.

Table 8. COUGH-COLD-FLU PRODUCTS (cont.)

Brand Name	Analgesic	Antihistamine	Decongestant	Cough Suppressant	Expectorant	Dose
Vicks 44 liquid *(Procter & Gamble)*				Dextromethorphan HBr 30mg/15mL		**Adults & Peds: ≥12 yrs:** 1 tbl (15mL) q6-8h. **Peds: 6-12 yrs:** 1.5 tsp (7.5mL) q6-8h. **Max:** 4 doses q24h.
Vicks BabyRub *(Procter & Gamble)*				Eucalyptus, petrolatum, fragrance, aloe extract, eucalyptus oil, lavender oil, rosemary oil		**Peds: ≥3 mth:** Apply q8h.
Vicks Cough Drops Cherry Flavor *(Procter & Gamble)*				Menthol 1.7mg		**Adults & Peds: ≥5 yrs:** 3 drops q1-2h.
Vicks Cough Drops Original Flavor *(Procter & Gamble)*				Menthol 3.3mg		**Adults & Peds: ≥5 yrs:** 2 drops q1-2h.
Vicks VapoRub *(Procter & Gamble)*				Camphor 5.2% Menthol 2.8% Eucalyptus 1.2%		**Adults & Peds: ≥2 yrs:** Apply q8h.
Vicks VapoRub Cream *(Procter & Gamble)*				Camphor 4.8% Menthol 2.6% Eucalyptus 1.2%		**Adults & Peds: ≥2 yrs:** Apply q8h.
Vicks VapoSteam *(Procter & Gamble)*				Camphor 6.2%		**Adults & Peds: ≥2 yrs:** 1 tbl/quart q8h.
COUGH SUPPRESSANT + ANTIHISTAMINE						
Coricidin HBP Cough & Cold tablets *(Schering-Plough)*		Chlorpheniramine Maleate 4mg		Dextromethorphan HBr 30mg		**Adults & Peds: ≥12 yrs:** 1 tabs q6h. **Max:** 4 tabs q24h.
Dimetapp Long-Acting Cold Plus Cough elixir *(Wyeth Consumer Healthcare)*		Chlorpheniramine Maleate 1mg/5mL		Dextromethorphan HBr 7.5mg/5mL		**Peds: ≥12 yrs:** 4 tsp (20mL) q6h. **6-12 yrs:** 2 tsp (10 mL) q6h. **Max:** 4 doses q24h.
Robitussin Cough & Cold Long-Acting liquid *(Wyeth Consumer Healthcare)*		Chlorpheniramine Maleate 2mg/5mL		Dextromethorphan HBr 15mg/5mL		**Adults: ≥12 yrs:** 2 tsp (10mL) q6h. **Max:** 4 doses q24h.
Triaminic Softchews Cough & Runny Nose *(Novartis Consumer Health)*		Chlorpheniramine Maleate 1mg		Dextromethorphan HBr 5mg		**Adults & Peds: ≥12 yrs:** 1 tabs q4-6h. **Max:** 6 tabs q24h.
Vicks Children's NyQuil liquid *(Procter & Gamble)*		Chlorpheniramine Maleate 2mg/15mL		Dextromethorphan HBr 15mg/15mL		**Adults: ≥12 yrs:** 2 tbl (30mL) q6h. **Peds: 6-11 yrs:** 1 tbl (15mL) q6h. **Max:** 4 doses q24h.
Vicks NyQuil Cough liquid *(Procter & Gamble)*		Doxylamine Succinate 6.25mg/15mL		Dextromethorphan HBr 15mg/15mL		**Adults & Peds: ≥12 yrs:** 2 tbl (30mL) q6h. **Max:** 8 tbl (120mL) q24h.
COUGH SUPPRESSANT + ANTIHISTAMINE + ANALGESIC						
Alka-Seltzer Plus Flu effervescent tablets *(Bayer Healthcare)*	Aspirin 500mg	Chlorpheniramine Maleate 2mg		Dextromethorphan HBr 15mg		**Adults & Peds: ≥12 yrs:** 2 tabs q6h. **Max:** 8 tabs q24h.

Table 8. COUGH-COLD-FLU PRODUCTS (cont.)

Brand Name	Analgesic	Antihistamine	Decongestant	Cough Suppressant	Expectorant	Dose
Alka-Seltzer Plus Nighttime Liquid Gels (Bayer Healthcare)	Acetaminophen 325mg	Doxylamine Succinate 6.25mg		Dextromethorphan HBr 15mg		**Adults & Peds: ≥12 yrs:** 2 tabs q6h. **Max:** 12 tabs q24h.
Coricidin HBP Maximum Strength Flu tablets (Schering-Plough)	Acetaminophen 500mg	Chlorpheniramine Maleate 2mg		Dextromethorphan HBr 15mg		**Adults & Peds: ≥12 yrs:** 2 tabs q6h. **Max:** 8 tabs q24h.
Triaminic Flu Cough & Fever liquid (Novartis Consumer Health)	Acetaminophen 160mg/5mL	Chlorpheniramine Maleate 1mg/5mL		Dextromethorphan HBr 7.5mg/5mL		**Adults & Peds: ≥12 yrs:** 1 tsp (5mL) q6h. **Max:** 4 doses (20mL) q24h.
Tylenol Nighttime Cough & Sore Throat Cool Burst liquid (McNeil Consumer)	Acetaminophen 1000mg/30mL	Doxylamine 12.5mg/30mL		Dextromethorphan HBr 30mg/30mL		**Adults & Peds: ≥12 yrs:** 2 tbl (30mL) q6h. **Max:** 8 tbl (120mL) q24h.
Vicks 44M liquid (Procter & Gamble)	Acetaminophen 162.5mg/5mL	Chlorpheniramine Maleate 1mg/5mL		Dextromethorphan HBr 7.5mg/5mL		**Adults & Peds: ≥12 yrs:** 4 tsp (20mL) q6h. **Max:** 16 tsp (80mL) q24h.
Vicks NyQuil liquicaps (Procter & Gamble)	Acetaminophen 325mg	Doxylamine Succinate 6.25mg		Dextromethorphan HBr 15mg		**Adults & Peds: ≥12 yrs:** 2 caps q6h. **Max:** 8 caps q24h.
Vicks NyQuil liquid (Procter & Gamble)	Acetaminophen 500mg/15mL	Doxylamine Succinate 6.25mg/15mL		Dextromethorphan HBr 15mg/15mL		**Adults & Peds: ≥12 yrs:** 2 tbl (30mL) q6h. **Max:** 8 tbl (120mL) q24h.
COUGH SUPPRESSANT + ANTIHISTAMINE + ANALGESIC + DECONGESTANT						
Alka-Seltzer Plus Cough & Cold Liquid Gels (Bayer Healthcare)	Acetaminophen 325mg	Chlorpheniramine Maleate 2mg	Phenylephrine HCl 5mg	Dextromethorphan HBr 10mg		**Adults & Peds: ≥12 yrs:** 2 tabs q4h. **Max:** 12 tabs q24h.
Alka-Seltzer Plus Nighttime effervescent tablets (Bayer Healthcare)	Acetaminophen 250mg	Doxlamine Succinate 6.25mg	Phenylephrine HCl 5mg	Dextromethorphan HBr 10mg		**Adults & Peds: ≥12 yrs:** 2 tabs q4h. **Max:** 8 tabs q24h.
Alka-Seltzer Plus Cough & Cold effervescent tablets (Bayer Healthcare)	Acetaminophen 250mg	Chlorpheniramine Maleate 2mg	Phenylephrine HCl 5mg	Dextromethorphan HBr 10mg		**Adults & Peds: ≥12 yrs:** 2 tabs q4h. **Max:** 8 tabs q24h.
Alka-Seltzer Plus Cough & Cold liquid (Bayer Healthcare)	Acetaminophen 162.5mg/5mL	Chlorpheniramine Maleate 1mg/5mL	Phenylephrine HCl 2.5mg/5mLmg	Dextromethorphan HBr 5mg/5mL		**Adults & Peds: ≥12 yrs:** 4 tsp q4h. **Max:** 24 tsp q24h.
Comtrex Cold & Cough Nighttime caplets (Novartis Consumer Healthcare)	Acetaminophen 500mg	Chlorpheniramine Maleate 2mg	Pseudoephedrine HCl 30mg	Dextromethorphan HBr 15mg		**Adults & Peds: ≥12 yrs:** 2 tabs q6h. **Max:** 8 tabs q24h.
Comtrex Nighttime Cold & Cough liquid (Novartis Consumer Healthcare)	Acetaminophen 1000mg/30mL	Chlorpheniramine Maleate 4mg/30mL	Pseudoephedrine HCl 60mg/30mL	Dextromethorphan HBr 30mg/30mL		**Adults & Peds: ≥12 yrs:** 2 tbl (30mL) q6h. **Max:** 8 tbl (240mL) q24h.
Dimetapp Children's Nighttime Flu liquid (Wyeth Consumer Healthcare)	Acetaminophen 160mg/5mL	Chlorpheniramine Maleate 1mg/5mL	Phenylephrine HCl 2.5mg/5mL	Dextromethorphan HBr 5mg/5mL		**Adults: ≥12 yrs:** 4 tsp (20mL) q4h. **Peds: 6-12 yrs:** 2 tsp (10mL) q4h. **Max:** 5 doses q24h.
Robitussin Cold Cough & Flu liquid (Wyeth Consumer Healthcare)	Acetaminophen 160mg/5mL	Chlorpheniramine Maleate 1mg/5mL	Phenylephrine HCl 2.5mg/5mL	Dextromethorphan HBr 5mg/5mL		**Adults: ≥12 yrs:** 4 tsp (20mL) q4h. **Peds: 6-12 yrs:** 2 tsp (10mL) q4h. **Max:** 5 doses q24h.

Table 8. COUGH-COLD-FLU PRODUCTS (cont.)

Brand Name	Analgesic	Antihistamine	Decongestant	Cough Suppressant	Expectorant	Dose
Tylenol Children's Plus Flu liquid *(McNeil Consumer)*	Acetaminophen 160mg/5mL	Chlorpheniramine Maleate 1mg/5mL	Phenylephrine HCl 2.5mg/5mL	Dextromethorphan HBr 7.5mg/5mL		**Peds: 6-11 yrs (48-95 lbs):** 2 tsp (10mL) q6-8h. **Max:** 4 doses q24h.
Tylenol Cold & Flu Severe Nighttime Cool Burst liquid *(McNeil Consumer)*	Acetaminophen 1000mg/30mL	Doxylamine 12.5mg/30mL	Pseudoephedrine HCl 60mg/30mL	Dextromethorphan HBr 30mg/30mL		**Adults & Peds: ≥12 yrs:** 2 tbl (30mL) q6h. **Max:** 8 tbl (120mL) q24h.
Tylenol Cold Head Congestion Nighttime caplets *(McNeil Consumer)*	Acetaminophen 325mg	Chlorpheniramine Maleate 2mg	Phenylephrine HCl 5mg	Dextromethorphan HBr 10mg		**Adults & Peds: ≥12 yrs:** 2 caps q4h. **Max:** 12 caps q24h.
Tylenol Cold Multi-Symptom Nighttime caplets *(McNeil Consumer)*	Acetaminophen 325mg	Chlorpheniramine Maleate 2mg	Phenylephedrine HCl 5mg	Dextromethorphan HBr 10mg		**Adults & Peds: ≥12 yrs:** 2 caps q4h. **Max:** 12 caps q24h.
Tylenol Cold Multi-Symptom Nighttime liquid *(McNeil Consumer)*	Acetaminophen 325mg/15mL	Doxylamine 6.25mg/30mL	Phenylephedrine HCl 5mg/15mL	Dextromethorphan HBr 10mg/15mL		**Adults & Peds: ≥12 yrs:** 2 tbl (30mL) q4h. **Max:** 12 tbl (180mL) q24h.
Tylenol Cold Nighttime Cool Burst caplets *(McNeil Consumer)*	Acetaminophen 325mg	Chlorpheniramine Maleate 2mg	Pseudoephedrine HCl 30mg	Dextromethorphan HBr 15mg		**Adults & Peds: ≥12 yrs:** 2 tabs q6h. **Max:** 8 tabs q24h.
COUGH SUPPRESSANT + ANTIHISTAMINE + DECONGESTANT						
Dimetapp DM Children's Cold & Cough elixir *(Wyeth Consumer Healthcare)*		Brompheniramine Maleate 1mg/5mL	Phenylephrine HCl 2.5mg/5mL	Dextromethorphan HBr 5mg/5mL		**Adults & Peds: ≥12 yrs:** 4 tsp (20mL) q4h. **Peds: 6-12 yrs:** 2 tsp (10mL) q4h. **Max:** 6 doses q24h.
Robitussin Allergy & Cough liquid *(Wyeth Consumer Healthcare)*		Chlorpheniramine Maleate 2mg/5mL	Phenylephrine HCl 5mg/5mL	Dextromethorphan HBr 10mg/5mL		**Adults & Peds: ≥12 yrs:** 2 tsp (10mL) q4h. **Peds: 6-12 yrs:** 1 tsp (5mL) q4h. **Max:** 6 doses q24h.
Robitussin Pediatric Cough & Cold Nighttime liquid *(Wyeth Consumer Healthcare)*		Chlorpheniramine Maleate 1mg/5mL	Phenylephrine HCl 2.5mg/5mL	Dextromethorphan HBr 5mg/5mL		**Adults & Peds: ≥12 yrs (≥ 96 lbs):** 4 tsp (20mL) q4h. **Peds: 6-12 yrs (48-95 lbs):** 2 tsp (10mL) q4h.
Robitussin Cough & Cold Nighttime liquid *(Wyeth Consumer Healthcare)*		Chlorpheniramine Maleate 1mg/5mL	Phenylephrine HCl 2.5mg/5mL	Dextromethorphan HBr 5mg/5mL		**Adults & Peds: ≥12 yrs:** 4 tsp (20mL) q4h. **Peds: 6-12 yrs:** 2 tsp (10mL) q4h. **Max:** 6 doses q24h.
Theraflu Cold & Cough Hot Liquid *(Novartis Consumer Health)*		Pheniramine Maleate 20mg/packet	Phenylephrine HCl 10mg/packet	Dextromethorphan HBr 20mg/packet		**Adults & Peds: ≥12 yrs:** 1 packet q4h. **Max:** 6 packets q24h.
COUGH SUPPRESSANT + DECONGESTANT						
PediaCare Children's Multi-Symptom Cold Liquid *(McNeil Consumer)*			Phenylephrine HCl 2.5mg/5mL	Dextromethorphan HBr 5mg/5mL		**Peds: 6-12 yrs:** 2 tsp (10mL) q4h. **2-6 yrs:** 1 tsp (5mL) q4h. **Max:** 6 doses q24h.
PediaCare Decongestant & Cough Infants' drops *(McNeil Consumer)*			Phenylephrine HCl 1.25mg/0.8mL	Dextromethorphan HBr 2.5mg/0.8mL		**Peds: 2-3 yrs:** 1.6mL q4h. **Max:** 6 doses q24h.

Table 8. COUGH-COLD-FLU PRODUCTS (cont.)

Brand Name	Analgesic	Antihistamine	Decongestant	Cough Suppressant	Expectorant	Dose
Vicks 44D Cough & Congestion Relief liquid (*Procter & Gamble*)			Phenylephrine HCl 10mg/15mL	Dextromethorphan HBr 30mg/15mL		**Adults: ≥12 yrs:** 1 tbl (15mL) q4h. **Peds: 6-12 yrs:** 1.5 tsp (7.5mL) q4h. **Max:** 6 doses q24h.
COUGH SUPPRESSANT + DECONGESTANT + ANALGESIC						
Alka-Seltzer Plus Day Cold liquid gels (*Bayer Healthcare*)	Acetaminophen 325mg		Phenylephrine HCl 5mg	Dextromethorphan HBr 10mg		**Adults & Peds: ≥12 yrs:** 2 tabs q4h. **Max:** 12 tabs q24h.
Alka-Seltzer Plus Day & Night liquid gels (*Bayer Healthcare*)	Acetaminophen 325mg		Phenylephrine HCl 5mg	Dextromethorphan HBr 10mg		**Adults & Peds: ≥12 yrs:** 2 tabs q4h. **Max:** 12 tabs q24h.
Alka-Seltzer Plus Day & Night effervescent tablets (*Bayer Healthcare*)	Acetaminophen 250mg		Phenylephrine HCl 5mg	Dextromethorphan HBr 10mg		**Adults & Peds: ≥12 yrs:** 2 tabs q4h. **Max:** 8 tabs q24h.
Alka-Seltzer Plus Day Cold Liquid (*Bayer Healthcare*)	Acetaminophen 162.5mg/5mL		Phenylephrine HCl 2.5mg/5mL	Dextromethorphan HBr 5mg/5mL		**Adults & Peds: ≥12 yrs:** 4 tsps q4h. **Max:** 6 doses q24h.
Sudafed PE Cold & Cough caplets (*McNeil Consumer*)	Acetaminophen 325mg		Phenylephrine HCl 5mg	Dextromethorphan HBr 10mg		**Adults & Peds: ≥12 yrs:** 2 caps q4h. **Max:** 12 tabs q24h.
Theraflu Daytime Severe Cold caplets (*Novartis Consumer Health*)	Acetaminophen 325mg		Phenylephrine HCl 5mg	Dextromethorphan HBr 5mg		**Adults & Peds: ≥12 yrs:** 2 tabs q6h. **Max:** 8 tabs q24h.
Tylenol Cold & Flu Severe Daytime Cool Burst liquid (*McNeil Consumer*)	Acetaminophen 1000mg/30mL		Pseudoephedrine HCl 60mg/30mL	Dextromethorphan HBr 30mg/30mL		**Adults & Peds: ≥12 yrs:** 2 tbl (30mL) q6h. **Max:** 8 tbl (120mL) q24h.
Tylenol Cold Daytime Cool Burst caplets (*McNeil Consumer*)	Acetaminophen 325mg		Pseudoephedrine HCl 30mg	Dextromethorphan HBr 15mg		**Adults & Peds: ≥12 yrs:** 2 tabs q6h. **Max:** 8 tabs q24h.
Tylenol Cold Head Congestion Daytime Capsules (*McNeil Consumer*)	Acetaminophen 325mg		Phenylephrine HCl 5mg	Dextromethorphan HBr 10mg		**Adults & Peds: ≥12 yrs:** 2 caps q4h. **Max:** 12 caps q24h.
Tylenol Cold Head Congestion Day/Night pack (*McNeil Consumer*)	Acetaminophen 325mg		Phenylephrine HCl 5mg	Dextromethorphan HBr 10mg		**Adults & Peds: ≥12 yrs:** 2 caps q4h. **Max:** 12 caps q24h.
Tylenol Cold Multi-Symptom Daytime Capsules (*McNeil Consumer*)	Acetaminophen 325mg		Phenylephrine HCl 5mg	Dextromethorphan HBr 10mg		**Adults & Peds: ≥12 yrs:** 2 caps q4h. **Max:** 12 caps q24h.
Tylenol Cold Multi-Symptom Day/Night pack (*McNeil Consumer*)	Acetaminophen 325mg		Phenylephrine HCl 5mg	Dextromethorphan HBr 10mg		**Adults & Peds: ≥12 yrs:** 2 caps q4h. **Max:** 12 caps q24h.
Tylenol Plus Cold & Cough Infants' drops (*McNeil Consumer*)	Acetaminophen 80mg/0.8mL		Phenylephrine HCl 1.25mg/0.8mL	Dextromethorphan HBr 2.5mg/0.8mL		**Peds: 2-3 yrs (24-35 lbs):** 1.6mL q4h. **Max:** 5 doses q24h.

Table 8. COUGH-COLD-FLU PRODUCTS (cont.)

BRAND NAME	ANALGESIC	ANTIHISTAMINE	DECONGESTANT	COUGH SUPPRESSANT	EXPECTORANT	DOSE
Tylenol Flu Daytime gelcaps (McNeil Consumer)	Acetaminophen 500mg		Pseudoephedrine HCl 30mg	Dextromethorphan HBr 15mg		**Adults & Peds: ≥12 yrs:** 2 caps q6h. **Max:** 8 caps q24h.
Vicks DayQuil liquicaps (McNeil Consumer)	Acetaminophen 325mg		Phenylephrine HCl 30mg	Dextromethorphan HBr 10mg		**Adults & Peds: ≥12 yrs:** 2 caps q4. **Max:** 6 caps q24h.
Vicks DayQuil liquid (McNeil Consumer)	Acetaminophen 325mg/15mL		Phenylephrine HCl 5mg/15mL	Dextromethorphan HBr 10mg/15mL		**Adults & Peds: ≥12 yrs:** 2 tbl (30mL) q4h. **Max:** 12 tbl (120mL) q24h.
COUGH SUPPRESSANT + DECONGESTANT + EXPECTORANT						
Robitussin CF liquid (Wyeth Consumer Healthcare)			Phenylephrine HCl 5mg/5mL	Dextromethorphan HBr 10mg/5mL	Guaifenesin 100mg/5mL	**Adults: ≥12 yrs:** 2 tsp (10mL) q4h. **Peds: 6-12 yrs:** 1 tsp (5mL) q4h. **2-6 yrs:** 1/2 tsp (2.5mL) q4h. **Max:** 6 doses q24h.
COUGH SUPPRESSANT + DECONGESTANT + EXPECTORANT + ANALGESIC						
Comtrex Chest Cold capsules (Novartis Consumer Healthcare)	Acetaminophen 250mg		Pseudoephedrine HCl 30mg	Dextromethorphan HBr 10mg	Guaifenesin 100mg	**Adults & Peds: ≥12 yrs:** 2 caps q4h. **Max:** 12 caps q24h.
Tylenol Cold Multi-Symptom Severe liquid (McNeil Consumer)	Acetaminophen 325mg/15mL		Phenylephrine HCl 5mg/15mL	Dextromethorphan HBr 10mg/15mL	Guaifenesin 200mg/15mL	**Adults & Peds: ≥12 yrs:** 2 tbs q4h. **Max:** 12 tbs q24h.
Tylenol Cold Multi-Symptom Severe caplets (McNeil Consumer)	Acetaminophen 325mg		Phenylephrine HCl 5mg	Dextromethorphan HBr 10mg	Guaifenesin 200mg	**Adults & Peds: ≥12 yrs:** 2 tabs q4h. **Max:** 12 tabs q24h.
Tylenol Severe Head Congestion caplets (McNeil Consumer)	Acetaminophen 325mg		Phenylephrine HCl 5mg	Dextromethorphan HBr 10mg	Guaifenesin 200mg	**Adults & Peds: ≥12 yrs:** 2 tabs q4h. **Max:** 12 tabs q24h.
COUGH SUPPRESSANT + EXPECTORANT						
Coricidin HBP Chest Congestion & Cough softgels (Schering-Plough)				Dextromethorphan HBr 10mg	Guaifenesin 200mg	**Adults & Peds: ≥12 yrs:** 1-2 caps q4h. **Max:** 12 caps q24h.
Mucinex DM extended-release tablets (Adams Respiratory Therapeutics)				Dextromethorphan HBr 30mg	Guaifenesin 600mg	**Adults & Peds: ≥12 yrs:** 1-2 tabs q12h. **Max:** 4 tabs q24h.
Robitussin Cough & Congestion liquid (Wyeth Consumer Healthcare)				Dextromethorphan HBr 10mg/5mL	Guaifenesin 200mg/5mL	**Adults: ≥12 yrs:** 2 tsp (10mL) q4h. **Peds: 6-12 yrs:** 1 tsp (5mL) q4h. **2-6 yrs:** 1/2 tsp (2.5mL) q4h. **Max:** 6 doses q24h.
Robitussin DM Infant drops (Wyeth Consumer Healthcare)				Dextromethorphan HBr 5mg/2.5mL	Guaifenesin 5mg/2.5mL	**Peds 2-6 yrs (24-47lbs):** 2.5mL q4h. 100mg/2.5mL **Max:** 6 doses q24h.
Robitussin DM liquid (Wyeth Consumer Healthcare)				Dextromethorphan HBr 10mg/5mL	Guaifenesin 100mg/5mL	**Adults: ≥12 yrs:** 2 tsp (10mL) q4h. **Peds: 6-12 yrs:** 1 tsp (5mL) q4h. **2-6 yrs:** 1/2 tsp (2.5mL) q4h. **Max:** 6 doses q24h.

Table 8. COUGH-COLD-FLU PRODUCTS (cont.)

Brand Name	Analgesic	Antihistamine	Decongestant	Cough Suppressant	Expectorant	Dose
Robitussin Sugar Free Cough liquid *(Wyeth Consumer Healthcare)*				Dextromethorphan HBr 10mg/5mL	Guaifenesin 100mg/5mL	**Adults: ≥12 yrs:** 2 tsp (10mL) q4h. **Peds: 6-12 yrs:** 1 tsp (5mL) q4h. **2-6 yrs:** 1/2 tsp (2.5mL) q4h. **Max:** 6 doses q24h.
Vicks 44E liquid *(Procter & Gamble)*				Dextromethorphan HBr 20mg/15mL	Guaifenesin 200mg/15mL	**Adults: ≥12 yrs:** 1 tbl (15mL) q4h. **Peds: 6-12 yrs:** 1.5 tsp (7.5mL) q4h. **Max:** 6 doses q24h.
Vicks 44E Pediatric liquid *(Procter & Gamble)*				Dextromethorphan HBr 10mg/15mL	Guaifenesin 100mg/15mL	**Adults: ≥12 yrs:** 2 tbl (30mL) q4h. **Peds: 6-12 yrs:** 1 tbl (15mL) q4h. **2-5 yrs:** 0.5 tbl (7.5mL) q4h. **Max:** 6 doses q24h.

DECONGESTANT

Brand Name	Analgesic	Antihistamine	Decongestant	Cough Suppressant	Expectorant	Dose
Contac-D Cold Decongestant tablets *(GlaxoSmithKline Consumer Healthcare)*			Phenylephrine HCl 10mg			**Adults & Peds: ≥12 yrs:** 1 tabs q4h. **Max:** 6 tabs q24h.
Dimetapp Children's Cold & Allergy Chewable tablets *(Wyeth Consumer Healthcare)*			Phenylephrine HCl 1.25mg			**Peds: 6-12 yrs:** 2 tabs q4h. **Max:** 6 tabs q24h.
Dimetapp Toddler's Drops Decongestant *(Wyeth Consumer Healthcare)*			Phenylephrine HCl 1.25mg/0.8mL			**Peds: 2-6 yrs:** 1.6mL q4h. **Max:** 6 doses q24h.
PediaCare Decongestant Infants' drops *(McNeil Consumer)*			Phenylephrine HCl 1.25mg/0.8mL			**Peds: 2-3 yrs:** 1.6mL q4h. **Max:** 6 doses q24h.
PediaCare Children's Decongestant liquid *(McNeil Consumer)*			Phenylephrine HCl 2.5mg/5mL			**Peds: 6-12 yrs:** 2 tsp (10mL) q4h. **2-6 yrs:** 1 tsp (5mL) q4h. **Max:** 5 doses q24h.
Sudafed 12 Hour tablets *(McNeil Consumer)*			Pseudoephedrine HCl 120mg			**Adults & Peds: ≥12 yrs:** 1 tab q12h. **Max:** 2 tabs q24h.
Sudafed 24 Hour tablets *(McNeil Consumer)*			Pseudoephedrine HCl 240mg			**Adults & Peds: ≥12 yrs:** 1 tab q24h. **Max:** 1 tab q24h.
Sudafed Children's liquid *(McNeil Consumer)*			Pseudoephedrine HCl 15mg/5mL			**Adults: ≥12 yrs:** 4 tsp (20mL) q4-6h. **Peds: 6-12 yrs:** 2 tsp (10mL) q4-6h. **2-6 yrs:** 1 tsp (5mL) q4-6h. **Max:** 4 doses q24h.
Sudafed PE tablets *(McNeil Consumer)*			Phenylephrine HCl 10mg			**Adults & Peds: ≥12 yrs:** 1 tab q4h. **Max:** 6 tabs q24h.
Sudafed PE Quick Dissolve Strips *(McNeil Consumer)*			Phenylephrine HCl 10mg			**Adults & Peds: ≥12 yrs:** 1 film q4h. **Max:** 6 films q24h.
Sudafed tablets *(McNeil Consumer)*			Pseudoephedrine HCl 30mg			**Adults: ≥12 yrs:** 2 tabs q4-6h. **Peds: 6-12 yrs:** 1 tab q4-6h. **Max:** 4 doses q24h.

Table 8. COUGH-COLD-FLU PRODUCTS (cont.)

Brand Name	Analgesic	Antihistamine	Decongestant	Cough Suppressant	Expectorant	Dose
Vicks Sinex 12-hour nasal spray (*Procter & Gamble*)			Oxymetazoline HCl 0.05%			**Adults & Peds: ≥6 yrs:** 2-3 sprays q10-12h. **Max:** 2 doses q24h.
Vicks Sinex nasal spray (*Procter & Gamble*)			Phenylephrine HCl 0.5%			**Adults & Peds: ≥12 yrs:** 2-3 sprays q4h. **Max:** 18 sprays q24h.
Vicks Sinex UltraFine Mist (*Procter & Gamble*)			Phenylephrine HCl 0.5%			**Adults & Peds: ≥12 yrs:** 2-3 sprays q4h. **Max:** 18 sprays q24h.
Vicks Sinex 12 Hour UltraFine Mist (*Procter & Gamble*)			Oxymetazoline HCl 0.05%			**Adults & Peds: ≥6 yrs:** 2-3 sprays q10-12h. **Max:** 2 doses q24h.
Vicks Vapor Inhaler (*Procter & Gamble*)			Levmetamfetamine 50mg			**Adults: ≥12 yrs:** 2 inhalations q2h. **Max:** 24 inhalations q24h **Peds: 6-12 yrs:** 1 inhalation q2h. **Max:** 12 inhalations q24h.

DECONGESTANT + ANALGESIC

Brand Name	Analgesic	Antihistamine	Decongestant	Cough Suppressant	Expectorant	Dose
Advil Children's Cold liquid (*Wyeth Consumer Healthcare*)	Ibuprofen 100mg		Pseudoephedrine HCl 15mg			**Peds: 6-11 yrs (48-95 lbs):** 2 tsp (10mL) q6h. **2-5 yrs (24-47 lbs):** 1 tsp (5mL) q6h. **Max:** 4 doses q24h
Advil Cold & Sinus caplets/liqui-gels (*Wyeth Consumer Healthcare*)	Ibuprofen 200mg		Pseudoephedrine HCl 30mg			**Adults & Peds: ≥12 yrs:** 1-2 caps q4-6h. **Max:** 6 caps q24h.
Alka-Seltzer Plus Cold & Sinus tablets (*Bayer Healthcare*)	Acetaminophen 250mg		Phenylephrine HCl 5mg			**Adults & Peds: ≥12 yrs:** 2 tabs q4h. **Max:** 8 tab q24h.
Alka-Seltzer Plus Cold & Sinus Effervescent tablets (*Bayer Healthcare*)	Acetaminophen 250mg		Phenylephrine HCl 5mg			**Adults & Peds: ≥12 yrs:** 2 tabs q4h. **Max:** 8 tab q24h.
Contac Cold & Flu Day & Night caplets (*GlaxoSmithKline Consumer Healthcare*)	Acetaminophen 500mg		Phenylephrine HCl 5mg			**Adults & Peds: ≥12 yrs:** 2 caps q4-6h. **Max:** 8 tab q24h.
Contac Cold & Flu Maximum Strength caplets (*GlaxoSmithKline Consumer Healthcare*)	Acetaminophen 500mg		Phenylephrine HCl 5mg			**Adults & Peds: ≥12 yrs:** 2 caps q4-6h. **Max:** 8 tab q24h.
Motrin Children's Cold suspension (*McNeil Consumer*)	Ibuprofen 100mg/5mL		Pseudoephedrine HCl 15mg/5mL			**Peds: 6-12 yrs (48-95 lbs):** 2 tsp (10mL) q6h. **2-6 yrs (24-47 lbs):** 1 tsp (5mL) q6h. **Max:** 4 doses q24h.
Sinutab Sinus tablets (*McNeil Consumer*)	Acetaminophen 500mg		Phenylephrine HCl 5mg			**Adults & Peds: ≥12 yrs:** 2 tabs q6h. **Max:** 8 tabs q24h.
Sudafed PE Sinus Headache caplets (*(McNeil Consumer)*)	Acetaminophen 325mg		Phenylephrine HCl 5mg			**Adults & Peds: ≥12 yrs:** 2 caps q4h. **Max:** 12 caps q24h.

Table 8. COUGH-COLD-FLU PRODUCTS (cont.)

Brand Name	Analgesic	Antihistamine	Decongestant	Cough Suppressant	Expectorant	Dose
Theraflu Daytime Severe Cold Hot liquid (*Novartis Consumer Health*)	Acetaminophen 650mg		Phenylephrine HCl 10mg			**Adults & Peds: ≥12 yrs:** 1 packet q4h. **Max:** 6 packets q24h.
Tylenol Sinus Congestion & Pain Daytime gelcaps (*McNeil Consumer*)	Acetaminophen 325mg		Phenylephrine HCl 5mg			**Adults & Peds: ≥12 yrs:** 2 caps q4h. **Max:** 12 caps q24h.
Tylenol Sinus Congestion & Pain Day/Night pack (*McNeil Consumer*)	Acetaminophen 325mg		Phenylephrine HCl 5mg			**Adults & Peds: ≥12 yrs:** 2 caps q4h. **Max:** 12 caps q24h.
Vicks DayQuil Sinus liquicaps (*Procter & Gamble*)	Acetaminophen 325mg		Phenylephrine HCl 5mg			**Adults & Peds: ≥12 yrs:** 2 caps q4h. **Max:** 6 caps q24h.

DECONGESTANT + EXPECTORANT

Brand Name	Analgesic	Antihistamine	Decongestant	Cough Suppressant	Expectorant	Dose
Robitussin PE Head & Chest liquid (*Wyeth Consumer Healthcare*)			Phenylephrine HCl 5mg/5mL		Guaifenesin 100mg/5mL	**Adults: ≥12 yrs:** 2 tsp (10mL) q4h. **Peds: 6-12 yrs:** 1 tsp (5mL) q4h. **Max:** 6 doses q24h.
Sinutab Non-Drying liquid caps (*McNeil Consumer*)			Pseudoephedrine HCl 30mg		Guaifenesin 200mg	**Adults & Peds: ≥12 yrs:** 2 cap q4h. **Max:** 12 q24h
Sudafed Non-Drying Sinus caps (*McNeil Consumer*)			Phenylephrine HCl 5mg		Guaifenesin 200mg	**Adults & Peds: ≥12 yrs:** 2 caps q4h. **Max:** 8 caps q24h.
Triaminic Chest & Nasal liquid (*Novartis Consumer Health*)			Phenylephrine HCl 2.5mg/5mL		Guaifenesin 50mg/5mL	**Adults & Peds: ≥12 yrs:** 1 tsp q 4h. **Max:** 6 doses q24h. **Peds: 6-12 yrs:** 2 tsp (10mL). **2-6 yrs:** 1 tsp (5mL).

DECONGESTANT + EXPECTORANT + ANALGESIC

Brand Name	Analgesic	Antihistamine	Decongestant	Cough Suppressant	Expectorant	Dose
Tylenol Sinus Congestion & Severe pain caplets (*McNeil Consumer*)	Acetaminophen 325mg		Phenylephrine HCl 5mg		Guaifenesin 200mg	**Adults & Peds: ≥12 yrs:** 2 caps q4h. **Max:** 12 caps q24h.

EXPECTORANT

Brand Name	Analgesic	Antihistamine	Decongestant	Cough Suppressant	Expectorant	Dose
Mucinex extended-release tablets (*Adams Respiratory Therapeutics*)					Guaifenesin 600mg	**Adults & Peds: ≥12 yrs:** 1-2 tabs q12h. **Max:** 4 tabs q24h.
Robitussin liquid (*Wyeth Consumer Healthcare*)					Guaifenesin 100mg/5mL	**Adults: ≥12 yrs:** 2-4 tsp (10-20mL) q4h. **Peds: 6-12 yrs:** 1-2 tsp (5-10mL) q4h. **2-6 yrs:** 1/2-1 tsp (2.5-5mL) q4h. **Max:** 6 doses q24h.

Table 9. HEADACHE/MIGRAINE PRODUCTS

BRAND NAME	INGREDIENT/STRENGTH	DOSE
ACETAMINOPHEN		
Anacin Aspirin Free tablets *(Insight Pharmaceuticals)*	Acetaminophen 500mg	**Adults & Peds: ≥12 yrs:** 2 tabs q6h. **Max:** 8 tabs q24h.
Tylenol 8 Hour caplets *(McNeil Consumer)*	Acetaminophen 650mg	**Adults & Peds: ≥12 yrs:** 2 tabs q8h prn. **Max:** 6 tabs q24h.
Tylenol 8 Hour geltabs *(McNeil Consumer)*	Acetaminophen 650mg	**Adults & Peds: ≥12 yrs:** 2 tabs q8h prn. **Max:** 6 tabs q24h.
Tylenol Arthritis caplets *(McNeil Consumer)*	Acetaminophen 650mg	**Adults:** 2 tabs q8h prn. **Max:** 6 tabs q24h.
Tylenol Arthritis geltabs *(McNeil Consumer)*	Acetaminophen 650mg	**Adults:** 2 tabs q8h prn. **Max:** 6 tabs q24h.
Tylenol Children's Meltaways tablets *(McNeil Consumer)*	Acetaminophen 80mg	**Peds: 2-3 yrs (24-35 lbs):** 2 tabs. **4-5 yrs (36-47 lbs):** 3 tabs. **6-8 yrs (48-59 lbs):** 4 tabs. **9-10 yrs (60-71 lbs):** 5 tabs. **11 yrs (72-95 lbs):** 6 tabs. May repeat q4h. **Max:** 5 doses q24h.
Tylenol Children's suspension *(McNeil Consumer)*	Acetaminophen 160mg/5mL	**Peds: 2-3 yrs (24-35 lbs):** 1 tsp (5mL). **4-5 yrs (36-47 lbs):** 1.5 tsp (7.5mL). **6-8 yrs (48-59 lbs):** 2 tsp (10mL). **9-10 yrs (60-71 lbs):** 2.5 tsp (12.5mL). **11 yrs (72-95 lbs):** 3 tsp (15mL). May repeat q4h. **Max:** 5 doses q24h.
Tylenol Extra Strength caplets *(McNeil Consumer)*	Acetaminophen 500mg	**Adults & Peds: ≥12 yrs:** 2 tabs q4-6h prn. **Max:** 8 tabs q24h.
Tylenol Extra Strength Cool caplets *(McNeil Consumer)*	Acetaminophen 500mg	**Adults & Peds: ≥12 yrs:** 2 tabs q4-6h prn. **Max:** 8 tabs q24h.
Tylenol Extra Strength gelcaps *(McNeil Consumer)*	Acetaminophen 500mg	**Adults & Peds: ≥ 12 yrs:** 2 caps q4-6h prn. **Max:** 8 caps q24h.
Tylenol Extra Strength liquid *(McNeil Consumer)*	Acetaminophen 1000mg/30mL	**Adults & Peds: ≥12 yrs:** 2 tbl (30mL) q4-6h prn. **Max:** 8 tbl (120mL) q24h.
Tylenol Extra Strength tablets *(McNeil Consumer)*	Acetaminophen 500mg	**Adults & Peds: ≥12 yrs:** 2 tabs q4-6h prn. **Max:** 8 tabs q24h.
Tylenol Infants' suspension *(McNeil Consumer)*	Acetaminophen 80mg/0.8mL	**Peds: 2-3 yrs (24-35 lbs):** 1.6 mL q4h prn. **Max:** 5 doses (8mL) q24h.
Tylenol Junior Meltaways tablets *(McNeil Consumer)*	Acetaminophen 160mg	**Peds: 6-8 yrs (48-59 lbs):** 2 tabs. **9-10 yrs (60-71 lbs):** 2.5 tabs. **11 yrs (72-95 lbs):** 3 tabs. **12 yrs (≥96 lbs):** 4 tabs. May repeat q4h. **Max:** 5 doses q24h.
Tylenol Regular Strength tablets *(McNeil Consumer)*	Acetaminophen 325mg	**Adults & Peds: ≥12 yrs:** 2 tabs q4-6h prn. **Max:** 12 tabs q24h. **Peds: 6-11 yrs:** 1 tab q4-6h. **Max:** 5 tabs q24h.
ACETAMINOPHEN COMBINATIONS		
Excedrin Extra Strength caplets *(Novartis Consumer Health)*	Acetaminophen/Aspirin/Caffeine 250mg-250mg-65mg	**Adults & Peds: ≥12 yrs:** 2 tabs q6h. **Max:** 8 tabs q24h.
Excedrin Extra Strength geltabs *(Novartis Consumer Health)*	Acetaminophen/Aspirin/Caffeine 250mg-250mg-65mg	**Adults & Peds: ≥12 yrs:** 2 tabs q6h. **Max:** 8 tabs q24h.
Excedrin Extra Strength tablets *(Novartis Consumer Health)*	Acetaminophen/Aspirin/Caffeine 250mg-250mg-65mg	**Adults & Peds: ≥12 yrs:** 2 tabs q6h. **Max:** 8 tabs q24h.
Excedrin Migraine caplets *(Novartis Consumer Health)*	Acetaminophen/Aspirin/Caffeine 250mg-250mg-65mg	**Adults:** 2 tabs prn. **Max:** 2 tabs q24h.
Excedrin Migraine geltabs *(Novartis Consumer Health)*	Acetaminophen/Aspirin/Caffeine 250mg-250mg-65mg	**Adults:** 2 tabs prn. **Max:** 2 tabs q24h.
Excedrin Migraine tablets *(Novartis Consumer Health)*	Acetaminophen/Aspirin/Caffeine 250mg-250mg-65mg	**Adults:** 2 tabs prn. **Max:** 2 tabs q24h.
Excedrin Sinus Headache caplets *(Novartis Consumer Health)*	Acetaminophen/Phenylephrine HCl 325mg-5mg	**Adults & Peds: ≥12 yrs:** 2 tabs q4h. **Max:** 12 tabs q24h.

Table 9. HEADACHE/MIGRAINE PRODUCTS (cont.)

BRAND NAME	INGREDIENT/STRENGTH	DOSE
Excedrin Sinus Headache tablets *(Novartis Consumer Health)*	Acetaminophen/Phenylephrine HCl 325mg-5mg	**Adults & Peds: ≥12 yrs:** 2 tabs q4h. **Max:** 12 tabs q24h.
Excedrin Tension Headache caplets *(Novartis Consumer Health)*	Acetaminophen/Caffeine 500mg-65mg	**Adults & Peds: ≥12 yrs:** 2 tabs q6h. **Max:** 8 tabs q24h.
Excedrin Tension Headache geltabs *(Novartis Consumer Health)*	Acetaminophen/Caffeine 500mg-65mg	**Adults & Peds: ≥12 yrs:** 2 tabs q6h. **Max:** 8 tabs q24h.
Excedrin Tension Headache tablets *(Novartis Consumer Health)*	Acetaminophen/Caffeine 500mg-65mg	**Adults & Peds: ≥12 yrs:** 2 tabs q6h. **Max:** 8 tabs q24h.
Goody's Extra Strength Headache Powders *(GlaxoSmithKline Consumer Healthcare)*	Acetaminophen/Aspirin/Caffeine 260mg-520mg-32.5mg	**Adults & Peds: ≥12 yrs:** 1 powder q4-6h. **Max:** 4 powders q24h.
Tylenol Sinus Congestion & Pain Daytime gelcaps *(McNeil Consumer)*	Acetaminophen/Phenylephrine HCl 325mg/5mg	**Adults & Peds: >12 yrs:** 2 caps q4h. Max:. 12 caps q24h.
Tylenol Sinus Congestion & Pain Daytime coolburst caplets *(McNeil Consumer)*	Acetaminophen/Phenylephrine HCl 325mg/5mg	**Adults & Peds: >12 yrs:** 2 caps q4h Max: 12 caps q24h.
Vanquish caplets *(Bayer Healthcare)*	Acetaminophen/Aspirin/Caffeine 194mg-227mg-33mg	**Adults & Peds: ≥12 yrs:** 2 tabs q6h. **Max:** 8 tabs q24h.
ACETAMINOPHEN/SLEEP AIDS		
Excedrin PM caplets *(Novartis Consumer Health)*	Acetaminophen/Diphenhydramine 500mg-38mg	**Adults & Peds: ≥12 yrs:** 2 tabs qhs.
Excedrin PM geltabs *(Novartis Consumer Health)*	Acetaminophen/Diphenhydramine citrate 500mg-38 mg	**Adults & Peds: ≥12 yrs:** 2 tabs qhs.
Excedrin PM tablets *(Novartis Consumer Health)*	Acetaminophen/Diphenhydramine citrate 500mg-38 mg	**Adults & Peds: ≥12 yrs:** 2 tabs qhs.
Goody's PM Powders *(GlaxoSmithKline Consumer Healthcare)*	Acetaminophen/Diphenhydramine 1000mg-76mg/dose	**Adults & Peds: ≥12 yrs:** 1 packet (2 powders) qhs.
Tylenol PM caplets *(McNeil Consumer)*	Acetaminophen/Diphenhydramine 500mg-25mg	**Adults & Peds: ≥12 yrs:** 2 tabs qhs.
Tylenol PM gelcaps *(McNeil Consumer)*	Acetaminophen/Diphenhydramine 500mg-25mg	**Adults & Peds: ≥12 yrs:** 2 caps qhs.
Tylenol PM geltabs *(McNeil Consumer)*	Acetaminophen/Diphenhydramine 500mg-25mg	**Adults & Peds: ≥12 yrs:** 2 tabs qhs.
Tylenol Sinus Night Time caplets *(McNeil Consumer)*	Acetaminophen/Pseudoephedrine HCl/ Doxylamine Succinate 500mg-30mg-6.25mg	**Adults & Peds: ≥12 yrs:** 2 tabs q4-6h. **Max:** 8 tabs q24h.
NONSTEROIDAL ANTI-INFLAMMATORY DRUGS (NSAIDs)		
Advil caplets *(Wyeth Consumer Healtcare)*	Ibuprofen 200mg	**Adults & Peds: ≥12 yrs:** 1-2 tabs q4-6h. **Max:** 6 tabs q24h.
Advil Children's Chewables tablets *(Wyeth Consumer Healthcare)*	Ibuprofen 50mg	**Peds: 2-3 yr (24-35 lb):** 2 tabs q6-8h. **4-5 yr (36-47 lb):** 3 tabs q6-8h. **6-8 yr (45-89 lb):** 4 tabs q6-8h. **9-10 yr (60-71 lb):** 5 tabs q6-8h. **11 yr (72-95 lb):** 6 tabs q6-8h. **Max:** 4 doses q24h.
Advil Children's suspension *(Wyeth Consumer Healthcare)*	Ibuprofen 100mg/5mL	**Peds: 2-3 yrs (24-35 lbs):** 1 tsp (5mL). **4-5 yrs (36-47 lbs):** 1.5 tsp (7.5mL). **6-8 yrs (48-59 lbs):** 2 tsp (10mL). **9-10 yrs (60-71lbs):** 2.5 tsp (12.5mL). **11 yrs (72-95 lbs):** 3 tsp (15mL). May repeat q6-8h. **Max:** 4 doses q24h.
Advil gelcaps *(Wyeth Consumer Healthcare)*	Ibuprofen 200mg	**Adults & Peds: ≥12 yrs:** 1-2 caps q4-6h. **Max:** 6 caps q24h.
Advil Infants' drops *(Wyeth Consumer Healthcare)*	Ibuprofen 50mg/1.25mL	**Peds: 6-11 months (12-17 lbs):** 1.25mL. **12-23 months (18-23 lbs):** 1.875mL. May repeat q6-8h. **Max:** 4 doses q24h.
Advil Junior Strength tablets *(Wyeth Consumer Healthcare)*	Ibuprofen 100mg	**Peds: 6-10 yrs (48-71 lbs):** 2 tabs. **11 yrs (72-95 lbs):** 3 tabs. May repeat q6-8h. **Max:** 4 doses q24h.

Table 9. HEADACHE/MIGRAINE PRODUCTS (cont.)

BRAND NAME	INGREDIENT/STRENGTH	DOSE
Advil liqui-gels (*Wyeth Consumer Healthcare*)	Ibuprofen 200mg	**Adults & Peds: ≥12 yrs:** 1-2 caps q4-6h. **Max:** 6 caps q24h.
Advil Migraine capsules (*Wyeth Consumer Healthcare*)	Ibuprofen 200mg	**Adults:** 2 caps prn. **Max:** 2 caps q24h.
Advil tablets (*Wyeth Consumer Healthcare*)	Ibuprofen 200mg	**Adults & Peds: ≥12 yrs:** 1-2 tabs q4-6h. **Max:** 6 tabs q24h.
Aleve caplets (*Bayer Healthcare*)	Naproxen Sodium 220mg	**Adults: ≥65 yrs:** 1 tab q12h. **Max:** 2 tabs q24h. **Adults & Peds: ≥12 yrs:** 1 tab q8-12h. **Max:** 3 tabs q24h.
Aleve gelcaps (*Bayer Healthcare*)	Naproxen Sodium 220mg	**Adults: ≥65 yrs:** 1 cap q12h. **Max:** 2 caps q24h. **Adults & Peds: ≥12 yrs:** 1 cap q8-12h. **Max:** 3 caps q24h.
Aleve tablets (*Bayer Healthcare*)	Naproxen Sodium 220mg	**Adults: ≥65 yrs:** 1 tab q12h. **Max:** 2 tabs q24h. **Adults & Peds: ≥12 yrs:** 1 tab q8-12h. **Max:** 3 tabs q24h.
Motrin Children's suspension (*McNeil Consumer*)	Ibuprofen 100mg/5mL	**Peds: 2-3 yrs (24-35 lbs):** 1 tsp (5mL). **4-5 yrs (36-47 lbs):** 1.5 tsp (7.5mL). **6-8 yrs (48-59 lbs):** 2 tsp (10mL). **9-10 yrs (60-71 lbs):** 2.5 tsp (12.5mL). **11 yrs (72-95 lbs):** 3 tsp (15mL). May repeat q6-8h. **Max:** 4 doses q24h.
Motrin IB caplets (*McNeil Consumer*)	Ibuprofen 200mg	**Adults & Peds: ≥12 yrs:** 1-2 tabs q4-6h. **Max:** 6 tabs q24h.
Motrin IB tablets (*McNeil Consumer*)	Ibuprofen 200mg	**Adults & Peds: ≥12 yrs:** 1-2 tabs q4-6h. **Max:** 6 tabs q24h.
Motrin Infants' Drops (*McNeil Consumer*)	Ibuprofen 50mg/1.25mL	**Peds: 6-11 months (12-17 lbs):** 1.25mL. **12-23 months (18-23 lbs):** 1.875mL. May repeat q6-8h. **Max:** 4 doses q24h.
Motrin Junior Strength chewable tablets (*McNeil Consumer*)	Ibuprofen 100mg	**Peds: 6-8 yrs (48-59 lbs):** 2 tabs. **9-10 yrs (60-71 lbs):** 2.5 tabs. **11 yrs (72-95 lbs):** 3 tabs. May repeat q6-8h. **Max:** 4 doses q24h.
Nuprin caplets (*CVS*)	Ibuprofen 200mg	**Adults & Peds: ≥12 yrs:** 1-2 tabs q4-6h. **Max:** 6 tabs q24h.
Nuprin tablets (*CVS*)	Ibuprofen 200mg	**Adults & Peds: ≥12 yrs:** 1-2 tabs q4-6h. **Max:** 6 tabs q24h.
NSAID COMBINATIONS		
Aleve Sinus & Headache caplets (*Bayer Healthcare*)	Naproxen Sodium/Pseudoephedrine HCl 220 mg-120 mg	**Adults & Peds: ≥12 yrs:** 1 tab q12h. **Max:** 2 tabs q24h.
Nuprin Cold and Sinus caplets (*CVS*)	Ibuprofen/Pseudoephedrine HCl 200mg-30 mg	**Adults & Peds: ≥12 yrs:** 1-2 tabs q4-6h. **Max:** 6 tabs q24h.
SALICYLATES		
Anacin 81 tablets (*Insight Pharmaceuticals*)	Aspirin 81mg	**Adults & Peds: ≥12 yrs:** 4-8 tabs q4h. **Max:** 48 tabs q24h.
Aspergum chewable tablets (*Schering-Plough*)	Aspirin 227mg	**Adults & Peds: ≥12 yrs:** 2 tabs q4h. **Max:** 16 tabs q24h.
Bayer Aspirin Extra Strength caplets (*Bayer Healthcare*)	Aspirin 500mg	**Adults & Peds: ≥12 yrs:** 1-2 tabs q4-6h. **Max:** 8 tabs q24h.
Genuine Bayer Aspirin safety coated tablets (*Bayer Healthcare*)	Aspirin 325mg	**Adults & Peds: ≥12 yrs:** 1-2 tabs q4h or 3 tabs q6h. **Max:** 12 tabs q24h.
Bayer Aspirin safety coated caplets (*Bayer Healthcare*)	Aspirin 325mg	**Adults & Peds: ≥12 yrs:** 1-2 tabs q4h or 3 tabs q6h. **Max:** 12 tabs q24h.
Bayer Children's Aspirin chewable tablets (*Bayer Healthcare*)	Aspirin 81mg	**Adults & Peds: ≥12 yrs:** 4-8 tabs q4h. **Max:** 48 tabs q24h.
Bayer Low Dose Aspirin tablets (*Bayer Healthcare*)	Aspirin 81mg	**Adults & Peds: ≥12 yrs:** 4-8 tabs q4h. **Max:** 48 tabs q24h.

Table 9. HEADACHE/MIGRAINE PRODUCTS (cont.)

BRAND NAME	INGREDIENT/STRENGTH	DOSE
Doan's Extra Strength caplets *(Novartis Consumer Health)*	Magnesium Salicylate Tetrahydrate 580mg	**Adults & Peds: ≥12 yrs:** 2 tabs q6h. **Max:** 8 tabs q24h.
Ecotrin Adult Low Strength tablets *(GlaxoSmithKline Consumer Healthcare)*	Aspirin 81mg	**Adults:** 4-8 tabs q4h. **Max:** 48 tabs q24h.
Ecotrin Enteric Low Strength tablets *(GlaxoSmithKline Consumer Healthcare)*	Aspirin 81mg	**Adults:** 4-8 tabs q4h. **Max:** 48 tabs q24h.
Ecotrin Enteric Regular Strength tablets *(GlaxoSmithKline Consumer Healthcare)*	Aspirin 325mg	**Adults & Peds: ≥12 yrs:** 1-2 tabs q4h. **Max:** 12 tabs q24h.
Ecotrin Maximum Strength tablets *(GlaxoSmithKline Consumer Healthcare)*	Aspirin 500mg	**Adults & Peds: ≥12 yrs:** 2 tabs q6h. **Max:** 8 tabs q24h.
Ecotrin Regular Strength tablets *(GlaxoSmithKline Consumer Healthcare)*	Aspirin 325mg	**Adults & Peds: ≥12 yrs:** 1-2 tabs q4h. **Max:** 12 tabs q24h.
Halfprin 162mg tablets *(Kramer Laboratories)*	Aspirin 162mg	**Adults & Peds: ≥12 yrs:** 2-4 tabs q4h. **Max:** 24 tabs q24h.
Halfprin 81mg tablets *(Kramer Laboratories)*	Aspirin 81mg	**Adults & Peds: ≥12 yrs:** 4-8 tabs q4h. **Max:** 48 tabs q24h.
St. Joseph Adult Low Strength chewable tablets *(McNeil Consumer)*	Aspirin 81mg	**Adults & Peds: ≥12 yrs:** 4-8 tabs q4h. **Max:** 48 tabs q24h.
St. Joseph Adult Low Strength tablets *(McNeil Consumer)*	Aspirin 81mg	**Adults & Peds: ≥12 yrs:** 4-8 tabs q4h. **Max:** 48 tabs q24h.
SALICYLATES, BUFFERED		
Ascriptin Maximum Strength tablets *(Novartis Consumer Health)*	Aspirin Buffered with Maalox/Calcium Carbonate 500mg	**Adults & Peds: ≥12 yrs:** 2 tabs q4h. **Max:** 8 tabs q24h.
Ascriptin Regular Strength tablets *(Novartis Consumer Health)*	Aspirin Buffered with Maalox/Calcium Carbonate 325mg	**Adults & Peds: ≥12 yrs:** 2 tabs q4h. **Max:** 12 tabs q24h.
Bayer Extra Strength Plus caplets *(Bayer Healthcare)*	Aspirin Buffered with Calcium Carbonate 500mg	**Adults & Peds: ≥12 yrs:** 1-2 tabs q4-6h. **Max:** 8 tabs q24h.
Bufferin Extra Strength tablets *(Novartis Consumer Health)*	Aspirin Buffered with Calcium Carbonate/Magnesium Oxide/ Magnesium Carbonate 500mg	**Adults & Peds: ≥12 yrs:** 2 tabs q6h. **Max:** 8 tabs q24h.
Bufferin tablets *(Novartis Consumer Health)*	Aspirin Buffered with Calcium Carbonate/Magnesium Oxide/ Magnesium Carbonate 325mg	**Adults & Peds: ≥12 yrs:** 2 tabs q4h. **Max:** 12 tabs q24h.
SALICYLATE COMBINATIONS		
Alka-Seltzer effervescent tablets *(Bayer Healthcare)*	Aspirin/Citric Acid/Sodium Bicarbonate 325mg-1000mg-1916mg	**Adults & Peds: ≥12 yrs:** 2 tabs q4h. **Max:** 8 tabs q24h.
Alka-Seltzer Extra Strength effervescent tablets *(Bayer Healthcare)*	Aspirin/Citric Acid/Sodium Bicarbonate 500mg-1000mg-1985mg	**Adults & Peds: ≥12 yrs:** 2 tabs q6h. **Max:** 7 tabs q24h.
Alka-Seltzer Morning Relief effervescent tablets *(Bayer Healthcare)*	Aspirin/Caffeine 500mg-65mg	**Adults & Peds: ≥12 yrs:** 2 tabs q6h. **Max:** 8 tabs q24h.
Anacin Pain Reliever caplets *(Insight Pharmaceuticals)*	Aspirin/Caffeine 400mg-32mg	**Adults & Peds: ≥12 yrs:** 2 tabs q6h. **Max:** 8 tabs q24h.
Anacin Extra Strength tablets *(Insight Pharmaceuticals)*	Aspirin/Caffeine 500mg-32mg	**Adults & Peds: ≥12 yrs:** 2 tabs q6h. **Max:** 8 tabs q24h.
Anacin tablets *(Insight Pharmaceuticals)*	Aspirin/Caffeine 400mg-32mg	**Adults & Peds: ≥12 yrs:** 2 tabs q6h. **Max:** 8 tabs q24h.
Bayer Back & Body Pain caplets *(Bayer Healthcare)*	Aspirin/Caffeine 500mg-32.5mg	**Adults & Peds: ≥12 yrs:** 2 tabs q6h. **Max:** 8 tabs q24h.
BC Arthritis Strength powders *(GlaxoSmtihKline Consumer Healthcare)*	Aspirin/Caffeine/Salicylamide 742mg-38mg-222mg	**Adults & Peds: ≥12 yrs:** 1 powder q3-4h. **Max:** 4 powders q24h.
BC Original powders *(GlaxoSmithKline Consumer Healthcare)*	Aspirin/Caffeine/Salicylamide 650mg-33.3mg-195mg	**Adults & Peds: ≥12 yrs:** 1 powder q3-4h.

Table 9. HEADACHE/MIGRAINE PRODUCTS (cont.)

Brand Name	Ingredient/Strength	Dose
SALICYLATES/SLEEP AIDS		
Alka-Seltzer PM Pain Reliever & Sleep Aid effervescent tablets *(Bayer Healthcare)*	Aspirin/Diphenhydramine Citrate 325mg-38 mg	**Adults & Peds: ≥12 yrs:** 2 tabs qpm.
Bayer PM Relief caplets *(Bayer Healthcare)*	Aspirin/Diphenhydramine 500mg-38.3mg	**Adults & Peds: ≥12 yrs:** 2 tabs qhs.
Doan's Extra Strength PM caplets *(Novartis Consumer Health)*	Magnesium Salicylate Tetrahydrate/ Diphenhydramine 580mg-25mg	**Adults & Peds: ≥12 yrs:** 2 tabs qhs.

Table 10. LAXATIVE PRODUCTS

BRAND NAME	INGREDIENT/STRENGTH	DOSE
BULK-FORMING		
Citrucel caplets (*GlaxoSmithKline Consumer Healthcare*)	Methylcellulose 500mg	**Adults:** ≥12 yrs: 2-4 tabs qd. **Max:** 12 tabs q24h. **Peds:** 6-12 yrs: 1 tabs qd. **Max:** 6 tabs q24h.
Citrucel powder (*GlaxoSmithKline Consumer Healthcare*)	Methylcellulose 2g/tbl	**Adults:** ≥12 yrs: 1 tbl (11.5g) qd tid. **Peds:** 6-12 yrs: 1/2 tbl (5.75g) qd.
Equalactin chewable tablet (*Numark Laboratories*)	Calcium Polycarbophil 625mg	**Adults & Peds:** ≥12 yrs: 2 tabs qd. **Max:** 8 tabs qd.
Fibercon caplets (*Lederle Consumer Health*)	Calcium Polycarbophil 625mg	**Adults & Peds:** ≥12 yrs: 2 tabs qd. **Max:** 8 tabs qd.
Fiber-Lax tablets (*Rugby Laboratories*)	Calcium Polycarbophil 625mg	**Adults & Peds:** ≥12 yrs: 2 tabs qd. **Max:** 8 tabs qd.
Konsyl Easy Mix powder (*Konsyl Pharmaceuticals*)	Psyllium 6g/tsp	**Adults:** ≥12 yrs: 1 tsp qd-tid. **Peds:** 6-12 yrs: 1/2 tsp qd-tid.
Konsyl Fiber tablets (*Konsyl Pharmaceuticals*)	Calcium Polycarbophil 625mg	**Adults & Peds:** ≥12 yrs: 2 tabs qd. **Max:** 8 tabs qd.
Konsyl Orange powder (*Konsyl Pharmaceuticals*)	Psyllium 3.4g	**Adults:** ≥12 yrs: 1 tsp qd-tid. **Peds:** 6-12 yrs: 1/2 tsp qd-tid.
Konsyl Original powder (*Konsyl Pharmaceuticals*)	Psyllium 6g/tsp	**Adults:** ≥12 yrs: 1 tsp qd-tid. **Peds:** 6-12 yrs: 1/2 tsp qd-tid.
Konsyl-D powder (*Konsyl Pharmaceuticals*)	Psyllium 3.4g/tsp	**Adults:** ≥12 yrs: 1 tsp qd-tid. **Peds:** 6-12 yrs: 1/2 tsp qd-tid.
Metamucil capsules (*Procter & Gamble*)	Psyllium 0.52g	**Adults & Peds:** ≥12 yrs: 5 caps qd-tid.
Metamucil Original Texture powder (*Procter & Gamble*)	Psyllium 3.4g/tbl	**Adults:** ≥12 yrs: 1 tbs qd-tid. **Peds:** 6-12 yrs: 1/2 tsp qd-tid.
Metamucil Smooth Texture powder (*Procter & Gamble*)	Psyllium 3.4g/tbl	**Adults:** ≥12 yrs: 1 tbs qd-tid. **Peds:** 6-12 yrs: 1/2 tsp qd-tid.
Metamucil wafers (*Procter & Gamble*)	Psyllium 3.4 g/dose	**Adults:** ≥12 yrs: 2 wafers qd-tid. **Peds:** 6-12 yrs: 1 wafer qd-tid.
HYPEROSMOTICS		
Fleet Children's Babylax suppositories (*C.B. Fleet*)	Glycerin 2.3g	**Peds:** 2-5 yrs: 1 supp. qd.
Fleet Glycerin suppositories (*C.B. Fleet*)	Glycerin 2g	**Adults & Peds:** ≥6 yrs: 1 supp qd.
Fleet Liquid Glycerin suppositories (*C.B. Fleet*)	Glycerin 5.6g	**Adults & Peds:** ≥6 yrs: 1 supp qd.
Fleet Mineral Oil enema (*C.B. Fleet*)	Mineral Oil 133mL	**Adults:** ≥12 yrs: 1 bottle (133mL). **Peds:** 2-12 yrs: 1/2 bottle (66.5mL).
HYPEROSMOTIC COMBINATION		
Fleet Pain Relief Pre-Moistened Anorectal Pads (*C.B. Fleet*)	Glycerin/Pramoxine HCl 12%-1%	**Adults & Peds:** ≥12 yrs: Apply to affected area five times daily.
SALINES		
Ex-Lax Milk of Magnesia liquid (*Novartis Consumer Health*)	Magnesium Hydroxide 400mg/5mL	**Adults & Peds:** ≥12 yrs: Take 2-4 tbl hs. **Peds:** 6-11 yrs: 1-2 tbl hs. 2-5 yrs: 1-3 tbl hs.
Fleet Children's Enema (*C.B. Fleet*)	Monobasic Sodium Phosphate/Dibasic Sodium Phosphate 9.5g-3.5g/66mL	**Peds:** 5-11 yrs: 1 bottle (66mL). 2-5 yrs: 1/2 bottle (33mL).
Fleet Enema (*C.B. Fleet*)	Monobasic Sodium Phosphate/Dibasic Sodium Phosphate 19g-7g/133mL	**Adults & Peds:** ≥12 yrs: 1 bottle (133mL).
Fleet Phospho-Soda (*C.B. Fleet*)	Monobasic Sodium Phosphate/Dibasic Sodium Phosphate 2.4g-0.9g/5mL	**Adults:** ≥12 yrs: 4-9 tsp qd. **Peds:** 10-11 yrs: 2-4 tsp qd. 5-9 yrs: 1-2 tsp qd.
Magnesium Citrate solution (*Various*)	Magnesium Citrate 1.75gm/30mL	**Adults:** ≥12 yrs: 300mL. **Peds:** 6-12 yrs: 90-210mL. 2-6 yrs: 60-90mL.
Phillips Antacid/Laxative chewable tablets (*Bayer Healthcare*)	Magnesium Hydroxide 311mg	**Adults:** ≥ 12 yrs: 6-8 tabs qd. **Peds:** 6-11 yrs: 3-4 tabs qd. 2-5 yrs: 1-2 tabs qd.

Table 10. LAXATIVE PRODUCTS (cont.)

BRAND NAME	INGREDIENT/STRENGTH	DOSE
Phillips Soft Chews, Laxative *(Bayer Healthcare)*	Magnesium/Sodium 500mg-10mg	**Adults & Peds: ≥12 yrs:** Take 2-4 tab qd. **Max:** 4 tab q24h.
Phillips Cramp-free Laxative caplets *(Bayer Healthcare)*	Magnesium 500mg	**Adults & Peds: ≥12 yrs:** Take 2-4 tab qd. **Max:** 4 tab q24h.
Phillips Milk of Magnesia Concentrated liquid *(Bayer Healthcare)*	Magnesium Hydroxide 800mg/5mL	**Adults: ≥12 yrs:** 15-30mL qd. **Peds: 6-11 yrs:** 7.5-15mL qd. **2-5 yrs:** 2.5-7.5mL qd.
Phillips Milk of Magnesia liquid *(Bayer Healthcare)*	Magnesium Hydroxide 400mg/5mL	**Adults: ≥12 yrs:** 30-60mL qd. **Peds: 6-11 yrs:** 15-30mL qd. **2-5 yrs:** 5-15mL qd.
SALINE COMBINATION		
Phillips M-O liquid *(Bayer Healthcare)*	Magnesium Hydroxide/Mineral Oil 300mg-1.25mL/5mL.	**Adults: ≥12 yrs:** 30-60mL qd. **Peds: 6-11 yrs:** 5-15mL qd.
STIMULANTS		
Alophen Enteric Coated Stimulant Laxative pills *(Newmark Laboratories)*	Bisacodyl 5mg	**Adults: ≥12 yrs:** Take 1-3 tab qd. **Peds: 6-12 yrs:** Take 1 tab qd.
Carter's Laxative, Sodium Free pills *(Carter-Wallace)*	Bisacodyl 5mg	**Adults: ≥12 yrs:** Take 1-3 tab (usually 2 tab) qd. **Peds: 6-12 yrs:** Take 1 tab qd.
Castor Oil *(Various)*	Castor Oil	**Adults: ≥12 yrs:** 15-60mL. **Peds: 2-12 yrs:** 5-15mL.
Correctol Stimulant Laxative Tablets For Women *(Schering-Plough)*	Bisacodyl 5mg	**Adults: ≥12 yrs:** Take 1-3 tab qd. **Peds: 6-12 yrs:** Take 1 tab qd.
Doxidan capsules *(Pharmacia Consumer Healthcare)*	Bisacodyl 5mg	**Adults: ≥12 yrs:** 1-3 caps (usually 2) qd. **Peds: 6-12 yrs:** 1 cap qd.
Dulcolax Overnight Relief Laxative tablets *(Boehringer Ingelheim Consumer Healthcare)*	Bisacodyl 5mg	**Adults: ≥12 yrs:** 1-3 tabs (usually 2) qd. **Peds: 6-12 yrs:** 1 tab qd.
Dulcolax suppository *(Boehringer Ingelheim Consumer Healthcare)*	Bisacodyl 10mg	**Adults: ≥12 yrs:** 1 supp qd. **Peds: 6-12 yrs:** ¹/₂ supp qd.
Dulcolax tablets *(Boehringer Ingelheim Consumer Healthcare)*	Bisacodyl 5mg	**Adults: ≥12 yrs:** 1-3 tabs (usually 2) qd. **Peds: 6-12 yrs:** 1 tab qd.
Ex-Lax Maximum Strength tablets *(Novartis Consumer Health)*	Sennosides 25mg	**Adults: ≥12 yrs:** 2 tabs qd-bid. **Peds: 6-12 yrs:** 1 tab qd-bid.
Ex-Lax tablets *(Novartis Consumer Health)*	Sennosides 15mg	**Adults: ≥12 yrs:** 2 tabs qd-bid. **Peds: 6-12 yrs:** 1 tab qd-bid.
Ex-Lax Ultra Stimulant Laxative tablets *(Novartis Consumer Health)*	Bisacodyl 5mg	**Adults: ≥12 yrs:** 1-3 tabs qd. **Peds: 6-12 yrs:** 1 tab qd.
Fleet Bisacodyl suppositories *(C.B. Fleet)*	Bisacodyl 10mg	**Adults: ≥12 yrs:** 1 supp qd. **Peds: 6-12 yrs:** ¹/₂ supp qd.
Fleet Stimulant Laxative tablets *(C.B. Fleet)*	Bisacodyl 5mg	**Adults: ≥12 yrs:** 1-3 tabs (usually 2) qd. **Peds: 6-12 yrs:** 1 tab qd.
Nature's Remedy caplets *(GlaxoSmithKline Consumer Healthcare)*	Aloe/Cascara Sagrada 100mg-150mg	**Adults: ≥12 yrs:** 2 tabs qd-bid. **Max:** 4 tabs bid. **Peds: 6-12 yrs:** 1 tab qd-bid. **Max:** 2 tabs bid. **2-6 yrs:** ¹/₂ tab qd-bid. **Max:** 1 tab bid.
Perdiem Overnight Relief tablets *(Novartis Consumer Health)*	Sennosides 15mg	**Adults: ≥12 yrs:** 2 tabs qd-bid. **Peds: 6-12 yrs:** 1 tab qd-bid.
Senokot tablets *(Purdue Products)*	Sennosides 8.6mg	**Adults: ≥12 yrs:** 2 tabs qd. **Max:** 4 tabs bid. **Peds: 6-12 yrs:** 1 tab qd. **Max:** 2 tabs bid. **2-6 yrs:** ¹/₂ tab qd. **Max:** 1 tab bid.
STIMULANT COMBINATIONS		
Perdiem powder *(Novartis Consumer Health)*	Senna/Psyllium 0.74g-3.25g/6g	**Adults: ≥12 yrs:** 1-2 tsp qd-bid. **Peds: 6-12 yrs:** 1 tsp qd-bid.
Peri-Colace tablets *(Purdue Products)*	Sennosides/Docusate 8.6mg-50mg	**Adults: ≥12 yrs:** 2-4 tabs qd. **Peds: 6-12 yrs:** 1-2 tabs qd. **2-6 yrs:** 1 tab qd.
SennaPrompt capsules *(Konsyl Pharmaceuticals)*	Sennosides/Psyllium 500mg/9mg	**Adults & Peds: ≥12 yrs:** 5 caps qd-bid.

Table 10. LAXATIVE PRODUCTS (cont.)

BRAND NAME	INGREDIENT/STRENGTH	DOSE
Senokot S tablets *(Purdue Products)*	Sennosides/Docusate 8.6mg-50mg	**Adults: ≥12 yrs:** 2 tabs qd. **Max:** 4 tabs bid. **Peds: 6-12 yrs:** 1 tab qd. **Max:** 2 tabs bid. **2-6 yrs:** ^{1}/₂ tab qd. **Max:** 1 tab bid.
SURFACTANTS (STOOL SOFTENERS)		
Colace capsules *(Purdue Products)*	Docusate Sodium 100mg	**Adults: ≥12 yrs:** 1-3 caps qd. **Peds: 2-12 yrs:** 1 cap qd.
Colace capsules *(Purdue Products)*	Docusate Sodium 50mg	**Adults: ≥12 yrs:** 1-6 caps qd. **Peds: 2-12 yrs:** 1-3 caps qd.
Colace Glycerin suppositories *(Purdue Products)*	Glycerin 2.1g; 1.2g	**Adults: ≥6 yrs:** 2.1g supp qd. **Peds: 2-6 yrs:** 1.2g supp qd.
Colace liquid *(Purdue Products)*	Docusate Sodium 10mg/mL	**Adults: ≥12 yrs:** 5-15mL qd-bid. **Peds: 2-12 yrs:** 5-15mL qd.
Colace syrup *(Purdue Products)*	Docusate Sodium 60mg/15mL	**Adults: ≥12 yrs:** 15-90mL qd. **Peds: 2-12 yrs:** 5-37.5mL qd.
Correctol Stool Softener Laxative soft-gels *(Schering-Plough)*	Docusate Sodium 100mg	**Adults: ≥12 yrs:** Take 1-3 cap qd. **Peds: 6-12 yrs:** Take 1 cap qd.
Docusol Constipation Relief, mini enemas *(Western Research Laboratories)*	Docusate Sodium 283mg	**Adults: ≥12 yrs:** Take 1-3 units qd. **Peds: 6-12 yrs:** Take 1 unit qd.
Dulcolax Stool Softener capsules *(Boehringer Ingelheim Consumer)*	Docusate Sodium 100mg	**Adults: ≥12 yrs:** 1-3 caps qd. **Peds: 2-12 yrs:** 1 cap qd.
Ex-Lax Stool Softener tablets *(Novartis Consumer Health)*	Docusate Sodium 100mg	**Adults: ≥12 yrs:** 1-3 caps qd. **Peds: 2-12 yrs:** 1 cap qd.
Fleet Sof-Lax tablets *(C.B. Fleet)*	Docusate Sodium 100mg	**Adults: ≥12 yrs:** 1-3 caps qd. **Peds: 2-12 yrs:** 1 cap qd.
Kaopectate Liqui-Gels *(Pharmacia Consumer Healthcare)*	Docusate Calcium 240mg	**Adults & Peds: ≥12 yrs:** 1 cap qd until normal bowel movement.
Phillips Stool Softener capsules *(Bayer Healthcare)*	Docusate Sodium 100mg	**Adults: ≥12 yrs:** 1-3 caps qd. **Peds: 2-12 yrs:** 1 cap qd.

Table 11. PSORIASIS PRODUCTS

Brand Name	Ingredient/Strength	Dose
COAL TAR		
Denorex Psoriasis Overnight Treatment cream *(Wyeth Consumer Healthcare)*	Coal Tar (strength NA)	**Adults & Peds:** Apply to affected area qhs prn.
Denorex Therapeutic Protection 2-in-1 shampoo *(Wyeth Consumer Healthcare)*	Coal Tar 2.5%	**Adults & Peds:** Use at least biw.
Denorex Therapeutic Protection shampoo *(Wyeth Consumer Healthcare)*	Coal Tar 2.5%	**Adults & Peds:** Use at least biw.
DHS Tar Shampoo *(Person & Covey)*	Coal Tar 0.5%	**Adults & Peds:** Use at least biw.
Ionil-T Plus Shampoo *(Healthpoint)*	Coal Tar 2%	**Adults & Peds:** Use at least biw.
Ionil-T Shampoo *(Healthpoint)*	Coal Tar 1%	**Adults & Peds:** Use at least biw.
MG217 Ointment *(Trenton)*	Coal Tar 2%	**Adults & Peds:** Apply to affected area qd-qid.
MG217 Tar Shampoo *(Trenton)*	Coal Tar 3%	**Adults & Peds:** Use at least biw.
Neutrogena T/Gel Shampoo Extra Strength *(Neutrogena)*	Coal Tar 1%	**Adults & Peds:** Use at least biw.
Neutrogena T/Gel Shampoo Orignial Formula *(Neutrogena)*	Coal Tar 0.5%	**Adults & Peds:** Use at least biw.
Neutrogena T/Gel Stubborn Itch Shampoo *(Neutrogena)*	Coal Tar 0.5%	**Adults & Peds:** Use at least biw.
PolyTar shampoo *(Stiefel)*	Coal Tar 0.5%	**Adults & Peds:** Use at least biw.
PolyTar soap *(Stiefel)*	Coal Tar 0.5%	**Adults & Peds:** Apply to affected area prn.
Psoriasin Multi-Symptom Psoriasis Relief Gel *(Alva-Amco Pharmacal)*	Coal Tar 1.25%	**Adults & Peds:** Apply to affected area qd-qid.
Psoriasin Multi-Symptom Psoriasis Relief Ointment *(Alva-Amco Pharmacal)*	Coal Tar 2%	**Adults & Peds:** Apply to affected area qd-qid.
CORTICOSTEROIDS		
Aveeno Anti-Itch Cream 1% *(Johnson & Johnson Consumer)*	Hydrocortisone 1%	**Adults & Peds: ≥2 yrs:** Apply to affected area tid-qid.
Cortaid Advanced 12-Hour Anti-Itch Cream *(Johnson & Johnson Consumer)*	Hydrocortisone 1%	**Adults & Peds: ≥2 yrs:** Apply to affected area tid-qid.
Cortaid Intensive Therapy Cooling Spray *(Johnson & Johnson Consumer)*	Hydrocortisone 1%	**Adults & Peds: ≥2 yrs:** Apply to affected area tid-qid.
Cortaid Intensive Therapy Moisturizing Cream *(Johnson & Johnson Consumer)*	Hydrocortisone 1%	**Adults & Peds: ≥2 yrs:** Apply to affected area tid-qid.
Cortaid Maximum Strength Cream *(Johnson & Johnson Consumer)*	Hydrocortisone 1%	**Adults & Peds: ≥2 yrs:** Apply to affected area tld-qid.
Cortaid Maximum Strength Ointment *(Johnson & Johnson Consumer)*	Hydrocortisone 1%	**Adults & Peds: ≥2 yrs:** Apply to affected area tid-qid.
Cortizone-10 Cream *(Chattem)*	Hydrocortisone 1%	**Adults & Peds: ≥2 yrs:** Apply to affected area tid-qid.
Cortizone-10 Maximum Strength Anti-Itch Ointment *(Chattem)*	Hydrocortisone 1%	**Adults & Peds: ≥2 yrs:** Apply to affected area tid-qid.
Cortizone-10 Ointment *(Chattem)*	Hydrocortisone 1%	**Adults & Peds: ≥2 yrs:** Apply to affected area tid-qid.
Cortizone-10 Plus Maximum Strength Cream *(Chattem)*	Hydrocortisone 1%	**Adults & Peds: ≥2 yrs:** Apply to affected area tid-qid.
Cortizone-10 Quick Shot Spray *(Chattem)*	Hydrocortisone 1%	**Adults & Peds: ≥2 yrs:** Apply to affected area tid-qid.
SALICYLIC ACID		
Denorex Psoriasis Daytime Treatment cream *(Wyeth Consumer Healthcare)*	Salicylic Acid 3%	**Adults & Peds:** Apply to affected area qd-qid.

Table 11. PSORIASIS PRODUCTS (cont.)

Brand Name	Ingredient/Strength	Dose
Dermarest Psoriasis Medicated Foam Shampoo *(Del Laboratories)*	Salicylic Acid 3%	**Adults & Peds:** Apply to affected area at least biw.
Dermarest Psoriasis Medicated Moisturizer *(Del Laboratories)*	Salicylic Acid 2%	**Adults & Peds:** Apply to affected area qd-qid.
Dermarest Psoriasis Medicated Scalp Treatment *(Del Laboratories)*	Salicylic Acid 3%	**Adults & Peds:** Apply to affected area qd-qid.
Dermarest Psoriasis Medicated Scalp Treatment mousse *(Del Laboratories)*	Salicylic Acid 3%	**Adults & Peds:** Apply to affected area qd-qid.
Dermarest Psoriasis Medicated Shampoo/Conditioner *(Del Laboratories)*	Salicylic Acid 3%	**Adults & Peds:** Apply to affected area at least biw.
Dermarest Psoriasis Skin Treatment Psoriasis Medicated *(Del Laboratories)*	Salicylic Acid 3%	**Adults & Peds:** Apply to affected area qd-qid.
Neutrogena T/Gel Conditioner *(Neutrogena)*	Salicylic Acid 2%	**Adults & Peds:** Use at least biw.
Psoriasin Therapeutic Body Wash With Aloe *(Alva-Amco Pharmacal)*	Salicylic Acid 3%	**Adults & Peds:** Use biw.
Psoriasin Therapeutic Shampoo With Panthenol *(Alva-Amco Pharmacal)*	Salicylic Acid 3%	**Adults & Peds:** Use biw.

Table 12. WOUND CARE PRODUCTS

Brand Name	Ingredient/Strength	Dose
NEOMYCIN/POLYMYXIN B/BACITRACIN COMBINATIONS		
Bacitracin ointment *(Various)*	Bacitracin 500 U	**Adults & Peds:** Apply to affected area qd-tid.
Bactine Pain Relieving Protective Antibiotic *(Bayer Healthcare)*	Neomycin/polymyxin B/bacitracin/pramoxine 3.5mg-10,000 U-500 U-1%	**Adults & Peds:** Apply to affected area qd-tid.
Neosporin ointment *(Johnson & Johnson Consumer)*	Neomycin/polymyxin B/bacitracin 3.5mg-5,000 U-400 U	**Adults & Peds:** Apply to affected area qd-tid.
Neosporin Plus Pain Relief cream *(Johnson & Johnson Consumer)*	Neomycin/polymyxin B/pramoxine 3.5mg-10,000 U-10mg	**Adults & Peds:** Apply to affected area qd-tid.
Neosporin Plus Pain Relief Ointment *(Johnson & Johnson Consumer)*	Neomycin/polymyxin B/bacitracin/pramoxine Relief ointment 3.5mg-10,000 U-500 U-10mg	**Adults & Peds:** Apply to affected area qd-tid.
Neosporin To Go ointment *(Johnson & Johnson Consumer)*	Neomycin/polymyxin B/bacitracin 3.5mg-5,000 U-400 U	**Adults & Peds:** Apply to affected area qd-tid.
Polysporin ointment *(Johnson & Johnson Consumer)*	Polymyxin B/bacitracin 10,000 U-500 U	**Adults & Peds:** Apply to affected area qd-tid.
BENZALKONIUM CHLORIDE COMBINATIONS		
Bactine First Aid Liquid *(Bayer Healthcare)*	Lidocaine HCl/benzalkonium chloride 2.5%-0.13%	**Adults & Peds: ≥2 yrs.:** Apply to affected area qd-tid.
Bactine Pain Relieving Cleansing Spray *(Bayer Healthcare)*	Lidocaine HCl/benzalkonium chloride 2.5%-0.13%	**Adults & Peds: ≥2 yrs.:** Apply to affected area qd-tid.
Bactine Pain Relieving Cleansing Wipes *(Bayer Healthcare)*	Benzalkonium chloride/pramoxine HCl 0.13%-1.0%	**Adults & Peds: ≥2 yrs.:** Use 1 wipe qd-tid.
Band-Aid Antiseptic Foam, One-Step Cleansing and Infection Protection *(Johnson & Johnson Consumer)*	Benzalkonim chloride 0.13%	**Adults & Peds: ≥3 yrs.:** Use tid.
BENZETHONIUM CHLORIDE COMBINATIONS		
Gold Bond First Aid Quick Spray *(Chattem)*	Menthol/benzethonium chloride 1%-0.13%	**Adults & Peds: ≥2 yrs.:** Apply to affected area tid-qid.
Lanacane Maximum Strength Cream *(Combe)*	Benzocaine/benzethonium chloride 20%-0.1%	**Adults & Peds: ≥2 yrs.:** Apply to affected area tid-qid.
CHLORHEXIDINE GLUCONATE		
Hibiclens *(Regent)*	Chlorhexidine gluconate 4%	**Adults & Peds:** Apply sparingly to affected area prn.
IODINE		
Betadine Skin Cleanser *(Purdue)*	Povidone-iodine 7.5%	**Adults & Peds:** Apply to affected area for 3 minutes and rinse. Repeat bid-tid.
Betadine solution *(Purdue)*	Povidone-iodine 10%	**Adults & Peds:** Apply to affected area qd-tid.
Betadine spray *(Purdue)*	Povidone-iodine 10%	**Adults & Peds:** Apply to affected area qd-tid.
Betadine Surgical Scrub *(Purdue)*	Povidone-iodine 7.5%	**Adults & Peds:** Apply to affected area for 5 minutes.
Betadine swab *(Purdue)*	Povidone-iodine 10%	**Adults & Peds:** Apply to affected area qd-tid.
MISCELLANEOUS		
Aquaphor Healing Ointment *(Beiersdorf)*	Petrolatum, mineral oil, ceresin, lanolin, alcohol, panthenol, glycerin, bisabolol	**Adults & Peds:** Apply to affected area prn.
Curad Spray Bandage *(Beiersdorf)*	Ethyl acetate, pentane, methylacrylate, menthol, carbon dioxide	**Adults & Peds:** Apply to affected area prn.
Proxacol Hydrogen Peroxide	Hydrogen peroxide 3%	**Adults:** Apply to affected area qd-tid.
Wound Wash Sterile Saline spray *(Blairex Laboratories)*	Sterile sodium chloride solution 0.9%	**Adults & Peds:** Apply to affected area prn.

The Go-to Guides for Prescribing Decisions

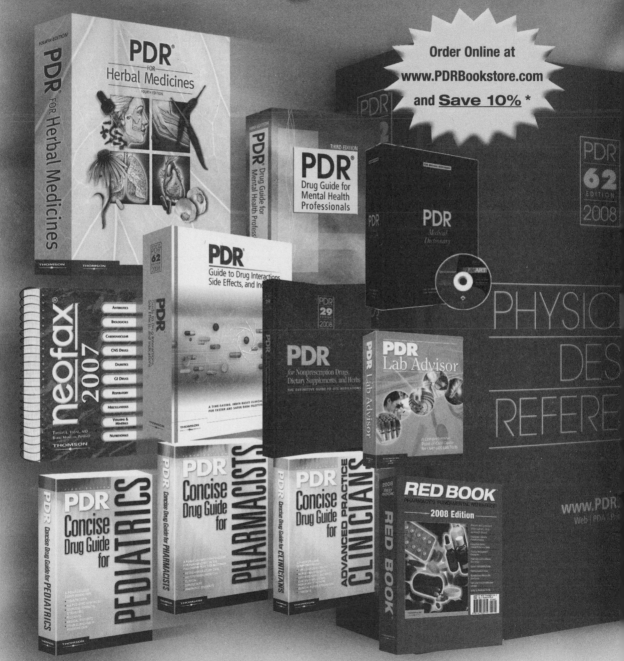

Order Online at www.PDRBookstore.com and **Save** 10% *

New and Updated Titles from Thomson Healthcare, Publisher of the PDR® and Other Trusted Healthcare References.

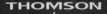